Practical General Practice

Practical General Practice
Guidelines for Effective Clinical Management

EIGHTH EDITION

Adam Staten, MA MBBS MRCGP MRCP (UK) DRCOG DMCC PGCertCE

General Practitioner
Milton Keynes, UK

Kate Robinson, MBChB (Hons) BMedSci DRCOG MRCGP PGCert Med Ed (Distinction)

General Practitioner
Cheshire, UK

ELSEVIER

First edition 1988
Second edition 1992
Third edition 1999
Fourth edition 2003
Fifth edition 2006
Sixth edition 2011
Seventh edition 2020
Eighth edition 2025

ISBN: 978-0-443-12359-7

Printed in India

Last digit is the print number: 9 8 7 6 5 4 3 2 1

Content Strategist: Trinity Hutton
Content Project Manager: Arpita Paul
Design: Vicky Pearson Esser
Marketing Manager: Deborah Watkins

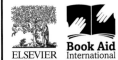

Working together
to grow libraries in
developing countries

www.elsevier.com • www.bookaid.org

Contents

Preface

It is now 35 years since Alex Khot and Andrew Polmear produced the first edition of *Practical General Practice* as a desktop companion for general practitioners dealing with the ever complex and nuanced presentations of primary care. Perhaps now more than ever before is there a need for a guide to cut through the noise of the multitudinous evolving guidelines produced in every area of medicine as our evidence base grows.

Since the publication of the seventh edition, the world has endured the COVID-19 pandemic, a wave of global illness such as had not been seen for a century. The pandemic was a seismic event, shaking healthcare systems all around the world at their foundations. As medical practitioners, we had to adapt in all kinds of unexpected ways, but as we emerge on the other side of the pandemic, what is somewhat surprising is the absence of the impact of COVID-19 in the guidelines from which this book draws its information. This may be a testament to the enduring nature of how we deliver care to our patients: despite a global pandemic, the principles of assessing, treating, and communicating with our patients hold firm.

For editors of a guidelines-based textbook, this is heartening. To some extent, a book such as this is at risk of becoming out of date even as the ink dries on the page, but despite frequent changes in the details of how we treat our patients, the principles and processes change hardly at all.

As ever, this book should be seen as a guide and template from which medical practitioners can derive their own ways of working. The chapters of the book are designed to mirror the mental process of the doctor during a general practice consultation and so help that doctor synthesise rational and safe treatment plans for their patients.

Adam Staten
Kate Robinson

The Structure of the Book

Bullets

Different coloured bullet points have been used to provide emphasis for different types of comment:

- Black bullets are for general information or explanation e.g. 'Treatment can be expected to….'
- Pink bullets are instructions for questions that should be asked, examinations that should be performed, or investigations and treatments that should be undertaken e.g. 'Ask the patient x, y and z', 'Examine for a, b and c'.
- Grey bullets are used where there is a subdivision of another heading.

Lists

Where we present a list in no particular order we use:

(a) chest pain; or
(b) hypotension; or
(c) heart failure.

Where the order is important we number the list:

1. Sit the patient up.
2. Give oxygen.
3. Give diamorphine …

Boxes

These are used to highlight information that might otherwise get lost in the text: guidelines, a list of tests as a 'work-up' for a patient with a particular condition, or patient organisations for example.

References

Our aim is to reference every statement of fact. Where such a statement is not accompanied by a reference, the reader can assume it is taken from the reference in a box at the start of that section.

Acknowledgements

First, we thank Alex Khot and Andrew Polmear, whose vision led to the creation of this book and whose drive led to the publication of the first seven editions. In particular, we acknowledge the enormous contribution to medicine made by Andrew Polmear, who sadly passed away in 2022. We hope he would approve of this new edition.

We thank Trinity Hutton and Arpita Paul at Elsevier, who held our hands through the production of this edition and enabled its production. We also give a huge thank you to all of our contributors, who have worked so hard to update each chapter in the face of COVID-19 recovery work, elongating NHS waiting lists, and strikes throughout the NHS. Your efforts are very much appreciated.

Adam thanks his wife Shiva for her support and his daughters Rose and Grace, whose father spends more time than he should at his laptop. Kate thanks her two cats Yara and Lykke, who have tried their best to contribute, whether invited to or not.

List of Contributors

Stewart Mercer, MBChB BSc (Hons) MSc PhD MRCGP FRCGP FRCPE FFPHM FRSE
Professor of Primary Care and Multimorbidity
University of Edinburgh
Scotland

Harry Wang, PhD
School of Public Health, Sun Yat-Sen University, PR China
Honorary Fellow, Usher Institute University of Edinburgh
Scotland

Ruth Bland, BSc MBChB MD FRCPCH
Consultant General Paediatrics and Honorary Associate Clinical Professor
Royal Hospital for Sick Children and University of Glasgow, Glasgow

Hilary Pearce, MBChB MRCPCH
Consultant Paediatrician
Medical Paediatrics
Royal Hospital for Children, Glasgow

Andy Potter, MBBS MRCGP FRCP
General Practitioner
Milton Keynes

Kristian Brooks, MBBS MRCP DTM&H
Respiratory Registrar
Gateshead

Vincent Cheung, MA MBBS MRCP (UK)
Consultant Gastroenterologist
Translational Gastroenterology Unit
John Radcliffe Hospital
Oxford

Lulia Al-Hillawi, BSc (Hons) MBBS MRCP (UK)
Senior Clinical Fellow
Translational Gastroenterology Unit
John Radcliffe Hospital
Oxford

Iain Wilson, MBBS BSc FRCS
Consultant in General and Upper GI Surgery
Frimley Health NHS Foundation Trust
Frimley

Jennifer Stevens, MBBS FRCS
Consultant in General and Upper GI Surgery
Ashford & St Peter's Hospitals NHS Foundation Trust
Chertsey

John MacLean, MB CHB FFSEM FRCPS (Glas) MRCGP DRCOG
Sports Medicine Physician
Honorary Clinical Professor University of Glasgow
Glasgow

Maria Panourgia, FRCP PhD MSc MBGS
Consultant Geriatrician
Milton Keynes University Hospital
Honorary Senior Lecturer of the University of Buckingham
Buckingham

Sarah Henry, MBBS MRCPsych DGM
Consultant Old Age Psychiatrist
North Tyneside

Soumyajit Sanyal, MBBS MD DM MRCPsych
Specialist Registrar Old Age Psychiatry
Health Education England North East

Robert Hone, MBBS MCh FRCS
ENT Consultant
East Kent Hospitals University NHS Trust

Shivun Khosla, MA (Cantab) MCh MBBChir FRCSEd (ORL-HNS)
ENT Registrar
East Kents Hospitals University Foundation Trust

Sana Rasool, MBChB MRes FRCOphth
Consultant Ophthalmologist
Sandwell & West Birmingham NHS Trust

Anchal Agarwal Goyal, MBBS MRCGP DRCOG DPD
Speciality Doctor in Dermatology
NHS Lanarkshire, Cardiff

Helen Dilworth, MBChB
Consultant Dermatologist
NHS Lanarkshire

Kieran Dinwoodie, MBChB FRCGP Dip Derm DRCOG DTM&H DGM
Calderside Medical Practice
GP Partner and Trainer

Rakhee Choukhany Gupta, MBBS DVD DNB Dermatology
University Hospital Monklands in NHS Lanarkshire

Mohit Kumar, MBChB (Hons) MRCP
Consultant
Diabetes and Endocrinology
WWL Teaching Hospitals
Wigan

Christopher Burton, MD FRCGP
Professor of Primary Medical Care
School of Medicine & Population Health, University of Sheffield
Sheffield

Ben Dietsch, MB BS DipPallMed PGCert Med Ed FHEA
Consultant in Palliative Medicine
Willen Hospice & Milton Keynes University Hospital NHS Foundation Trust
Honorary Senior Clinical Lecturer
University of Buckingham
Buckingham

1

Principles and Practice of Primary Care

Adam Staten

CHAPTER CONTENTS

Challenges of Primary Care

Population Challenges

- The provision of holistic care is at the heart of primary care, and providing this care is increasingly challenging with a global population that is increasing in size, age, and morbidity.
- The increasing capability to diagnose and treat disease leads to increasing patient demand and increasing resource cost in terms of both time and finance.
- Particularly in developed nations, the rise of illnesses related to lifestyle factors such as smoking, alcohol consumption, and obesity has created a burden on the healthcare system and are a complicating factor in many other illnesses. Globally, infectious diseases such as human immunodeficiency virus/acquired immunodeficiency syndrome (HIV/AIDS) contribute to the increasing burden on primary healthcare (and the wider healthcare system).
- An increasing emphasis on maintaining 'wellness' rather than simply treating ill health has put primary care at the forefront of screening programmes, education programmes, and primary preventive treatment.
- The increasing capabilities of modern medicine, the emphasis on keeping people well, and wider public access to healthcare information (via the internet and so on) all contribute to rising patient expectations and managing these expectations in a resource-limited environment can prove very challenging. In the United Kingdom, the General Medical Council (GMC) found that this rise in expectations is a key contributing factor to increasing rates of complaint against doctors (GMC, 2014). Rising patient expectations is also frequently cited as a reason for doctors leaving their role in primary care (Leese et al, 2002).

The Challenge of External Factors

- Healthcare is expensive and funding for primary care is not always adequate to meet the needs of the population it serves. For example, in many developing countries funding is diverted away from the provision of comprehensive primary care in favour of providing 'vertical care' programmes targeting specific issues such as HIV/AIDs or childhood immunisations (De Maeseneer et al, 2008).

- The provision of healthcare can become highly politicised, and interference in healthcare from politicians for political purposes, rather than to improve patient care, can be a source of real frustration and dissatisfaction for doctors.
- Doctors now practice in the full glare of the media (and social media) spotlight. Not only can this be intimidating and exposing, but doctors working in general practice are also often left to undo the damage done by inaccurate messages promulgated by the media.
- A worldwide tendency to increasing litigation and, in some circumstances, the criminalisation of medical error add to the pressures of working within primary care and medicine in general.

The Evolving Primary Care Team

- Whereas general practitioners (GPs) are usually considered to be central to the provision of primary care services, the primary care team includes all professionals who contribute to the health and well-being of patients in the community.
- With the increasing complexity of healthcare provision and the increasing complexity of the patients who receive treatment in the community, any attempt for GPs to practice in isolation, without recourse to the wider primary healthcare team, is likely to result in frustration for the GP and poor quality, possibly dangerous, care for patients.
- The roles and responsibilities of the primary care team are to some extent limitless. It is characteristic of primary care that practitioners working in the community are expected to be able to deal to some extent with every problem that a patient may present. Often these problems are not simply medical, and they may be complicated by, or indeed may primarily be, psychological or social problems.
- Many tasks in primary care are as well, and often better, performed by members of the primary care team other than GPs.
- The structure of primary care teams varies from country to country. For example, in the United Kingdom, dentists usually work separately from GPs, but in other European countries, it is common for doctors and dentists to be co-located. Similarly, professionals such as social workers and mental health nurses are located alongside GPs in many countries.
- As coordinating patient care becomes ever more complex, it is vital that the extended primary care team works coherently to avoid patient neglect or duplication of effort to deliver effective, rational care to patients.

- Workforce problems in primary care in many countries have led to the innovation of new roles for established healthcare professionals within primary care and the creation of entirely new types of healthcare professionals.
- The primary care team in any community should be tailored to suit the healthcare needs of the local population; therefore, it is essential for everyone involved with workforce planning to be familiar with the variety of professionals who can contribute to providing primary healthcare.
- To deal with the demands of modern healthcare, doctors should see themselves as having a key role in driving healthcare policy towards establishing the most effective primary care teams for their particular populations.

Nurse Practitioners

- Nurse practitioners, or advanced nurse practitioners, are nurses trained beyond the usual competences of registered nurses so they are able to practice autonomously and assess and diagnose undifferentiated problems to synthesise treatment plans (Royal College of Nursing, 2012). Key to this is their ability to prescribe independently.
- Nurse practitioners work in many different areas of healthcare, but within primary care, they provide care both for acute illness (usually by providing consultations for minor illness) and chronic disease (such as performing routine reviews in respiratory illness or diabetes).
- Nurse practitioners are well established in anglophone countries, where they are seen as key resources in helping to manage patient demand, but they are less well recognised in other parts of the world.
- Training to become an advanced nurse practitioner varies from country to country and depends on the area of healthcare in which the nurse is working. In the United Kingdom, the Royal College of Nursing provides accredited training courses to upskill nurses and prepare them for an advanced role.
- Evidence suggests that nurse practitioners provide good levels of patient satisfaction and good patient outcomes, but the evidence of cost-effectiveness remains equivocal (Martin-Misener et al, 2015).

Physiotherapists

- Up to 30% of primary care consultations relate to musculoskeletal problems, many of which are best dealt with by physiotherapists. However, direct access to physiotherapists for patients is not necessarily the norm within primary care.
- Direct access is usually available to patients in Australia, absent in the United States, and patchy throughout the European Union. This variability in access exists even though the majority of countries, particularly within

Europe, have the requisite legislation and train their physiotherapists to have the requisite competencies to practice independently. Often the barriers to enabling direct access come from within the medical profession itself despite the potential reduction in workload that physiotherapists can provide (Chartered Society of Physiotherapists, 2013). Where direct access is not available, patients must usually come via their primary care physicians to get access to physiotherapy.

- The provision of direct access physiotherapy has been shown to be both clinically effective and cost effective (Mallett et al, 2014).

Clinical Pharmacists

- Clinical pharmacists are pharmacists with an extended role that involves direct patient facing activity with particular respect to medicines management. Their key roles are in optimising medication and dosage regimens, deconflicting medications that may interact, and ensuring the cost-effectiveness of medications. Many are also involved in the management of patients with minor ailments and chronic disease.
- As polypharmacy in an ageing population becomes more common, expertise in medicines management will be increasingly important and will become an increasing workload burden for GPs.
- The role is perhaps best established in the United States, where clinical pharmacists have been working and evolving their role over a period of decades. However, in 1997, the WHO published a policy statement that envisaged an expanded future role for pharmacists that would benefit patients in healthcare systems globally. Since then, the role has become increasingly recognised in the Anglosphere and across Europe. Clinical pharmacists are also invaluable in bolstering primary care teams in countries where doctor numbers are low.

Physician Associates

- In the United Kingdom, to train as a physician associate, the trainee must already have a degree in a life or healthcare science subject. Physician assistants then undergo an intense period of training in the medical model to enable them to interview, examine, and diagnose patients; order and interpret tests; and perform procedures according to competency. They may work in a variety of settings from surgery to emergency medicine, but many work in primary care.
- A physician associate is a dependent medical practitioner who works under the supervision of a physician. In the United Kingdom, physician associates cannot currently prescribe medications, and prescriptions must be authorised by the supervising physician.
- Physician associates fulfil a range of roles within primary care, including acute illness management, chronic disease

management, and home visiting. They are also increasingly common in a wide range of roles in secondary care.

Physician Assistant

- Despite the similarity in job title, the role of a physician assistant is different to that of a physician associate.
- The physician assistant is a US invention, and they have been established in the United States for more than 50 years with more than 120,000 of them currently practising.
- Physician assistants have been shown to be cost effective and acceptable to patients, and a number of other countries throughout the world have developed training programmes to produce physician assistants to alleviate pressure on primary care doctors (Legler, Cawley, & Fenn, 2007).
- The ability to prescribe and the autonomy with which they practice vary from country to country.

Mental Health Professionals

- Mental health problems are an enormous part of primary care, either as the presenting problem or as a complicating factor for other problems. Up to one-third of all general practice appointments are thought to involve a mental health component.
- Given this workload and the economic burden of mental health in primary care, the WHO has produced policy emphasising the importance of providing good-quality primary mental healthcare. However, it remains unusual for mental health nurses or other mental health professionals who are capable of delivering psychological treatments to be embedded within the primary care team. In the United Kingdom, this is now changing with the provision of mental health staff to primary care networks.
- Since 2014 in the Netherlands, there has been a deliberate shift in the provision of mental healthcare from secondary to primary care. This has been largely facilitated by increasing the number of mental health nurses working alongside GPs such that between 2010 and 2014, the proportion of practices in the Netherlands with a mental health nurse increased from 20% to more than 80%. This has not reduced GP workload but has increased the number of long appointments available in the community to patients with mental health problems (Magnée et al, 2016).
- A Cochrane review of the effectiveness of counselling provided within primary care found that it was clinically more effective in the short term than usual care (although not in the long term) and was associated with similar costs to usual care (Bower et al, 2011).

Medical Assistants

- Medical assistants primarily work within primary care teams in the United States. They are allied health professionals who work in both administrative and clinical roles. Their duties may include scheduling appointments, handling correspondence, and updating patient notes, as well as clinical procedures such as performing electrocardiography, taking blood, assisting the physician during procedures, and preparing patients for examination.

- It is suggested that medical assistants are a key means by which doctors can relieve themselves of their administrative workload, enabling themselves to focus more on direct patient care (Sinsky et al, 2013).
- The equivalent role of 'GP assistant' is now emerging in the United Kingdom.

Social Prescribers

- Social prescribers are employed within primary care networks within the United Kingdom and aim to address the various social issues that often complicate medical problems.
- They are intended to be a key liaison between patients, healthcare services, social services, and third-sector sources of support.

Use of Technology

- The use of technology within medicine has the potential to improve patient care and make the working life of primary healthcare professionals easier and less stressful. As technologies develop, it is important that those working within primary care stay alert to new ways in which this technology can be applied to their own working environments.
- The COVID-19 pandemic rapidly accelerated the use of technology, particularly with regards to remote consultations.

Telemedicine

- Telemedicine (or telehealth) relates to the remote monitoring of patients and the transfer of biometric data from the patient's home to their doctor. It has perhaps been most often used when dealing with cardiovascular or respiratory disease to enable early detection of decompensation of the monitored illness and proactive, early management.
- As technology advances and equipment (e.g., blood pressure monitors and oxygen saturation probes) becomes cheaper, it is likely that this will be seen as a convenient and cost-effective means of managing patients. It has the added advantage of engaging patients with their own care and empowering them to take responsibility for managing their illnesses.
- There is good evidence that telemedicine can be a safe and effective way to manage certain conditions, but good evidence of overall effectiveness and of overall cost-effectiveness remains patchy (Eze et al, 2020).

Communications Technology

- The use of communications technology, such as text message, email, and video calling, expanded rapidly during the COVID-19 pandemic, leading to greater comfort with its use for both patients and clinicians.
- Younger patients in particular are comfortable with communicating electronically. For example the use of virtual clinics that employed email and text messaging to communicate with young patients with diabetes dramatically improved attendance rates (Mayor, 2016).
- Video phone applications (e.g., Skype) have been used in a variety of settings such as providing remote care for refugees, orthopaedic follow-up, and psychiatric consultation and for conducting remote ward rounds in nursing homes.
- Numerous email- and phone-based systems can be used to enable GPs to access specialist advice rapidly. These systems may obviate the need for an acute admission or a referral for specialist advice. They are increasingly being used as ways to manage demand on secondary care and to streamline patient care.

Models of Care

- As the burden of caring for enlarging and ageing populations increases, the way in which patients are seen in primary care will need to be adapted to increase capacity within the system.
- GPs need to adapt the ways in which they see their patients to suit their particular patient populations. Some of these varied models of seeing patients will be reliant on the technologies discussed earlier; others require a fresh approach to the traditional medical consultation.

Telephone Triage

- Telephone triage is a means by which patient demand and flow can be managed. Before the COVID-19 pandemic, telephone triage had already become popular, particularly in the United Kingdom, as a way to reduce the number of patients who need to be seen face to face. The pandemic resulted in universal use of telephone triage for a period in UK primary care, which increased both patient and clinician familiarity with it.
- Some who advocate the system estimate that up to 60% of primary care problems can be resolved over the phone, and there is evidence suggesting that patients find this means of interacting with their GPs satisfactory.
- However, the ESTEEM trial was a large-scale trial of telephone triage that found that although clinician contact time on the day of the appointment request was reduced, overall clinician contact time was no different

to usual care, which to some extent undermines its purpose (Holt et al, 2016).

Shared Medical Appointments

- Shared medical appointments are part medical consultation, part education session. Groups of patients with the same condition are seen together for an extended appointment and are educated about their condition and how it can be managed. This saves overall clinician time whilst increasing the contact time patients have with the clinician. Other benefits include empowering patients to self-manage and the creation of a peer support network for patients.
- Shared medical appointments have been used in a range of settings, including diabetes, maternity, physiotherapy, and liver disease. Patients report higher levels of satisfaction with shared medical appointment care than with usual care (Heyworth et al, 2014).

The General Practitioner Consultant

- This is a model of care which relies on the GP having a team of varied allied health professionals around them.
- This model of care relies on central triage, which directs patients towards the relevant professional (e.g., the physiotherapist, mental health nurse, or physician associate). The GP is not directly involved in the initial patient contact but is called in to consult on cases that are beyond the capability of the allied health professional.
- Theoretically, this frees the GP up to dedicate time to patients with the most complex conditions who require the most skilled input albeit at the expense of the regular and recurrent patient contacts that many argue provide job satisfaction in primary care.

The Virtual Ward

- The virtual ward is a concept designed to manage patients, often housebound patients, who require intense, proactive, and multidisciplinary input. It is an elaboration on the concept of the multidisciplinary team and may or may not make use of telehealth data.
- Versions of the virtual ward that have been trialled usually involve a team consisting of community nurses, GPs, geriatricians, and possibly representatives from social services. This team meets at regular intervals to discuss a case load of complex patients.
- By meeting regularly and having input from a number of disciplines, this approach aims to improve proactive care therefore reduce the risk of an acute decompensation in illness requiring hospital admission. It should also reduce duplication of effort by improving communication between all those involved in the patient's care.

Caring for the Doctor

The Burnout Syndrome

- The world of general practice is without doubt stressful and continues to become more stressful as a result of the challenges detailed in this chapter. A Commonwealth Fund survey of primary care in 10 developed nations in 2022 found that doctors in all countries reported increasing workloads and stress levels. In the United Kingdom, 71% of GPs reported that they found their jobs 'very' or 'extremely' stressful (Beech et al, 2023).
- The phenomenon of physician burnout is well recognised but often not well dealt with. The three key features of burnout are usually described as:
  1. Emotional exhaustion
  2. Depersonalisation
  3. An absent sense of personal accomplishment
- The burnout syndrome overlaps with and is complicated by anxiety and depression and shares key features with these issues such as social withdrawal, absenteeism from work, and problems with drug and alcohol abuse.
- Doctors are at high risk of burnout because they are selected based on personality traits such as perfectionism, high achievement, a sense of responsibility, and competitiveness, which all put them at higher risk of burning out.
- Work within medicine exposes people to extended periods of extreme emotional stress (both their own and that of other people), which contributes to burnout.
- A perceived stigma to mental illness amongst doctors also means that doctors tend to seek help late by which point the damage may well be significant, including suicidality.

Finding Help and Treatment

- It is important that those working within general practice recognise the signs of stress and burnout both in themselves and in their colleagues and feel able to seek help or suggest that their colleagues seek help.
- Treatment for the burnout syndrome or for depression or substance misuse problems in general is along standard lines and includes cognitive-behavioral therapy, medication, and counselling. These can be sought via the doctor's own GP, although many GPs are reluctant to seek help in this way for themselves. Alternatively, many countries have mental health programmes specifically for medical professionals that operate on an anonymous basis.
- Self-help techniques such as mindfulness also have a good evidence base amongst doctors working in primary care, and many simple mindfulness techniques can be learnt via online apps.
- GPs also have the opportunity to tackle the source of their distress either by changing the way in which they

work or by changing the type of work that they do within the varied world of primary care.

Further Reading

Staten, A., & Lawson, E. (2017). *GP wellbeing: Combatting burnout in general practice.* London: CRC Press.

References

Beech, J., Fraser, C., Gardner, T., Buzelli, L., Williamson, S., & Alderwick, H.(2023). *Stressed and overworked: What the Commonwealth Fund's 2022 International Health Policy Survey of primary care physicians in 10 countries means for the UK.* Retrieved from https://www.health.org.uk/sites/default/files/upload/publications/2023/Stressed%20and%20overworked_WEB.pdf.

Bower, P., Knowles, S., Coventry, P. A., & Rowland, N. (2011). Counselling for mental health and psychosocial problems in primary care. *Cochrane Database of Systematic Reviews 2011*:(9), CD001025.

Chartered Society of Physiotherapists. (2013). Direct access and patient/client self-referral to physiotherapy: A review of contemporary practice within the European Union. *Physiotherapy, 99*(4), 285–291.

De Maeseneer, J., van Weel, C., Egilman, D., Mfenyana, K., Kaufman, A., Sewankambo, N., & Flinkenflögel, M. (2008). Funding for primary health care in developing countries. *BMJ, 336*(7643), 518–519.

Eze, N. D., Mateus, C., & Cravo Oliveira Hashiguchi, T. (2020). Telemedicine in the OECD: An umbrella review of clinical and cost-effectiveness, patient experience and implementation. *PLoS One, 15*(8), e0237585. doi:10.1371/journal.pone.0237585.

General Medical Council. (2014). *What's behind the rise in complaints about doctors from members of the public?* Retrieved from https://gmcuk.wordpress.com/2014/07/21/whats-behind-the-rise-in-complaints-about-doctors-from-members-of-the-public/.

Heyworth, L., Rozenblum, R., Burgess, J. F., Jr, Baker, E., Meterko, M., Prescott, D., Neuwirth, Z., & Simon, S. R. (2014). Influence of shared medical appointments on patient satisfaction: A retrospective 3-year study. *Annals of Family Medicine, 12*(4), 324–330.

Holt, T. A., Fletcher, E., Warren, F., Richards, S., Salisbury, C., Calitri, R., Green, C., Taylor, R., Richards, D. A., Varley, A., & Campbell, J. (2016). Telephone triage systems in UK general practice: Analysis of consultation duration during the index day in a pragmatic randomised controlled trial. *British Journal of General Practice, 66*(644), e214–e218.

Kringos, D. S., Boerma, W., van der Zee, J., & Groenewegen, P. (2013). Europe's strong primary care systems are linked to better population health but also to higher health spending. *Health Affairs (Project Hope) 32*(4), 686–694. doi:10.1377/hlthaff.2012.1242.

Leese, B., Young, R., & Sibbald, B. (2002). GP principals leaving practice in the UK. *European Journal of General Practice, 8*, 62–68.

Legler, C. F., Cawley, J. F., & Fenn, W. H. (2007). Physician assistants: Education, practice and global interest. *Medical Teacher, 29*(1), e22–e25.

Magnée, T., de Beurs, D. P., de Bakker, D. H., & Verhaak, P. F. (2016). Consultations in general practices with and without mental health nurses: An observational study from 2010 to 2014. *BMJ Open, 6*(7), e011579.

Mallett, R., Bakker, E., & Burton, M. (2014). Is physiotherapy self-referral with telephone triage viable, cost-effective and beneficial to musculoskeletal outpatients in a primary care setting? *Musculoskeletal Care, 12*(4), 251–260.

Martin-Misener, R., Harbman, P., Donald, F., Reid, K., Kilpatrick, K., Carter, N., Bryant-Lukosius, D., Kaasalainen, S., Marshall, D. A., Charbonneau-Smith, R., & DiCenso, A. (2015). Cost-effectiveness of nurse practitioners in primary and specialised ambulatory care: Systematic review. *BMJ Open, 5*, e007167.

Mayor, S. (2016). Use texts, apps, and Skype to keep young people with diabetes engaged with services, says guidance. *BMJ, 352*, i394.

Royal College of Nursing. (2012). Advanced Nurse Practitioners: An RCN Guide to advanced nursing practice, advanced nurse practitioners and programme accreditation.

Sinsky, C. A., Willard-Grace, R., Schutzbank, A. M., Sinsky, T. A., Margolius, D., & Bodenheimer, T. (2013). In search of joy in practice: A report of 23 high-functioning primary care practices. *Annals of Family Medicine, 11*(3), 272–278.

World Health Organization. (2003). *The World Health report: Shaping the future.*

World Health Organization. (1978). *Declaration of International Conference on Primary Health Care, Alma-Ata, USSR, 6–12 September 1978.*

2

Long-Term Conditions

Harry Wang & Stewart Mercer

CHAPTER CONTENTS

Prevalence of Long-Term Conditions

- Prevalence rates of individual long-term conditions (LTCs) vary considerably between different countries and populations, though in most countries, including developing countries, LTCs are increasing rapidly in the population. This is true in all age groups, although certain conditions affect certain age groups more than others.
- It should be borne in mind that all prevalence estimates of LTCs are based on data collection methods that have some flaws. Thus, prevalence estimates vary according to how the condition is defined and measured and how well documented these are in routine healthcare records.

Comorbidity and Multimorbidity

- International studies have demonstrated that many people living with chronic disorders have multiple chronic health problems simultaneously. The cooccurrence of one or more additional LTCs to a person with an index condition (a condition of primary concern) is termed *comorbidity*. For example, a patient with diabetes and asthma, being cared for by a diabetologist, may be considered by the specialist physician as a diabetic with comorbidity. It is a term mainly used by specialists reflecting their own area of expertise.

- In general practice, patients commonly have two or more LTCs without one being clearly an index condition, and indeed the extent to which different conditions affect patients often varies over time. Thus, in primary care, the term *multimorbidity* is preferred to comorbidity.
- Multimorbidity is common and has been rising in prevalence over recent years. For example, a Canadian study of 21 family practices in Quebec reported a multimorbidity prevalence of 69% in 18- to 44-year-old adults, 93% in 45- to 64-year-old adults, and 98% in those aged older than 65 years, with the number of chronic conditions varying from 2.8 in the youngest to 6.4 in the oldest (Fortin et al, 2005). In the United Kingdom, a large, nationally representative study in Scotland found that more than 40% of the whole population (all ages included) had at least one LTC, and almost 25% of the entire population had multimorbidity (Barnett et al, 2012).
- The prevalence of multimorbidity increases substantially with age and is present in most people aged 65 years or older. However, the Scottish study also found that the absolute number of people with multimorbidity was higher in those younger than 65 years than those older than 65 years. Therefore, LTCs and multimorbidity should not be considered simply a problem of old age.

Global Burden

- Over recent decades, life expectancy has improved dramatically and currently exceeds the age of 75 years on average in nearly 60 countries. This is attributed to improved living circumstances, greater access to universal education, and rapid advances in clinical medicine and public health.
- The ageing of the global population is regarded as the most crucial driver of increases in the burden of chronic diseases. It is particularly evident in wealthier countries, where many people are living much longer now than ever, though not necessarily healthier in their extra years. However, there is increasing evidence of the growing burden of multimorbidity in low- and middle-income countries.

Deprivation Effects

- Health is seldom distributed evenly across populations, and in most (if not all) countries of the world, the poorest health is found in those living in situations of poverty. This is also true of multimorbidity, which tends to be worse in those of the lowest socioeconomic status. The study in Scotland (discussed earlier) revealed an astonishingly precise relationship between multimorbidity and deprivation. Multimorbidity in those living in the most deprived areas also develops some 10 to 15 years younger than in the least deprived decile of the population.
- Many (though not all) studies have found that multimorbidity is commoner in females than in males.

Effects of Multimorbidity

- Many LTCs are associated with increased mortality or morbidity (or both), and this is exacerbated by increasing levels of multimorbidity. There is a clear linear relationship between levels of multimorbidity and death rate.
- Multimorbidity also increases hospital admission rates, even for those with potentially avoidable admissions, and has a major negative impact on quality of life.
- Multimorbidity also increases the need for social care, though there are limited data on this in most countries.

Healthcare Utilisation

- Patients with LTCs and multimorbidity may have higher overall vulnerability to diseases and less resistance to acute health threats (e.g., higher susceptibility to influenza). These interacting influences lead to a complex pattern in the demand and utilisation of health services.
- Multimorbidity leads to an increased likelihood of referrals between different providers of healthcare (often in a vertical manner, i.e., general practitioner [GP] to

several specialists but also between specialists, especially in centres of 'excellence'). Excessive use of specialist care leads to a rapid increase in healthcare expenditure. Multimorbidity has become one of the most salient influences on cost of healthcare because of the heavy burden on the healthcare utilisation.

Mental and Physical

- LTCs span both mental and physical conditions, and commonly patients have both. This relationship is bidirectional in that patients with mental health problems commonly go on to develop physical health problems, and patients with a wide-range of LTCs are more likely to go on to develop mental health problems than the general population.

Polypharmacy

- A common problem in patients with LTCs is polypharmacy, which is usually defined as taking five or more regular medications. In patients with multimorbidity, polypharmacy is even more common. This has serious implications for iatrogenesis. Indeed, common reasons for hospital admission, especially in older adults, are medication side effects and interactions. Not only are these harmful to patients, but they also put a huge financial drain on healthcare systems.
- A second problem with polypharmacy is adherence to medication regimens. Research has shown that when patients get to five or more medications per day, their adherence begins to decline. That's not to say that patients stop taking all their tablets, but they do tend to be creative in developing their own regimens, especially skipping tablets that have effects that they don't like such as loop diuretics.
- Patients often have strong perceptions of which tablets may be giving them side effects (even if this is unlikely to be the case), which can be influenced by a whole host of things such as pill size, colour, taste, and so on. It has been suggested that 'polypills' (combination pills with several ingredients, e.g., for cardiovascular disease) may enhance adherence by reducing the number of tablets required each day, though at present, there is little evidence to support this.

Clinical Guidelines

- A likely major driver of polypharmacy is guidelines. The development of clinical guidelines based on evidence collated from randomised controlled trials (RCTs) has been one of the major advances in the delivery of evidence-based medicine over the past 20 years. However, guidelines are invariably single-disease focused. They give good advice on when to start medications in single LTCs, though seldom give advice on when to stop them. This, combined with the fact that most patients with LTCs have multimorbidity, means that most patients rapidly accumulate new prescriptions and thus polypharmacy.

Evidence-Based General Practice

- The rise of evidence-based medicine (EBM) has been one of the greatest achievements in medical research, and the implementation of EBM into general practice has resulted in huge improvements in the management of LTCs. Statin prescribing for hypercholesterolaemia, antihypertensive prescribing for hypertension, and achievement of glycaemic control in diabetes through insulin or drug interventions are just a few examples of EBM. The gold standard research method that underpins EBM is the RCT.
- It is such evidence of benefit from RCTs that underpin clinical guidelines. However, there is a danger of over extrapolating findings from RCTs on specific populations (e.g., males younger than 65 years) to a much wider population (e.g., both sexes, older adults). It is also important to realise that most RCTs on LTCs are done on patients with single conditions, and most trials actively exclude patients with comorbidity or multimorbidity from taking part in such trials. A recent Cochrane review of interventions specifically for patients with multimorbidity found only a handful of RCTs published worldwide.
- Care must thus be taken not to blindly apply guidelines to all multimorbid patients without consideration of the individual patient's needs, circumstances, and priorities. Clinical judgement and shared decision making based on informed choice are vital tools in the management patients with LTCs, alongside clinical guidelines.

Management

- The management of patients with LTCs is a large and important part of the work of general practice and primary care. In the United Kingdom, about 80% of patients who consult their GPs or practice nurses have an LTC, and as we have seen, most of these patients are likely to have more than one LTC.
- The majority of care for most patients with LTCs can safely be undertaken in primary care, especially after any acute phase has been dealt with by secondary care (e.g., myocardial infarction in patients with CHD, initiation of insulin in a person newly diagnosed with type 1 diabetes) and the diagnosis is confirmed.
- In the United Kingdom, practice nurses and other members of the multidisciplinary team such as physiotherapists, pharmacists, and advanced practitioners are increasingly involved in the routine care of patients with LTCs, for example, in conducting annual reviews of patients with hypertension, asthma, and so on. These staff require suitable training and supervision, and it is important to emphasise that they are not

working autonomously but in partnership with GPs, who remain the key clinicians in dealing with patients with complex LTCs.

Organisational

- The effective management of patients with LTCs in primary care depends on a well-organised and strong primary care system. The work of the late Barbara Starfield, a preeminent primary care clinical researcher, has shown that countries with strong primary care systems deliver a higher quality of care and are more cost-effective.
- So, a well-funded and well-developed primary care system is a basic requisite for the cost-effective management of the vast numbers of patients with LTCs.
- Many models exist with regards to how the management of patients with LTCs is best organised, but one of the best known and most widely used is the chronic care model developed by Wagner and colleagues in the United States. The chronic care model defines a range of important factors which they suggest need to be addressed to promote effective management of chronic disease. These factors include:
  a. Clinical information systems (e.g., disease registers so that patients with known LTCs can be identified and recalled)
  b. Delivery system design (e.g., annual review at a planned visit, with members of the primary care team working in a coordinated and complementary way)
  c. Decision support (e.g., evidence-based practice guidelines, access to specialist advice)
  d. Self-management support (e.g., by giving information, coaching, and motivation to support patients to manage their own conditions better)
- These four factors are thought to work together to improve patients' functional and clinical outcomes as a result of prepared and proactive primary care staff having productive interactions with informed and activated patients.
- Although the chronic care model is intuitively appealing and gives a comprehensive overview of how best care may be achieved, it should be noted that evidence of its effectiveness outside the United States is limited, and achieving certain aspects of it can be very difficult in practice.
- The model envisages self-management support as being not just a function of the healthcare system but also a collaborative function of communities. Although this makes good sense in theory, as primary care is imbedded within communities, and communities often have a range of assets that could help people with LTCs (e.g., charitable organisations, faith groups, lunch clubs, exercise facilities, etc.), effective linkages between primary healthcare providers and local community resources are hard to achieve in practice. A recent development has been 'social prescribing' involving community link workers who work alongside primary care teams to link patients to local community resources.

Inverse Care Law

- An important issue compounding the effective management of patients with LTCs in primary care is the continuing existence of the 'inverse care law' in many (if not all) countries around the world. The term was first introduced in the 1970s by Julian Tudor Hart, a GP working in a socioeconomically deprived population in Wales. The inverse care law states that the availability of good medical care tends to vary inversely with the need for it in the population served. In general terms, this means that the poorest patients have the worst healthcare.

- This is, of course, abundantly clear within healthcare systems that are largely privately run. However, it is sadly also true of systems that have a national health service, such as the United Kingdom. The reason for this is that within the United Kingdom, primary care services (and the number of GPs in an area) are not distributed according to health need but according to population size.

- Although health need rises two- to threefold from the most affluent to the most deprived patients, the distribution of GPs is flat across deprivation deciles. In practice, this means that patients who live in poorer areas have worse access to high-quality care (longer waiting times to see a GP, shorter consultation length) with primary care practitioners in deprived areas being more stressed because of the greater need, demand, and clinical complexity of the patients.

- The inverse care law is, of course, not a law as such; rather, it is a situation brought about by policy decisions by governments as the funders of healthcare. Such policies could, of course, be changed, and doctors themselves can be active advocates of such change. In Scotland, for example, the GPs working in the 100 most deprived areas of the country formed an informal group, called GPs at the Deep End, which has been active in vocalising the problems they and their patients face. The GPs at the Deep End movement has now spread to other parts of the United Kingdom and internationally, with new groups being established as far away as Japan.

What Do Patients With Long-Term Conditions Need From General Practice?

- *Practice organisation.* Practices need to be well organised in caring for patients with LTCs, with effective means of identifying patients (e.g., electronic disease registers) and arranging proactive anticipatory care rather than simply reacting to problems that patients present with in an unplanned way. The best way to organise such anticipatory care depends on the practice resources and the patient population. For example, in more affluent areas, patients with LTCs are more likely to be proactive in their self-management and attend booked reviews. However, patients in deprived areas more commonly have additional social and psychological problems and may fail to attend for booked appointments for reviews; therefore, more anticipatory care may need to be done within the 'reactive' consultation. This, of course, has implications for consultation length, but some practices in deprived areas are able to give longer consultations (e.g., 15–20 minutes) when it is needed by having spare time slots within booked sessions that can be moved so that a 10-minute slot can be changed immediately into a 20-minute one.

- *Empathic, person-centred care.* The encounter between doctor and patient should never be reduced to a dry tick box exercise in which the GP blandly follows protocol. General practice defines itself as a discipline that provides holistic, generalist medicine. Holism means taking a biopsychosocial (and at times spiritual) approach to care. General practice is community based and community facing. Nowhere else in medicine is whole-person care so possible on a population level and so needed. We have the opportunity to get to know our patients and their families over time and thus provide much needed continuity of care. Our care is comprehensive and coordinated and is delivered with compassion and caring. Empathy is important in all therapeutic relationships, and empathic care is supported by values of altruism. Empathy is especially valued by patients with multimorbidity. Empathy leads to higher patient and practitioner satisfaction and better outcomes; research has shown that patients never feel enabled in consultations without GP empathy. Empathy has also been linked to better adherence with treatment regimens, reduction in symptom severity, and improved well-being. The effects of empathy can be direct and immediate or indirect and longer term.

- *Generalism.* GPs need to be expert generalists, which not only requires excellent technical clinical skills and knowledge and effective communication skills but also being skilled in 'interpretive medicine', integrating multiple sources of knowledge (including biomedical, biographical, and professional) in a dynamic exploration and interpretation of the individual illness experience. Practising interpretive medicine leads to decisions about what is wrong, and what is needed to intervene, which supports an outcome of health as a resource for living, with the patient as an active partner in 'coproducing' health.

Conclusions

- As the population ages, the dramatic rise in the prevalence of LTCs is the major challenge facing the world and most of its countries. It is also the major challenge facing general practice and primary care.
- Multimorbidity is the norm, not the exception, yet guidelines and EBM are largely derived from research that excludes patients with multimorbidity.
- In managing patients with single or multiple LTCs, general practice and primary care teams need to be well organised to care for such patients and to be

proactive and anticipatory rather than simply reactive. This requires a strong primary care system with adequate resources.

- Patients with multiple complex needs must be at the centre of care, not the round pegs in the square holes of single-disease focused approaches. Holism lies at the heart of good management, and empathic, patient-centred care is a key requirement of the two facets of high-quality primary care for patients with LTCs, generalism and interpretive medicine.

References

Barnett, B., Mercer, S. W., Norbury, M., Watt, G., Wyke, S., & Guthrie, B. (2012). The epidemiology of multimorbidity – authors reply. *The Lancet, 380*(9851), 1383–1384.

Fortin, M., Bravo, G., Hudon, C., Vanasse, A., & Lapointe, L. (2005). Prevalence of multimorbidity among adults seen in family practice. *Annals of Family Medicine, 3*(3), 223–228.

Wagner, E. H. (1998). Chronic disease management: what will it take to improve care for chronic illness? *Eff Clin Pract.* 1, 2–4.

3

Communication Skills

Adam Staten

CHAPTER CONTENTS

Professional Requirement

- The professional requirements related to communication skills are outlined in the General Medical Council's (GMC's) (2013) Good Medical Practice as:
  a. Treat patients as individuals and respect their dignity.
  b. Treat patients politely and considerately.
  c. Respect patients' right to confidentiality.
  d. Work in partnership with patients.
  e. Listen to and respond to patients' concerns and preferences.
  f. Give patients the information they want or need in a way they can understand.
  g. Respect patients' right to reach decisions with you about their treatment and care.
  h. Support patients in caring for themselves to improve and maintain their health.
  i. Work with colleagues in the ways that best serve patients' interests.
- The Royal College of General Practitioners curriculum statement in 2023 describes how expert communication and consultation skills lie at the heart of true patient-centred care (Royal College of General Practitioners, 2023).

Communication Skills

Verbal Communication

- During consultations it is important to use a mixture of question types, which include:
  a. Open questions
  b. Closed questions
  c. Focused questions
  d. Indirect questions
- Question types to avoid include:
  a. Leading questions
  b. Compound or double questions
- As well as questions, language is used for other purposes:
  a. Social exchanges ('good morning' or comments on the weather)
  b. Facilitations ('go on' or 'uh uh')
  c. Repetition or restatement (repeating back what has just been said)

d. Confrontation (confronting with an observation: 'You look worried/sad/angry')
e. Clarification or interpretation (clarifying what the patient has said: 'So, the tiredness started after your sleep pattern was disturbed?')
f. Judgemental statements (responses that state the value judgement of the doctor: 'Anyone who smokes cigarettes is foolish')
g. Reassurance, explanation, instruction, or advice

Nonverbal Communication

- This includes:
  a. Dress and appearance
  b. Facial expression
  c. Gaze and eye contact
  d. Gestures
  e. Posture
  f. Proximity (comfort zones)
  g. Body contact and touch
  h. Mirroring
  i. Pacing

Paralinguistics

- This is the term given to those aspects of vocalisation, such as the speed, loudness, and pitch of the voice. These may convey information about emotions, attitudes, or personality (e.g., whereas a soft, slow hesitant voice is associated with depression, a more rapid, loud voice suggests anger or excitement).

Rapport

- Some of the most common mistakes in communication are to talk too much and listen too little. In listening to patients, it is important to really listen and let the patient know that you are listening to them. This establishes trust and rapport.
- Rapport can be established and maintained at four levels.
  Level 1: nonverbal level—by matching body language; posture, gestures, facial expressions, and eye contact
  Level 2: paralinguistics or voice level—by matching breathing rate, tone, pitch, and tempo
  Level 3: language level—by matching or using another's words
  Level 4: values level—by connecting with shared beliefs and values
- Sensitivity to the patient's cues (Silverman, Kurtz & Draper, 2013):
  1. Be alert to the patient's verbal cues (prompts, throw-away comments) and nonverbal cues (body language, facial expression, vocal cues) to elicit emotional content of the illness, ideas, effect on daily living, and expectations.
  2. Clarify the emotions that the patient is hinting at (e.g., by repeating or checking out a verbal cue: 'You said that the cough worries you, especially at night. What do you think it might be?' or a nonverbal cue:

'Am I right in thinking that you are puzzled by the information that I gave you?').
  3. Explicitly acknowledge cues as appropriate.
- Demonstrating empathy to help develop rapport involves (Derksen et al, 2013):
  1. Understanding (or reconstruct and imagine) the patient's situation, perspective, and feelings
  2. Verbally communicating the understanding to check its accuracy (e.g., 'I can see that you are very worried about the test results')
  3. Acting on the understanding in a helpful therapeutic way
- Empathy does not require you to have experienced the same problem as the patient or to like the patient.
  Research shows that patients consider empathy to be a key component of quality of care and that empathy is linked to patient enablement (Mercer et al, 2012; Derksen et al, 2013).

Ideas, Concerns, Effect, and Expectations

- These include obtaining an understanding of how the patient sees the situation and experiences the illness. As well as exploring the disease, inquire about (Stewart et al, 2003):
  a. Feelings that reflect the emotional content of the illness (e.g., 'Do you have any concerns about … ?')
  b. Ideas about what the patient thinks the cause is (e.g., 'What do think is causing it?')
  c. The effect on the patient's daily life (e.g., how illness limits daily activities and impairs their capacity to fulfil certain responsibilities)
  d. Expectation of the consultation (e.g., 'What were you expecting from seeing me today?')
- By taking other factors into account, such as age, culture, the physical environment, or people affected by the illness, the patient's experience of the illness is put into the context of the person's life (e.g., 'Who is at home with you?')
- This can be summarised as the ICEE framework, in which the doctor explores:
  a. The patient's ideas (I) about what is wrong
  b. The patient's feelings or concerns (C) about the illness
  c. The impact or effect (E) of the patient's problems
  d. The patient's expectations (E) about what should be done

Sharing Information

- The GMC states that you must 'give patients the information they want or need to know in a way they can understand'.
- Tailor the explanation to the patient by taking into account the patient's needs and beliefs (e.g., 'You mentioned depression and tiredness. I think tiredness is more likely because … ')
  - Observe the patient's reactions to check if the explanation needs refinement.

- Find out what and how much the patient wants to know to match the amount and type of information to the patient's needs and preferences (e.g., the diagnosis, coping techniques or support available, the causes of the illness, or side effects of treatment).
- Check what the patient already knows, e.g., 'I don't know how much you know about high blood pressure already'.
- Avoid jargon or check the patient's understanding of the technical term used.
- Back up verbal information with written information, if appropriate, and ensure it is in the relevant language.
- Check the patient's understanding.

Depending on the patient, Thistlethwaite and Morris (2006) suggest that the explanation is based on three domains:

Type of Explanation	Type of Questions	Purpose
Interpretive	What	To interpret or clarify
	What is diabetes?	
Descriptive	How	To describe a concept or process
	How do my kidneys work?	
Giving reasons	Why	To give reason based on principle, motives, or values
	Why did this happen to me?	

Shared Decision Making

- 'Shared decision making is an approach in which clinicians and patients make decisions together using the best available evidence' (Elwyn et al, 2010).
- The shared decision-making process includes (Thistlewaite & Morris, 2006):
  a. Giving information to the patient on treatment options, possible risks, and benefits in a way that the patient understands
  b. Helping the patient to balance the risks and benefits and make sure that their choice is based on fact rather than misconception

Informed Consent

- The GMC (2013) states that it is the responsibility of the person providing treatment or undertaking an investigation to obtain consent.
- According to the GMC, you must give patients the information they want or need about:
  a. The diagnosis and prognosis
  b. Any uncertainties, including options for further investigations
  c. Options for treating and managing the condition, including the option not to treat
  d. The purpose of proposed treatments and what these will involve

  e. The potentials risks, burdens, and likelihood of success of each option
  f. Whether a proposed investigation or treatment is experimental (part of research or innovative)
  g. Who is responsible for the treatment, the roles of those involved, the involvement of students
  h. Their right to refuse to take part in research or teaching
  i. Their right to seek a second opinion
  j. Any bills they will have to pay
  k. Any conflicts of interest that you may have
  l. Information on any treatments with potential greater benefit than the ones offered by you or your organisation
- Before accepting a patient's consent, you must consider whether they have been given the information they want or need and how well they understand the details and implications of what is proposed. This is more important than how their consent is expressed or recorded.
- Patients can give consent orally or in writing, or they may imply consent by complying with the proposed examination or treatment, for example, by rolling up their sleeve to have their blood pressure taken.
- In the case of minor or routine investigations or treatments, if you are satisfied that the patient understands what you propose to do and why, it is usually enough to have oral or implied consent.
- In cases that involve higher risk, it is important that you get the patient's written consent. This is so that everyone involved understands what was explained and agreed.
- By UK law, you must get written consent for certain treatments, such as fertility treatment. You must follow the laws and codes of practice that govern these situations.

Confidentiality

- The GMC (2009), in the discussion of confidentiality, states the principles of confidentiality and respect for patients' privacy. This includes:
  a. Making sure that any personal information about patients that you hold or control is effectively protected at all times against improper disclosure.
  b. Instances when personal information can be disclosed, including if it is required by law, the patient consents to this disclosure (either implicitly for the sake of their own care or expressly for other purposes), or if it justified in the public interest.
- Data protection is a highly legislated area, and the specific laws around data protection vary from region and country. Therefore, all medical professionals should ensure that they are familiar with and comfortable with the laws with which they must comply. For example, in the European Union, the General Data Protection Regulation (GDPR) came into effect in 2016 and made widespread changes to how personal data were handled. The GDPR has been retained within UK law after the UK's departure from the European Union.

- Inevitably in medicine, there are times when information must be shared to ensure patient safety. In the United Kingdom, the Caldicott principles are used to guide clinicians with regards to information sharing. These are:
  1. Justify the purpose for sharing confidential information.
  2. Use confidential information only when necessary.
  3. Use the minimum necessary confidential information.
  4. Access to confidential information should be on a strict need-to-know basis.
  5. Everyone with access to confidential information should be aware of their responsibilities.
  6. Comply with the law.
  7. The duty to share information for individual care is as important as the duty to protect patient confidentiality.
  8. Inform patients and service users about how their confidential information is used and what choice they have. There should be no surprises.

Working With Interpreters

- The GMC states that you should make sure that arrangements are made, whenever possible, to meet patients' language and communication needs.
- Ask that the interpretation should be in the first person without omissions, editing, polishing, or outside conversations.
- Ask the interpreter to clarify (in their own words) any misunderstandings that occur because of cultural differences.
- Position yourself so you face and speak directly to the patient rather than the interpreter.
- Talk with the patient in the first person (using 'I').
- Maintain direct eye contact with the patient.
- Do not direct your questions or inquiries to the interpreter.
- Ask the patient to repeat any instructions and explanations given to ensure that they are understood.
- Issues to be aware of (Lloyd & Bor, 2004) include:
  - Meanings can be altered in the translation process.
  - The patient can be embarrassed by the presence of interpreter because of the sensitive of problem, especially when they are of same nationality.
  - The patient's ideas can be reinterpreted by interpreter or translated in a shortened version.

Adherence and Compliance

- Tate (2010) states several reasons why patients follow or do not follow the treatment:
  a. Some patients adhere because they are told by the doctor to do so.
  b. If the patient understands and believes the explanation given to them by the doctor, then the patient is more likely to adhere to treatment.
  c. If the patient's own understanding matches that of the doctor and their agenda is shared, then the patient is most likely to adhere.

  d. Shared decision making and linking the management plan with the patient's beliefs are key to ensuring adherence and compliance.

Physical Arrangement of the Room

- The physical arrangement of the room can facilitate or hinder communication (Lloyd & Bor, 2004).
- Arrangement of seats
  - Turning away and facing a computer can indicate disinterest, so the patient may not give information critical to the consultation.
  - Arrangements such as sitting sideways or facing each other without a desk in the middle and being at the same eye level facilitate communication.
  - Usually, the patient's chair is stable with four legs, and the doctor's chair is often a swivel seat on wheels, which helps to complete the various tasks and to face the patient and the computer at different times.
- Use of a computer: Communication guides (Silverman, Kurtz & Draper, 2013) suggest:
  a. Waiting until the patient has finished their opening statement before looking at the computer
  b. Turning your attention back to the patient if they start to speak whilst you are looking at the computer
  c. Explaining to the patient what you are doing so that the patient understands the process

The Structure of the Consultation

The ability to select from different consultation styles and skills to navigate through the consultation facilitates the need to meet patients with different expectations and preferences.

The Consultation

- Pendleton et al (1984) defined seven doctor's tasks, which form the aims for each consultation. It is not suggested that all tasks should be completed in every consultation, though they argue that continued omission of one or more tasks will negatively impact on consultation outcome. Tasks 1 to 5 identify what the doctor needs to achieve. Tasks 6 to 7 relate to the entire consultation and highlight the use of time and resources and the development of an effective doctor–patient relationship.
- The seven tasks are as follows:
  1. Define the reason for the patient's attendance, including:
     a. The nature and history of the problem(s)
     b. The aetiology (or cause) of the problem (i.e., the interaction of the physical, psychological, and social factors)
     c. The patient's ideas, concerns, and expectations
     d. The effects of the problems (on daily living)
  2. Consider other problems that are present but not presented by the patient:

a. Continuing problems (e.g., previous problems discussed at earlier consultations or social conditions relevant to the current problem)
b. Modifiable risk factors (health promotion)

3. Choose with the patient an appropriate action for each problem.
4. Achieve a shared understanding of the problems with the patient (including giving explanations that relate to patient's ideas about the problem).
5. Involve the patient in the management and encourage them to accept appropriate responsibility. The level of involvement that is appropriate will vary from patient to patient and from problem to problem.
6. Use time and resources appropriately.
   a. In the consultation
   b. In the long term
7. Establish or maintain a relationship with the patient that helps to achieve the other tasks (e.g., the doctor–patient relationship encourages the sharing of decisions).

The Inner Consultation

- Neighbour (1987) uses five checkpoints (subgoals) in the consultation alongside an awareness of 'minimal cues' (verbal and nonverbal) to help discover the unspoken agenda. He emphasises the importance of the start of the consultation in which the patient conveys more information than often is realised. Ideally, a checkpoint is reached before moving to the next one.
- The five-stage model includes:
  1. Connecting—with the patient and developing rapport
  2. Summarising—your understanding of the problem (events and emotional content)
  3. Handing over—the management plan that is understood, accepted, and agreed with the patient. Strategies for handing over include:
     a. Negotiating
     b. Influencing
     c. Gift wrapping
  4. Safety netting—and planning for the unexpected to manage uncertainty (e.g., using a specific time frame such as 'Come back in 2 weeks if it doesn't get better'). Neighbour (1987) points to three safety netting questions:
     a. If I am right, what do I expect to happen?
     b. How will I know if I am wrong?
     c. What would I do then?
  5. Housekeeping and taking care of yourself through stress prevention. Various options are given on what to do about job stress during and outside the consultation.

The Calgary Cambridge Method

- The Calgary Cambridge method (2013) integrates the tasks of the consultation and skills for communication. Silverman et al (2013) analysed 71 communication skills, which are grouped under six headings. The skills needed

depend on the context and the outcomes that the doctor and patient want to achieve.
- These skills include:
  1. Initiating the session
     - Establishing initial rapport
     - Identifying the reason(s) for attendance
  2. Gathering information
     - Exploring the patient's problems
     - Additional skills for understanding the patient's perspective
  3. Providing structure to the consultation
     - Making organisation overt
     - Attending to flow
  4. Building the relationship
     - Using appropriate nonverbal behaviour
     - Developing the rapport
     - Involving the patient
  5. Explaining and planning
     - Providing the right amount and type of information
     - Aiding accurate recall and understanding
     - Achieving a shared understanding: incorporating the patient's perspective
     - Planning: shared decision making
  6. Closing the session
     - Forward planning
     - Ensuring appropriate point of closure

The CARE Approach

- The Consultation and Relational Empathy (CARE, 2011) approach aims to foster the achievement of empathic, patient-centred communication in healthcare encounters and is based on the CARE measure, a patient-rated experience measure. It is a broad set of guiding principles to be applied flexibly depending on the situation and circumstance.
- It consists of four interacting components that form an integrated cyclical process
  a. Connecting: Actively engaging with the patient to create or deepen rapport and to facilitate open communication in a safe environment
  b. Assessing: Listening and taking a holistic approach to fully understand the patient's situation, perspective, and feelings (and their attached meanings)
  c. Responding: Communicating your understanding (and checking its accuracy) in a caring and compassionate way and responding positively with clear explanations if appropriate
  d. Empowering: Helping patients to feel more in control according to their abilities, preferences, and values and planning their treatment in partnership with them

How to React to a Complaint

- The GMC states that 'you must respond promptly, fully and honestly to complaints and apologise when appropriate'.

- The Medical and Dental Defence Union of Scotland recommends:
  a. Ask colleagues for support.
  b. If you are the person who is being complained about, make sure someone else in the practice deals with the complaint.
  c. Keep good contemporaneous notes; this is absolutely critical!
  d. Be open to accepting that something may have gone wrong.
  e. Share learning from complaints with the whole practice.
  f. Let the complainant know what the practice plans to do to put things right.

Telephone and Video Consultations

- The use of telephone and video consultation is now very widespread and generally has a high degree of acceptance amongst patients.
- In general, the communication skills required to conduct remote consultations are much the same as those used for face-to-face consultations.
- The same standards of care, confidentiality, and safety must apply to both in-person and remote consultations.
- If care cannot be safely delivered remotely, the consultation must be converted to a face-to-face consultation.

Communication Skills for Telephone Consultations

- Car and Sheikh (2003) suggest using the same skills as in face-to-face consultations and being systematic in covering the following:
  a. Active listening (including verbal facilitation, e.g., 'Mmm, I see', 'Tell me a bit more') and increased questioning or detailed history taking (e.g., 'What does the rash look like?') to compensate for the lack of visual cues
  b. Frequent clarifying and paraphrasing (to ensure that the messages have been sent and received in both directions)
  c. Picking up verbal (red flag words or warning signs) and nonverbal cues (e.g., pace, pauses, change in voice intonation, e.g., 'I can hear from your voice that you are not sure about …')
  d. Offering opportunities to ask questions
  e. Offering patient education
  f. Documentation
- Check the provided number with the number on the patient's record. If it does not match, additional care might be needed.
- Telephone consulting is considered to have some additional risk with respect to confidentiality with the risk of a conversation being overheard as the area of most concern, so always check when phoning a patient that they are in an environment where they can speak comfortably and confidentially.
- Always confirm identity, ideally with three points of data (e.g., name, date of birth, and first line of address).
- Avoid getting involved with third-party consultations; always ask to speak directly to the patient if possible.
- If asking patients to provide details of a problem, receptionists should explain 'why' they are asking (e.g., so the doctor can prioritise) and explain that the patient does not have to give any information if they do not wish to.
- Practices should have caller identification switched off.
- If messages are left on an answering machine, they should be confined to confirmation that the clinician called and a request to call back.
- If in doubt, ask to see the patient.

Guidance on Remote Prescribing

- The GMC (2013) states that to prescribe, 'You must satisfy yourself that you can make an adequate assessment, establish a dialogue and obtain the patient's consent' and that 'You may prescribe only when you have adequate knowledge of the patient's health, and are satisfied that the medicines serve the patient's needs'.

Email and Text Message Consultations

- Email and text messaging can be highly effective means of communicating both with patients and colleagues.
- With the phasing out of fax machines in many healthcare services and an environmental drive towards using less paper, email in particular is now a core means by which healthcare is coordinated.
- Points to note regarding to email:
  - Email between secure email addresses such as those with governmental or health service domain names is a secure and effective means of communication.
  - Patient emails should only be used with the patient's consent, and the patient should be informed that you cannot guarantee the security of *their* email accounts.
  - Exercise extreme caution with regards to personal data when there are multiple recipients or a bulk email list.
  - Do not write anything in an email that you would not be happy to see recorded in the patient's notes.
  - Remember the Caldicott principles with regards to the information shared.
- Points to note regarding text messaging:
  - Text messaging should only be used with patient consent.
  - Take care to ensure the number to which the message is being sent matches that in the patient notes.

Recordings and Photography

- The transfer and receipt of photographs and recordings has increased with the increasing use of remote consultation.

- The GMC has issued guidance, the principles of which include:
  - Recordings and photographs must be treated with the same degree of data security as other components of the patient record.
  - Images should only be taken with patient consent. The patient may withdraw that consent at any time.
  - Any secondary use of the recording (e.g., for research purposes) must be made clear to the patient at the point of consent and should be on an anonymised basis.
  - The patient's privacy and dignity should be respected at all times.
- In general, taking photographs of intimate areas should be avoided.

References

Car, J., & Sheikh, A. (2003). Telephone consultations. *British Medical Journal, 326*(7396), 966–969.

Derksen, F., Bensing, J., & Lagro-Janssen, A. (2013). Effectiveness of empathy in general practice: A systematic review. *British Journal of General Practice, 63*(606), e76–e84.

Elwyn, G., Laitner, S., Coulter, A., Walker, E., Watson, P., Thomson, R. (2010). Implementing shared decision making in the NHS. *British Medical Journal, 341*, c5146.

General Medical Council. (2009). *Confidentiality: Good practice in handling patient information*. Retrieved from https://www.gmc-uk. org/professional-standards/professional-standards-for-doctors/confidentiality. (Accessed 28 August 2024).

General Medical Council. (2013). *Good medical practice*. London, England: GMC. Retrieved from www.gmc-uk.org/gmp.

Lloyd, M., & Bor, R. (2004). *Communication skills for medicine* (2nd ed.). London: Harcourt.

Mercer, S. W., Jani, B. D., Maxwell, M., Wong, S. Y. S., & Watt, G. C. M. (2012). Patient enablement requires physician empathy: A cross-sectional study of general practice consultations in areas of high and low socioeconomic deprivation in Scotland. *BMC Family Practice, 13*, 6.

Neighbour, R. (1987). *The inner consultation*. Int: Kluwer Academic Publishers.

Pendleton, D., Schofield, T., Tate, P., & Havelock, P. (1984). *The consultation: An approach to learning and teaching*. Oxford: Oxford University Press.

Royal College of General Practitioners. (2023). *The RCGP Curriculum: Being a General Practitioner*. Retrieved from https://www.rcgp.org.uk/getmedia/38f37bbe-f677-429f-90e9-37f855b0ae16/curriculum-being-a-gp-rcgp_26-10-22.pdf.

Silverman, J. D., Kurtz, S., & Draper, J. (2013). *Skills for Communicating with Patients* (3rd Ed.). CRC Press.

Stewart, M., Brown, J. B., Weston, W., McWhinney, I. R., McWilliam, C. L., & Freeman, T. R. (2013). *Patient Centred Medicine: Transforming the Clinical Method* (3rd Ed.). CRC Press.

Tate, P. (2010). *The doctor's communication handbook*. Oxon: Radcliffe Publishing.

Thistlewaite, M., & Morris, P. (2006). *The Patient-Doctor Consultation in Primary Care: Theory and Practice*. Royal College of General Practitioners.

4

Disability

Adam Staten

Disabilities is an umbrella term, covering impairments, activity limitations, and participation restrictions. An impairment is a problem in body function or structure; an activity limitation is a difficulty encountered by an individual in executing a task or action; whilst a participation restriction is a problem experienced by an individual in involvement in life situations.

Disability is thus not just a health problem. It is a complex phenomenon, reflecting the interaction between features of a person's body and features of the society in which they live. Overcoming the difficulties faced by people with disabilities requires interventions to remove environmental and social barriers.

People with disabilities have the same health needs as non-disabled people – for immunisation, cancer screening, etc. They also may experience a narrower margin of health, both because of poverty and social exclusion, and because they may be vulnerable to secondary conditions, such as pressure sores or urinary tract infections. Evidence suggests that people with disabilities face barriers in accessing the health and rehabilitation services they need in many settings (World Health Organization, 2011).

CHAPTER CONTENTS

Effect of Impairment on Carrying Out Normal Day-to-Day Activities

- Complete or substantial dependence on another.
- Time taken may be significantly longer (e.g., dressing and toileting) (Office for Disability Issues UK, 2010).
- May affect a person's ability to sustain an activity for long periods of time or carry out the activity repeatedly. A person may be able to carry out an activity (e.g., walking) but have significant pain in doing so, which in turn may limit the performance of that activity (Office for Disability Issues UK, 2010).
- May have a cumulative effect on the day as difficulties are experienced with a sequence of activities.
- Interruption of normal day-to-day activities such as a frequent need to go to the toilet.
- May have a circadian rhythm such as rheumatoid arthritis (i.e., joint pain, morning stiffness, and functional disability in the early morning hours).

- May affect a person's ability to estimate or assess danger (e.g., road safety, touching very hot things, or an inability to protect themselves from potential exploitation or violence).
- May cause a person to modify their behaviour (e.g., a person with rheumatoid arthritis may limit their activities first thing in the morning to avoid pain or to wait for prescribed medications to take effect). Equally, a person may use an avoidance strategy if there is a risk of considerable embarrassment in social situations such as faecal incontinence or facial disfigurement.
- Physical impairments can cause mental effects and vice versa (e.g., a person with fatigue or pain, may experience difficulties in remembering or concentrating). Similarly, mental impairments can have physical manifestations, for example, a person with a mental impairment such as depression may experience difficulty in carrying out physical activities.

Prevalence of Disability

Disability is common and becomes more so as populations age. Approaches to measuring disability vary, but it is estimated that 16% of the world's population, one in six people, have a disability (World Health Organization [WHO], 2022).

Human Rights and Disability

People with disabilities experience inequalities and social injustice, including rejection, isolation, discrimination, harassment, stigma, segregation, and institutionalisation. They also experience barriers in accessing education and employment opportunities and timely and appropriate healthcare and services.

Rehabilitation

- The WHO defines rehabilitation as 'a set of measures that assist individuals who experience, or are likely to experience, disability to achieve and maintain optimal functioning in interaction with their environments'.
- The term *rehabilitation* is also a process aimed at enabling disabled people 'to reach and maintain their optimal physical, sensory, intellectual, psychological and social functional levels thus providing them with the tools they need to attain independence and self-determination'.
- The aims of rehabilitation are:
  - Prevent loss of function
  - Improve or restore function
  - Compensate for lost function
  - Halt or slow decline in function
  - Maintain function

Physical and Rehabilitation Medicine

Physical and rehabilitation medicine doctors (physiatrists) are involved in the diagnosis of health conditions, assessment of functioning, and prescription of medical and technological interventions that manage health conditions and optimise functional capacity.

Therapy

Therapy may be done by occupational therapists, physiotherapists, orthotists and prosthetists, speech and language therapists, rehabilitation nurses, audiologists, psychologists, social workers, and rehabilitation technologists.
- Interventions include:
  - Manual therapy, specific exercises, manipulation, the use of electrotherapeutic and mechanical agents, acupuncture, and specific therapies such as reminiscence therapy and compensatory strategies such augmentative and alternative communication
  - Promotion of a healthy lifestyle and physical activity
  - Education
  - Support and counselling
  - Task and environmental modification
  - Provision of equipment, products, and technologies

Assistive Technologies

An assistive technology is a product or service designed to enable persons with a disability to achieve and maintain optimal functioning in interaction with their environments.
- Examples of assistive technologies include:
  - For people with mobility impairments: wheelchairs, prostheses, orthoses, scooters, bath boards and seats, ramps, grab rails, and stair lifts
  - For people with visual impairments: Braille-based typewriters (braillers) and embossers, access technology such as screen reader programmes, high-contrast spectacles, and radios for people with visual impairment
  - For people with hearing impairments: cochlear implants, amplified telephones and mobiles, vibrating alarm clocks, products to relieve the effect of tinnitus, and hearing aids
  - For people with cognitive impairment: computer-based technology for recording of information, text-to-speech apps or programmes that assist people with writing and reading difficulties, pictorial-based electronic timetables, and GPS devices
  - For people with speech impairments: speech synthesisers, communication boards, modified typewriters, and text-to-voice software
  - Equipment for activities of daily living: modified eating utensils, dressing aids, adapted personal hygiene equipment, emergency call systems, and dosette boxes for medications
- Rehabilitation services can be delivered in a variety of settings, including hospitals, clinics, general practitioner (GP) surgeries, patients' homes, residential or nursing care homes, school, and work (WHO, 2011).

Evidence-Based Rehabilitation

- Examples include:
  - Multidisciplinary rehabilitation for acquired brain injury in adults of working age
  - Home-based versus centre-based cardiac rehabilitation
  - Physical rehabilitation for older people in long-term care
  - Multidisciplinary rehabilitation for older people with hip fractures
  - Multidisciplinary rehabilitation for adults with multiple sclerosis
  - Multidisciplinary biopsychosocial rehabilitation for neck and shoulder pain among working age adults
  - Multidisciplinary biopsychosocial rehabilitation for subacute low back pain among working age adults
  - Pulmonary rehabilitation after exacerbations of COPD
  - Vocational rehabilitation for people with severe mental illnesses
  - Exercise-based cardiac rehabilitation for patients with coronary heart disease
  - Cognitive rehabilitation for people with schizophrenia and related conditions

EVIDENCE-BASED PRACTICE RESOURCES FOR GENERAL PRACTITIONERS, PATIENTS, AND CARERS

Cochrane systematic reviews are published online in The Cochrane Library. http://www.cochrane.org

The Royal College of Physicians London National Clinical Guidelines for Stroke. https://www.strokeaudit.org/Guideline/Full-Guideline.aspx

Royal National Institute for the Blind. http://www.rnib.org.uk/Pages/Home.aspx

Action on Hearing Loss. https://actionhearingloss.org.uk/

Stroke Association. http://www.stroke.org.uk

Chest Heart & Stroke Scotland. http://www.chss.org.uk

Parkinson's UK. http://www.parkinsons.org.uk

Multiple Sclerosis Society UK. http://www.mssociety.org.uk

Alzheimer's Society. http://www.alzheimers.org.uk

Versus Arthritis. https://www.versusarthritis.org

National Rheumatoid Arthritis Society UK. https://nras.org.uk/

Motor Neurone Disease Association. https://www.mndassociation.org/

The British Heart Foundation. http://www.bhf.org.uk

Muscular Dystrophy UK. http://www.muscular-dystrophy.org

Intellectual Disability, Learning Disability, and Developmental Disability

Terminology

- *Learning disability* is synonymous with *intellectual disability* and is a significant general impairment in intellectual functioning (typically an IQ of <70) that is acquired during childhood (Emerson & Heslop, 2010). *Developmental disability* includes motor impairments (cerebral palsy), social impairments (autism spectrum disorders), and sensory impairments (vision and hearing) as well as cognitive impairment (intellectual disability).
- There are three key features in the definition of intellectual disability:
  - IQ below 70
  - Deficits in two or more adaptive skills (self-care, home living, social skills, leisure, health and safety, self-direction, functional academics, community use and work)
  - Present at birth or acquired in childhood (before 18 years of age)
- People with intellectual disability have a significantly reduced ability to understand new or complex information and to learn and apply new skills. This results in a reduced ability to cope independently.
- It is estimated that 1% to 3% of the population has an intellectual disability (depending on definitions and methods of ascertainment).

The Importance of Language

Language reflects the attitudes of the speaker and influences the attitudes of others. Inappropriate language can cause hurt and offense to people with disabilities and their families and friends. People with disabilities are people first. Their disability impacts on their life experience, but it does not define them.

Health and Learning Disability: The Evidence

- People with learning disabilities experience:
  - Higher rates of morbidity and premature death than their non–learning-disabled peers, a significant proportion of which is avoidable (Emerson & Baines, 2010)
  - Chronic and complex health and social needs
  - Barriers to accessing healthcare
  - Fewer opportunities for preventive health and health promotion interventions
  - More undiagnosed and undertreated health conditions.
- *Standardised health assessments* are effective in the detection of previously unrecognised or unmet health needs, including life-threatening conditions, and lead to targeted actions to address health needs (Lennox et al, 2007; Robertson et al, 2011; Sullivan et al, 2018).
- The Canadian Consensus Guidelines in the Primary Care of Adults with Intellectual and Developmental Disabilities (Sullivan et al, 2018) provide evidence under the headings
  - Approaches to Care
  - Assessments and Considerations Important for All Care
  - Physical Health
  - Mental Health
- Care should be delivered to people with disabilities as part of a collaborative team.
- The aetiology of the disability should be established.

- Be aware of the communicative role of behaviour and the behavioural manifestations of illness, pain or discomfort (physical and mental), and environmental stressors.
- Disease prevention is essential.
- Avoid the unnecessary or inappropriate use of medications that may cause harm.
- Be aware of the increased prevalence in people with disabilities of:
  - Vision and hearing impairment
  - Dental disease
  - Cardiac disorders (congenital and acquired)
  - Musculoskeletal disorders, including spasticity, scoliosis, osteopenia or osteoporosis, and osteoarthritis
  - Respiratory disorders, particularly aspiration pneumonia, which are among the most common causes of death for people with developmental disability
  - Epilepsy. Seizures are a prominent cause of death
  - Gastrointestinal disease, particularly reflux and constipation, and the impact of these on quality of life and behaviour. *Helicobacter pylori* infection is more common in people with developmental disabilities
  - Endocrine disorders such as thyroid disease, hypogonadism, and diabetes
  - Disorders of mental health can be difficult to identify when people have communication difficulties. Effective treatment depends on an accurate diagnosis

Providing Healthcare

- *Person-first approach.* Think first of them as a female or male of a particular age, background, and physique. What care would you provide to them if they did not have a disability? Is there any reason to modify that care? If so, why?
- *Then consider their disability.*
  - How does their intellectual disability affect their health and healthcare? Consider their life experiences and opportunities, their communication and cognitive ability, and their ability to make considered decisions and plan and anticipate consequences.
  - What is the cause of their disability, and does this aetiologic diagnosis inform healthcare? For example, people with Down syndrome are at increased risk, throughout their lives, of thyroid dysfunction, hearing and vision impairment, immune deficiency. and respiratory infection. In their teens, 20s, and 30s, they are at risk of depression and anxiety, and in their 40s and beyond, they are at risk of Alzheimer disease.
- *Demonstrate respect.*
  - Address the person directly and use a tone of voice consistent with their age, raising your voice only if they have a hearing impairment.
  - Ask the person's permission before inviting the accompanier into the consultation or asking questions of them but ensure the focus remains on the person.

- *Support the person to understand.* Many people with intellectual and associated developmental disabilities have communication difficulties.
  - Address the person by name and use eye contact, touch, or both to get their attention.
  - Assume competence when unsure of someone's ability to understand and then adjust accordingly. A person's ability to understand may be better than their ability to express themselves (and vice versa).
  - Speak slowly in short, clear sentences.
  - Explain what will happen in the consultation to help the person know what to expect.
  - Ask one question at a time and provide adequate time for the person to think about your question and formulate their reply. Avoid leading questions and check responses by asking again in a different way.
  - Understanding and using abstract concepts such as time may be difficult. Use significant events such as meals, social or sporting events, or birthdays or celebrations rather than hours, days, or months when asking questions related to time.
  - Use visual information, including pictures, diagrams, signs, and gestures, to aid comprehension.
  - Check understanding by asking them to demonstrate or repeat what you have said in their own words.
  - Some people may have limited literacy, so they may have difficulty reading patient information or appointment letters. The person may wish to involve support workers or family members to assist them with these tasks.
- *Support the person to express her- or himself.* Cognitive impairment makes identifying and verbalising difficult, and the person's physical condition may have impact on their speech.
  - If you do not know, ask the person how they communicate (i.e., how they indicate yes or no, use of communication aids).
  - If the person uses a communication device, ensure they have access to it, read the directions (usually on or in the device or book), and use it with them.
  - Use visual cues, such as objects, pictures, or diagrams.
- *If you can't understand, then ask for help.* There may be times when you do not understand what the person is saying. In this situation, it may be helpful to ask the person:
  - To repeat what they have just said
  - To say it another way (using different words, for instance)
  - To show you how they say 'yes' and 'no' and then ask yes-or-no questions to identify what it is they are saying
  - To ask an accompanier to help you understand
- *Never pretend to understand when you do not* because this devalues the person's communication. If you can't understand after using these strategies, acknowledge the importance of their message by apologising and expressing regret at not understanding.

- *All people communicate.* People communicate through facial expression, body language, and behaviour. It may be clear that someone finds a sensation unpleasant from their grimace, is cold when they shiver, or want to leave when they become agitated and look at the door. Acknowledging their experience and communication demonstrates that they have been heard and are valued and respected.

Reasonable Adjustments

- Reasonable adjustments are those required under the Disability Discrimination Act to ensure services are as accessible and effective for people with disabilities, including intellectual disabilities, as they would be for people without disabilities (Turner & Robinson, 2011).
- Knowing a patient has an intellectual disability provides guidance to the GP as to the reasonable adjustments to care that may be required to ensure equity. A person may:
  - Require more time for a consultation to enable them to understand the information presented and have a chance to ask questions.
  - Wish to have a family member, paid carer, or advocate present during the consultation.
  - Have difficulty reading and writing and may need information presented in easy English or in audio form.
  - Find it difficult to wait in a waiting room; therefore, it may be more appropriate that they wait with their carer in comfortable surroundings nearby and be rung a few minutes before their appointment.

Advocacy

People with intellectual disabilities require their doctors to be advocates in negotiating the health system and making sure their rights to equity in healthcare are upheld.

Principles of Practice

1. Take a person-centred approach by seeking to understand the perspective, personality, experiences, and strengths of each person.
2. Support empowerment of the person to make as many decisions as possible about their own life.
3. Enable choice by providing information about choices and support for the person to choose which suits them best.
4. Treat each person with dignity and respect, recognising the inherent shared humanity in all people.

Legal Issues of Consent and Capacity

- For children, parents generally hold legal power to make decisions on their behalf.
- For adults, it is presumed that they can make their own decisions about healthcare. If this is in doubt, it is up to the health practitioner to establish the person's 'legal capacity' and ability to:
  1. Understand the information provided.
  2. Believe and retain the information provided.
  3. Evaluate the relevant information.
  4. Express their choice.
- People who do not have capacity will require someone to assist them or to make decisions on their behalf. Whatever their capacity, the person concerned should be as actively involved in the decision-making process as possible.

Comprehensive Healthcare

- Holistic healthcare is that in which the person's physical and mental health are understood and supported in the context of the person's social context and life experiences.
- All doctors should adopt a proactive approach to their patients' healthcare.
- Comprehensive health assessments should always include a systems review and a medication review, and for those in whom the cause of their intellectual disability is unknown, consideration of an aetiologic review every few years is recommended. Understanding of the genetic causes of disability is growing rapidly, and referral to a genetic services provider could be enlightening.
- Comprehensive care includes a focus on disease prevention (e.g., immunisation, cancer screening) and health promotion (e.g., adequate exercise, healthy diet, not smoking).

Mental Health Issues

- People with intellectual disabilities have a higher rate of mental health issues.
- Depression, anxiety, mania, and psychosis all occur in people with intellectual disabilities. When people have cognitive or communication impairments, they express their symptoms through changes in their behaviour. Depression may present as social withdrawal, irritability, changes in appetite and sleep; mania as increased activity, vocalisation, and sleep disturbance; and psychosis as an unexplained fear or appearing to respond to visual or auditory hallucinations.
- Treatment of disorders of mental health is the same as in the general population. Effective treatment depends on an accurate diagnosis. Vigilance by both the GP and family or support staff with respect to response to medication and side effects is vital because the patient is likely to have difficulty reporting these.
- Principles of medication use include:
  a. Effective treatment depends on an accurate diagnosis.
  b. Start at a low dosage and increase slowly (start low, go slow).
  c. Always use the lowest effective dose.
  d. Review medications regularly with particular regard to indications and side effects.

HEALTHCARE FOR PEOPLE WITH INTELLECTUAL DISABILITIES

Some Tips for Consultations

	Challenge	One Possible Solution
Before an appointment	A required appointment may not be made.	A general practitioner or nurse initiates the appointment and reminds the patient.
	The person, family, or staff may not know what information is required.	Surgery to contact person and/or carer and detail information required at appointment.
	Waiting time may be an issue.	Arrange for a person to wait nearby in comfortable surroundings (park, coffee shop, car). Ring them a few minutes before the appointment.
At consultation	The person may feel anxious or frightened.	Greet the person warmly and establish rapport by chatting about something of interest to person.
	The person may become irritated.	Speak to the person concerned. Remember they are your patient, not the family member or paid carer.
	The person may get bored, become anxious, or want to leave.	Include the person in the discussion, both verbally and nonverbally, no matter what their capacity.
	Information given at consultation may not be retained or passed on accurately to those involved in the person's care.	Write a summary of outcomes of consultation, the next steps in their care, and who is responsible.
After consultation	The person may be anxious next time.	Discuss with patient and carer what went well and how to improve for next time. Record in notes.

RESOURCE FOR HEALTH PROFESSIONALS

Understanding Health and Intellectual Disability. www.intellectualdisability.info

Down Syndrome

- People with Down syndrome still experience significant barriers to the receipt of high-quality healthcare, and health outcomes compare unfavourably with those of the general population.
- People with Down syndrome are at increased risk of a range of physical and mental health conditions, often live with multiple unrecognised health issues, and have limited access to disease prevention and health promotion interventions.

Healthcare for Children With Down Syndrome

- *General care.* As for all children, primary care has responsibility for monitoring health and development. Health promotion and disease prevention should focus on diet, exercise, weight management, and immunisations.
- *Neonatal examination and investigation* can identify congenital anomalies, including cardiac and gastrointestinal effects.
- *Nutrition.* Dieticians can also offer information and support (note: calcium and vitamin D for osteoporosis prevention).
- *For families.* Link to services and supports, including early intervention services; dental services; allied health services; and support services, including the Down Syndrome Association.
- *Hearing.* Auditory brainstem evoked response should be done at 0 to 6 months. An audiology examination should be performed annually from 1 to 5 years; twice yearly from age 5 to 18 years; and at any time concern regarding hearing loss is raised by parents, carers, or screening tests.
- *Vision.* Ophthalmologic examination should be performed at 0 to 6 months; annually to age 5 years; twice yearly to age 18 years; and at any time concern regarding vision is raised by parents, carers, or screening tests.
- *Endocrine.* Check thyroid function at birth and then annually throughout childhood and again if suggestive symptoms or signs are noted. Assess specifically for undescended testes and hypogonadism.
- *Dental and oral health.* Dental review should be done 3 to 6 monthly from eruption of the first teeth for monitoring development plus prevention and treatment of oral disease.
- *Gastrointestinal.* Monitor diet and weight. Consider gastro-oesophageal reflux disease (GORD), *H. pylori* infection, coeliac disease, and constipation because these are all more common in children with Down syndrome.
- *Atlantoaxial instability.* Monitor for signs and symptoms of cord compression.
- *Haematologic and immunologic.* Be alert to increased risk of infections and leukaemia.

Healthcare for Adolescents With Down Syndrome

- *Sexuality.* Girls require education and support to manage periods (see Resources for Carers). Both sexes require additional advice about sex and contraception. Teenagers with Down syndrome are more vulnerable to sexual exploitation and abuse. They require education about appropriate behaviours (themselves and others), how to keep themselves safe, and how to get help if needed. For those who are unable to advocate for themselves, adequate protection and supervision are required to ensure their safety.

- *Skin.* Folliculitis or acne may affect self-esteem and interactions with others. Proactive treatment is required.
- *Mental health.* Biological, psychological, and social factors contribute to increased risk of disorders of mental health, especially anxiety and depression.
- *Transition from paediatric to adult services.* Consider all services used by the child and their family, including recreation, respite services, school and postschool options (employment, education, other), and mental health services. The GP has an important role in providing support and guidance through this time of change. Encourage the adolescent to take an increasingly active role in their health management.

Healthcare for Adults With Down Syndrome

- *Health monitoring.* Risk factor identification (e.g., cardiovascular disease) is important.
- *Health promotion and disease prevention* include diet, exercise, weight management, cancer screening (may include smear test, mammography, bowel cancer screening), and immunisations.
- *Annual health assessments* underpin proactive healthcare and enable early detection, health promotion, and disease prevention.
- *Behaviour change.* A change in behaviour is a communication; consider disorders of physical, dental, or mental health, as well as environmental causes.
- *Dental and oral health.* Dental review should be done every 6 months.
- *Cardiovascular.* Mitral valve prolapse may develop during adulthood (50% of adults); therefore, regular cardiac examination or echocardiography (or both) is required.
- *Atlantoaxial instability.* Cervical cord compression occurs in about 2% of people with Down syndrome. Symptoms and signs include neck pain, torticollis, limb weakness, increased reflexes, change in gait or bladder or bowel function, and sensory changes.
- *Hearing.* Audiologic examination should be done every 3 years and if suspicion of hearing loss is raised by carers or screening.
- *Vision.* Ophthalmologic review should be done at age 30 years, every 5 years thereafter, and if suspicion of visual loss is raised by carers or screening.
- *Thyroid function.* This should be done annually and whenever suggestive symptoms or signs are noted.
- *Mental health.* Biological, psychological, and social factors contribute to increased risk of disorders. Anxiety and depression are more common.
- *Alzheimer disease.* The average age of diagnosis in people with Down syndrome is the early 50s; it is rare before 45 years of age. Physical and mental causes of functional decline should be excluded.
- *Gastrointestinal.* People with Down syndrome have an increased risk of GORD, coeliac disease, and chronic constipation.
- *Osteoporosis.* Bone mineral density testing should be done in early adulthood and repeated at menopause in females and at about 40 years of age for hypogonadal males. Discuss and implement prevention strategies, including diet, exercise, and calcium and vitamin D supplementation, if levels are low or the person is taking an anticonvulsant.
- *Medications.* Regular review should be done (at least very 12 months). Response and side effects should be monitored. Reevaluate indications and efficacy (cease if ineffective), ensure the lowest effective dose, and educate the patient and carers about expected response and side effects. Consider prepackaging of medication by a pharmacy to ensure accurate dosing and safety. Be aware of sensitivity to psychoactive medication. 'Start low, go slow' and be vigilant for side effects. (Behaviour change may be an early symptom.)

Healthcare for Older People With Down Syndrome

- The increasing lifespan of people with Down syndrome means more people experience the conditions of ageing, including menopausal symptoms, arthritis, cardiovascular disease, osteoporosis, sensory loss, and dementia.
- Alzheimer disease occurs earlier in people with Down syndrome, with an average age of diagnosis in the early to mid-50s. Symptoms may be difficult to differentiate from physical disease (e.g., hypothyroidism, anaemia), medication effects (e.g., nausea, confusion, dizziness), mental illness (e.g., depression, psychosis), and sensory deterioration (e.g., hearing and vision).
- Proactive assessment and investigation are required to exclude treatable causes of functional decline.

RESOURCES FOR PARENTS AND PROFESSIONALS

Down Syndrome Association of Australia. http://www.downsyndrome.org.au

Down Syndrome Association UK. http://www.downs-syndrome.org.uk

Down Syndrome Association Scotland. www.dsscotland.org.uk

Down Syndrome Association Ireland. http://downsyndrome.ie/campaigns-and-projects/person-first-language

Carers

- In Australia, around 10% identify as carers (Australian Bureau of Statistics, 2019); 70% of primary carers are female, and 83% of carers were caring for someone in their household. Figures are similar in the United Kingdom (Carers UK, 2022).
- When a person comes to their medical practitioner accompanied by a carer, it is important to:
  - Establish the relationship between the person and carer.
  - Clarify the carer's role.
  - Ensure the person's consent for the carer to be present.
  - Speak directly to the person, not to the carer. If the person finds it difficult to express themselves or if you have trouble understanding them, ask them if you may ask questions of the carer. Always involve and

include the person in the consultation through verbal and nonverbal communication.

- Write down the key outcomes of the consultation, any follow-up tasks that are required (e.g., investigations, further information, monitoring for response to treatment and side effects of medication), and arrangements for review. This information must be given to the person or the carer (or both) to ensure it is relayed accurately to other carers involved.

Caring for the Carers

- Family members who care for a relative tend to have lower rates of workforce participation, lower incomes, and reduced connection with their social group and communities.
- They may find aspects of care difficult and struggle to make the time to address their own physical and mental health issues.
- It may therefore be helpful if the GP invites the carer to come for their own consultation to discuss ways in which they may be assisted in their caring role (e.g., services, equipment, therapy, local activity groups for people requiring care, respite).
- The consultation also provides an opportunity to review the carer's physical and mental health status and needs and to address current and potential issues.

Resources for Carers

- *Carer organisations* provide advice, peer support, and access to information and resources. Examples include:
  - Carers UK. https://www.carersuk.org
  - Carers Australia. http://www.carersaustralia.com.au
  - *Local councils and authorities* provide information about services, resources, support, and activities.
- *Therapy services* such as occupational therapists, physiotherapists, speech therapists may also help.

Cycle of Good Healthcare: A Shared Responsibility

- Optimal healthcare for someone with a disability requires a cycle (Fig. 4.1) (Tracy, 2013). At each step, there is a risk that the next may not occur.
- GPs, support staff, and family members have a shared responsibility to work collaboratively with the person with an intellectual disability to ensure the steps of the cycle are worked through and completed to ensure the person concerned achieves and maintains optimal health and function.

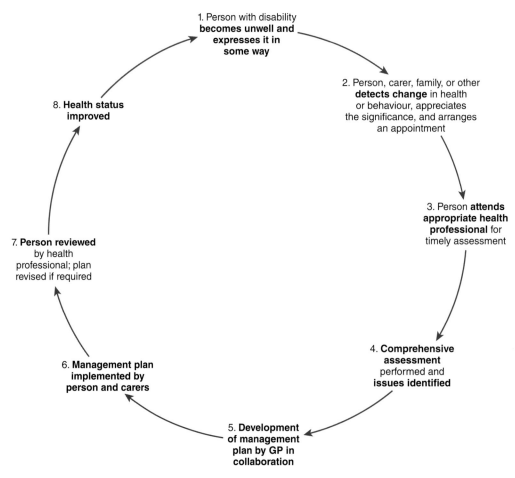

- **Fig. 4.1** Cycle of good healthcare. *GP,* General practitioner.

References

Australian Bureau of Statistics. (2012). *Disability, Ageing and Carers.* Australia: Australian Bureau of Statistics. Retrieved from http://www.abs.gov.au/ausstats/abs@.nsf/Lookup/A813E50F4C45A338CA257C21000E4F36?opendocument. Accessed Nov 2013.

Australian Bureau of Statistics. (2019). *Disability, Ageing and Carers,* Australia: Summary of findings. https://www.abs.gov.au/statistics/health/disability/disability-ageing-and-carers-australia-summary-findings/latest-release#key-statistics

Emerson, E., & Heslop, P. (2010). *A working definition of learning disabilities.* Durham: Improving Health & Lives: Learning Disabilities Observatory.

Emerson, E., & Baines, S. (2010). *Health inequalities and people with learning disabilities in the UK: 2010.* Durham: Improving Health & Lives: Learning Disabilities Observatory.

Lennox, N., Bain, C., Rey-Conde, T., Purdie, D., Bush, R., & Pandeya, N. (2007). Effects of a comprehensive health assessment programme for Australian adults with intellectual disability: A cluster randomized trial. *International Journal of Epidemiology, 36,* 139–146.

Office for Disability Issues UK. (2013). *UK Equality Act 2010 Guidance. HM Government.* Available: https://www.gov.uk/guidance/equality-act-2010-guidance

Robertson, J., Roberts, H., Emerson, E., Turner, S., & Greig, R. (2011). The impact of health checks for people with intellectual disabilities: A systematic review of evidence. *Journal of Intellectual Disabilities Research, 55*(11), 1009–1019. doi:10.1111/j.1365-2788.2011.01436.x.

Tracy, J. (2013). Disability in the mainstream: Improving healthcare provided to people with intellectual disability and the role of mainstream and specialist services. In C. Bigby & C. Fyffe (Eds.), *Making mainstream services accessible and responsive to people with intellectual disability: What is the equivalent of lifts and Labradors? Proceedings of the Seventh Annual Roundtable on Intellectual Disability Policy.* Bundoora: Living with Disability Research Group, Faculty of Health Sciences, La Trobe University.

Turner, S., & Robinson, C. (2011). *Reasonable adjustments for people with learning disabilities – implications and actions for commissioners and providers of healthcare.* Learning Disabilities Observatory. Retrieved from http://www.improvinghealthandlives.org.uk/uploads/doc/vid_11084_IHAL%202011%20-01%20Reasonable%20adjustments%20guidance.pdf. (Accessed Nov 2013).

World Health Organization. (2011). *World report on disability 2011.* Geneva: World Health Organization.

World Health Organization. (2022). *Global report on health equity for persons with disabilities.* Available: https://www.who.int/health-topics/disability

5

Childhood Problems

Ruth Bland & Hilary Pearce

CHAPTER CONTENTS

The Child With a Tic
What to Ask About the Child
What to Look for on Examination
What to Do

The Child With Dysuria and Abdominal Pain
What to Ask About the Child
What to Look for on Examination
What to Do

The Child With Bedwetting (Nocturnal Enuresis)
What to Ask About the Child
What to Look for on Examination
What to Do

The Child With Protein in Their Urine
What to Ask About the Child
What to Look for on Examination
What to Do

The Child With Blood in Their Urine
What to Ask About the Child
What to Look for on Examination
What to Do

The Child With an Itchy Perineum
What to Ask About the Child
What to Look for on Examination
What to Do

The Child With Worms in Their Stool
What to Ask About the Child
What to Look for on Examination
What to Do

The Child With a Painful Penis
What to Ask About the Child
What to Look for on Examination
What to Do

The Child With a Groin Swelling
What to Ask About the Child
What to Look for on Examination
What to Do

The Child With a Painful Scrotum
What to Ask About the Child
What to Look for on Examination
What to Do

The Child With a Nonblanching Rash
What to Ask About the Child
What to Look for on Examination
What to Do

The Child With Cervical Lymphadenopathy
What to Ask About the Child
What to Look for on Examination
What to Do

The Child With Pica
What to Ask About the Child
What to Look for on Examination
What to Do

The Child Who Is Short
What to Ask About the Child
What to Look for on Examination
What to Do

The Child Who Is Tall
What to Ask About the Child
What to Look for on Examination
What to Do

The Child With Precocious Puberty
What to Ask About the Child
What to Look for on Examination
What to Do

The Child With Excess Body Hair
What to Ask About the Child
What to Look for on Examination
What to Do

The Child With a Painful Limp
What to Ask About the Child
What to Look for on Examination
What to Do

The Infant Who Screams or Vomits When Feeding
What to Ask About the Child
What to Look for on Examination
What to Do

The Infant Who Has Weight Faltering in the First 6 Months of Life
What to Ask About the Child
What to Look for on Examination
What to Do

The Infant Who Has Weight Faltering After 6 Months of Age
What to Ask About the Child
What to Look for on Examination
What to Do

The Child Who Is Suspected of Having a Nonaccidental Injury
What to Ask About the Child
What to Look for on Examination
What to Do

The Child With a Fever

GUIDELINE

National Institute for Health and Clinical Excellence. (2019). *Fever in under 5s: Assessment and initial management. NICE clinical guideline 143.* Available at https://www.nice.org.uk/guidance/ng143.

PATIENT INFORMATION

NHS Inform. Fever in children. Available at www.nhsinform.scot/illnesses-and-conditions/infections-and-poisoning/fever-in-children.

- Fever is one of the most common reasons for seeking medical help. There are many causes of acute fever, and it is important to take a thorough history and examine the child carefully.
- On average, young children experience three to six febrile episodes per year, mostly self-limiting viral illnesses.
- The challenge for the general practitioner (GP) is identifying the child with a potentially serious bacterial infection. If a child is acutely unwell, they should be referred to hospital immediately, particularly if there is no obvious source for the fever, in which case the child requires further investigation.
- Classical signs of particular infections, such as the stiff neck and headache of meningitis, may not be present in infants, who often present with fever, pallor, and irritability, so the GP needs to maintain a high index of suspicion for underlying serious infection.

What to Ask About the Child

- It is important to ask how long the fever has been present. A fever of more than 8 days' duration, with no source, requires further paediatric assessment and possible investigation (see later). A history of fever described by a parent should always be taken seriously even if a pyrexia is not recorded by the examining doctor, particularly if the pyrexia is obtained by a digital thermometer rather than a forehead strip thermometer.
- Ask about how long the fever has been present and whether the child is getting better or worse.
- In all cases of fever, ask specifically about a rash. A blanching rash is often present with viral infections, but a nonblanching rash may indicate an underlying serious bacterial infection.
- Explore how the child is feeding and whether they are refusing feeds or vomiting. Ask specifically about symptoms that may point to a cause of the fever, including vomiting and diarrhoea (possible gastroenteritis), cough and coryzal symptoms (pneumonia or other respiratory infection), and pulling at an ear (possible otitis media). In an older child, ask about pain passing urine (possible urinary tract infection (UTI)), painful joints (possible septic arthritis), and seizures (possible meningitis or herpes encephalitis).
- Ask if other members of the family have been unwell and whether there has been any recent travel abroad.

What to Look for on Examination

- The National Institute of Clinical Excellence (NICE) has produced a traffic light system for signs and symptoms that predict the risk of serious illness in children younger than 5 years of age, which is familiar to most GPs in the United Kingdom.

National Institute for Health and Clinical Excellence Assessment of Risk of Serious Illness

	High Risk: Refer Urgently	Intermediate Risk: Refer	Low Risk: Manage at Home
Colour: skin, lips, and tongue	Pale, mottled, ashen, or blue	Pallor	Normal colour
Activity	Appears ill to health professional	Not responding normally to social cues	Responds normally to social cues
	Does not wake if roused	No smile	Content and smiles
	Weak, high-pitched or continuous cry	Wakes only with prolonged stimulation	Strong normal cry or not crying
		Decreased activity	
Respiratory	Grunting	Nasal flaring	
	Respiratory rate >60 breaths/min	Respiratory rate: 6–12 months of age >50 breaths/min; older than 12 months of age >40 breaths/min	
	Moderate to severe chest indrawing	Oxygen saturation ≤95%	
		Crackles in chest	
Circulation and hydration	Reduced skin turgor	Tachycardia: younger than 12 months: 160 beats/min; 12–24 months of age: 150 beats/min; 2–5 years of age: >140 beats/min	Normal skin and eyes
		Capillary return time ≥3 s	Moist mucous membranes
		Dry mucous membranes	
		Poor feeding in infant	
		Reduced urine output	

National Institute for Health and Clinical Excellence Assessment of Risk of Serious Illness—Cont'd

	High Risk: Refer Urgently	Intermediate Risk: Refer	Low Risk: Manage at Home
Other	3 months of age or younger: temperature ≥38°C Nonblanching rash Bulging fontanelle Neck stiffness Status epilepticus Focal neurologic signs Focal seizure	Age 3–6 months: temperature ≥39°C Fever ≥5 days Rigors Swelling limb or joint Non–weight-bearing limb, not using an extremity	

- In addition to these clinical findings, examine the child for specific signs that could indicate the source of the fever, including examining for pus on the tonsils, inflammation of the tympanic membranes, swelling and inflammation of the joints, enlargement of the lymph nodes, and tenderness in the abdomen.

What to Do

- The priority is to decide whether to refer the child for further investigations and whether it needs to be done urgently (see NICE guidelines for children younger than 5 years of age).
- In children older than 5 years of age who are not acutely unwell and in whom no source of acute fever can be found, the following investigations are useful: urinalysis and urine culture, full blood count, and C-reactive protein (CRP).
- For these older children, a normal or mildly increased white blood cell count or CRP and negative urinalysis results are reassuring, and it is unlikely that there is any serious pathology underlying the fever.
- It is not advisable to prescribe antibiotics to children without a source for their fever, in particular giving antibiotics for a possible UTI without a urine culture being sent. Most children who are not acutely unwell with fever do not have underlying bacteraemia.
- If an unwell child presents with a nonblanching rash and fever, suspect meningococcal disease and give intramuscular (IM) antibiotics before urgent transfer to hospital.

Pyrexia of Unknown Origin

- Pyrexia of unknown origin is defined as a fever above 38°C present most days with an unclear diagnosis for at least 3 weeks with an uncertain diagnosis after initial investigations.
- These children should be referred for further investigation. The list of causes is vast, including infectious bacterial diseases (*Salmonella* spp.), viral illnesses (Epstein–Barr virus), fungal and parasitic diseases, connective tissue diseases, and malignancy.

The Child With a Cough

> **GUIDELINES**
>
> British Thoracic Society. (2019). *Paediatric community acquired pneumonia—Quality improvement tool*. Available at Brit-thoracic.org.uk/quality-improvement/clinic-resources/paediatric-community-acquired-pneumonia.
> National Institute for Health and Clinical Excellence Clinical Knowledge Summaries. (2023). *Cough: Acute with chest signs in children*. Available at cks.nice.org.uk/topics/cough-acute-with-chest-signs-in-children.

- Cough is a common symptom in children. It can be acute (<3 weeks) or chronic (3–12 weeks). In infants, consider pertussis and bronchiolitis. Most acute coughs in older children are caused by viruses, but if a child is unwell with fever and tachypnoea, pneumonia must be excluded.
- Causes of chronic cough include asthma, pertussis, viruses (including adenovirus), bacteria (including *Mycoplasma* spp.), and postnasal drip.

What to Ask About the Child

- Ask about the duration of the cough to find out if it is acute or chronic. Most acute coughs are caused by viruses and are self-limiting. However, viruses such as adenoviruses can cause coughs that last up to 3 months.
- Ask if there is a pattern to the coughing. Children with pertussis have paroxysmal spells of coughing but are generally well with no respiratory symptoms between the episodes of spasmodic coughing. A child with asthma may have exercise induced or nocturnal cough. An infant with gastro-oesophageal reflux (GOR) may experience coughing after feeding or when prone, for example, when put into their cot to sleep, when the parents might report a nighttime cough.
- Ask about the onset of the cough. If it started suddenly with no prodromal symptoms, ask about a history of choking and consider the possibility of an inhaled foreign body.

- Ask whether the cough sounds 'wet' or 'dry'. Whereas the cough associated with asthma sounds 'dry', the cough associated with a respiratory infection sounds 'wet' and may be productive of sputum. Whereas a barking cough associated with stridor is typical of croup, a harsh paroxysmal cough is suggestive of pertussis.
- Check whether there are associated symptoms that might point to the aetiology of the cough, for example, whether the child has fever, nasal discharge, increased work of breathing, reduced exercise tolerance, anorexia, fatigue, or weight loss. If the child has a persistent cough associated with fever and night sweats, ask whether the child has been exposed to tuberculosis (TB).
- For infants and young children, ask whether the caregivers have noted any episodes of apnoea, which may be associated with pertussis, bronchiolitis, and GOR.
- Children with sinusitis may present with persistent cough and tenderness over the sinuses, and the child may present with facial pain.
- Ask about feeding, appetite, and weight gain. In infants, vomiting and cough may suggest a diagnosis of GOR.
- In the family history, specifically ask about atopy, asthma, and a TB contact.
- Take the child's immunisation status, in particular bacillus Calmette–Guérin and pertussis.
- Ask about recent travel abroad, and if relevant, consider TB.

What to Look for on Examination

- Assess if the child is acutely unwell (see earlier discussion), in particular looking for cyanosis or pallor and signs of respiratory distress, including nasal flaring, grunting, chest indrawing, or an increased respiratory rate (>50 breaths/min in children 0–12 months of age; >40 breaths/min in children older than 12 months of age). Refer urgently as appropriate if these signs are present.
- In young children, most information is gained by observation. However, it is useful to auscultate the chest for crackles and wheeze if the child is not distressed and crying. If there are crackles, determine whether they are generalised (e.g., in an infant with bronchiolitis) or localised (e.g., in a child with lobar pneumonia).
- Examine the upper respiratory tract, including the tonsils, ears, and nose.
- Palpate the face over the region of the sinuses because tenderness over these areas may suggest sinusitis.
- Look for evidence of a chronic respiratory illness, including a chest deformity (e.g., sulci, or an increased anteroposterior diameter) and finger clubbing.
- Weigh the child, plot the weight on an appropriate growth chart, and compare it with previous measurements to assess growth. Failure to thrive associated with a cough needs further investigation.

What to Do

- Have a low threshold for referring infants with a clinical diagnosis of a lower respiratory illness, bronchiolitis, or pertussis to secondary care if they were born preterm (because they can deteriorate quickly), have had apnoeic episodes with this illness, or have been admitted to hospital previously with a respiratory illness. For children older than 1 year of age with pneumonia, if they are not acutely unwell, they may be managed at home with an oral antibiotic and antipyretic.
- A child with a sudden onset of cough and a possible history of choking should be referred urgently for investigation of an inhaled foreign body. These children may also have stridor.
- If a child has a persistent nocturnal cough, that you think might be asthma, give a trial of an inhaled steroid for 4 to 6 weeks. If they do not respond to this, refer to outpatient secondary care.
- Refer all children with a persistent cough for more than 1 month who are not improving.
- Refer all children with a cough and failure to thrive for further investigations, which may include imaging, assessment of immune function, and bronchoscopy.
- In infants with a possible diagnosis of GOR, try an antireflux medication.

The Child With Wheeze

GUIDELINES

BTS/SIGN. (2019). *British guideline on the management of asthma.* Available at brit-thoracic.org.uk/quality-improvement/guidelines/asthma.
    National Institute for Health and Clinical Excellence Clinical Knowledge Summaries. (2023). *Asthma management.* Available at https://cks.nice.org.uk/topics/asthma/management.

PATIENT INFORMATION

Allergy UK. Childhood asthma and wheeze. Available at https://www.allergyuk.org/resources/childhood-asthma-wheeze-factsheet.
    Asthma + Lung UK. Asthma and your child. Available at asthmaandlung.org.uk/conditions/asthma/child.

- Wheeze within the context of a viral illness is common in preschool children. One-third of children have at least one episode of wheeze before they are 3 years old. This is defined as an episode of viral-induced wheeze. If children experience episodes of wheeze with further viral infections, it is defined as episodic viral wheeze.
- The diagnosis of asthma is a clinical one based on the presence of interval symptoms.

- In older children, asthma is diagnosed if more than one of the following symptoms is present: recurrent wheeze, cough, difficulty breathing, and chest tightness. The diagnosis should be supported with spirometry in children old enough to comply with assessment (older than the age of 5 years, but this is often not possible until they are around 7 or more years).
- A trial of a β_2 agonist may demonstrate reversibility of bronchospasm, but in children younger than 2 years of age, the response to bronchodilator therapy is not always consistent. The diagnosis should be considered if there are other features, including nocturnal cough or exercise-induced symptoms. A family or personal history of atopy may also be helpful.

What to Ask About the Child

- Ask about the pattern and frequency of episodes of wheeze. Is the wheeze frequent and episodic, with definite triggers such as exercise or cold weather, suggestive of asthma? Or does the wheeze only occur with upper respiratory tract infections and is therefore more likely to be viral-induced wheeze, particularly in a younger child?
- Ask if the child has associated symptoms, including a dry cough, respiratory symptoms with exercise, disturbed sleep, or snoring. Children with asthma may have a nocturnal or early morning cough. A 'wet' cough is less likely to be asthma.
- Ask about family history. A diagnosis of asthma is more likely if there is a family or personal history of atopy, including eczema, hay fever, or other allergies.
- Ask if the wheeze has been present since birth; if it has, consider a diagnosis of tracheobronchomalacia.
- Check if the child was born prematurely and if they were intubated and ventilated because these children may be more likely to deteriorate quickly with respiratory illnesses and may need referral to secondary care more promptly than children born at term with no neonatal complications.
- Always ask whether the child is exposed to cigarette smoke and check their growth.

What to Look for on Examination

- Assess if the child is acutely unwell, particularly looking for cyanosis or pallor and signs of respiratory distress.
- In a child with known asthma, look out for a 'silent chest' with no wheeze; this is a dangerous sign because it indicates little air movement.
- Be aware of children who are so breathless that they cannot talk in sentences; this is a dangerous sign indicating severe respiratory distress. Children who are agitated or exhausted should also be referred urgently.
- Auscultate for wheeze. A generalised wheeze is present in asthma and in infants with bronchiolitis and for crackles, which may suggest lower respiratory tract infection.

- If the child is old enough, measure a peak expiratory flow and compare the results with reference charts and, if available, with previous measurements of the child.
- Look for evidence of a chronic respiratory condition, including a chest deformity (e.g., sulci) and finger clubbing.
- Weigh the child, plot the weight on an appropriate growth chart, and compare the result with previous measurements. Failure to thrive associated with a cough or wheeze needs further investigation; consider referring these children to secondary care.

What to Do

- Management of acute wheeze in a child who is unwell includes oxygen therapy, a β_2 agonist via a nebuliser or multidosing with an inhaler through a spacing device, oral steroids, and referral to secondary care if indicated. For longer term management of asthma, refer to guidelines, including the British Guideline on the Management of Asthma, which provides a stepwise approach to the medical management of patients with asthma.

For children with viral-induced wheeze who are well in between episodes, treatment with a β_2 agonist for acute symptoms may be beneficial. However, β_2 agonists are often ineffective for children younger than 1 year of age.

- For all children, it is useful to provide advice to the families about related triggers, including avoidance of smoke, pollen, and animal dander when appropriate.

Refer children to secondary care if they have wheeze and are not growing well or have recurrent chest infections or a chronic cough.

The Child With Constipation

PATIENT INFORMATION

Bowel and Bladder UK. Available at https://www.bbuk.org.uk. ERIC, The Children's Bowel and Bladder Charity. Helpline: 0800 169 9949. Available at https://eric.org.uk.

- Constipation is one of the commonest reasons for referral to secondary care. Parents are often concerned that the children have underlying pathology and may come to hospital expecting that investigations, including imaging, will be carried out.
- More than 90% of cases of constipation are idiopathic (i.e., no underlying anatomic or physiological cause are found). It is important to provide a clear explanation to the parent and child (when appropriate), implement a management plan, and arrange regular follow-up to ensure that the child responds to treatment.

What to Ask About the Child

- Ask about the frequency and consistency of the stools. (Use the Bristol Stool Chart to help children and caregivers to identify the type of stools they are passing.) Fewer than three formed stools per week and stools that are hard or like 'rabbit droppings' are features of constipation.
- Explore whether the child has abdominal pain while passing stool and between episodes of stooling. Children with constipation often experience regular lower abdominal pain and pain on defecation, particularly if the stools are large and hard.
- Ask if there has ever been blood coating the stool, suggesting a fissure caused by constipation.
- Ask about episodes of diarrhoea. Sometimes children with constipation present with diarrhoea, but this is overflow diarrhoea, passed with no sensation and often with an offensive odour. Caregivers often report that the child is 'lazy' and fails to go to the toilet in time, and caregivers are often concerned about treating their child with laxatives (see later) because they believe it is 'making the diarrhoea worse'. However, overflow diarrhoea will not resolve until any impacted faeces are passed.
- Ask about stool withholding behaviours, including passage of numerous small stools during the day.
- In the past history, ask whether the child passed meconium within the first 48 hours after delivery. Failure to pass meconium or constipation beginning in the first few weeks of life may indicate an underlying pathology (e.g., Hirschsprung disease). However, it is important to stress that most cases of constipation are idiopathic, and these children require no investigations.
- As with all children, check that the child is thriving and otherwise well.

What to Look for on Examination

- Assess if the child is acutely unwell. A distended abdomen, especially in a child who is also vomiting, requires urgent referral to secondary care. Palpate the abdomen for faecal masses, which are most often felt above the pelvic rim in children with constipation. Check the child's height and weight and plot the information on a chart, comparing with previous measurements. A child who is failing to thrive with constipation should be referred to secondary care for exclusion of other disorders, including coeliac disease and hypothyroidism.
- There is no need to perform a rectal examination in a child with constipation in primary care. This will cause distress to the child and not help with the diagnosis. However, it is useful to check the external appearance of the anus. In a young infant, check that the anus is patent; in rare cases, an imperforate anus may have been missed on neonatal examination. Check if there is an anal fissure, which may be the cause of bleeding per rectum, or multiple fissures or a fistula, which may be suggestive of other pathology such as Crohn's disease. Bruising around the anus may indicate possible child abuse.
- Neuromuscular causes of constipation are rare but check that there is no obvious deformity of the spine; that the child does not have a sacral dimple (and if they do, check the base is visible); and that the child has normal tone, power, gait, and reflexes. In toddlers, check for delayed walking, which could indicate an underlying neuromuscular problem.

What to Do

- Investigations are not normally required, and idiopathic constipation can usually be managed in primary care. The key points of management are reassurance, a clear management plan, and follow-up to check response to treatment.
- It is important to explain that constipation is common and that diet alone is unlikely to solve the problem, particularly in the short term. Explain the importance of starting a laxative to soften the stools, with the goal of passing a soft stool at least once per day. Explain that it is preferable to have stools that are 'too loose' rather than 'too hard' at this stage.
- Ensure the child has an adequate fluid intake because many children underdrink. How much a child should drink depends on their age, sex (for older children), and exercise and activities. A rough guide is:
  - Ages 1 to 3 years: 900 to 1000 mL
  - Ages 4 to 8 years: 1000 to 1400 mL
  - Ages 9 to 13 years, females: 1200 to 2100 mL
  - Ages 9 to 13 years, males: 1400 to 2300 mL
  - Ages 14 to 18 years, females: 1400 to 2500 mL
  - Ages 14 to 18 years, males: 2100 to 3200 mL
- Explain that if a child is soiling (likely because of impaction and overflow diarrhoea) that they are not doing this deliberately and should not be punished. It is often a relief to caregivers and children to understand that overflow diarrhoea will stop after the constipation resolves.
- Treatment includes regular treatment with laxatives. Some children require disimpaction first followed by maintenance treatment. A macrogol is the laxative of choice for children. Clear guidance on doses for disimpaction and maintenance doses are given in the *British National Formulary for Children* and in the *NICE guidelines*.
- Explain how to make up the macrogols using the correct amount of water (or diluting juice) per sachet as per the instructions on the medication.
- Give clear instructions on how to take the laxative, explaining that it should not be stopped and started and that some abdominal pain and loose stools are experienced during the first days of administration. Caregivers often stop giving laxatives as the child passes loose stools, but explain that this is to be expected in the first few days.

- Children are often fearful of sitting on the toilet and attempting to pass stool. When the stools are soft, encourage the child to sit on the toilet for 5 to 10 minutes after their breakfast and evening meals. Giving a school-aged child balloons to blow up whilst on the toilet and providing them with a foot stool if they cannot reach the floor are strategies to encourage children to push.
- Arrange follow-up for the child to check on response to treatment and to suggest modifications in laxative doses as required. If the child has faecal impaction, arrange follow-up after 1 week. Discuss with the local paediatric team if a child does not respond to a disimpaction regimen.

The Child With Abdominal Pain

> **GUIDELINE**
>
> BMJ Best Practice. (2023). *Assessment of abdominal pain in children*. Available at bestpractice.bmj.com/topics/en-gb/787.

- At least 10% of school-aged children experience abdominal pain regularly. There are many causes, and the challenge is to identify children with underlying pathologies and to avoid unnecessary tests on children with functional abdominal pain who do not require them.

What to Ask About the Child

- Ask at what age the pain started. Take seriously abdominal pain commencing in young children (younger than 5 years) in whom constipation has been excluded.
- Explore about the frequency and pattern of the pain. Pain that regularly interferes with play, education, or normal activities requires further evaluation.
- Ask if the pain wakes the child at night; functional pain does not tend to cause nocturnal wakening.
- Explore if there is a relationship to eating. *Helicobacter pylori* disease may be associated with upper abdominal and retrosternal pain on eating.
- Ask if any particular foods aggravate the pain. Pain can occur in coeliac disease after eating gluten. Some children may have a non–immunoglobulin E (IgE)–mediated dairy allergy, and a 4-week exclusion diet may be helpful to identify this as a cause of pain (improvement of pain on the dairy-free diet and recurrence when challenged again with dairy).
- Ask if the pain is associated with pallor, nausea, or a family history of migraine. Children can get 'abdominal migraine', which presents with nonspecific abdominal pain but not necessarily headache.
- Ask specifically about vomiting. Bilious vomiting usually has a surgical cause, and children should be referred to secondary care. Children with an acute surgical cause for their vomiting are usually unwell; for example, a child with acute appendicitis usually presents with listlessness and anorexia in addition to abdominal pain.

- Ask about the stools and whether defecation is associated with pain. Diarrhoea and blood or mucous per rectum may be indicative of underlying pathology (e.g., inflammatory bowel disease (IBD)). However, constipation with a fissure may also cause blood that coats the stools and is a common cause of abdominal pain.
- Check whether the child has other symptoms that may indicate underlying pathology. For example, mouth ulcers, joint pains, anal skin tags are associated with Crohn's disease.
- Explore for factors in the social history that may be sources of anxiety, including problems at school, difficulties with parents, parental separation, or divorce.
- Ask about dysuria, which may suggest a UTI.

What to Look for on Examination

- Examine for an acute abdomen or surgical cause for abdominal pain. Check for acute or rebound tenderness on palpation, a distended abdomen, fever, lethargy, and a furred tongue.
- Functional abdominal pain or irritable bowel syndrome is nonspecific. Children often vaguely point to their umbilicus when trying to localise the pain and do not usually complain of tenderness when their abdomens are palpated.
- Measure and plot the child's weight and height on a growth chart and compare them with previous measurements. A child with abdominal pain associated with weight faltering needs further investigations to rule out conditions such as IBD and coeliac disease.
- Check the anus externally for skin tags, fissures, fistulae, and ulceration (there is no need to do a per rectum (PR)). A fissure may be present with constipation. Skin tags, multiple fissures, and fistulae may suggest IBD and should be further investigated.
- Finger clubbing in a child with abdominal pain is suggestive of underlying pathology, including IBD. Similarly, mouth ulcers may indicate Crohn's disease (but may also be an incidental finding or be associated with iron deficiency).

What to Do

- If you are concerned that there is underlying pathology, the following investigations may be helpful in distinguishing between functional and nonfunctional pain:
  - Faecal calprotectin: Levels greater than 200 μg/g *may* be suggestive of IBD, and these children should be referred.
  - Blood tests: A ferritin blood test, ferritin, inflammatory markers (CRP, erythrocyte sedimentation rate), liver function tests, and coeliac antibody screen should be done. (Ensure that the child has been having gluten in their diet for 6 weeks before testing.)
  - Faecal *H. pylori* antigen may be helpful in children with upper abdominal or retrosternal pain and pain on eating.

- Urine culture should be performed to exclude a UTI.
- Normal investigations are often reassuring to parents.
- If the child is constipated, manage appropriately. Drug treatment may be helpful in the following conditions: serotonin antagonists in abdominal migraine and mebeverine in irritable bowel syndrome. For debilitating functional abdominal pain, psychology input may be required.

The Child With Diarrhoea

- It is important to distinguish between acute (<2 weeks) and chronic (>2 weeks) diarrhoea.
- Acute diarrhoea is often associated with vomiting and is usually caused by viruses including: rotavirus, adenovirus, and calicivirus. Rarely, acute diarrhoea is caused by bacteria (*Salmonella, Shigella, Yersinia,* or *Campylobacter* spp.) or protozoa (*Giardia* and *Cryptosporidium* spp.).

What to Ask About the Child

- Ask about the duration of the diarrhoea and distinguish between acute and chronic diarrhoea.
- Enquire whether the child has vomiting; gastroenteritis causes acute diarrhoea and vomiting.
- Specifically ask whether the child has blood in the diarrhoea. This is found in infections (also see the discussion of haemolytic uraemic syndrome (HUS)) and in IBD if the diarrhoea is chronic.
- Ask about recent travel abroad because this may indicate the cause of the diarrhoea (e.g., *Salmonella* spp).
- Ask if the child lives on a farm or if they have had contact with animals and consider whether they could have *Campylobacter* infection.
- Ask whether the child has ongoing abdominal pain or other symptoms suggestive of IBD or coeliac disease. If the child has constipation, consider whether the diarrhoea is overflow diarrhoea.
- Ask about the child's diet because fruit juices, diluting juice, fizzy drinks, and sugar-free chewing gum may cause osmotic diarrhoea.

What to Look for on Examination

- Assess whether the child is acutely unwell and whether they need acute admission for treatment of severe dehydration or severe underlying infection.
- Check for petechiae, which are present in HUS and sepsis.
- Examine the abdomen for tenderness, masses, and organomegaly.
- Plot the child's current weight and height on a growth chart and compare them with previous measurements. (Remember that if the child is dehydrated, their weight will be lower than normal.)
- Check whether the child has finger clubbing, suggestive of underlying chronic pathology.

- Check the anus externally for skin tags, fissures, fistulae, and ulceration (there is no need to do a PR examination), particularly if you suspect a chronic underlying cause. A fissure may be present with constipation. Skin tags, multiple fissures, and fistulae may suggest IBD and should be further investigated.
- Check the mouth for ulcers, which may indicate underlying pathology (e.g., Crohn's disease) but may also be an incidental finding.

What to Do: Acute Diarrhoea

- Acutely unwell children should be referred.
- For children with acute bloody diarrhoea, immediate referral is recommended to rule out HUS, which requires blood tests, including a blood count, electrolytes, glucose, and renal function.
- Send stool for culture if the child has recently travelled abroad or the diarrhoea is persistent.
- Antibiotics may be required in the following specific circumstances to treat diarrhoea (if in doubt discuss with local microbiology or public health departments):
  - If *Giardia* spp. are isolated from the stool, give metronidazole for 3 days. Asymptomatic patients do not require treatment.
  - If *Campylobacter* spp. are isolated from the stool, give erythromycin if there is systemic upset or persistent blood in the stools, though many cases resolve without antibiotic treatment.
  - If *Salmonella* or *Shigella* spp. are isolated from the stool of the child, consider referral to secondary care for treatment and management, particularly if the child is systemically unwell or younger than 1 year old.
- If any of the following organisms are cultured from the stool, notify the environmental health department: *Shigella, Salmonella, Giardia, Campylobacter,* or *Cryptosporidium* spp. or *Escherichia coli* 157.

What to Do: Chronic Diarrhoea

- In cases of chronic diarrhoea and failure to thrive or other symptoms, consider further investigations, referral, or both.
- IBD and coeliac disease may present with diarrhoea in children.
- If a dietary cause for osmotic diarrhoea has been found, suggest relevant dietary modifications.

What to Do: Fluid and Diet Management in Diarrhoea

- It is important to provide appropriate advice for feeding a child who has diarrhoea.
- Caregivers may think that it is important to 'starve the child' and only provide them with water, which is not helpful.

- Practical tips about feeding include the following:
  - For breastfed infants, encourage continued breast-feeding, which provides both calories and water.
  - For nonbreastfeeding infants, it is rarely necessary to withdraw feeds; doing so may delay recovery.
  - It is rarely necessary to restrict lactose in the diet.
  - Oral rehydration solution (ORS) may be prescribed in patients with moderate dehydration for replacement of fluids during the first 4 hours (50 mL/kg over 4 hours). After this, recommence normal feeds. ORS is intended to replace fluid losses if the child is dehydrated. Do not keep children on ORS for prolonged periods of time.

The Child With a Murmur

- Most murmurs are innocent.
- The majority of pathological heart murmurs are picked up in infancy or have been found on an antenatal scan. Because many infants are now discharged from hospital a few hours after birth, they may present to primary care in the first few days of life with either heart failure or cyanosis. These children require urgent referral to hospital for investigation and management.
- Murmurs are often picked up at the routine 6-week baby check. These murmurs should also be referred to secondary care for assessment.
- The key features of an innocent murmur are the seven Ss (Frank and Jacobe, 2011):
  1. Sensitive (change with position and respiration)
  2. Short duration
  3. Single (no associated clicks or gallops)
  4. Small (nonradiating)
  5. Soft (low amplitude)
  6. Sweet (not harsh but 'musical')
  7. Systolic

What to Ask About the Child

- Ask about cardiac symptoms, including chest pain, syncope, impaired exercise tolerance, colour changes, and cyanosis.
- Ask whether the murmur has ever been noted previously.
- Enquire about the child's feeding, appetite, and growth; all children with failure to thrive who have a murmur should be further investigated.
- Check if there is a family history of cardiac disease. Children have an increased risk of congenital heart disease if they have a first-degree relative with a history of congenital heart disease.

What to Look for on Examination

- Assess if the child is acutely unwell.
- Check for cyanosis and pallor and whether there are signs or symptoms that could indicate heart failure, including tachycardia, an enlarged liver, sweating, and difficulties with feeding (particularly in infants).
- Feel for the femoral pulses. Decreased or absent femoral pulses and a short systolic murmur may indicate coarctation of the aorta, a murmur that may not be picked up in early childhood.
- The commonest murmur is an innocent one. On auscultation, an innocent murmur changes with the child's position (often being loudest when the child is lying down), has a short duration, does not radiate to the precordium or back, has a soft quality often described as 'musical', and is systolic with no associated clicks or gallops.

What to Do

- Refer urgently all children with a murmur who have cyanosis or signs of heart failure (i.e., tachycardia, sweating, poor feeding, tachypnoea, enlarged liver, or failure to thrive).
- Also refer urgently all children noted to have a murmur in the first 48 hours of life.
- Refer children whose murmurs are not consistent with the findings of an innocent murmur, including a widely radiating, or particularly loud, murmur.
- Refer those who have cardiac symptoms, including syncope, chest pain, or concerns regarding growth.
- If you think the murmur is an innocent one:
  1. Document your findings.
  2. Arrange to review the child again to reassess the murmur. (If the child is currently unwell, arrange review after the acute illness has resolved.)
  3. If the child is well and the murmur has the characteristics of an innocent murmur, there is no need to refer to secondary care.

The Child Who Collapses

> **PATIENT INFORMATION**
>
> STARS (Syncope Trust and Reflex anoxic Seizures). Reflux anoxic seizures patient information. Available at heartrhythmalliance.org/stars/uk/reflex-anoxic-seizures-ras-syncope-in-the-young.

- Syncope is a temporary loss of consciousness, resulting in 'collapse', caused by reduction in oxygenation to the brain. There are a number of causes, the most common of which are vasovagal episodes ('fainting') and reflex anoxic seizures (RASs). RASs are most common in the toddler age group.
- RASs are a common nonepileptic paroxysmal event in infants and preschool-aged children, but they can occur at any age. They are provoked by a sudden noxious stimulus followed by a loss of consciousness and brief clonic movements of the limbs.
- Rare cardiac causes of syncope include arrhythmias (long QT syndrome, Wolff–Parkinson–White syndrome) and

cardiac abnormalities (aortic or pulmonary stenosis). Because syncope may result in abnormal movements, including stiffening of the body or limbs, convulsive jerking, or drowsiness, after the event, syncope may sometimes be confused for epilepsy.

- Breathholding attacks also occur in the toddler age group. During these events, the child gets cross, starts to cry, holds their breath, turns blue, and collapses. The cyanosis is caused by the glottis being held closed. These events are respiratory in origin, and an electrocardiogram (ECG) taken at the time would not show asystole.

What to Ask About the Child

- Obtain a detailed history of the event, including what happened before, during, and after the 'collapse'. Try to obtain a history from a witness and, if old enough, the child themself. In vasovagal episodes, the child often has prodromal features, including sweating, dizziness, and pallor.
- Ask about the frequency of episodes and if the child has had more than one episode, whether they all have similar features. Enquire whether there are specific triggers to the events. Whereas breathholding attacks occur when a child is crying, RAS occurs in response to a noxious stimulus. Events during exercise or whilst supine are unusual in benign cases of syncope, and children with these features should be referred to secondary care.
- Check if there a history of sudden death in a family member younger than 30 years of age or a family history of sudden infant death syndrome; refer children with a positive family history for further assessment. If possible, ask the family to capture one of these events on video.

What to Look for on Examination

Usually the child presents with a history of collapse rather than immediately after the collapse. In most cases, the child will have a normal examination. However:
- Examine the cardiovascular system, including taking the blood pressure (take whilst the child is sitting and standing and look for a postural decrease in the pressure, which might be the cause of a vasovagal episode).
- Examine the neurologic system, looking for cranial nerve abnormalities, asymmetry of tone or power, and an abnormal or unstable gait, suggestive of an underlying neurologic condition, which would be a rare cause of collapse.
- In reflex anoxic seizure, check the conjunctivae and palmar creases for signs of iron-deficiency anaemia.

What to Do

- All children with unexplained or recurrent syncope should have an ECG to rule out a rare, but potentially fatal, cardiac problem. Ideally, the ECG should be read by an experienced paediatrician.

- For classical breathholding attacks in which the child is seen to cry, hold their breath, and turn blue, an ECG is not routinely required unless there is a family history of cardiac arrhythmias or early or sudden death.
- An electroencephalogram (EEG) is not usually required in cases of syncope.
- A clear explanation and reassurance are required for parents and children. Prevention of vasovagal episodes includes the following strategies:
  - Children can learn to recognise the prodromal symptoms and sit with their arms folded and legs crossed to maintain their blood pressure and prevent syncope.
  - Suggest increasing fluids and dietary salt.
- It is difficult to prevent RAS or breathholding attacks. Sometimes advising the parents to blow gently on the face of a child about to have a breathholding attack may abort the event.

The Child With Chest Pain

- Chest pain is a common reason for 10- to 16-year-old children and teens to attend the emergency department (ED). It can cause significant concern to parents and children but in the majority of cases is noncardiac in origin.
- The most common cause is a musculoskeletal problem, but also consider respiratory causes, including asthma and pneumonia; gastrointestinal (GI) causes, including oesophagitis; and anxiety associated with hyperventilation.

What to Ask About the Child

- Ask about the duration, frequency, location, and description of the pain.
- Enquire whether the pain occurs at rest, on exertion, or during the night.
- Check whether there are associated symptoms, including syncope, pallor, sweating, or palpitations, all of which are concerning.
- Ask whether there are respiratory or GI symptoms, including asthma or GOR.
- Check whether analgesia helps the pain. Antiinflammatory medication helps ease pain caused by costochondritis or musculoskeletal problems.
- If the child has been partaking in new exercises or lifting or if they carry heavy books to school, consider a possible musculoskeletal cause.
- Ask if there is a family history of sudden death in young adults because there may be a history of hypertrophic obstructive cardiomyopathy or long QT syndrome.
- Check if the child has a history of Kawasaki disease because this may result in later cardiac problems, including a coronary aneurysm.

What to Look for on Examination

- Assess for local tenderness, found in costochondritis and musculoskeletal problems.

- Examine the cardiovascular system. Check the peripheral pulses and auscultate for a murmur. If possible, check the blood pressure.
- Examine the respiratory and GI systems to look for alternative causes of chest pain.

What to Do

- Patients with musculoskeletal causes should be managed with rest and antiinflammatory medication.
- Indications for immediate referral to a paediatric cardiologist include:
  - Chest pain on exertion
  - Chest pain with palpitations
  - Chest pain with syncope
  - A cardiac abnormality found on examination (e.g., a murmur)
  - A family history of sudden death or cardiac problems in a young adult
- If features suggest a diagnosis of GOR, a trial of an acid-blocking drug might be worthwhile.
- Treat patients with respiratory conditions as appropriate.
- Manage anxiety-induced episodes with behavioural techniques.

The Child Who Does Not Walk at Age 15 Months

> **GUIDELINE**
>
> National Institute for Health and Clinical Excellence Clinical Knowledge Summaries. (2019). *Scenario: Delayed walking in children*. Available at cks.nice.org.uk/topics/developmental-rheumatology-in-children/management/delayed-walking-in-children.

- Delays in walking (beyond 18 months) may be from a variety of causes ranging from simple bottom shuffling to cerebral palsy (children have spasticity); neuromuscular disorders, including Duchenne muscular dystrophy (children have weakness); and rarely, a missed developmental dysplasia of the hip (DDH).

What to Ask About the Child

- Ask about the birth history, including maternal health during pregnancy and prematurity. Check the records for the Apgar scores. Cerebral palsy has many causes, but the insult is usually prenatal. DDH is more common in breech deliveries and when there is a family history.
- Ask if the child appears unwell or in pain and whether there is a local cause of the delayed walking (e.g., a swollen or painful joint).
- Assess whether the child has met their other gross developmental milestones:

- Was reaching or grasping delayed (after 5 months)?
- Was sitting delayed (after 7 months)?
- Did the child dislike lying prone (more likely in bottom shufflers)?
- Did the child crawl? (Bottom shufflers tend not to crawl.)
- Ask if the child bottom shuffles and if there is a family history of delayed walking or bottom shuffling.

What to Look for on Examination

- Look for dysmorphic features and assess the general development of the child, including vision, hearing, speech, and social and fine-motor skills.
- Check the child's truncal tone. Pick up the child under the arms. If they slide through your hands ('like a rag doll'), they have truncal hypotonia.
- Check for asymmetry in tone or power in the legs or arms. (This may point to an underlying neuromuscular problem.)
- Check for tenderness on palpation of the legs or joints.
- Undertake a hip examination to exclude DDH and refer urgently to paediatric orthopaedics if found.

What to Do

- For children who are bottom shufflers and have otherwise normal examination results, reassure the parents that the child is likely to walk eventually. However, if the child does not walk by 20 months of age, refer them for further assessment to ensure there are no other issues.
- For children who are not bottom shufflers and who are not walking by 15 months, refer for further assessment. There may be a delay between your referral and the child's being seen, so referring before 18 months will ensure the child is seen at an appropriate time. A physiotherapy assessment is often useful if you are not sure whether there is an underlying problem.

The Child With a Small Head

- Microcephaly is defined as an occipital–frontal circumference (OFC) more than 2 standard deviations below the mean. This indicates a small brain, or microcephaly.
- Microcephaly can be caused by a variety of genetic and environmental causes. It is important to distinguish between 'primary' microcephaly in which an abnormal OFC has been present since birth (corrected appropriately for gestational age and weight and length) and secondary or 'acquired' microcephaly, which is caused by deceleration in the growth of the brain after birth.

What to Ask About the Child

- Ask about the pregnancy and whether the mother was well, whether she had any infections (e.g., cytomegalovirus, rubella, toxoplasmosis), and whether she took any drugs during pregnancy. Consider whether there could have been a prenatal insult.

- Ask about the delivery, including the type of delivery and the Apgar scores, and consider whether there could have been an insult during delivery.
- Enquire whether the parents are consanguineous and consider whether there could be a metabolic or genetic cause. (Microcephaly may be autosomal recessive.)
- Ask whether the infant was unwell during the first 6 weeks of life (e.g., with a serious bacterial infection such as meningitis) and consider whether there has been a postnatal insult.
- Ask about recent travel of the mother whilst pregnant because congenital Zika virus is a cause of microcephaly.
- Ask about appropriate developmental milestones, including whether the child smiles (at 6 weeks), reaches or grasps (by 5 months), and sits (by 7 months).

What to Look for on Examination

- Take careful measurements of the weight, length, and OFC and plot the information on appropriate charts.
- Measure the OFC of the parents and any siblings and plot the information on appropriate charts.
- Look for any dysmorphic features. Syndromes associated with microcephaly include primordial dwarfism and Dubowitz syndrome.
- Check if the child is hyper- or hypotonic.

What to Do

- All children with microcephaly should be referred to secondary care for further assessment.

The Child With a Large Head

- Macrocephaly is defined as an OFC more than 2 standard deviations above the mean.
- Macrocephaly does not always indicate a large brain (megalencephaly); for example, children with hydrocephalus have large heads, but their brains are not enlarged.
- It is important to distinguish between an infant who has always has a large head and whose OFC is tracking appropriately without deviating upward away from previous measurements and an infant whose OFC was on a lower centile and is now accelerating and crossing centiles in an upward direction.
- A large head may be familial. Other causes include congenital problems, infections, subdural bleeds, metabolic storage and degenerative diseases, and cranioskeletal dysplasias.

What to Ask About the Child

- Ask about the child's development and whether normal milestones have been reached.

- Check if there are any signs of increased intracranial pressure (ICP), including poor feeding or irritability.
- Explore whether other members of the family have large heads.
- Enquire whether the child has had any serious illnesses (e.g., meningitis).
- Finally, ask if the parents have any concerns about the child.

What to Look for on Examination

- Take careful measurements of the child's weight, length, and OFC and plot them on appropriate charts.
- If possible, measure the parents' OFCs and plot them on an appropriate chart. (Plot at age 18 years on female and male charts as appropriate.)
- Assess the child's development and whether it is appropriate for their age. In familial macrocephaly, the child's development is normal.
- Palpate the anterior and posterior fontanelles. The anterior fontanelle usually closes by 12 to 18 months and the posterior fontanelle by 2 months. If they are open beyond these times, consider whether the child has increased ICP.
- Check whether the child's anterior fontanelle is tense and bulging, suggesting increased ICP.
- Check whether the child has any depigmented or pigmented patches because neurofibromatosis and tuberous sclerosis are both causes of macrocephaly.

What to Do

- A normally developed child whose OFC is tracking parallel to the 99th centile without deviating in an upward direction and with a family history of macrocephaly does not need further investigations. Reassure the parents.
- A child with signs suggesting increased ICP or an OFC crossing centiles in an upward direction should be referred immediately.

The Child With a Febrile Seizure

- Febrile seizures occur when there is a rapid increase in the temperature of a young child, usually between the ages of 1 and 3 years.
- Children who have a seizure before 6 months of age, even if it is associated with fever, should be referred to secondary care for further management and investigation of the source of the fever.
- First febrile seizures do not usually occur in those older than 6 years of age.
- The prevalence of first febrile seizures is around 1 in 20 children; approximately one-third of children who have a febrile seizure go on to have another febrile seizure.
- Most commonly, the duration of febrile seizures ranges from a few seconds to 15 minutes.

What to Ask About the Child

- Ask for a description of the seizure. Febrile seizures may involve a variety of abnormal movements or posturing. Children with focal seizures should be referred to hospital.
- Ask about the length of the seizure and the recovery time. Any child who has not regained consciousness or whose conscious level is not clearly improving after 30 minutes should be assumed to have increased ICP and referred for further management.
- Ask about a family history of epilepsy or febrile seizures. If one or both parents have a history of febrile seizures, the risk of recurrent febrile seizures for the child increases.
- Try to find a source of the fever by asking about respiratory symptoms, vomiting, diarrhoea, rash, and illness in other family members.

What to Look for on Examination

- Refer all children at high or intermediate risk of a serious illness (see the NICE traffic light system for fever in children younger than 5 years of age).
- Take the temperature and give an antipyretic, either orally or per rectum.
- Look for a source of the infection. Specifically, examine the throat, ears, chest, abdomen, and skin.

What to Do

- The priority is to manage the seizure. Check airway, breathing, and circulation. If the seizure has lasted for more than 5 minutes, give buccal midazolam or rectal diazepam and refer the child to hospital.
- You will often be consulted after a seizure, and your priority is to determine the cause of and to treat when appropriate the underlying cause of the fever. See 'The Child With a Fever' section to guide whether the child should be referred to hospital.
- For children being managed at home, reassure the parents that:
  - Febrile seizures are common.
  - Most children will not have another one.
  - Longitudinal studies show that children with febrile seizures have normal school achievement, comparable with their siblings who have not had febrile seizures.
  - The majority of children with febrile seizures do not go on to develop epilepsy.
- Refer the child to hospital if there are unusual features associated with the seizure, including a prolonged duration (>15 minutes), asymmetrical movements, or a long time (>30 minutes) to return to a normal conscious level.

The Child With Seizures

- There are numerous forms of epilepsy, including generalised seizures, focal seizures, absence seizures, infantile spasms, and myoclonic seizures.

- In all children with a seizure, a detailed description of the episode is critical to making a diagnosis. If possible, ask the caregivers to capture the event on video. Providing a detailed description helps to classify the seizure and determine the drugs to use. Approximately 40% of children presenting with a first seizure have nonepileptic events. These include syncope, migraine-related disorders, and self-gratification events. (Masturbation is normal in infants, although it is sometimes shocking for the parents.)
- Seizures may also be the first indication of increased ICP and may occur in children with meningitis or with a metabolic derangement, including low blood sugar. These children are unwell.
- Infants sometimes present with a history of myoclonic jerks. These usually occur either when the child is asleep or when they are going into or out of sleep. The parents describe rhythmic movements of the limbs. This is not a seizure and does not require investigation or treatment, and the parents should be reassured.

What to Ask About the Child

- Document events preceding the episode(s), including at what time of day or night the events occur, if there are any obvious triggers, and what the child was doing before the seizure.
- Ask for a description of the seizure from the events preceding the episode to the child recovering completely.
- Ask the caregivers to describe any movements or sounds. Explore whether the movements were symmetrical and if there were any lateralising signs, including eye deviation and tonic-clonic movements of one side of the body only.
- Ask about the length of the episode and whether the child had bladder or bowel incontinence during or after the episode.
- If the child is old enough, ask them about the events and what they remember.
- Ask how the child appeared after the episode, what they did, and how they behaved.

What to Look for on Examination

- Usually the patient will present to you after the seizure, so you are unlikely to witness it.
- If the child has a fever or looks unwell, assess for signs of meningitis or another cause of febrile illness that may have precipitated the seizure.
- Examine the tone and power and check for symmetry. Examine for signs of increased ICP.

What to Do

- If the child is having a seizure, your priority is to manage the seizure. Check airway, breathing, and circulation. If the seizure has lasted for more than 5 minutes, give

buccal midazolam or rectal diazepam and refer the child to hospital in an ambulance.
- You will often be consulted after the seizure, and your priority is to determine whether the child needs to be urgently referred to hospital (e.g., child not regained consciousness, signs of a serious bacterial infection, seizure was associated with a fever with no obvious cause, or there are signs of increased ICP) or whether they can be referred nonurgently for a clinic appointment.
- If a child is being referred nonurgently, ask the parents to try to video any further events.
- It is advisable not to start a discussion about epilepsy, including the prognosis and consequences for lifestyle, until the child has had further assessment and possible investigations (e.g., an EEG) and a diagnosis has been made. Some children may not be started on medication immediately.
- Most neonates with seizures require urgent referral for investigation because they are often caused by an acute event, including hypoglycaemia, an electrolyte imbalance, or infection.
- Myoclonic jerks are not seizures and do not require investigations or treatment.

The Child With Headaches

GUIDELINES AND RESOURCES

Headsmart. Available at headsmart.org.uk.
National Institute for Health and Care Excellence. (2019). *Suspected neurological conditions recognition and referral guidance for children under 16. NICE clinical guideline 127.* Available at http://www.nice.org.uk.
National Institute for Health and Care Excellence (2021). *Headaches in over 12s: Diagnosis and management. NICE clinical guideline 153.* Available at http://www.nice.org.uk.

PATIENT INFORMATION

The Migraine Trust, 7-14 Great Dover Street, London, SE1 4YR. Helpline: 0800 802 0066 Available at http://migrainetrust.org.

Headaches are common in school-aged children and are usually benign. The challenge is to identify the very small group of children who have serious underlying pathology, including brain tumours.

What to Ask About the Child

- Ask when the headaches first began. A long history of intermittent headaches and a child who is well in between suggest a benign aetiology.
- Ask about the frequency of headaches and whether the child is well in between episodes of headache.

A headache caused by meningeal stretching (i.e., increased ICP) is more likely to be constant rather than intermittent.
- Ask about nature of the headaches:
  - Throbbing headaches are typical of migraines.
  - Feeling as though there is a 'band' around the scalp is typical of tension headaches.
  - Tenderness over the face may suggest inflammation of the sinuses.
- Check whether there are any symptoms suggesting increased ICP, including:
  - Have there been recent changes in behaviour?
  - Is the headache made worse on coughing, sneezing, bending over (e.g., to touch the toes), or squatting down?
  - Is the headache worse in the mornings, and is it associated with vomiting?
  - Does the headache wake the child from sleep?
- Enquire whether there have there been problems with unsteadiness of the gait and ask whether the child has had seizures. If the child wears glasses, enquire whether they have had their eyes tested recently.
- Explore the social history for any issues that may be causing the child anxiety, including recent separation of parents, change in school, or bullying.

What to Look for on Examination

- Assess whether the child looks well or unwell. A short history of headaches in an unwell child with fever may indicate an infective cause.
- Ideally, check the blood pressure because increased blood pressure can be a cause of headaches. Refer all children with hypertension urgently to secondary care.
- Conduct a neurologic examination. In particular, examine for unsteadiness of the gait and examine the cranial nerves. Specifically assess whether the child can maintain an upward gaze and whether there is 'sun setting' of the eyes.
- Examine whether the child's eyes move laterally in both directions and whether there is diplopia.
- Check whether the child has an abnormal head position (e.g., a new head tilt).
- Examine the optic fundi for papilloedema. It is often difficult to get a good view of the fundi in young children.
- Palpate the area over the sinuses to check for tenderness.

What to Do

- If the child is acutely unwell, refer immediately. This includes children with fever.
- If the child has abnormalities of their cranial nerves, gait, or neurologic examination, refer immediately because these signs are suggestive of raised ICP.
- If the history and examination are not suggestive of serious underlying pathology, management will depend on the

type of headache. However, discussion of some lifestyle issues is useful for all headaches.

a. Adequate fluid intake (many children underdrink). A rough guide is:
   - Ages 1 to 3 years: 900 to 1000 mL
   - Ages 4 to 8 years: 1000 to 1400 mL
   - Ages 9 to 13 years, females: 1200 to 2100 mL
   - Ages 9 to 13 years, males: 1400 to 2300 mL
   - Ages 14 to 18 years, females: 1400 to 2500 mL
   - Ages 14 to 18 years, males: 2100 to 3200 mL
b. Sleep hygiene and an appropriate bedtime
c. Eating regularly and not missing meals
d. Avoiding caffeine in the diet
e. Reducing screen time, particularly before sleep
f. Avoiding taking too many pain relievers for headaches because these can cause a 'medication overuse headache' if they are taken more than two to three times weekly

- For migraine headaches, reassure. Suggest simple analgesia or a triptan, and if vomiting is a feature, an antiemetic may be useful. For children with frequent and debilitating migraine, a trial of a migraine prophylaxis (pizotifen or propranolol, which should be avoided if the child has asthma) may be helpful.
- For tension headaches, reassure, offer advice about avoidance of triggers, and suggest simple analgesia.
- For sinusitis, offer a trial of decongestants.
- If headaches are debilitating, refer to secondary care.
- For all children with headaches, recommend an optician review.

The Child With a Tic

The appearance of facial tics in children is common but is a source of concern to parents.

What to Ask About the Child

- Ask if there were there any triggers for the facial tics, including events that occurred before the ticking starting.
- Enquire whether the tics can be suppressed. Often children can suppress a tic if they are outside the home environment, including at school.
- Ask if the tic is associated with motor or vocal tics. This is suggestive of Tourette syndrome, and the child may benefit from psychology or psychiatry input.

What to Look for on Examination

- If possible, observe the tics or ask the parents to capture them on video.
- Observe for motor and vocal tics.
- Conduct a neurologic examination, particularly ensuring the cranial nerves are normal.

What to Do

- Reassurance is the most important management strategy for children with facial tics.

- Advise parents to ignore the tics and do not ask the child to try to stop the tics.
- Suggest the parents discuss their child's tics with their school.
- If the tics are causing excessive distress, psychological interventions may be helpful.
- Suggest that the parents (and teachers) do not reprimand the child or try to stop them from ticking because this is likely to make the tics worse.
- Explain to the parents that the ticking often resolves, although it is difficult to predict if and when the tics may get better.

The Child With Dysuria and Abdominal Pain

> **GUIDELINE**
>
> National Institute for Health and Clinical Excellence. (2022). *Urinary tract infection in under 16s: Diagnosis and management*. NICE clinical guideline 224. Available at https://www.nice.org.uk/guidance/ng224.

What to Ask About the Child

- In older children, ask about fever, dysuria, and abdominal and loin pain.
- Infants with a UTI present with nonspecific symptoms, including fever, vomiting, lethargy, irritability, and sometimes poor feeding and failure to thrive.
- In all children with a fever and no obvious source of infection, a clean-catch urine sample should be obtained for urinalysis and culture (see later).
- Ask about a history of previous confirmed or unconfirmed UTIs.
- Explore the antenatal history and ask about any antenatal ultrasound scan results.
- Ask about a history of constipation because children who are constipated are prone to UTIs.
- Ask if there a family history of renal disease, including vesicoureteric reflux (VUR).
- Ask about the child's development and if there are any concerns that the child has a neurologic problem.
- Ask if the child has a history of dysfunctional voiding, including poor urine flow or diurnal or nocturnal enuresis.
- Ask about hygiene, including how the child wipes their bottom. (Encourage children to wipe their bottoms from front to back.)
- Assess the child's fluid intake and check that they are taking enough for their age. Many children underdrink. A rough guide is:
  - Ages 1 to 3 years: 900 to 1000 mL
  - Ages 4 to 8 years: 1000 to 1400 mL
  - Ages 9 to 13 years, females: 1200 to 2100 mL
  - Ages 9 to 13 years, males: 1400 to 2300 mL
  - Ages 14 to 18 years, females: 1400 to 2500 mL
  - Ages 14 to 18 years, males: 2100 to 3200 mL

What to Look for on Examination

- In most cases, the examination results are normal.
- Take the child's temperature.
- Plot their weight and height on a chart and compare them with previous measurements to assess growth.
- Examine the abdomen for tenderness or an enlarged bladder.
- Examine the spine and assess tone and power in the lower limbs and observe the child's gait. Rarely, the child may have an underlying neurologic condition.
- If appropriately sized cuffs are available, take the child's blood pressure.

What to Do

- Refer febrile children to secondary care if appropriate according to the NICE guidelines. Children, particularly infants, may need to be referred urgently before you are able to obtain a urine sample if they have a fever and are unwell looking.
- Obtain a clean-catch urine sample:
  - Undertake urinalysis looking for leucocyte esterase and nitrites. The presence of nitrites with or without leucocyte esterase is indicative of a UTI, and the child should be treated with antibiotics whilst awaiting the result of a urine culture (see later).
  - Send the urine for culture if the child has symptoms indicative of a urine infection or if the urinalysis is positive for nitrites or leucocytes.
- Try to distinguish between:
  - An upper UTI (acute pyelonephritis): bacteriuria and fever of 38°C or above with or without loin pain
  - A lower UTI: bacteriuria with no systemic features
- If the child can be managed at home, treat with antibiotics if the urinalysis is positive for nitrites (whilst awaiting results of the urine culture).
- If the urinalysis is negative for nitrites but positive for leucocyte esterase, only start the antibiotics if there are clinical symptoms of a UTI (whilst awaiting results of the urine culture).
- If urinalysis is negative for both nitrites and leucocyte esterase, then do not assume that this is a UTI; send urine for culture but also search for alternative causes to explain the symptoms.
- Be cautious of interpreting urinalysis in children younger than 12 months of age because urinalysis may be nitrite negative even in the presence of a UTI because they void frequently.
- Management of a confirmed UTI:
  - Refer all infants younger than 3 months of age with either upper or lower UTI for parenteral antibiotics.
  - Refer all infants older than 3 months of age for parenteral antibiotics if they are in the high- or intermediate-risk group (see NICE assessment of risk of serious illness) or they are unable to tolerate oral fluids or medication.
  - Refer all children with recurrent UTIs (two upper UTIs or three lower UTIs in the previous 12 months).
  - Infants older than 3 months old with lower UTIs who are not unwell should be managed at home with 3 days of an oral antibiotic (usually trimethoprim or a cephalosporin, but this should be guided by local antibiotic policy).
  - Refer infants older than 3 months of age who are unwell with suspected upper UTIs for further management.
  - Infants who are managed at home need an early review to ensure they are responding to treatment. Review the choice of antibiotics when the urine culture and sensitivity results are available.
  - It is not necessary to repeat urine culture at the end of a course of antibiotics if the child responded well.
- Further investigations for children younger than 3 years of age with a proven UTI:
  - Children younger than 3 years of age are most at risk of renal damage after a UTI. In addition, they are more likely to have underlying pathology leading to the UTI (e.g., VUR).
  - These depend on your local guidelines and referral hospital.
  - Children younger than 6 months of age usually have a renal ultrasound examination within 6 weeks. Further imaging depends on local guidelines, whether the child responded to treatment within the first 48 hours, and whether the UTI was upper or lower should guide further imaging.
- For older children, give advice about:
  - Cleaning themselves after toileting
  - Encouraging complete bladder emptying and a good fluid intake
  - Management of constipation when appropriate
- Prophylactic antibiotics are required only in special circumstances (e.g., infants with underlying structural issues).
- Most children who require prophylactic antibiotics will have been referred to secondary care, and the antibiotics will have been started there.
- Counsel parents on recognition of the symptoms associated with UTIs, particularly in infants who may have nonspecific symptoms.

The Child With Bedwetting (Nocturnal Enuresis)

GUIDELINE

National Institute for Health and Care Excellence. (2010). *Bedwetting in under 19s. NICE clinical guideline 111.* Available at http://nice.org.uk/guidance/cg111.

PATIENT INFORMATION

Bowel and Bladder UK. https://www.bbuk.org.uk.
ERIC, The Children's Bowel and Bladder Charity. Helpline: 0800 169 9949. https://eric.org.uk.

- Nocturnal enuresis is a distressing condition with significant impact on the lives of children and their families.
- The prevalence improves with age: 21% at age 4 years, decreasing to 1.5% at age 9 years.
- It is important to establish whether the enuresis is primary (the child has never been dry at night) or secondary (there has been a recent loss of acquired nighttime control).

What to Ask About the Child

- Establish whether the child has primary or secondary enuresis.
- If the child has secondary enuresis, consider systemic illness (including UTIs and diabetes mellitus) and emotional issues.
- Ask about the pattern of the wetting, including how many nights and how many times per night. The latter might be difficult to ascertain if the child does not wake up. Multiple episodes of wetting per night are suggestive of an overactive bladder.
- Enquire the time of night when wetting happens. Wetting often happens after 1 to 2 hours of sleep if the diagnosis is enuresis.
- Ask if the child wakes on wetting.
- Ask about associated daytime symptoms:
  - Ask about daytime wetting, the frequency of micturition (more than seven times per day), and urgency of micturition suggestive of an irritable bladder.
  - Enquire whether the child has dysuria or other symptoms of a UTI.
  - Explore symptoms that would suggest diabetes mellitus (if the child drinking more than usual or passing more urine than previously or has secondary enuresis).
- If diabetes mellitus is considered in a child, do an immediate capillary blood test and do not wait for a fasting blood sugar result or a urine sample.
- Check if the child is having an appropriate or excessive fluid intake. Recommended intakes are:
  - Ages 1 to 3 years: 900 to 1000 mL
  - Ages 4 to 8 years: 1000 to 1400 mL
  - Ages 9 to 13 years, females: 1200 to 2100 mL
  - Ages 9 to 13 years, males: 1400 to 2300 mL
  - Ages 14 to 18 years, females: 1400 to 2500 mL
  - Ages 14 to 18 years, males: 2100 to 3200 mL
- Finally, explore whether the child has learning difficulties, developmental delay, behavioural or emotional problems, or a family history of diabetes mellitus.

What to Look for on Examination

- In the majority of cases, examination results are normal.
- Examine the abdomen for tenderness (possible UTI) and masses and the spine for abnormalities.
- Observe the child's gait because rarely, enuresis may be secondary to a neurologic cause.
- Plot the weight and compare it against previous measurements. A child with secondary enuresis and weight loss may have diabetes mellitus.

What to Do

- Investigations are not normally required unless the child has symptoms of a UTI (check urinalysis with or without urine culture) or diabetes mellitus (check capillary blood glucose).
- Manage UTIs appropriately.
- General management for nocturnal enuresis includes the following:
  - The child should never be penalised for wetting. A supportive approach should be encouraged.
  - Optimise fluid intake and avoid caffeine.
  - Manage constipation if present.
  - Waking the child to go to the toilet, before the time they usually wet (if this time is known), may be helpful in the short term but does not influence long-term resolution.
  - Star charts may be helpful for all aspects of management, including adequate fluid intake, regular toileting, and engaging in practical steps such as changing bed sheets.
  - If the child is younger than 5 years of age, a trial of 2 consecutive nights without wearing a nappy or pull-up is worthwhile to assess the success of any intervention.
- Alarm systems are often used in children with nocturnal enuresis. They have a high long-term success rate and may be useful if there has been no response to toileting and reward systems. They are less useful if the wetting is infrequent (one to two times per week). Assess the response after 1 month and, if successful, continue until the child has had 2 weeks of uninterrupted dry beds.
- A trial of medication may be used in children from age 5 years. Desmopressin may be used (a) in the short term (e.g., occasional sleepovers), (b) in conjunction with an alarm system, and (c) if an alarm system is undesirable. Treat for 3 months and then withdraw for 1 week to check if dryness has been achieved. If used longer term, withdraw to assess success every 3 months.

The Child With Protein in Their Urine

- Proteinuria may be an incidental finding in a well child but may also be a clue to underlying renal disease.
- A trace of protein is not usually significant.
- Persistent proteinuria is suggestive of a glomerular lesion, and if associated with haematuria, the likelihood of underlying renal disease increases.

What to Ask About the Child

- In a child with an incidental finding of proteinuria, ask if the child has had a recent illness and whether they have undertaken strenuous exercise. Both are triggers for benign proteinuria.

- For a child with oedema and proteinuria, ask if there has been a previous history of oedema, suggesting that the child has had previous episodes of proteinuria.
- Ask if there is a history of a recent upper respiratory infection because glomerulonephritis may follow a recent infection.
- Check if the child is taking any medications because some drugs, such as penicillamine, gold, and ethosuximide, may be associated with nephrotic syndrome.
- Ask about a family history of renal disease.

What to Look for on Examination

- Check the child's temperature, blood pressure (if the appropriately sized cuff is available), heart rate, and capillary return. And assess if the child is haemodynamically stable or acutely unwell.
- Assess for oedema in dependent sites, including the feet, lower back, and face, when the child has been recumbent.
- Examine the abdomen for pain.
- If possible, test for orthostatic proteinuria (i.e., check a urinalysis in the recumbent and standing positions). The standing sample will have two to four times more protein in it than the recumbent sample. Orthostatic proteinuria may also be diagnosed if an early morning urine specimen is negative for protein but samples taken later in the day are positive.

What to Do

- If there is an incidental finding of proteinuria (≥2+), repeat urinalysis three times over a period of 2 to 3 weeks using an early morning urine sample. If proteinuria is persistent, obtain an early morning urine sample and send to the laboratory for a protein-to-creatinine ratio. The normal range for children aged 2 years or older is less than 20 mg/mmol; for those aged 6 to 24 months, it is less than 50 mg/mmol.
- If the child has intermittent proteinuria, reassess in 3 to 6 months. If still present, refer to secondary care.
- If the child has orthostatic proteinuria, reassure and repeat urinalysis in 1 year. If the child has nonorthostatic proteinuria, refer for further evaluation.
- If the child has associated haematuria or oedema or a increased protein-to-creatinine ratio, refer to secondary care.

The Child With Blood in Their Urine

GUIDELINE

Dalrymple, R., & Ramage, I. (2017). Fifteen-minute consultation: The management of microscopic haematuria. Education and practice edition. *Archives of Disease in Childhood, 102,* 230–234.

- Microscopic haematuria is not visible to the naked eye but is diagnosed on urinalysis and seeing red blood cells on microscopy.
- Macroscopic haematuria is visible to the naked eye.
- It is important to confirm the presence of red blood cells in the urine because there are other reasons the urine might appear red or brown in colour, including ingestion of some food substances, urates, and the presence of myoglobin or haemoglobin.

What to Ask About the Child

- Ask about the colour of the urine:
  - Bright red or pink urine is suggestive of bleeding from the urinary tract (e.g., a UTI, trauma or a renal calculus).
  - Brown or cola-coloured urine is suggestive of a glomerular source of bleeding (e.g., poststreptococcal glomerulonephritis, Henoch–Schönlein purpura (HSP), HUS).
- Ask if there are symptoms of a UTI (dysuria, frequency or urgency of micturition, fever, abdominal or loin pain).
- Enquire whether the child has had a recent upper respiratory tract infection because glomerulonephritis may follow an infection.
- Ask if the child has had a rash, which is present in HSP and HUS.
- Ask about any medications and whether the child is taking rifampicin, which can cause pink urine.
- Ask about the ingestion of specific foods, including beetroot.
- Check if there is a family history of deafness (Alport syndrome), renal disease, or haematuria and whether the child has had previous documented episodes of haematuria. Consider benign familial haematuria.
- Enquire whether the child has a history of easy bruising or bleeding and consider a haematologic cause.

What to Look for on Examination

- There will be little to find in children with an incidental finding of haematuria.
- Check for oedema suggesting proteinuria.
- Examine the abdomen for a mass (Wilms tumour presents with a mass in a young child) and tenderness (may be present with a UTI).
- Examine for a rash, bruising, petechiae, and purpura, which are present in those with HSP and HUS.
- Check the joints. Swollen and painful joints may be present in those with HSP.
- Take the temperature, and if possible, measure the blood pressure, ensuring the correct size cuff is used.

What to Do

- In an asymptomatic child with isolated microscopic haematuria, repeat urinalysis with microscopy in 2 weeks. If the haematuria persists, check the blood pressure, send urine for a protein-to-creatinine ratio, arrange to repeat the urinalysis, and ask family members to bring in urine samples for urinalysis (considering a diagnosis of benign familial haematuria).

- If haematuria is present on three occasions, refer to secondary care for further investigations.
- If there are symptoms suggestive of a UTI, manage appropriately.
- Children with macroscopic haematuria should have a renal ultrasound examination performed to exclude a Wilms tumour.
- Refer all children with persistent haematuria to secondary care for further assessment.
- In the absence of a UTI, refer children with *both* haematuria (>2+) and proteinuria (>2+) to secondary care because this is suggestive of glomerulonephritis.

The Child With an Itchy Perineum

- Inflammation or irritation of the vulva is common in young females and improves at puberty.
- It results from a lack of oestrogen and a thin vaginal or vulval lining that is easily irritated.
- Girls have often had the symptoms for some time before presenting to medical staff.

What to Ask About the Child

- Ask about the frequency and pattern of symptoms (e.g., itch and discharge, both of which are features of vulvovaginitis).
- Ask about urinary symptoms, including burning or stinging on passing urine. If these are present, obtain a clean-catch urine specimen for urinalysis and culture. Lichen sclerosus is an uncommon condition in children that can present with itch and dysuria, but it has distinct clinical findings (see later).
- Ask about the following, which might be triggers for vulvovaginitis:
  - Irritants, including soap, bubble bath, or shampoo
  - Toilet hygiene, including whether bottom is wiped from front to back
  - Wearing of tight clothing, including jeans and tights
- Ask whether threadworms have been noted. Threadworms cause itch and scratching, which may be the cause of the symptoms or may have exacerbated an episode of vulvovaginitis.
- Explore carefully whether there are any concerns around child abuse, including whether the child has demonstrated any change in their behaviour, if there have been previous social work concerns, how the child is doing at school, and who regularly looks after the child.

What to Look for on Examination

- Examine the external vulval and vaginal area for erythema, discharge, skin changes, and labial adhesions.

Vulvovaginitis presents with an erythematous vulva or vagina. Lichen sclerosus also presents with erythema and white patches in a distinctive 'figure of 8' pattern.

- Observe the external anal margin for threadworms.
- Examine for other skin conditions, including eczema.
- Observe for any features of potential concern, including bruising around the perineal area or bleeding.

What to Do

- Investigations are not necessary or helpful in most cases.
- Vaginal thrush is very unusual in an immune-competent, prepubescent female. If a child has vaginal thrush, consider type 1 diabetes mellitus and undertake urinalysis and a nonfasting capillary blood glucose (refer immediately if the capillary glucose is >8 mmol/L because this is abnormal).
- If the child has symptoms suggestive of a UTI, obtain a clean-catch urine for urinalysis and urine culture.
- Advice to prevent recurrence of vulvovaginitis includes:
  - Do not overwash the area.
  - Avoid shampoo, soap, and bubble bath; soap substitutes can be used.
  - Suggest showers rather than baths, particularly for washing the hair.
  - Suggest nonbiologic laundry powders for washing their clothes and no fabric softeners.
  - Avoid tight clothing and change wet clothing quickly.
  - Use cotton underwear and change it regularly.
  - Encourage regular toileting and complete emptying of the bladder.
  - Use soft toilet paper and encourage good toilet hygiene (wipe from front to back).
  - Treat constipation.
  - Avoid prolonged sitting if experiencing symptoms (e.g., horse riding or cycling).
  - Chlorine in swimming pools can irritate; applying a barrier cream before swimming can be helpful. Ensure washing and drying the area afterwards.
  - Avoid hot tubs.
- Suggest strategies to manage an episode of vulvovaginitis:
  - Cool compress may soothe the area.
  - Barrier creams (particularly those used for napkin dermatitis, e.g., Vaseline) are usually effective.
  - Some experts suggest urinating with the knees open and rinsing with water afterwards.
  - Advise to avoid tight clothing and suggest wearing nightdresses rather than pyjamas at night. The exception is a child with threadworms in which pyjamas can decrease the chance of eggs being spread to bedclothes or fingers during the night.
  - Prescribing antibiotic or antifungal treatment is not necessary.
  - If the problem is persistent, it would be worth a trial of a mild steroid ointment such as Daktacort ointment once daily for 7 days. If the symptoms persist despite this management, consider a referral to paediatric dermatology.

- Management of lichen sclerosus:
  - The earlier measures for treating vulvovaginitis may be helpful.
  - Have a low threshold for referral to a paediatric dermatologist or paediatrician to confirm the diagnosis.
  - A steroid cream may be helpful.

The Child With Worms in Their Stool

- Threadworms affect both preschool- and school-aged children, with often more than one family member affected.
- They are spread by the faecal–oral route, and the eggs can survive for up to 2 weeks, so repeat infection is common.
- Other worms may be present in the stools, particularly in children who have travelled to areas where other varieties of worms are prevalent.

What to Ask About the Child

- Ask about itch, particularly intense nocturnal perineal itching, which is common with threadworms.
- Ask about previous episodes.
- Ask about sleep disturbance and irritability at night.
- For females, ask about symptoms of vulvovaginitis.
- Ask if other family members have been affected.
- Note that recurrent abdominal pain in a child with no evidence of threadworms should not be assumed to be caused by worms; other causes should be sought.

What to Look for on Examination

- Look for small white worms on the perineum or in the stools.
- Examine for evidence of perineal or vulval erythema or irritation.

What to Do

- Investigation for threadworms is not usually necessary. The worms are readily seen at night or in the early morning on the perineum or visible in the stools.
- If the diagnosis is unclear, the 'Sellotape test' can be conducted. Tape a piece of Sellotape over the perineum and then remove it. The worms will be seen on the tape.
- Management includes treating all family members because worms are readily spread within households.
- Prescribe mebendazole for children older than 6 months of age. All household members, including adults, should be treated. (Note: Mebendazole is not recommended for pregnant females.) A second dose in 2 weeks may be required. Mebendazole kills the threadworms but not the eggs, which can live for up to 2 weeks outside the body.
- Ask all family members to shower every morning and wash all bedclothes, sleepwear, towels, and soft toys in a hot water wash. Vacuum all carpets and floors and disinfect kitchen and bathroom surfaces. Ensure children are wearing underwear at night and changing it in the morning.
- Ensure that fingernails are cut short, encourage good hand washing (including scrubbing of the nails), and avoid thumb sucking.
- Avoid shaking clothing or bedding to prevent eggs from spreading.
- Rinse toothbrushes before use.

The Child With a Painful Penis

- Balanitis affects prepubescent males, mostly those who are preschool aged.
- There is inflammation of the glans of the penis, which is painful and sometimes associated with swelling.
- The non- or partially retractile foreskin present in males of this age results in poor hygiene and infection.
- Most males only experience a single episode, but balanitis can be chronic or recurrent.
- The cause may be grouped into nonspecific dermatitis, infection, irritant or allergic, dermatologic (including eczema), and caused by manipulation of the foreskin.

What to Ask About the Child

- Ask about penile pain, itch and odour, and any penile discharge suggestive of an infective cause.
- Enquire about penile swelling and difficulties with urination and check for a normal urine stream.
- Ask about previous episodes.
- Explore hygiene practices and exposure to irritants, including bubble baths.
- Ask about associated skin conditions, including eczema, and check for symptoms of a UTI (dysuria, abdominal or loin pain).

What to Look for on Examination

- Observe for redness of the glans and foreskin with possible swelling.
- Observe for penile exudate and odour.
- Ask an older child to retract the foreskin for you to assess for phimosis.
- Assess for urinary flow if there is a history of problems and ask about ballooning of the foreskin upon micturition caused by a tight meatus.
- In severe phimosis, there may be obstruction to the urinary flow.

What to Do

- If there are symptoms of a UTI, obtain a clean-catch urine for urinalysis and culture.
- Refer for a urologic assessment if the child has recurrent episodes of balanitis or phimosis because circumcision may be required.

- A subpreputial swab is only required if symptoms are severe or persistent.
- General management of balanitis includes:
  - Avoidance of potential irritants, including soap, bubble bath, and wipes.
  - Encouragement of good hygiene, including washing the area twice daily with warm water and patting (not rubbing) dry.
  - Thorough hand washing.
  - In younger children, encourage frequent nappy changes.
  - If the foreskin is free, gently retract it during washing but do not forcefully retract the foreskin of an infant.
- Specific management of balanitis is related to the underlying cause.
- Patients with nonspecific dermatitis are treated with a topical hydrocortisone with imidazole cream twice daily for 1 week only.
- If there is no improvement after 1 week, stop the cream and send a swab from the affected area.
- For allergic or irritant balanitis, treat with topical hydrocortisone.
- If a swab has shown *Candida* infection, treat with imidazole cream but do not treat blindly with an antifungal cream.
- For bacterial infections, treat with a 1-week course of oral flucloxacillin with or without hydrocortisone cream depending on the level of discomfort.

The Child With a Groin Swelling

- The two commonest causes of a groin swelling (apart from inguinal lymphadenopathy) are an inguinal hernia and a hydrocele.
- Inguinal hernias may occur in females but are rare and present as a lump in the groin.

What to Ask About the Child

- Ask when the swelling was first noticed. Inguinal hernias are usually noticed during the second or third month of life.
- Enquire whether the swelling 'comes and goes'. Often hernias appear during coughing or crying and reduce spontaneously in between times.

What to Look for on Examination

- Transillumination helps to identify a hydrocele. However, testicular tumours also transilluminate, so they may be misdiagnosed as hydrocele.
- Check for cellulitis of the scrotum and groin area, which may indicate an incarcerated hernia. If so, do not try to reduce the hernia but refer immediately to secondary care.

What to Do

- Refer all children with a groin swelling for a surgical opinion (except for a swelling caused by enlarged inguinal lymph nodes).
- Urgently refer children with a suspected incarcerated hernia.

The Child With a Painful Scrotum

- It is important not to miss a torsion of the testis in a child presenting with a painful scrotum.
- Other causes include epididymo-orchitis, idiopathic scrotal oedema, trauma, tumour, and varicocele.

What to Ask About the Child

- Ask whether the pain is in the scrotum and testis or also in the abdomen. A torsion of the testis presents with a painful, swollen testis and often with pain in the lower abdomen and groin.

What to Look for on Examination

- A painful, swollen testis indicates a torsion of the testis until proven otherwise.
- Examine the scrotum whilst the child is standing up. Do the veins of the testis feel like a 'bag of worms'? If so, the child may have a varicocele.
- Check whether the scrotum and perineal area is red and swollen, with a nontender testis; this may be caused by idiopathic scrotal oedema.

What to Do

- Refer all cases of a painful scrotum for surgical review. Patients with torsion of the testis should be referred urgently to a paediatric surgeon.

The Child With a Nonblanching Rash

GUIDELINE

National Institute for Health and Care Excellence. (2015). *Meningitis (bacterial) and meningococcal septicaemia in under 16s: Recognition, diagnosis and management.* NICE clinical guideline CG102. Available at http://www.nice.org.uk.

- The most common causes of a nonblanching rash (petechiae and purpura) include:
  - Meningococcal disease
  - Idiopathic thrombocytopenic purpura (ITP)
  - HSP
  - Haematologic malignancy

- Viral illnesses, streptococcal infections, connective tissues disorders, and HUS may also cause nonblanching rashes.
- All children with a nonblanching rash need urgent assessment and investigation.
- HSP affects the skin, joints (most commonly the knees and ankles), abdomen, kidneys, and GI tract. (Children may present with GI bleeding.) Approximately 1% of children develop end-stage renal disease, but the nephritis is usually self-limiting.
- ITP is an immune-mediated thrombocytopenia that is usually acute. Children are usually well and of preschool age.
- HUS presents with thrombocytopenia, anaemia, and renal failure. The child often has bloody diarrhoea, most commonly caused by *E. coli, Shigella* spp., or echovirus.

What to Ask About the Child

- Ask how long the rash been present; a rapidly spreading rash in an unwell child suggests meningococcal disease and requires urgent management.
- Check if the child has a fever, which would suggest an infectious cause but may also be present in those with malignancy and connective tissue disorders.
- Enquire whether the child had a preceding upper respiratory tract infection because this is often a prodrome to HSP and ITP.
- Ask if the child has bleeding from mucous membranes (e.g., the nose) because this may be present in those with malignancy and ITP.
- Enquire whether there is a family history of bruising, which is suggestive of a familial form of thrombocytopenia.
- A history of joint pain, weight loss, or fever may indicate a malignancy or connective tissue disease.
- Abdominal pain and arthritis are common presentations of HSP.
- Check if the child has had bloody diarrhoea because abdominal pain and bloody diarrhoea are often the prodrome to HUS.

What to Look for on Examination

- Assess if the child is acutely unwell. Measure the temperature; a high fever is suggestive of a bacterial infection (e.g., meningococcal or streptococcal disease).
- Check the pattern of petechiae, purpura, or bruising:
  - Meningococcal: There is no specific distribution. This is a widespread, rapidly progressing rash in an ill child.
  - HSP's typical distribution is on the lateral malleoli, ventral aspects of feet, buttocks, and extensor aspects of legs. The rash is a palpable, purpuric rash sometimes with preceding urticaria. The child often has associated joint swelling or inflammation and a tender abdomen on palpation.

- ITP: This includes widespread petechiae and purpura in a child who is not acutely unwell. (Note: Children with meningococcal disease are acutely unwell.)
  - Does the child have a petechial rash that is only present in the distribution of the superior vena cava (i.e., above the clavicles)? In a child with vomiting or a cough, petechiae may be present in this distribution.
- Check for lymphadenopathy, hepatomegaly, and splenomegaly, which may indicate a malignancy.
- Check for signs of a nonaccidental injury, including unusual or unexplained patterns of bruising and petechiae, particularly in infants, who are unable to give a history. If you have any concerns, discuss them with a paediatrician.

What to Do

- Most children with a nonblanching rash should be referred for further investigation and management. Exceptions are when the child has a known respiratory illness, is not acutely unwell, and has petechiae in the distribution of the superior vena cava.
- If the child is acutely unwell, give IM antibiotics before transfer.
- In a child with suspected HSP, check the urine for blood and protein and, if possible, check the blood pressure. If HSP is confirmed, it is important to monitor the blood pressure and urine protein at regular intervals to detect any renal damage. Check your local guidelines for follow-up for these children.

The Child With Cervical Lymphadenopathy

- Cervical lymphadenopathy is extremely common in children, a cause of great concern to parents, and a common reason for referral to secondary care.
- The main causes are benign lymphadenopathy secondary to infections and, rarely, granulomatous disease (i.e., TB) and malignancy.
- The commonest malignancies causing lymphadenopathy include Hodgkin disease, non-Hodgkin lymphoma, and leukaemia.

What to Ask About the Child

- Ask if the child has had any recent infections, particularly of the throat, ear, nose, or scalp. Benign lymphadenopathy is typically secondary to a recent infection.
- Ask if any of the lymph nodes have recently increased in size. Rapid enlargement of the lymph nodes may need further investigation.
- Enquire whether there has been any contact with TB or recent travel to a TB endemic area and if the child has night sweats. Night sweats are present with TB and malignancy.
- Ask whether the child has been more lethargic than usual. Unusual lethargy may suggest TB or malignancy.

- Ask if the child has a chronic cough that may suggest TB.
- Ask about eczema because this is a common cause of localised lymphadenopathy.

What to Look for on Examination

- Assess the pattern of the enlarged lymph nodes. Are they only in the cervical region, or are they also in the axillary and inguinal regions?
- Check the appearance of the nodes. Are they red, tender, or fluctuant (which suggests infection and possibly an abscess)?
- Check for supraclavicular nodes. A supraclavicular node is not usually associated with a recent infection and is more suggestive of malignancy.
- Nodes that are hard, matted together, or nonmobile (i.e., fixed to underlying structures) are more suggestive of nonbenign lymphadenopathy.
- Examine for hepatosplenomegaly, which may be present in malignancies and in some viral infections, including Epstein–Barr virus (glandular fever).
- Measure the weight and compare against previous weights. Benign lymphadenopathy does not present with weight loss, and further investigation to rule out TB and malignancy should be undertaken in a child with acute weight loss.
- Examine the mouth for dental caries.

What to Do

- If the child is well, with mobile, small lymph nodes (<1 cm in diameter) and a recent infection, reassure the parents.
- If you are suspicious of TB or malignant disease, refer the patient for further investigations.

The Child With Pica

- Pica (eating substances with no nutritive value) is a common reason for referral to secondary care.
- The main cause of pica is iron deficiency.
- Iron-deficiency anaemia is common in children and is usually caused by a combination of a limited diet, large milk intake, and a period of rapid growth.
- Lead poisoning can be a result of pica and the ingestion of toxic substances such as paint.

What to Ask About the Child

- Take a good dietary history, specifically asking about the amount of milk in the child's diet. Sources of iron that are palatable to children include fortified breakfast cereals and fortified bread, eggs, pulses (including beans and lentils), dried fruit, and meat.
- Ask about the child's gestational age. Preterm infants require supplemental iron because iron is transferred transplacentally during the last trimester of pregnancy, and there is little iron in milk. The iron in breastmilk is more available than that in formula milk.

- Ask if there has been any history of blood loss (e.g., melena, blood in vomit, or menorrhagia in pubertal females). This is to exclude other causes of iron deficiency, particularly in a child with an apparently good diet.
- Enquire whether the family home is old and consider whether the child has developed lead poisoning from old paint work.
- Check if there is a family history of β-thalassaemia, which also causes low haemoglobin and low mean corpuscular volume (MCV).

What to Look for on Examination

- Examine for pale conjunctivae and pale palmar creases.
- Always examine for lymphadenopathy and hepatosplenomegaly to ensure that the child does not have an underlying pathology accounting for the iron deficiency.
- Examine for a systolic flow murmur often present in iron deficiency.
- Examine the mouth for glossitis or angular cheilitis, both suggesting iron deficiency.

What to Do

- It is often difficult to take blood tests in primary care, so children are often referred to secondary care. If blood testing is possible, take a full blood count and film, ferritin, iron studies, and lead level.
  - In iron-deficiency anaemia, there will be a low MCV and low haemoglobin.
  - In lead poisoning, the blood is normochromic or slightly hypochromic with characteristic basophilic stippling on the film.
- If relevant for ethnicity, also send blood for a haemoglobinopathy screen.
- Usually patients with iron deficiency are treated with oral iron supplements after the diagnosis is confirmed.
- Children with lead poisoning require referral to secondary care for assessment and management.
- Premature infants should take prophylactic oral iron supplements as per local guidelines.

The Child Who Is Short

GUIDELINE

Scottish Paediatric Endocrine Network. (2023). *Short stature guideline*. Available at http://www.speg.scot.nhs.uk.

- Short stature is defined as a height below the 0.4th centile on a growth chart or less than 2 standard deviations below the mean for gender and age.
- Short stature may be a source of emotional and social distress to both children and parents, who often ask for referral to secondary care.

- The vast majority of those referred to secondary care have common variations of normal physiological growth. These include familial short stature and constitutional short stature (also known as constitutional delay).
- Pathological causes are unusual and include endocrine problems; syndromes, including Turner and Noonan syndromes; chronic disease; and malnutrition.

What to Ask About the Child

- Ask for the parents' and siblings' heights and ages of pubertal onset:
  - Children with familial short stature have short parents, a normal growth velocity and pubertal onset, and no signs of physical disease. These children look short but normal.
  - Children with constitutional short stature have parents with normal stature, but one of them may have had a delay in growth and late puberty. These children look short and normal and have delayed puberty with a late growth spurt but achieve a final height within the parental target range.
- Ask about nutrition and assess whether the dietary intake is adequate for growth.
- Ask about symptoms of chronic diseases, including diarrhoea, abdominal pain (IBD, coeliac disease), and uncontrolled asthma.
- Enquire about inhaled steroid therapy and the length and dose of steroid treatment, which may affect growth.
- Explore the social history and whether there are concerns about psychosocial deprivation.
- If relevant, ask about signs of puberty.

What to Look for on Examination

- Plot all weight and height measurements on an appropriate chart.
- If the child is younger than 2 years of age, also plot the OFC.
- It is useful to measure the height at 4-month intervals to assess the height velocity.
- Conduct a systemic examination examining for signs of chronic disease.
- Assess if there are any dysmorphic signs, such as skeletal disproportion.
- Plot the parents' heights on a growth chart at 'age 18 years'. This is useful information to provide if you are referring to secondary care because both parents may not attend the hospital appointment.
- The mean expected adult height is approximately calculated as follows:
  - Males: the mean of the parents' heights plus 7 cm
  - Females: the mean of the parents' heights minus 7 cm
- Most growth charts explain how to calculate the midparental height centile and the target range around this mean value.

What to Do

- If you or the parents have concerns about the child, then refer to secondary care. However, in most cases, monitoring the height velocity and reassurance are the mainstays of management.
- If referring to secondary care, it is useful to provide a detailed history, including measurements of the child, their siblings, and their parents.

The Child Who Is Tall

GUIDELINE

Davies, J. H., & Cheetham, T. (2014). Investigation and management of tall stature. *Archives of Disease in Childhood, 99*, 772–777.

- Tall stature, defined as a height greater than 2 standard deviations above the mean for gender and age, is more accepted by society than in previous generations.
- Concern is often expressed by parents about females who are tall, although most cases do not require investigation. However, repeated measurements to assess growth over a 6- to 12-month period are important.
- Rarely, tall stature is caused by endocrine problems such as hyperthyroidism or precocious puberty.

What to Ask About the Child

- Ask about parental heights and the heights of any siblings. Most growth charts explain how to calculate the midparental height centile and the target range around this mean value. Assess whether the child's height is out with the expected parental target range. The mean expected adult height is calculated as follows:
  - Males: the mean of the parents' heights plus 7 cm
  - Females: the mean of the parents' heights minus 7 cm
- Ask when the parents noticed that their child was tall and try to assess whether the child has been growing constantly or if the growth has accelerated recently.
- Ask about signs of puberty in the child and whether the parents had early puberty:
  - In normal genetic tall stature, one or both parents are tall, and the child looks normal and tall.
  - In constitutional tall stature, the child has early puberty and grows to their final height earlier than their peers.
- Ask about symptoms suggestive of hyperthyroidism and whether the child has headaches or visual problems suggestive of a cranial lesion.

What to Look for on Examination

- Measure and weigh the child, plot the information on an appropriate chart, and compare it with previous measurements.

- If the child is younger than 2 years, measure and plot the OFC.
- Assess if there are features of hyperthyroidism, including:
  - Weight loss
  - Goitre
  - Tachycardia
  - Exophthalmos
- Plot parental heights on a chart and calculate the expected adult height.
- Check for features of early puberty.

What to Do

- If the cause is thought to be normal genetic tall stature or constitutional tall stature, monitor the growth over 6 to 12 months and reassure the parents and child.
- If the history and examination are not consistent with a normal variant tall stature, refer to secondary care.
- If obesity is an associated issue, provide guidance on weight management.

The Child With Precocious Puberty

- The age of onset of puberty is subject to much variation. Definitions of precocious puberty vary in the literature, but features of sexual development in females younger than 8 years and males younger than 9 years require assessment.
- The impact of early sexual development can be detrimental to children both physically and emotionally.
- Precocious puberty can be 'true' (i.e., early puberty but under normal hypothalamic control) or 'pseudo' (i.e., independent of hypothalamic control).
- True precocious puberty is common in females but rare in males. Therefore, it is important to investigate and identify a cause for precocious puberty in all males.

What to Ask About the Child

- Ask about growth and pubertal onset in the parents and any siblings.
- Ask specifically about different aspects of puberty, including:
  - Breast enlargement
  - Penile enlargement
  - Development of pubic hair
  - Vaginal bleeding
  - Body odour
  - Mood swings
- Ask about a history of headaches, vomiting, visual disturbance, and polydipsia; all are suggestive of a brain tumour in the presence of precocious puberty.

What to Look for on Examination

- Measure the child, plot the weight and height on an appropriate chart, and compare with previous measurements.

- If you are confident, perform Tanner staging on the child.
- Examine the optic fundi and the cranial nerves and observe the gait. (Very rarely, precocious puberty is caused by a brain tumour.)
- Neurofibromatosis and McCune–Albright syndrome are both associated with precocious puberty, so check the skin for café-au-lait spots (neurofibromatosis and McCune–Albright syndrome) and axillary freckling (neurofibromatosis).

What to Do

- Refer to secondary care all females younger than 8 years and males younger than 9 years with signs of sexual development.

The Child With Excess Body Hair

GUIDELINE

Scottish Paediatric Endocrine Group National Managed Clinical Network. (February 2022). *Adrenarche*. Available at http://www.speg.scot.nhs.uk.

- Excessive or premature hair development can cause significant anxiety and distress for children, particularly females.
- It is important to establish whether there are associated concerns regarding precocious puberty.
- Adrenarche, the adrenal stage of puberty, results in body odour, greasy skin and hair, weight gain, and pubic and axillary hair development without breast development. It is usually seen from age 8 years and is considered 'premature' if it occurs before 6 years of age. An exaggerated form can be seen between 6 and 8 years of age.
- Hirsutism (androgen-dependent areas) and hypertrichosis (generalised) are forms of excessive or inappropriate hair growth. They predominate in certain ethnic groups but can also be indicative of polycystic ovary syndrome (PCOS).

What to Ask About the Child

- Ask about growth and pubertal onset in the parents and any siblings.
- Ask about features of adrenal excess, including greasy skin and hair and body odour.
- Enquire about mood swings or behavioural disturbance.
- Explore whether the child has had a recent growth spurt or gain in weight.
- Ask about other pubertal features, including breast and penile enlargement, and in females, ask about features suggestive of PCOS, including menstrual disturbance and weight gain.

What to Look for on Examination

- Measure and plot the height and weight and compare the information with previous measurements. Check the height velocity. Is the child deviating away from their previous centile line?
- Look for tall stature.
- Assess the amount and distribution of hair growth.
- If you are confident, perform Tanner staging.
- Observe for greasy hair and skin as well as body odour.
- Examine the abdomen for masses.
- Check the optic fundi and perform a general neurologic examination.

What to Do

- If pubic or axillary hair is present before 6 years of age, refer for investigation.
- If hair is present at 6 to 8 years and is sparse, refer for assessment. The hair growth should be reviewed every 3 to 4 months over a period of 1 year to ensure that hair growth is appropriate and there is no pubertal development.
- If hair growth is excessive and causing emotional distress, refer for assessment and advice about hair removal, including chemical and laser therapy.
- If features are suggestive of PCOS, manage as appropriate.

The Child With a Painful Limp

> **GUIDELINE**
>
> Foster, H., Jandial, S., & Whyte, S. (2017). Assessment of gait disorders in children. *BMJ Best Practice*. Available at http://bestpractice.bmj.com.

- The most common cause of limp from hip pain is transient synovitis, which is the most between the ages of 4 and 10 years.
- About 90% of cases resolve in 7 days, but because it cannot be reliably distinguished from more serious causes of hip pain, all children should be referred to secondary care.
- The child who presents with a painful limp and complains of pain in the knee should be assumed to have a problem in the hip until proved otherwise.
- An unwell child who is non–weight bearing is likely to have a more serious underlying pathology such as septic arthritis, osteomyelitis, or leukaemia.

What to Ask About the Child

- Check the child's age because many causes occur in specific age ranges; for example, synovitis tends to affect preschool-aged children.
- Ask whether the onset was acute or chronic and whether there was a prodromal illness. Transient synovitis typically presents after a viral illness.

- Ask about a history of trauma and consider a Toddler's fracture in a young child.
- Enquire if there has been a history of systemic upset, such as fever, lethargy, pallor, weight loss, or easy bruising or bleeding, and think about diagnoses, including leukaemia, septic arthritis, and osteomyelitis.
- If there is pain at rest or at night, consider osteomyelitis, septic arthritis, or malignancy.
- If the child is unable to weight bear, has pain at rest, and is also febrile, consider septic arthritis or osteomyelitis.
- Take a careful history of the presentation of any injury. If the history is not consistent with the injury, consider a possible nonaccidental injury.

What to Look for on Examination

- Assess whether the child looks well or unwell.
- Take the temperature and observe the level of comfort of the child. Children with septic arthritis are in pain at rest.
- Examine for restricted movement, bony tenderness, joint swelling, tenderness, erythema, or deformity and assess the child's gait and their spine.
- Remember to examine the feet. Check if there is a local cause of the limp such as a foreign body.
- Examine for a rash. HSP may present with joint swelling and pain.
- Check for pallor, lymphadenopathy, bruising, and hepatosplenomegaly, which may suggest a malignancy.

What to Do

- Refer to secondary care all children with a painful limp to exclude serious pathology.

The Infant Who Screams or Vomits When Feeding

> **GUIDELINE**
>
> National Institute for Health and Care Excellence. (2019). *Gastro-oesophageal reflux disease in children and young people: diagnosis and management. NICE clinical guideline NG1.* Available at http://www.nice.org.uk.

- The complaint of distress or vomiting with feeds is very common in general practice.
- Causes range from relatively benign to more serious, and the cause can often be elicited through a careful history.
- GOR is relatively common in infants, and often an explanation and reassurance are all that is needed.
- Gastro-oesophageal reflux disease (GORD) is less common, can cause significant distress in the infant, and may need treatment.

What to Ask About the Child

- For breastfeeding infants, ask about:
  - The duration and frequency of feeds. In the first few weeks of life, infants feed at least 8 times per 24 hours and usually more frequently than this.
  - Whether the infant appears satisfied after feeding from one breast. If infants are taken off one breast after a few minutes and then offered the second breast, they will only receive foremilk (containing water and lactose) and no hindmilk (containing more fat). These infants may feel hungry again soon after feeding.
- For formula-feeding infants, ask about:
  - The number and volume of feeds per day.
  - The volume of feeds the infant is receiving. If the total volume of feeds is greater than 150 mL/kg/24 hours and the infant is thriving, suggest reducing the volume per feed, particularly if the infant is vomiting.
- Ask about vomiting, including the frequency and timing of vomits in relation to feeds and whether the vomit contains blood or bile. In GOR, the infant vomits effortlessly during, after, and sometimes between feeds. Feeding relaxes the lower gastro-oesophageal sphincter. The vomit in infants with GOR does not contain bile and rarely contains blood.
- Ask if the vomiting is projectile and only occurs immediately after a feed. Consider pyloric stenosis and ask about a family history of pyloric stenosis. Infants with pyloric stenosis may have dehydration and failure to thrive, but if diagnosed early enough, the only sign may be projectile vomiting. These infants are hungry and often wish to feed again immediately after vomiting.
- Ask about the behaviour of the infant. Infants with GORD often display certain posturing, including arching of the back, straightening out of their legs, and becoming very distressed when they are put in a supine or prone position.

What to Look for on Examination

- Assess whether the infant is thriving. Plot the infant's current weight on a chart and compare it with previous weights. Infants with GORD are usually thriving. If the infant is not thriving, consider other diagnoses.
- Examine for pallor, cyanosis, and dehydration. Infants with GORD are usually well looking, normally developed, and thriving. Parents report that these infants are often unsettled and miserable and cry when being fed but are not acutely unwell looking.
- Always try to observe a feed.
- Conduct a full systematic examination of the infant, including auscultation of the heart and palpation of the abdomen.

What to Do

- If the infant has fever and is unwell, refer to secondary care. (See the guidelines for fever in children younger than 5 years of age.)
- If you suspect that the infant has pyloric stenosis, refer to secondary care.
- If you think the infant has GORD, try the following:
  - Reduced volume but more frequent feeds.
  - Thickened feeds in formula-fed babies (e.g., Instant Carobel).
  - Gaviscon. This is easy to give to formula-feeding infants; it is added to bottles. For breastfeeding infants, it is not as easy because it needs to be given before the feed, ideally mixed with breastmilk.
  - A trial of an acid-blocking medication may be useful (omeprazole). Give the medication for 4 weeks and explain to the parents that they may not see a beneficial effect for at least 1 week. Doses are given in the *British National Formulary for Children*. Explain to the parents how to prepare and administer the medication to a young infant.
- Arrange for someone to review the infant in a few days' time. GORD can be extremely upsetting for parents even though they can see that their infants are thriving, and they usually need a lot of support. It is easy for breastfeeding mothers to become discouraged and to stop breastfeeding.
- If the vomiting and screaming do not settle, refer to secondary care.
- It is not sensible to switch formula milks without a clear reason to do so.
- Non–IgE-mediated cow's milk protein allergy presents as excessive crying, vomiting, and sometimes diarrhoea and blood in the stool. Occasionally, the infant may have constipation. There is no diagnostic test, but other causes of crying should also be sought. For breastfed infants, the mother could trial a dairy-free diet. For formula-fed infants, a short trial of a hydrolysed formula will result in a dramatic improvement and reintroduction of cow's milk in resumption of symptoms. Local guidelines are usually available about the brand of milk to prescribe and at what age to rechallenge with cow's milk.
- IgE-mediated cow's milk protein allergy presents with an urticarial rash or anaphylaxis. There is often a personal or family history of atopy. It is appropriate to refer these children to secondary care for advice. For breastfed infants, their mothers should undertake a dairy-free diet. Formula-fed infants need a hydrolysed formula and a milk-free diet for at least the first year of life.

The Infant Who Has Weight Faltering in the First 6 Months of Life

GUIDELINE

National Institute for Health and Care Excellence. (2017). *Faltering growth: Recognition and management of faltering growth in children.* NICE clinical guideline NG75. Available at http://www.nice.org.uk.

What to Ask About the Child

- Weight faltering is when the weight falls downward through the centiles. An infant who is born petite (e.g., on the second centile) and continues to track along the second centile is not weight faltering but gaining weight appropriately.
- Ask if the mother thinks her baby is unwell. A baby who is failing to thrive may have sepsis.
- Take a thorough feeding history:
  - For breastfed infants:
    a. Frequency of breastfeeds. A young infant who is exclusively breastfed should be taking a minimum of 8 feeds per 24 hours (and usually many more in the first weeks of life).
    b. Duration of breastfeeds. Is the baby being offered one breast until they are satisfied and come off the breast themself? Is the baby offered the second breast? (Coming off the breast too soon may mean the infant is getting the foremilk but not the hindmilk, which contains a lot of fat and is more calorie dense).
    c. Is the baby feeding overnight, or do they sleep through the night? (Young infants should feed overnight because their stomach volumes are small, and they need frequent feeds.)
    d. Is the baby being given additional fluids or feeds? For example, is the infant given drinks of water (with empty calories) between feeds?
    e. Does breastfeeding feel comfortable for the mother? (If not, this could indicate a difficulty with positioning and attachment.)
  - For formula-fed infants, ask about:
    a. The frequency of feeds and volume of each feed taken
    b. The type of milk and how the milk is prepared. If milk is prepared incorrectly and made too dilute, this could be a reason for failure to gain weight.
- In all children, ask about vomiting, diarrhoea, and lethargy. Young infants who were initially jaundiced and sleepy are sometimes slower to establish feeding routines.
- Ask about the mother's health in pregnancy, the birth, and the delivery.
- Check the mother's antenatal record and make sure that she was screened for infections, including human immunodeficiency virus (HIV). Ask about any infections in the family, including TB.

What to Look for on Examination

- Check the infant thoroughly for symptoms and signs suggestive of a serious infection. If you have any concerns about the infant's general health, refer to secondary care.
- Plot weights on an appropriate chart (if the infant was preterm, adjust for gestational age). Use growth charts based on the World Health Organization growth charts that show the growth of children who have been optimally fed from birth. Also plot the length and head circumference. (Is the infant proportionally small?)
- Check the infant's mouth for thrush and the nappy area for rashes.
- Check the infant's tone. Infants who are floppy with poor tone should be referred to secondary care.
- Auscultate the heart and check for a heart murmur.
- Check for signs of a respiratory problem, including indrawing, tachypnoea, and nasal flaring.

What to Do

- A well infant whom you think has a feeding problem can be dealt with in primary care with support from an experienced health visitor and, if relevant, breastfeeding expert.
- If possible, check for a UTI. UTIs may present with failure to thrive in an infant who has few other symptoms.
- If there are concerns about the infant's general health or no obvious cause can be found for the failure to thrive, refer to secondary care.
- Regular review of infants is needed, and their families need support and encouragement.

The Infant Who Has Weight Faltering After 6 Months of Age

- Most cases of failure to thrive or weight faltering are caused by poor oral intake and not underlying pathology. However, sometimes the child has poor intake because of an underlying condition (e.g., children with a UTI may not feed well).
- It is always important to take a detailed dietary history.

What to Ask About the Child

- Take a detailed feeding history, starting from how the child was fed in the first months of life (see 'The Child With Weight Faltering in the First 6 Months of Life').
- Assess whether there were any problems with feeding in the first few weeks of life.
- Ask about the frequency of complementary feeds and snacks in children older than 6 months of age. By 10 months of age, children should be eating three meals and two snacks per day.
- Ask about the content and consistency of the complementary feeds. Some children are offered very dilute complementary feeds because their parents are concerned about their choking. Some children may be given a diet that is low in nutrients and low in calories.
- Ask about the quantity of feeds taken and whether they are only taking a mouthful or managing to finish a small bowl of food.
- Ask if there were any problems in transitioning from a full-milk diet to a diet containing solids.

- Find out what milk the child is taking. Ideally, breastfeeding should continue after the introduction of complementary feeds. If formula milk is being given, ask about the volume and frequency; too much formula may interfere with solid intake. After the patient is 1 year of age, ask about the volume and frequency of cow's milk.
- Ask about other symptoms the child may have, including fever and dysuria, suggestive of a UTI.
- Ask if the child has abdominal pain suggesting a possible GI problem (e.g., coeliac disease).
- Ask about stool patterns and whether the child has constipation (children with constipation often have poor appetites) or diarrhoea.
- Explore whether the child has been drinking more than usual or passing large quantities of urine because diabetes mellitus may be the cause of weight loss.
- Ask whether the child has a chronic cough (suggestive of a chronic respiratory condition) or if they snore at night with interruptions in breathing (suggestive of obstructive sleep apnoea).
- Check that the mother was tested for HIV in pregnancy.
- Explore whether there are there any concerns about the child's psychosocial well-being and if there have been previous social work concerns.

What to Look for on Examination

- Weigh and measure the child, including the OFC; plot the information on an appropriate chart; and compare it with previous measurements. Check if the child is tracking appropriately along their centile line. If the child's weight and height have always been on the 0.4th centile since birth and the child is well, they are not failing to thrive; rather, they have always been small.
- When assessing a child's weight, a rough rule of thumb is:
  - A child doubles their birth weight by 4 to 6 months.
  - A child triples their birth weight by 12 to 13 months.
- Examine for pale conjunctivae and palmar creases (suggestive of iron deficiency).
- Examine for loose skin folds (suggestive of recent weight loss).
- Assess whether the child looks neglected, if they are dirty and ill-kempt, and if there is severe nappy dermatitis.
- Examine the abdomen for masses, including faecal masses, and hepatosplenomegaly.
- Examine the respiratory system to assess if the child has chest signs suggestive of a chronic respiratory problem.
- Examine the tonsils and assess whether the child is a mouth breather. Children with obstructive sleep apnoea are often poor eaters with weight faltering.
- Examine whether the child has any signs suggestive of nonaccidental injury, including bruises and assess how the parent or caregiver interacts with the child. Observe how the child behaves during the consultation, whether they are withdrawn or active, and how the caregiver controls the child.

What to Do

- If the problem is a dietary, one address it.
- If possible, a home visit by a health visitor may be helpful.
- Give clear counselling around the quantities and frequency of foods to be offered.
- Explain that the child should not be forced to feed but should be fed responsively.
- All children older than 1 year of age in the United Kingdom should take a multivitamin supplement (e.g., Healthy Start Vitamins).
- Always encourage a mother who is breastfeeding to continue. It is easy for mothers to lose confidence in the value of her breastmilk if their children have weight faltering.
- Further management depends on the history and examination:
  - It is useful to obtain a clean-catch urine for urinalysis with or without culture to rule out a UTI.
  - Consider type 1 diabetes mellitus if there is history of lethargy, increased thirst, or polyuria (increased frequency of nappies or heavier nappies in young children). If diabetes mellitus is suspected, check a nonfasting capillary blood glucose sample and immediately refer all children with blood sugar greater than 8 mmol/L or with a very suggestive history.
  - Treat constipation.
  - If you suspect the child has obstructive sleep apnoea, refer to an ear, nose, and throat surgeon.
  - If you have concerns about neglect or nonaccidental injury, refer to secondary care and contact the social work department.
  - Refer children whom you think may have underlying pathology for further investigations.

The Child Who Is Suspected of Having a Nonaccidental Injury

GUIDELINE

National Institute for Health and Care Excellence. (2017). *Child maltreatment: When to suspect maltreatment in under 18s. NICE clinical guideline CG89.* Available at http://www.nice.org.uk.

- Children can sustain a multitude of injuries during normal active play. The challenge is to identify those who are at risk of nonaccidental injury and those whose clinical presentation or history is suggestive of nonaccidental injury.
- A thorough history and examination is essential.
- Information from other professionals, including health visitors, social workers, and school personnel, who know the family is useful in identifying vulnerable children.

What to Ask About the Child

- Obtain a detailed history of the injury:
  - Was it a witnessed fall or trauma?
  - Is the history describing how the injury occurred consistent with the clinical findings?
  - When did the injury occur, and has there been a delay in presentation to medical services?
  - Explore the past medical history, including the perinatal history. Have there been previous injuries, illnesses, or visits to the hospital ED?
  - Does the child have a history of bleeding or easy bruising, and is there a family history of bleeding disorders?
  - Take a detailed social history, including who lives in the house, who has contact with the child or children, and whether previous concerns have been raised about the family from the social work department.
  - Ask about the other siblings and how they are growing and developing.
  - Explore whether there have been any recent events in the family that could have caused stress, including financial difficulties or separation of the parents.

What to Look for on Examination

- Assess whether the child is thriving. Measure the child and plot their weight and height on appropriate charts.
- Observe whether the child is clean and appropriately dressed or unkempt, dirty, and inappropriately clad.
- Examine for features of potential neglect, including untreated skin conditions, severe nappy rash, and lice.
- Assess any injuries, document them carefully, and consider whether the injuries are in keeping with the history of how they occurred.
- Injuries of concern include:
  - Bruises in the shape of fingers, grip marks, or possibly caused by an implement
  - Any injury in a nonmobile child (unless it was an accident, e.g., a parent falling whilst holding the child)
  - Burns or scalds that appear to have been caused by direct contact being applied to the skin, including immersion in hot water or a cigarette burn
  - A torn frenulum in the mouth of an infant
  - Injuries on nonbony prominences of the head, neck, back, or buttocks
  - Multiple unexplained, lacerations, abrasions, or scars
- In young infants, feel the anterior fontanelle. An infant who has been shaken may have a tense, bulging fontanelle and signs of increased ICP (irritability, crying, vomiting, poor feeding).
- Assess the child's emotional state and interaction with the parents or caregivers. Is the child wary (frozen watchfulness), or is parental hostility or detachment noted?

What to Do

- Every child who presents with an unexplained injury or unexplained delay in presentation or whose history is inconsistent with the presentation should be referred for assessment. Local guidelines will dictate further management, but usually this includes:
  - An assessment by a senior paediatrician (including examination and history from the referrer and accompanying adult)
  - Consent for taking clinical photographs of any injuries
  - Investigations, including blood tests, cranial imaging, and radiographs
  - Liaising with other professionals, including social workers and police, as required on an individual case basis
- If you have concerns about any child whom you feel is being neglected or hurt, discuss the case with a social worker and senior paediatrician or local child protection team.

Reference

Frank, J. E., & Jacobe, K. M. (2011). Evaluation and management of heart murmurs in children. *American Family Physician, 84*(7), 793–800.

6

Cardiovascular Problems

Andy Potter

CHAPTER CONTENTS

Hypertension

GUIDELINE

National Institute for Health and Clinical Excellence. (2022). *Hypertension in adults: diagnosis and management. NICE clinical guideline 136.* Retrieved from https://www.nice.org.uk/guidance/ng136.

- Hypertension is one of the commonest conditions treated in primary care in the United Kingdom and one of the most important preventable causes of death worldwide (Krause et al, 2011). It is the main risk factor for development of stroke and ischaemic heart disease (IHD) and is strongly associated with the development of chronic kidney disease (CKD) and cognitive impairment.

- Hypertension, defined as the presence of persistently raised clinic blood pressure ($\geq$140/90 mm Hg) or daytime ambulatory blood pressure or home blood pressure ($\geq$135/85 mm/Hg) (Box 6.1), affects more than 25% of all adults in the United Kingdom and 50% of those older than 65 years of age (Health and Social Care Information Centre, 2011). The adult prevalence of high blood pressure is even higher in other parts of the world, with more than 40% of adults affected in Africa, for example (World Health Organization [WHO], 2023).

- Most people with hypertension have no symptoms or clinical findings on examination, and their hypertension is identified incidentally or as a result of complications such as angina, myocardial infarction (MI), stroke, or arrhythmias.

- The rule of halves was described in the United States in 1972 (Wilber & Barrow, 1972). It states that half of people with hypertension are not known to have a raised blood pressure; of those with known hypertension, half are not on treatment, and half of those on treatment have poorly controlled blood pressure. The figures for

detection and treatment of hypertension have improved in recent years, but this remains a useful reminder of the challenge posed by hypertension.

Detection

- All adults should have their blood pressure measured at least every 5 years up to the age of 80 years and at least annually thereafter (Hodgkinson et al, 2011).

- The 2011 National Institute for Health and Clinical Excellence (NICE) guidelines recommended a major shift in how blood pressure measurements are taken and hypertension diagnosed, centring on the use of ambulatory blood pressure monitoring (ABPM) and home blood pressure monitoring (HBPM) to complement clinic measurements (Box 6.2). This is in part a response to the overtreatment of people with 'white coat' hypertension.

- The guidelines recommend the following steps to diagnose hypertension.
  1. If a clinic blood pressure is greater than 140/90 mm Hg, take a second reading in the consultation.
  2. If the second reading is very different from the first, take a third reading.
  3. Record the lowest reading. If it is greater than 140/90 mm Hg, offer 24-hour ABPM to confirm the diagnosis (Hodgkinson et al, 2011).
  4. HBPM should be used as an alternative if ABPM is declined or not tolerated and for practices that lack ABPM equipment (Ritchie et al, 2011).

• BOX 6.2 Definitions of Ambulatory Blood Pressure Monitoring and Home Blood Pressure Monitoring

Ambulatory blood pressure monitoring (ABPM) is a noninvasive method of measuring blood pressure in a patient's own environment. At least two measurements per hour should be taken during the patient's usual waking hours (e.g., between 8 a.m. and 10 p.m.). The readings are taken automatically to minimise interference with everyday activities and sleep patterns. By taking regular readings throughout the day, a more accurate estimate of blood pressure can be obtained.

The average value of at least 14 measurements is needed to confirm a diagnosis of hypertension. Patients are most commonly referred to appropriately equipped hospital clinics, though it is possible for general practitioners to establish their own system of ABPM.

Home blood pressure monitoring (HBPM) requires the patient to measure their own blood pressure using an automatic blood pressure monitor, either supplied by the local health service or purchased privately. To confirm a diagnosis of hypertension, it is advised that:
1. Two consecutive measurements are taken at least 1 minute apart, twice daily (ideally in the morning and evening), with the patient seated, for 4 to 6 days.
2. Measurements taken on the first day should be discarded, and the average value of all remaining measurements should be used.

• BOX 6.1 Definition of Hypertension (NICE, 2011)

Stage 1 Hypertension

- Clinic blood pressure $\geq$140/90 mm Hg and subsequent ABPM or HBPM $\geq$135/85 mm Hg

Stage 2 Hypertension

- Clinic blood pressure $\geq$160/100 mm Hg and subsequent ABPM or HBPM $\geq$150/95 mm Hg

Severe Hypertension

- Clinic blood pressure $\geq$180/110 mm Hg

^{a}When a threshold or target level of blood pressure is given, e.g., 160/100 mm Hg (see Box 6.2), it means that action should be taken if the systolic blood pressure is 160 mm Hg or over or the diastolic blood pressure is 100 mm Hg or over. *ABPM,* Ambulatory blood pressure monitoring; *HBPM,* home blood pressure monitoring.

- Other recent research has suggested that blood pressure should be measured in both arms and that subsequent blood pressure monitoring should be done in the arm with the highest reading (Clarke et al, 2011, 2012).
- If a blood pressure difference of more than 10 mm Hg is found, peripheral artery disease is likely, and further evaluation (e.g., ankle-brachial pressure measurement) is warranted.

Blood Pressure Targets

- The target of hypertension treatment is to reduce clinic blood pressure levels to below 140/90 mm Hg in people younger than 80 years and below 150/90 mm Hg in people 80 years and older.
- Previous guidance focused on treating those younger than 80 years, but more recent evidence has shown that treatment is well tolerated and reduces total mortality and cardiovascular events in those older than 80 years as well (Beckett et al, 2008, 2011).
- Two points should be made about these targets:
  a. *Any* reduction in blood pressure carries benefit even if the target is not reached (Czernichow et al, 2011).
  b. The lower the blood pressure, the greater the benefit, at least down to 115/75 mm Hg (Nash, 2007). Below this, there is no evidence either way.

Practicalities of Blood Pressure Measurement

a. The patient should be seated, but in older patients and in those with diabetes, the blood pressure should be checked when they are both standing and sitting.
b. The patient should be as relaxed as possible with an empty bladder and should not have had caffeine or nicotine within 30 minutes.
c. On the first occasion, measure the blood pressure in both arms. A significant difference is found in 20% of those with hypertension. If there is a difference of more than 15 mm Hg, use the arm with the higher reading for future measurements.
d. Measure the systolic and diastolic pressures (phase V) to the nearest 2 mm. If it is greater than 140/90 mm Hg, repeat the measurement towards the end of the consultation. If the readings are markedly different from each other, take at least one more. Take the average. Repeated readings by a nurse give the most reliable clinic results and occasional readings by a doctor the least (Little et al, 2002).
e. Measure standing blood pressures in patients with type 2 diabetes, symptoms of postural hypotension, and older than 80 years. The effects of postural hypotension might not results in a blood pressure drop immediately; check the standing blood pressure after at least 2 minutes of standing. If there is a drop of 20 mm Hg or more on standing, use this reading
f. *Timing.* In mild uncomplicated hypertension, do not start treatment until three readings have been taken over

a 3-month period. About 25% of blood pressures settle in that time. Those that settle to below treatment levels need lifelong annual follow-up. If the initial diastolic blood pressure is greater than 200/110 mm Hg or there is evidence of end-organ damage, cardiovascular disease (CVD), or diabetes, three readings over 2 weeks would be more appropriate. Consider immediate treatment if the blood pressure is greater than 220/120 mm Hg.
g. Follow up every 6 months after the patient is established on treatment. This is as good as monthly.

Workup

a. Check for a history of family and personal risk factors for stroke or coronary heart disease (CHD). Check whether relevant drugs (e.g., nonsteroidal antiinflammatory drugs [NSAIDs], mirabegron, venlafaxine) or excess alcohol is taken.
b. Examination, including:
  - Fundi (essential only in severe hypertension) (van den Born, 2005)
  - Femoral pulses
  - Palpation of the kidneys and auscultation for the presence of bruit
  - Signs of left ventricular hypertrophy
c. Urinalysis for protein and blood (albumin-to-creatinine ratio [ACR])
d. Blood
  - Creatinine and electrolytes
  - Fasting blood sugar (haemoglobin A1c [HbA1c])
  - Serum lipids
e. Look for left ventricular hypertrophy using electrocardiography (ECG) and chest radiography.
f. Calculate the patient's 10-year CVD risk using a recognised calculator, such as the QRISK2-2013 CVD risk calculator (available at http://www.qrisk.org). A 20% 10-year CVD risk means that the lower threshold for treatment applies and that primary prevention of CVD is needed.

Nondrug Treatment

Nondrug treatment can lower the systolic pressure by 4 to 10 mm Hg (Stevens, Obarzanek, & Cook, 2001; Writing Group of the PREMIER Collaborative Research Group, 2003). It lowers the risk of CVD and should be offered to all patients with hypertension, whether or not drugs are being prescribed.
Consider the following:
a. *Smoking.* Ask about smoking. If appropriate offer, advise and refer to smoking cessation services. Stopping will not reduce the blood pressure, but it will lower the cardiovascular risk.
b. *Exercise.* Physical activity lowers the risk of developing hypertension and is an effective treatment for those with established hypertension. Brisk walking for 30 minutes every day is as beneficial as more vigorous exercise three

times a week. After only 2 weeks of aerobic exercise, the mean decrease in blood pressure is 5/4 mm Hg (Whelton et al, 2002).

c. *Weight.* Encourage weight loss if the patient is overweight (body mass index [BMI] >25 kg/m^2). Being overweight is a significant and independent predictor of the level of blood pressure (Cox et al, 1996). A 10-kg weight loss promotes a reduction of 5 to 20 mm Hg in blood pressure (Chobanian et al, 2003).

d. *Alcohol.* There is a direct dose–response relationship between alcohol intake and the risk of hypertension, particularly when alcohol intake exceeds two drinks per day (Xin et al, 2001). Support patients to reduce excessive consumption.

e. *Salt.* Reduce intake of salt to less than 5.8 g/day or less than 2.4 g of sodium. A 2011 Cochrane review was unable to confirm whether reducing dietary salt had significant effects on mortality or cardiovascular morbidity (Taylor et al, 2011), but a subsequent meta-analysis found a significant reduction in cardiovascular events (He & MacGregor, 2011), supporting longstanding public health recommendations to reduce salt consumption in the population. Common sources of salt are nuts, crisps, canned foods, table sauces, and bread. Many processed foods are high in salt; avoid those with more than 1.5 g per 100 g of food. Also note that many labels use sodium rather than salt content: 1 g of sodium = 2.5 g of salt, so more than 0.6 g of sodium per 100 g of food is high.

f. *The Dietary Approaches to Stop Hypertension (DASH) diet.* This is a diet rich in fruit, vegetables, and oily fish and low in sodium and total and saturated fat. It has been shown in a number of trials to reduce blood pressure by up to 11/5 mm Hg (Appel et al, 1997). It is similar to a Mediterranean-style diet (Sacks & Campos, 2010).

g. *Coffee.* Coffee is known to acutely raise blood pressure, but a 2012 systematic review and meta-analysis found no significant effect on blood pressure or the risk of hypertension (Steffen et al, 2012). However, standard advice remains to discourage *excessive* coffee drinking.

h. *Contraceptive pills.* Consider stopping but not until other adequate contraceptive measures are in place.

i. *Stress.* The relationship between stress and blood pressure is not well understood, yet anecdotally, patients often blame a stressful life for their hypertension. This is an area of ongoing research, with some promising results for stress reduction interventions (Hughes, 2013).

Drug Management

Primary Prevention

- *Aspirin.* The use of low-dose aspirin (75 mg/day) AP in primary prevention is controversial, with ongoing debates about the benefits (reducing cardiovascular events) versus risks (bleeding events) (Barnett, Burrill, & Iheanacho, 2010). At the time of writing, aspirin is not licensed for primary prevention in the United Kingdom and should not be routinely started even in those with risk factors such as hypertension and diabetes (Scottish Intercollegiate Guidelines Network [SIGN], 2010).

- *Statins.* Prescribe statins if the patient has CVD or diabetes or has a risk of CVD that is sufficiently high. Offer a high-intensive statin (e.g., atorvastatin 20 mg AP) for patients with an estimated 10-year risk of developing CVD is 10% or greater using the QRISK assessment tool (NICE).

Antihypertensives

- About half of patients fail to take their antihypertensives as prescribed. Patients have many reservations about drug treatment (Benson & Britten, 2002). Getting them to voice their reservations gives the clinician a chance to alter any erroneous ideas they may have. A study of Black Caribbean patients in London found that common misconceptions were:
  - When the blood pressure was controlled, they were cured and didn't need the medication.
  - They could sense when their blood pressure was increased, so they could judge when they needed to take the medication (Connell, McKevitt, & Wolfe, 2005).
- Commonly used drugs produce a similar average decrease of 9.1/5.5 mm Hg at standard doses (Law et al, 2003). Most patients with hypertension therefore need more than one antihypertensive drug.
- Combining two drugs from different classes reduces the blood pressure five times more than doubling the dose of one drug (Wald et al, 2009).
- The timing of medication was previously thought to be important. Recent evidence suggests there is no benefit to taking medication at a specific time (Mackenzie et al, 2022).
- The choice of drugs should be influenced by age, comorbidity, adverse effects, possible synergistic effects between classes of drugs, and the individual's response to each drug. Ethnic origin also influences the choice of medication: whereas younger White patients tend to have high levels of renin and angiotensin II, older patients and those of African origin tend to have low renin levels and so respond less well to drugs that block the renin–angiotensin system, although the differences are thought to be small.
- Follow the scheme outlined in (Table 6.1) but do not persevere with a drug that has produced no benefit (i.e., a decrease in blood pressure of <5 mm Hg.). Instead switch to a drug with a different mode of action (e.g., from A to C or D). Persevere with a drug that shows some but inadequate benefit; it may be synergistic with a drug from a different group.
- Divide drugs into those that suppress the renin system ('A' for angiotensin-converting enzyme [ACE] inhibitors and angiotensin II receptor blockers [ARBs] Known as both Angiotensin receptor blockers and angiotension II receptor blockers) and those that work independently of it ('C' for calcium channel blockers [CCBs] and 'D' for diuretics) (Brown et al, 2003). The following steps

TABLE 6.1	Drug Management in Hypertension	
Step	Age Younger Than 55 Years and Non-Black	Age 55 Years or Older or Black
1	A	C
2	A and C or D	C + A or D
3	A and C and D	C + A + D
4	Add an alpha-blocker, a beta-blocker, or spironolactone or another diuretic or refer	

A, Angiotensin-converting enzyme inhibitor or angiotensin II receptor blocker; *C*, calcium channel blocker; *D*, thiazide diuretic.

are recommended, but they should be tailored to the needs of the individual patient.

- Discuss starting step 1 treatment to people aged younger than 80 years with stage 1 hypertension and one or more of:
- Target organ damage
- Established CVD
- Renal disease
- Diabetes
- 10-year cardiovascular risk equivalent to 20% or more (NICE, 2022)

A 2012 Cochrane review of randomised controlled trials of treatment of mild hypertension in those without preexisting CVD found that treatment did not reduce morbidity or mortality (Diao et al, 2012).

- Offer step 1 treatment to people of any age with stage 2 hypertension.
- Offer people aged younger than 55 years an ACE inhibitor or a low-cost ARB. If an ACE inhibitor is prescribed and not tolerated (e.g., because of cough), offer a low-cost ARB.
- Offer people aged older than 55 years and Black people of African or Caribbean family origin of any age a CCB. If a CCB is not suitable (e.g., because of oedema or intolerance) or there is evidence or risk of heart failure, offer a thiazide-like diuretic.

Drug Treatment of Patients With Other Medical Problems

Most individuals (about four of five in one study (Barnett et al, 2012)) with hypertension have additional chronic diseases.

a. *Angina.* Use a beta-blocker or a CCB.
b. *Heart failure.* Use a diuretic, an ACE inhibitor, a beta-blocker, and then an alpha-blocker.
c. *Diabetics.* Use an ACE inhibitor, a low-dose thiazide, an alpha-blocker, or a CCB.
d. *Smokers.* Do not use a beta-blocker.
e. *Migraine.* Use a beta-blocker, an ARB, or both and then all other alternatives.

f. *Those active in sports.* Avoid beta-blockers.
g. *Raynaud's syndrome.* Use a CCB.
h. *Renal failure.* Get specialist advice. ACE inhibitors may improve renal function but need to be given in lower doses.
i. *Gout.* Avoid thiazides.
j. *Asthma.* Avoid beta-blockers.

Other Points About the Drugs

Thiazides

- Indapamide (2.5 mg/day AP) and chlortalidone (12.5–25 mg/day AP) have been suggested by NICE to be preferential to bendroflumethiazide.
- Recheck creatinine and electrolytes 1 month after starting a thiazide; then repeat annually. Repeat more frequently if the patient is unwell or is taking digoxin or another drug that might affect renal function. An increase of creatinine of up to 30% is acceptable provided it remains below 200 µmol/L (Martin & Coleman, 2006).
- Diabetes is not a contraindication. In the SHEP The Systolic Hypertension in the Elderly Program study, a thiazide was associated with the development of diabetes in an extra 4.3% of patients over 4 years, but it protected those who developed diabetes against an increase in cardiovascular death (Kostis et al, 2005).
- Ask specifically about erectile difficulties in males. The incidence in patients taking thiazides is double that in those taking a placebo (17% vs 8%), but patients rarely volunteer this information.

Calcium Channel Blockers

- Use a long-acting preparation (e.g., diltiazem 120–180 mg AP slow release twice a day [bd] or verapamil 120–240 mg bd or 240–480 mg slow release daily AP). Their hypotensive effect is the same as nifedipine, with fewer side effects. Use brand names. Different generic products have different bioavailabilities.
- Use a dihydropyridine (CCB, e.g., nifedipine slow release or amlodipine) if:
  a. Beta-blockers are also being given.
  b. The patient has peripheral vascular disease with skin ischaemia. It will not, however, help intermittent claudication.
  c. There is a risk of heart failure, which might be worsened by a nondihydropyridine.

Angiotensin-Converting Enzyme Inhibitors and Related Drugs

- When starting them:
  a. The first dose should be taken at night. Even then, first-dose hypotension caused by once-daily agents may not occur until 6 to 8 hours after the first dose and may last for 24 hours.
  b. Recheck serum creatinine and electrolytes 1 week after starting the drug and after all dose increases; then recheck annually.
- An increase of serum creatinine of less than 30% is acceptable provided it remains less than 200 µmol/L (Martin &

Coleman, 2006). A greater increase suggests renal artery stenosis or CKD. Above this, reduce or stop the drug and recheck weekly until the creatinine has returned to its previous level. Look for underlying renal disease.

- An increase of serum K^+ to 5.5 to 5.9 mmol/L is acceptable but recheck more frequently. Stop the drug if the level reaches 6 mmol/L and refer (WHO, 2023).
- Use them in patients with insulin-dependent diabetes; they improve insulin resistance (whereas thiazides and beta-blockers may worsen it).
- Avoid them in patients with peripheral vascular disease.
- Use an angiotensin II receptor antagonist in patients who need an ACE inhibitor but cannot tolerate it because of cough.

Beta-Blockers

- Perform a peak flow before and after starting treatment if the history suggests the possibility of chronic obstructive pulmonary disease (COPD). If there is a significant decrease, stop the drug. However, cardioselective beta-blockers may be tolerated in mild to moderate reversible airway obstruction (Salpeter et al, 2005).
- Warn the patient not to stop a beta-blocker suddenly, especially one without intrinsic sympathomimetic activity. Even those without known CHD have a fourfold increased risk of MI or angina in the subsequent 4 weeks.

Alpha-Blockers

- Total cholesterol (TC) Incorrect section - needs to be with lipid management section decreases by an average of 4%, with a beneficial increase in high-density lipoprotein (HDL) cholesterol.
- Start with a low dose (e.g., terazosin 1 mg AP or doxazosin 1 mg AP), taken at night in case of first-dose hypotension.
- Use with caution in older adults, who may experience continued postural hypotension.

Poor Control

- Gently ask about adherence. A question such as, 'How difficult do you find it to take all of your tablets'? is more likely to elicit a truthful answer than 'Do you ever forget to take them'?
- Consider the white coat effect. If the blood pressure seems to fluctuate or the patient seems tense, arrange for home readings.
- Consider trying small doses and build up very gradually; this might improve tolerance for some patients (e.g., amlodipine 2.5 mg AP on alternate days for 2 weeks; then daily).
- If none of these applies, consider the patient to have resistant hypertension (see later).

Resistant Hypertension

- Resistant hypertension is common, found in 20% to 30% of patients.
- It is defined as hypertension not controlled by three drugs, at best tolerated doses, when the patient is taking them and the blood pressure is increased at home as well as at the clinic.
- It is important because patients with resistant hypertension are very high risk: they are 50% more likely to experience an adverse cardiovascular event than other patients with hypertension (Myat et al, 2012).
- Before a diagnosis of resistant hypertension can be made, check that it is true resistance, not poor adherence or white coat hypertension.
- Resistant hypertension is likely to be multifactorial. Consider the following:
  a. *Lifestyle factors*, including obesity, excess alcohol intake, excess dietary sodium, cocaine, and amphetamines misuse. Of these, obesity is the most common feature of patients with resistant hypertension. One study of more than 45,000 primary care patients in Germany found that obese individuals (BMI >40 kg/m^2) were more than five times more likely to need three antihypertensive drugs and three times more likely to require four antihypertensive drugs to achieve blood pressure control compared with individuals with a normal BMIs (≤25 kg/m^2) (Sharma et al, 2004).
  b. *Medication-related causes.* These include NSAIDs, selective cyclooxygenase (COX)-2 inhibitors, steroids, sympathomimetics (e.g., decongestants), oral contraceptives, and liquorice ingestion in sweets or chewed tobacco.
  c. *An underlying medical cause.* Up to 10% of these patients have a previously undiagnosed secondary cause:
     - *Renal disorders.* These are the commonest overall cause and the least amenable to treatment. They include diabetic kidney disease, glomerulonephritis, chronic pyelonephritis, obstructive uropathy, and polycystic kidney disease.
     - *Primary hyperaldosteronism.* This is the commonest single cause of secondary hypertension, accounting for 5% to 13% of all cases of hypertension (Grasko et al, 2010). It should be suspected in patients with low potassium and high sodium, although in many patients, these are normal. The ratio of plasma aldosterone to renin is increased and warrants referral to confirm the diagnosis and the underlying cause (Conn adenoma or idiopathic). Note that spironolactone, eplerenone, amiloride, and dihydropyridine CCBs (e.g., amlodipine) should be stopped before doing these tests (Grasko et al, 2010).
     - *Obstructive sleep apnoea.* Ask about snoring, episodes of apnoea at night, and daytime sleepiness. High nighttime blood pressure readings on an ABPM might point to this.
     - *Vascular disorders.* These include coarctation of the aorta (suspect if there is a significant interarm difference in blood pressure; check for radioradial or radiofemoral delay) and renal artery stenosis (common in older patients with hypertension; suspect if there is evidence of peripheral vascular disease; check for abdominal bruit).

- *Thyroid diseases.* Hyperthyroidism usually increases systolic blood pressure, whereas hypothyroidism usually increases diastolic blood pressure.
- *Cushing disease.* Look for the typical clinical features (e.g., centripetal obesity, moon facies, abdominal striae).
- *Phaeochromocytoma.* This is suggested by a history of episodic headaches, sweating, and palpitations associated with an often dramatic increase of blood pressure. Check 24-hour urinary catecholamines.
- If a cause of resistance is found that can be managed in primary care, continue management even if it means proceeding to step 4. Otherwise, refer. Hypertension clinics are capable of controlling half of those referred with resistant hypertension.

Referral

- Refer patients in whom there is reason to suspect secondary hypertension, including those with onset before 40 years of age, fluctuating blood pressure levels, evidence of renal disease, or resistant hypertension.
- Refer urgently all patients with accelerated hypertension (grade IV retinopathy).

Chest Pain of Recent Onset

GUIDELINE

National Institute for Health and Clinical Excellence. (2016). *Chest pain of recent onset. NICE clinical guideline 95.* Retrieved from https://www.nice.org.uk/guidance/cg95.

- Chest pain is very common, accounting for about 1% of all patient encounters in general practice, 5% of visits to emergency departments, and 25% of all emergency hospital admissions (Goodacre et al, 2005). These encounters represent just a fraction of the number of episodes of chest pain experienced in the community, for which medical attention is not always sought (Elliot et al, 2011).
- *The challenge for general practitioners (GPs) is to identify serious cardiac disease while also protecting patients from unnecessary investigations and hospital admissions.*
- The 2010 NICE guidelines (updated 2016) focus on the assessment and diagnosis of recent onset chest pain or discomfort of suspected cardiac origin (NICE, 2010). They present two separate diagnostic pathways: one for people with acute chest pain in whom an acute coronary syndrome (ACS) is suspected and the other for those with intermittent stable chest pain in whom stable angina is suspected (Cooper et al, 2010). Medical history taking and physical examination determine which of these pathways to follow, as described in the following sections.

Unstable Angina (Acute Coronary Syndrome)

GUIDELINES

Scottish Intercollegiate Guidelines Network. (2016). *Acute coronary syndromes. SIGN publication no.148.* Available at http://www.sign.ac.uk.
National Institute for Health and Clinical Excellence. (2013). *Unstable angina and NSTEMI: The early management of unstable angina and non-ST-segment-elevation myocardial infarction. NICE clinical guideline 94.* Retrieved from http://www.nice.org.uk/guidance/CG94.

- The definition of ACS, which includes unstable angina and MI, depends on the specific characteristics of each element of the triad of:
  - Clinical presentation (including a history of coronary artery disease [CAD])
  - ECG changes
  - Biochemical cardiac markers (SIGN, 2013).
- Symptoms and signs that may indicate an ACS include the following:
  - Chest pain lasting more than 15 minutes (may be in the arms, back, or jaw)
  - Chest pain with associated nausea and vomiting, sweating, or breathlessness
  - Chest pain associated with haemodynamic instability
  - New-onset chest pain or abrupt deterioration in previously stable angina, with recurrent pain occurring at rest; at significantly lower levels of activity; or in which the frequency, duration, or severity of the attacks has substantially worsened.
- Subsequent management depends on timing of presentation:
  - If the patient is presenting with current chest pain, proceed with immediate management as outlined in Box 6.3.
  - If the chest pain was in the previous 12 hours but the patient is currently pain free, perform ECG. Arrange emergency admission if the ECG is abnormal or if ECG is unavailable; if ECG is normal, arrange urgent same-day assessment.
  - If the chest pain was 12 to 72 hours ago, arrange urgent same-day assessment.

Myocardial Infarction

- *Defibrillation.* Defibrillate a patient who develops ventricular fibrillation while awaiting transfer to hospital. If no defibrillator is available, perform cardiopulmonary resuscitation (CPR) while waiting for one to arrive. Out-of-hospital defibrillation has been shown to save lives.
- *Thrombolysis.* Make an initial judgement about the patient's suitability (see later for contraindications). All

- Admit by emergency ambulance any patient with cardiac pain lasting more than 15 minutes despite GTN with an abnormal or unavailable ECG. Start management immediately but **do not delay transfer to hospital.**
- While awaiting admission, give:
  - Pain relief:
    1. GTN, e.g., three sprays over 15 minutes if pain continues
    2. Consider an IV opioid if available: diamorphine 1 mg/min AP (maximum, 5 mg AP) or morphine 2 mg/min (maximum, 10 mg). Administer with an IV antiemetic such as metoclopramide 10 mg AP or cyclizine 50 mg AP.
  - Aspirin 300 AP mg (unless allergic): Provide a written record of administration to go with the patient.
  - 12-lead ECG
  - Do not do ECG if it will delay hospital transfer.
  - Do not exclude ACS if the ECG is normal.
  - Pulse oximetry. Offer oxygen only if O_2 saturation is below 94%. Aim for 94% to 98%.
  - Monitor the patient until diagnosis.

ACS, Acute coronary syndrome; *ECG,* electrocardiogram; *GTN,* glyceryl trinitrate; *IV,* intravenous.

patients with a typical history of MI and ST-segment elevation or left bundle branch block should be considered for thrombolysis regardless of age if their quality of life warrants it and if local policy does not prefer acute percutaneous coronary intervention (PCI).

- Thrombolysis is of benefit in the 24 hours after the onset of symptoms, with more benefit the sooner it is given. Thrombolysis involves hospital admission, whether or not it is given at home first.
- GPs need special training. It should be given outside hospital only if all of the following apply:
  a. There is strong clinical suspicion of acute MI.
  b. Chest pain, unrelieved by glyceryl trinitrate (GTN) spray, has been present for at least 20 minutes and for no more than 12 hours.
  c. The ECG shows ST-segment elevation or left bundle branch block.
  d. A defibrillator is available because of the small but significant increase in risk of ventricular fibrillation after thrombolysis.
  e. No contraindications exist.
  f. Local protocols do not favour acute PCI.

Contraindications to Thrombolysis (Lip, Chin, & Prasad, 2002)

Absolute

a. Aortic dissection
b. Previous cerebral haemorrhage
c. Known cerebral aneurysm or arteriovenous malformation
d. Intracranial neoplasm
e. Any cerebrovascular accident in the previous 6 months
f. Active internal bleeding (other than menstruation)

g. Streptokinase should not be given to a patient who has received it more than 4 days previously. The development of antibodies may reduce its effectiveness.

Relative

a. Uncontrolled hypertension (blood pressure >180/110 mm Hg) or chronic severe hypertension
b. On anticoagulants or known bleeding diathesis
c. Trauma within past 2 to 4 weeks, including head injury and prolonged (>10 minutes) CPR
d. Aortic aneurysm
e. Recent (within 3 weeks) major surgery, organ biopsy, or puncture of a noncompressible vessel
f. Recent (within 6 months) gastrointestinal (GI), genitourinary, or other internal bleeding
g. Pregnancy
h. Active peptic ulcer

Cardiac Rehabilitation

- After MI, most patients are now routinely enrolled in a cardiac rehabilitation programme. This should be a comprehensive package of support, including exercise, education, and psychological support.
- *Exercise.* Encourage the continuation of exercise, which will continue to improve cardiac performance and survival and reduce the risk of another MI by 20%. Exercise can be playing tennis, jogging, cycling, swimming, or circuit training. NICE recommends 20 to 30 minutes each day, increasing slowly so that it is sufficiently vigorous to make the patient slightly breathless (NICE, 2007).
- *Smoking.* Encourage smokers to stop with the news that stopping even at this late stage probably reduces the mortality risk by 50%.
- *Weight.* Advise obese patients to lose weight.
- *Diet.* Whether the patient needs to lose weight or not, recommend a Mediterranean diet. The elements of the diet that seem to be associated with a lower mortality rate are moderate alcohol; low meat intake; and high intake of vegetables, fruit, nuts, olive oil, and legumes.
- *Alcohol.* Check that safe limits are not being exceeded.
- *Lipids.* Arrange a test for serum lipids at 3 months after MI unless the lipids were assessed within 24 hours of the onset of the infarct. After blood has been taken, start a statin regardless of the baseline value and continue it long term.
- *Diabetes.* Unless known to have diabetes or to have had an assessment of glucose metabolism in hospital, check the fasting plasma glucose.
- *Depression.* Look again for depression. Even at 1 year, 25% of these patients are depressed.
- *Other drugs*
  a. Check that the patient continues to take an ACE inhibitor (or an ARB if not tolerated).
  b. A beta-blocker should be taken for at least 12 months after MI in people without left ventricular dysfunction

or heart failure unless contraindicated. A beta-blocker should be taken indefinitely in those the left ventricular dysfunction.
  c. Dual antiplatelet therapy is usually advised for up to 12 months after an MI. This is usually aspirin plus a second antiplatelet drug such as clopidogrel or ticagrelor. Aspirin is usually taken lifelong. Clopidogrel can be used for those who are intolerant of aspirin.
- Recommend an annual influenza immunisation.
- Check that the patient has a cardiology follow-up appointment for an assessment of the coronary arteries and suitability for invasive treatment (PCI), as well as for an assessment of left ventricular function.

Other Advice

- Sedentary workers may return to work at 4 to 6 weeks, light manual workers at 6 to 8 weeks, and heavy manual workers at 3 months after MI.
- Patients should not fly for 2 weeks and then only if they are able to climb one flight of stairs without difficulty. A more cautious policy is to advise against flying for 6 weeks.
- Drivers should not drive for 1 month but do not now need to notify the Driver and Vehicle Licensing Agency (DVLA). They should inform their insurance companies. HGV (Heavy Goods Vehicle) and PSV (Public Service Vehicle) licence holders must notify the DVLA and may only continue vocational driving after individual assessment.

Stable Angina

GUIDELINES

National Institute for Health and Clinical Excellence. (2016). *Management of stable angina. NICE clinical guideline 126.* Retrieved from https://www.nice.org.uk/guidance/cg126.
  Scottish Intercollegiate Guidelines Network. (2018). *Management of stable angina: A national clinical guideline.* SIGN guideline no. 151. Retrieved from www.sign.ac.uk.

- Angina is the main symptom of myocardial ischaemia and is usually caused by atherosclerotic CAD restricting blood flow (and therefore oxygen delivery) to the heart muscle.
- Stable angina is common, affecting about 8% of males and 3% of females aged 55 to 64 years and about 14% of males and 8% of females aged 65 to 74 years in England (O'Flynn et al, 2011). The diagnosis is clinical, based on the history.
- The history is of pain or constricting discomfort that typically occurs in the front of the chest but can radiate to the neck, shoulders, jaw, or arms (NICE, 2012). It is usually brought on by physical exertion or emotional stress, but some people can have atypical symptoms, such as GI discomfort, breathlessness, or nausea.
- Stable angina is unlikely if the pain is any of the following:
  - Continuous or very prolonged
  - Unrelated to activity
  - Brought on by breathing in

- Associated with dizziness, palpitations, tingling, or difficulty swallowing
In such cases, consider other causes of chest pain, such as GI or musculoskeletal pain.
- The NICE guidelines present a table to help estimate the likelihood of CAD in people presenting with symptoms of angina, but such tables are not yet routinely used in general practice. Put simply, the likelihood of angina increases with age and with the presence of additional cardiovascular risk factors, including:
  - Smoking
  - Hypertension
  - Diabetes
  - Family history of CHD (first-degree relative: male younger than 55 years or female younger than 65 years)
  - Increased cholesterol (>6.5 mmol/L) and other lipids
- As well as these risk factors, also assess for:
  a. BMI
  b. Hypo- or hyperthyroidism
  c. Anaemia or polycythaemia
  d. Arrhythmias
  e. Valvular disease. All patients with aortic systolic murmur need assessment for aortic stenosis.
  f. Depression and social isolation
  g. Physical activity levels (Box 6.4)

Referral

- Patients with suspected angina should be referred to a cardiologist (e.g., fast-track chest pain clinic) for definitive diagnosis.
- Further investigations depend on local arrangements but may include exercise ECG or other forms of noninvasive functional testing.

Management

- Information and support
  - Explain stable angina and its long-term course and management, including factors that can provoke an attack (e.g., cold, exertion, stress, heavy meals).

• BOX 6.4 Workup: Investigations for Patients Presenting with Stable Angina

a. Haemoglobin
b. Thyroid function tests
c. Fasting blood sugar
d. Fasting lipid profile
e. Resting ECG. A normal ECG does not exclude the diagnosis, but an abnormal ECG makes it more likely.
ECG features consistent with coronary artery disease include:
- Pathological Q waves
- Left bundle branch block
- ST-segment and T-wave abnormalities (e.g., flattening or inversion)

ECG, Electrocardiogram.

- Explore fears and misconceptions about angina (e.g., around physical exertion, including sexual activity).
- Encourage self-management skills (e.g., pacing activities and goal setting).
- Preventing and treating episodes of angina
  - Advise patients to use a short-acting nitrate (e.g., GTN) spray or buccal tablets during episodes of angina and immediately before any planned exertion, including intercourse (except if the patient has just taken Viagra or a similar drug).
  - Explain that side effects, such as flushing, headache, and lightheadedness, may occur. Patients should sit down or hold onto something if they feel lightheaded or dizzy.
  - Advise patients to repeat the dose after 5 minutes if the pain has not gone and to call 999 if the pain persists for a further 5 minutes.
- Patients with stable angina should seek professional help if they have a sudden worsening in the frequency or severity of their angina.

Drug Treatment of Stable Angina

- Patients require optimal drug treatment with one or two antianginal drugs as necessary to treat symptoms plus drugs for secondary prevention of CVD.
- Explain the purpose of the drug treatment, why it is important to take the drugs regularly, and how side effects of drug treatment might affect the person's daily activities.
- Titrate the drug dosage against the person's symptoms up to the maximum tolerable dosage.
- Review the person's response to treatment, including any side effects, 2 to 4 weeks after starting or changing drug treatment (O'Flynn et al, 2011).

Cardiovascular Risk Reduction

a. Encourage lifestyle change (i.e., diet, exercise, smoking, alcohol).
b. Consider 75 mg/day of aspirin.
c. Offer statin treatment and treat AP high blood pressure in line with NICE guidelines.
d. Consider ACE inhibitors or low-cost ARBs for people with stable angina and diabetes.

Selecting Drugs

1. Offer either a beta-blocker (e.g., atenolol 100 mg, metoprolol 50–100 mg bd, or bisoprolol 5–20 mg AP) or CCB (use a rate-limiting CCB, e.g., diltiazem, unless the patient has heart failure or heart block, in which case use amlodipine) as the first-line treatment.
   - If either is not tolerated, switch to the other.
   - If either is ineffective, switch to the other or combine both. (Avoid verapamil or diltiazem in combination with beta-blocker.)

2. If the person cannot tolerate beta-blockers or CCBs or if both are contraindicated, consider monotherapy with one of the following:
   - A long-acting nitrate
   - Ivabradine
   - Nicorandil
   - Ranolazine
3. If not satisfactorily controlled on two drugs, refer for consideration of revascularisation.

Revascularisation

- Coronary intervention such as PCI or coronary artery bypass graft (CABG) surgery should only be considered if symptoms are not optimally controlled with medical treatment.
- Refer to cardiology for further assessment, which may include noninvasive investigations, coronary angiography, or both.
- Coronary angiography is the traditional investigation for establishing the nature, anatomy, and severity of CHD. It is an invasive investigation and carries a mortality risk of around 0.1% for elective procedures (SIGN, 2013).
- The main purpose of revascularisation is to improve the symptoms of stable angina:
  - CABG surgery and PCI are effective in relieving symptoms, but repeat revascularisation may be necessary after either procedure. The rate is lower after CABG surgery.
  - Stroke is an uncommon complication of each of these two procedures. (The incidence is similar.)
  - There is a potential survival advantage with CABG surgery for some people with multivessel disease.
  - In those for whom both percutaneous and surgical revascularisation are feasible, percutaneous revascularisation is a more cost-effective approach.

Noncardiac Chest Pain

- Fewer than half of patients referred to cardiac clinics and accident and emergency departments with chest pain are found to have CAD (Bass & Mayou, 2002). Many of these patients continue to have pain and long-term functional impairment. Their management is often inadequate after the diagnosis of cardiac disease is excluded.
- There is a clinical prediction rule called the Marburg Heart Score to assist GPs in ruling out chest pain caused by CHD (Haasenritter et al, 2012). Based on five findings from the patient history and examination, the score has a high negative predictive value, but further research is needed to assess its use in routine practice.
- Be clear from the history, investigations, and specialist assessment that the pain is noncardiac. Then resist requests for further cardiac referral.
- Try to make a positive diagnosis of the cause of the pain, such as musculoskeletal disorders, panic attacks, reflux, or depression.

- If a clear diagnosis is possible, treat accordingly (e.g., with NSAIDs for musculoskeletal pain, a proton pump inhibitor [PPI] for reflux, antidepressants for depression).
- If no clear diagnosis is possible, attempt an explanation along the following lines: the symptoms are real; the symptoms do not arise from the heart or from any other specific illness; and the brain normally disregards sensations that it receives from all over the body but that for some reason, in this patient, it is sensitised to sensations from the chest. This explanation might lead on to discussion of how such sensitisation may have occurred. The patient may volunteer the memory of some event that seemed to trigger the chest pain.
- Ask who else in the family is worried about the pain and try to see them as well.
- Refer to a psychologist or counsellor patients who accept this explanation but who still find themselves bothered by the pain.
- Consider a trial of a tricyclic antidepressant or selective serotonin reuptake inhibitor (SSRI) in patients who are sufficiently troubled by pain even in the absence of depression.

Heart Failure

GUIDELINE

National Institute for Health and Clinical Excellence. (2018). *Chronic heart failure in adults: Diagnosis and management. NICE clinical guideline 106*. Retrieved from https://www.nice.org.uk/guidance/ng106.

- Heart failure is a complex syndrome of symptoms and signs caused by structural or functional abnormalities of the heart (NICE, 2018). It is often divided into heart failure caused by left ventricular systolic dysfunction (LVSD; associated with a reduced left ventricular ejection fraction) or heart failure with preserved ejection fraction (HF-PEF), although some cardiac societies have subdivided this further. Most of the evidence on treatment is for heart failure caused by LVSD. The most common causes of heart failure in the United Kingdom are CAD and hypertension, and many patients have had an MI in the past.
- Both the incidence and prevalence of heart failure increase steeply with age, and the prevalence is expected to increase in the future as a result of a combination of ageing population, improved survival of people with IHD, and more effective treatments for patients with heart failure (Owan et al, 2006).
- The prognosis remains poor despite improvements in outcomes in the past decade. In one community-based study, 10-year survival rates ranged from 12% in those with multiple-cause heart failure to around 31% in those with LVSD (Taylor et al, 2012).

Diagnosis

- Making the diagnosis of heart failure can be challenging. Patients may present with a range of symptoms, including fatigue, breathlessness, and ankle swelling, and they may also have other conditions such CHD, diabetes, hypertension, and COPD, which can confuse the picture (SIGN, 2016).
- Careful history taking and examination help to guide further assessment. The following clinical signs add to the suspicion of heart failure, though none are diagnostic in isolation:
  - Raised jugular venous pressure (JVP)
  - Presence of a third heart sound (S3)
  - Basal crepitations
  - Tachycardia
  - Peripheral oedema
- Initial investigations should help to rule out other causes of symptoms and should include a full blood count, fasting glucose, thyroid function tests, serum urea and creatinine, urinalysis, ECG, and chest radiography. NICE guidelines recommend the widespread use of serum natriuretic peptides as an aid to diagnosis of heart failure.

Serum Natriuretic Peptides

- B-type natriuretic peptide (BNP) and N-terminal pro b-type natriuretic peptide (NT-proBNP) are peptide hormones produced in the heart. They are increased with increasing left ventricular volume and pressure, and concentrations tend to increase with New York Heart Association (NYHA) class (Table 6.2). Very high levels indicate a worse prognosis and should prompt urgent referral. It is important to note the values for BNP and NT-proBNP differ and are not comparable. NICE and other international societies (as well as most research studies) favour the use of NT-proBNP.
- If the test result is negative, heart failure is very unlikely (i.e., it has high sensitivity). False-negative results may be caused by obesity and by drugs used to treat patients with heart failure (i.e., diuretics, ACE inhibitors, ARBs, and beta-blockers).

TABLE 6.2	New York Heart Association Classification of Heart Failure Symptoms
Class	**Description**
I: asymptomatic	No limitations of ordinary activity
II: mild	Slight limitation of physical activity but comfortable at rest
III: moderate	Marked limitation of physical activity; comfortable at rest but symptomatic on less than ordinary physical activity
IV: severe	Inability to carry on any physical activity without discomfort; symptoms present at rest

- If the test result is positive, it does not diagnose heart failure but should prompt referral for echocardiography (i.e., it has relatively low specificity). False-positive results occur with cardiac ischaemia from any causes (e.g., left ventricular hypertrophy, tachycardia, hypoxia) and in some other chronic conditions (e.g., diabetes, CKD, COPD, cirrhosis) (Al-Mohammad et al, 2010).

How to Use NT proBNP or BNP

- If heart failure is suspected based on symptoms and clinical signs, the NTproBNP (or BNP) should be measured, whether or not the patient has a history of CVD.
  - If the patient has a very high BNP (>400 pg/mL [116 pmol/L]) or NTproBNP (>2000 pg/mL [236 pmol/L]), refer them urgently (to be seen within 2 weeks).
  - If the patient has an increased BNP (100–400 pg/mL [29–116 pmol/L]) or NTproBNP (400–2000 pg/mL [47–236 pmol/L]), refer them within 6 weeks.
- If levels are normal (BNP <100 pg/mL [29 pmol/L] or NTproBNP <400 pg/mL [47 pmol/L]), a diagnosis of heart failure is unlikely in an untreated patient, and alternative diagnoses should be sought. Some guidelines, such as the European Society of Cardiology (ESC), use a much lower cutoff of less than 125 pg/mL to help exclude heart failure.

Management of Confirmed Congestive Heart Failure

Pharmacologic management of patients with heart failure depends on whether the person has LVSD or preserved ejection fraction (most research has been done on the former), and each is considered in turn in this section. First, a number of general measures apply to both forms of heart failure.

General Measures

- *Information.* Explain what is going on and what to do if things get worse.
- *Weight.* Encourage patients to reduce weight if they are obese. Recommend daily weighing at roughly the same time and in similar clothes. Patients should report if they gain more than 2 kg over 2 days. Use diuretics flexibly, guided by weight (Arroll et al, 2010).
- *Diet.* Advise a diet with no added salt.
- *Fluid.* Restrict fluid intake to 2 L/day unless the patient is losing fluids from sweat, diarrhoea, or vomiting.
- *Alcohol.* Keep alcohol intake low. In patients with alcoholic heart disease, recommend complete cessation.
- *Smoking.* Stop smoking; it causes vasoconstriction. Refer to smoking cessation services.
- *Exercise.* Rest in the acute phase but exercise when stable. Regular low-intensity physical activity improves mortality and morbidity. Refer to the heart failure rehabilitation service if it exists.
- *Sexual activity.* Be prepared to broach sensitive issues with patients, such as sexual activity, because they may not be raised by patients.

- *Vaccination.* Recommend influenza vaccination annually and pneumococcal vaccination once.
- *Air travel.* Air travel is possible for the majority of patients with heart failure, depending on their clinical condition at the time of travel
- *Driving regulations.* Advise patients to check with the DVLA, particularly drivers of large goods vehicles (https://www.gov.uk/government/organisations/driver-and-vehicle-licensing-agency).
- *Depression.* Check for depression. It is present in one-third and should be treated as thoroughly as if it was not associated with heart failure. Warn patients not to buy St John's wort over the counter (OTC) because of its interaction with prescribed medication, specifically digoxin and warfarin.
- *NSAIDs.* Stop NSAIDs (including COX-2 inhibitors) if taken unless they are essential. Warn the patient not to buy them OTC.
- *Carers.* Identify the carer or carers and involve them in the management.

Chronic Heart Failure With Left Ventricular Dysfunction

- LVSD, assessed by measuring the left ventricular ejection fraction by echocardiography, refers to impaired left ventricular pump (contractile) function. Most evidence to guide management of heart failure is in this group of patients, which make up around half of all heart failure cases (Arroll et al, 2010).
- All patients should be offered *both* ACE inhibitors and beta-blockers unless there are contraindications.

Angiotensin-Converting Enzyme Inhibitors and Angiotensin II Receptor Blockers

- ACE inhibitors increase the ability to exercise, improve well-being, and prolong life in patients with all degrees of heart failure (Dargie & McMurray, 1994).
- ARBs (e.g., candesartan and valsartan) may be used in patients who are intolerant of ACE inhibitors (e.g., with ACE inhibitor–related cough).
- If there is a high probability of congestive heart failure (CHF), start treatment before waiting for echocardiography unless valve disease is suspected, in which case wait.
- Exclude the absolute contraindications of allergy to ACE inhibitors and pregnancy.
- Start at a low dose and titrate upwards at short intervals (e.g., every 2 weeks) until the optimal tolerated or target dose is achieved.
- Measure serum urea, creatinine, electrolytes, and estimated glomerular filtration rate (GFR) when a patient is starting an ACE inhibitor and after each dose increment. Also check blood pressure.
  - ACE inhibitors (and ARBs) should not normally be started if the pretreatment serum potassium concentration is significantly above the normal reference range (typically >5.0 mmol/L) (NICE, 2021). Stop

ACE inhibitor and ARB therapy if the serum potassium concentration increases to above 6.0 mmol/L and other drugs known to promote hyperkalaemia have been discontinued.
  - If there is a decrease in eGFR of 25% or more or an increase in plasma creatinine of 30% or more, investigate other causes of a deterioration in renal function such as volume depletion or concurrent medication (e.g., NSAIDS). If no other cause is found, stop the ACE inhibitor or ARB or reduce the dose to a previously tolerated level.
- Advise the patient to take the first dose before going to bed to reduce the effect of first-dose hypotension.
- When the dose is stable, repeat creatinine and electrolytes at 3 months and then every 6 months or sooner if further dose titration is necessary or there is intercurrent infection.
- Warn the patient to avoid dehydration, for instance, in gastroenteritis or in hot weather, because this can cause a sudden deterioration in renal function. If the weight drops by more than 1 kg because of dehydration, the patient should stop the diuretic and drink more fluid.

Beta-Blockers

- All patients with LVSD should be started on a licensed beta-blocker (e.g., bisoprolol, carvedilol, nebivolol) after heart failure is controlled, provided there are no absolute contraindications (e.g., heart block or asthma).
- In patients already taking another beta-blocker (e.g., atenolol for angina) who develop heart failure, advise switching to one of the above. A study in British general practice found that switching to bisoprolol or carvedilol, mainly from atenolol, was the single most valuable manoeuvre in patients with left ventricular dysfunction (Mant et al, 2008).
- NICE guidelines suggest you should not be put off prescribing beta-blockers in individuals with what were previously considered to be relative contraindications, such as older adults and those with peripheral vascular disease, erectile dysfunction, diabetes mellitus, interstitial pulmonary disease, or COPD without reversibility.
- Take a 'start low, go slow' approach. Start at a low dose (e.g., bisoprolol 1.25 mg/day or carvedilol 3.125 mg bd) and double the dose every 2 to 4 weeks until the target dose is reached (bisoprolol 10 mg/day; carvedilol 25 mg bd).
- Monitor heart rate, blood pressure, and clinical status at each dose titration. If the pulse is greater than 50 beats/min and symptoms have worsened, halve the dose. Stop and seek specialist advice if symptoms have become severe.
- If at any stage it is necessary to stop the beta-blocker, tail it off gradually to avoid rebound ischaemia and arrhythmias.

Sodium Glucose Transport-2 Inhibitors

- This group of medications are now recommended for patients with heart failure with reduced ejection fraction (HF-REF) and possible HF-PEF. They act on the kidneys to cause glucosuria and were developed as a novel diabetes agent. In safety trials, reduced heart failure diagnosis and improved outcomes were noted. This led to large randomised trials (e.g., EMPEROR PRESERVED) The Empagliflozin Outcome Trial in Patients with Chronic Heart Failure with Preserved Ejection Fraction (EMPEROR-Preserved) using sodium-glucose cotransporter 2 (SGLT-2)s in patients with heart failure, both with and without diabetes.
- These agents should be started early in the management of heart failure
- They have a diuretic effect, and patients must be warned to seek medical attention if they feel unwell with other dehydrating illness (diarrhoea, vomiting, infection.)

Sacubitril Valsartan

- This agent is recommended for patients with symptomatic heart failure despite already taking other medications and an ejection fraction lower than 35%.
- These should be started by a heart failure specialist with titration and monitoring usually by a member of a heart failure specialist team.

Diuretics (Other Than Spironolactone)

- Diuretics should be routinely used for the relief of congestive symptoms and fluid retention in patients with heart failure and should be titrated (up and down) according to need after the initiation of first-line heart failure therapies. Their only function is symptom relief.
- Avoid overtreatment, which can lead to dehydration and renal dysfunction, particularly with loop diuretics. Hypovolaemia is a common cause of dizziness and lightheadedness.
- Monitor blood pressure and renal function after 4 weeks and then every 6 months.
- Use a loop diuretic (e.g., furosemide or bumetanide) in patients with moderate to severe heart failure. They cause less hypokalaemia and impotence than a high-dose thiazide (e.g., bendroflumethiazide). Increase the dose gradually until diuresis occurs.
- When stable, reduce the dose to as low as possible without oedema or breathlessness occurring. Alternatively, consider stopping or reducing to a thiazide diuretic.
- The addition of a thiazide diuretic or a potassium-sparing diuretic such as spironolactone (or both) to loop diuretics can be useful if pulmonary or ankle oedema persists because the different classes of diuretic are thought to have an additive effect. However, even with short-term combined use, the diuresis can be excessive and can cause hypokalaemia. Check creatinine and electrolytes after 3 days.

Second-Line Pharmacologic Management

- If a patient remains symptomatic despite optimal treatment with ACE inhibitor and beta-blocker, refer for specialist advice on second-line treatment, which might include:
  - Aldosterone antagonists
  - An ARB

- Hydralazine plus nitrate (especially for patients of African or Caribbean descent with moderate to severe heart failure)
- Ivabradine
- Digoxin

Aldosterone Antagonists

- Hyperkalaemia is a potentially fatal adverse effect and is most likely in those with impaired renal function. Only give spironolactone if the creatinine is less than 220 µmol/L.
- Warn the patient to avoid salt substitutes with a high potassium content. Warn males about gynaecomastia.
- If potassium reaches 5.5 to 5.9 mmol/L or creatinine increases to 200 µmol/L, reduce the dose, and monitor closely. If these levels are exceeded, stop and seek specialist advice.

Ivabradine

- Ivabradine was approved by NICE in November 2012 and is an option for patients (NICE, 2012):
  - With symptomatic stable heart failure (NYHA class II–IV) with LVSD and an ejection fraction of 35% or less
  - Who are in sinus rhythm with a resting heart rate greater than 75 beats/min
  - Who are also receiving standard therapy including beta-blockers, ACE inhibitors, and aldosterone antagonists
- Ivabradine should be initiated by a heart failure specialist (e.g., specialist nurse) with access to a multidisciplinary heart failure team.

Digoxin

Consider for patients in sinus rhythm if still symptomatic despite all the above.

- See the section on atrial fibrillation (AF) for the use of digoxin in patients with AF.

Heart Failure With Preserved Ejection Fraction

- As noted earlier, it is thought that up to 50% of patients with heart failure have a preserved ventricular ejection fraction. It has the same symptoms and signs as heart failure with LVSD and carries a similar mortality risk but has a less clear evidence base for treatment (Jong et al, 2010).
- Patients with HF-PEF are more likely than those with LVSD to be older and female and to have hypertension and AF but are less likely to have CAD.
- NICE recommends the use of diuretics for symptomatic relief.
- ACE inhibitors and beta-blockers should be considered, particularly when there are other compelling indications for their use (e.g., CAD, hypertension, and diabetes mellitus).
- If AF is present, digoxin may be added for rate control, and anticoagulation should be considered.

Grounds for Admission

a. Severe symptoms (e.g., severe dyspnoea or hypotension)
b. Acute MI
c. Severe complicating medical illness (e.g., pneumonia)
d. Inadequate social support
e. Failure to respond to treatment
f. Uncontrolled arrhythmia

Referral for Specialist Review

- Refer patients to the specialist multidisciplinary heart failure team for:
  - The initial diagnosis of heart failure
  - The management of:
    a. Severe heart failure (NYHA class IV)
    b. Heart failure that does not respond to treatment
    c. Heart failure that can no longer be managed effectively in the home setting
- Consider specialist review:
  a. When renal function continues to deteriorate or deteriorates rapidly
  b. When there are concerns about low blood pressure
  c. When the patient is pregnant or considering pregnancy

End-Stage Heart Failure

- Issues of sudden death and living with uncertainty are pertinent to all patients with heart failure. The opportunity to discuss these issues should be available at all stages of care.
- Deciding on prognosis in heart failure is difficult, and the advice of a cardiologist may be needed. The palliative needs of patients and carers should be identified, assessed, and managed at the earliest opportunity. There should be access to professionals with palliative care skills within the heart failure team.
- Nonessential treatment should be stopped.
- The focus should be on symptom control, as discussed next.

Breathlessness

- Morphine is the most effective palliation. Give a low oral dose (2.5–5 mg every 4 hours) AP because peak plasma levels are higher in patients with heart failure.
- If the patient is breathless at rest, then consider oxygen therapy at home (40%–80% if the patient does not have COPD).
- Refer for relaxation, breathing exercises, and anxiety management if available.

Weakness and Fatigue

- Weakness and fatigue are usually secondary to a low cardiac output.
- *Drug reduction.* Consider reducing ACE inhibitors, beta-blockers, and diuretics if the patient is dehydrated.
- *Depression.* Avoid tricyclics; SSRIs may be of value.

- *Social factors.* Increase social care if possible and ensure support for the carer(s).

Anorexia and Nausea

- *Digoxin.* Check serum level and renal function.
- Consider increasing diuretics if there is hepatic congestion.
- *Diet.* Advise the patient to have small, appetising meals more frequently. Allow small amounts of alcohol before meals.
- *Antiemetics.* Use levomepromazine 12.5 mg at night. Avoid cyclizine.

Oedema

- *Mobilisation* is advisable in theory but rarely practicable at this stage.
- *Diuretics.* Avoid increasing diuretics at this stage unless doing so gives symptomatic relief. They are unlikely to have much effect on the oedema.
- Be cautious about advising the patient to raise their feet. This may increase the venous return to the heart and worsen the dyspnoea.
- *Compression stockings and bandages.* These may increase tissue damage and are uncomfortable.

Acute Pulmonary Oedema

- When called urgently to the patient in extremis, get someone else to dial for an ambulance while you:
  1. Sit the patient up with the legs down.
  2. Give oxygen if available.
  3. Give a GTN tablet or spray sublingually (for its immediate vasodilator effect).
  4. If available, give intravenous (IV) diamorphine 1 mg AP per minute up to 5 mg or IV morphine 2 mg per minute up to 10 mg, mixed with metoclopramide 10 mg AP IV. Do not use cyclizine; it increases systemic arterial pressure.
  5. If available, give a loop diuretic (IV furosemide 50 mg or IV bumetanide 1 mg AP).
- Look for causes of the heart failure that may need treatment in their own right, especially MI.
- Admit when the patient is sufficiently stable for fuller assessment and for continuing treatment.
- Note: Digoxin and aminophylline should not be used in acute failure outside the hospital.

Right Heart Failure

Acute Right Heart Failure

- The clinical picture of a low-output state, no pulmonary oedema, and increased JVP may be caused by massive pulmonary embolism or acute right heart failure as in a right ventricle MI or acute cor pulmonale.
- Admit urgently. Position the patient however is most comfortable. Do not give morphine; respiratory depression and hypotension are very likely to follow. Do not give diuretics because they may precipitate shock.

Chronic Cor Pulmonale

- Treat the lung disease. Consider:
  a. Antibiotics for exacerbations of infection
  b. Inhaled bronchodilators and steroids via a spacing device
  c. Physiotherapy
  d. Long-term oxygen therapy
  e. Nasal intermittent positive-pressure ventilation for those with thoracic deformities and obstructive sleep apnoea
- Admit readily all patients with an acute exacerbation. Oxygen will dilate the pulmonary vessels and so reduce the pulmonary artery pressure. The danger of hypercapnoea makes this hazardous in the acute situation at home.
- Use diuretics carefully because they may further reduce renal blood flow. They are only required if oedema becomes troublesome.
- Use digoxin only if the patient is in AF.
- Do not start ACE inhibitors outside the hospital.

Palpitations and Arrhythmias

- Palpitations are a common presentation in general practice and a frequent reason for cardiology referrals. They often cause considerable distress and anxiety for the patient; however, more often than not, they are often benign, with fewer than half of patients with palpitations having an arrhythmia and not every identified arrhythmia being of clinical or prognostic significance (Mayou et al, 2003).
- Furthermore, not all arrhythmias present with palpitations. Some may cause no symptoms; in other cases, symptoms include tachycardia, bradycardia, chest pain, breathlessness, lightheadedness, and fainting (syncope) or near fainting.
- As well as arrhythmias, palpitations can be caused by structural heart diseases, psychosomatic disorders, systemic diseases, and the effects of medical and recreational drugs (Raviele et al, 2011).
- Careful history taking and physical examination are important, but further investigation is invariably required (Hoefman et al, 2007).

History

- Ask what the patient means by palpitations. It may be more like a pulsatile tinnitus or a chest discomfort.
- Ask about the rate, frequency, and duration of palpitations, as well as exacerbating and relieving factors. The patient may be able to tap out the rate on the consulting desk.
- Are there any associated symptoms, such as sweating, breathlessness, or chest pain? If any of these are present and the patient has palpitations at that time, refer to hospital immediately by 999 ambulance.
- Ask about smoking, alcohol, caffeine consumption, and use of illicit substances such as cocaine, methylenedioxymethamphetamine, and amphetamines.

- Ask about general well-being. In particular, assess for any life stressors and ask about personal or family history of anxiety or heart problems.

Examination

- Assess for tremor, which may indicate thyrotoxicosis or anxiety. Ask the patient to hold their arms outstretched in front of them with the palms down and to spread their fingers.
- Assess pulse rate and rhythm and check blood pressure. Is the pulse rate regularly irregular, suggesting ectopic beats, or irregularly irregular, suggesting AF or atrial flutter?
- Examine the heart, assessing for evidence of structural heart disease, such as murmurs, abnormal heart sounds, and signs of heart failure.

Investigations

- Blood tests should include full blood count (to exclude anaemia), urea and electrolytes, and thyroid function tests.
- Arrange a 12-lead electrocardiogram (ECG). ECG abnormalities to look for include:
  - AF
  - Second- and third-degree atrioventricular (AV) block
  - Signs of previous MI
  - Left ventricular hypertrophy and left ventricular strain patterns
  - Left bundle branch block
  - Abnormal T-wave inversion and ST-segment changes
  - Signs of preexcitation (short PR interval and delta waves)
  - Abnormal QTc interval and T-wave morphology

Next Steps

- There is no validated risk stratification tool that is widely used in practice, although some authors have proposed a traffic light system to guide further management (Wolff & Cowan, 2009).
- Patients with the following features should be referred *urgently* to cardiology:
  - Palpitations with syncope or near syncope
  - Palpitations during exercise
  - Family history of inheritable heart disease
  - High-risk structural heart disease
  - High-degree AV block
- Patients with the following features should be referred routinely to cardiology or to a local palpitations assessment service:
  - Palpitations with associated symptoms
  - Abnormal ECG findings
  - History suggestive of recurrent tachyarrhythmia
  - Structural heart disease
- Patients with the following features may not require referral:
  - History in keeping with extrasystoles or ectopic beats *and*

- Normal ECG findings *and*
- No family history *and*
- No evidence of IHD or structural heart disease

Ectopic Beats in a Normal Heart

- Explain their benign nature to the patient.
- Advise against caffeine, fatigue, smoking, and alcohol.
- *Beta-blockers* should be used only if the patient is unable to tolerate the ectopics.
- *Frequent ventricular ectopics (>100 per hour)* may be grounds for referral. Patients may have a prolapsing mitral valve, or older patients may have unsuspected IHD.
- For those still troubled by their symptoms, consider referral for cognitive-behavioural therapy or similar (Mayou et al 2002).

Atrial Fibrillation

> **GUIDELINE**
>
> National Institute for Health and Clinical Excellence. (2021). *Atrial fibrillation: Diagnosis and management. NICE clinical guideline 196.* Retrieved from https://www.nice.org.uk/guidance/ng196.

- AF is the most common disorder of heart rhythm with a prevalence that increases with age from about 6% in people aged 65 to 74 years to 12% in people aged 75 to 84 years to 16% in people aged 85 years and older (Fitzmaurice et al, 2007) (Box 6.5).
- It is associated with a fivefold increased risk of stroke and a threefold increased incidence of heart failure, with a higher mortality rate as a result (Camm et al, 2012).

• BOX 6.5   Workup of Atrial Fibrillation

a. History of alcohol intake (either chronic or bingeing)
b. Blood pressure (half of all cases of AF are hypertensive)
c. Thyroid function tests, creatinine, and electrolytes
d. Examine for heart failure, valvular heart disease, congenital heart disease, and acute pericarditis or myocarditis
e. ECG (looking for IHD, left ventricular strain, and delta waves)
f. NICE recommend performing an echocardiogram in patients for whom:
  - A baseline echocardiogram is important for long-term management
  - A rhythm control strategy which includes cardioversion is being considered
  - In whom there is a high risk or a suspicion of underlying structural or functional heart disease (e.g., heart failure or heart murmur) that influences their subsequent management (e.g., choice of antiarrhythmic drug)
  - Refinement of clinical risk stratification for antithrombotic therapy is needed

AF, Atrial fibrillation; *ECG,* electrocardiogram; *IHD,* ischaemic heart disease; *NICE,* National Institute for Health and Clinical Excellence.

- AF also increases the risk of sudden cardiac death (Chen et al, 2013).
- Oral anticoagulation can reduce the risk of stroke by two-thirds (Aguilar & Hart, 2005). However, current evidence suggests that only about half of patients with AF identified as being at high risk are receiving anticoagulants (Holt et al, 2012).
- The older a person is, the more dangerous AF becomes, with strokes being more common and more disabling. Yet underuse of anticoagulation is highest in older people, who have most to gain from treatment (Hobbs et al, 2011).
- Primary care has considerable potential to further reduce the risk of stroke in AF by identifying high-risk patients and lowering the threshold for offering anticoagulation, as recommended in the guidelines.

Identification of Atrial Fibrillation

- In 2005, the SAFE A randomised controlled trial and cost-effectiveness study of systematic screening (targeted and total population screening) versus routine practice for the detection of atrial fibrillation in people aged 65 and over: The SAFE study showed that opportunistic screening (by pulse palpation followed by ECG if the is pulse irregular) of patients older than 65 years is cost-effective for detecting AF (Hobbs et al, 2005). Opportunistic screening is endorsed by the ESC guidelines.
- Some have gone further, suggesting that a new national screening programme should be introduced, using this approach for all patients older than 65 years of age (James & Campbell, 2012).
- Screening of such patients while attending annual influenza vaccination clinics has been piloted but with mixed results (Gordon et al, 2012; Rhys et al, 2013).
- Admit if rapid AF is associated with:
  a. Chest pain
  b. Hypotension
  c. More than mild heart failure
- Refer urgently if seen within 48 hours of the onset of AF and the patient is a candidate for cardioversion (see later).

Cardioversion Versus Rate Control

- *Rate control* is recommended as the treatment of choice in most patients. It has advantages over rhythm control, including fewer hospital admissions, fewer adverse drug reactions, and possibly a lower mortality rate (Atrial Fibrillation Follow-up Investigation of Rhythm Management investigators, 2002), and it is more cost-effective (Hagens et al, 2004).
- *Referral for cardioversion is more appropriate for certain patients*, either because it is more likely to succeed than in others (the first three categories) or because sinus rhythm offers greater chance of clinical benefit than rate control (the last two categories):
  - Younger patients
  - Those presenting for the first time with lone AF
  - Those with AF secondary to a cause that has now been treated

- Those who are symptomatic
- Those with CHF (restoration of sinus rhythm may improve left ventricular function)
- The decision as to whether to use chemical or electrical cardioversion should be made in discussion between the patient and cardiologist. Vernakalant is an IV antiarrhythmic agent approved for cardioversion of AF of 7 days' duration or less. Other agents include ibutilide, flecainide, propafenone, and amiodarone.
- Rate control is more appropriate in those in whom cardioversion is less likely to succeed:
  - Those who are older than 65 years old
  - Those with structural heart disease or CHD
  - Those whose AF is longstanding (e.g., >12 months)
  - Those in whom previous attempts at cardioversion have failed or been followed by relapse
  - Those in whom an underlying cause (e.g., thyrotoxicosis) has not yet been corrected
  - Those with a contraindication to antiarrhythmic drugs
- Aim for lenient (heart rate <110 beats/min) rather than strict (heart rate <80 beats/min) rate control unless the patient is symptomatic.
- Use:
  a. A beta-blocker first line (e.g., atenolol, bisoprolol, metoprolol)
  b. A rate-limiting CCB second line (e.g., diltiazem or verapamil). Avoid both in heart failure and avoid the combination of verapamil and a beta-blocker.
  c. Digoxin if still symptomatic. If digoxin is contraindicated, add diltiazem to the beta-blocker. The usual concern about causing bradycardia or AV block is less of a problem in AF because this is the aim of the treatment.

Risk Stratification for Anticoagulation

- A risk factor–based approach to stroke risk stratification has been promoted for many years (e.g., CHADS2: CHF, hypertension, age 75 years or older, diabetes, stroke [doubled]; Gage et al, 2001), but recent evidence has prompted a shift in focus towards identification of 'truly low-risk' patients who *do not* need any antithrombotic therapy.
- The CHADS2 score has been replaced by CHA_2DS_2-VASc score, which has been found to be more accurate (Olesen et al, 2011) (Table 6.3, 6.4).
- Using the CHA_2DS_2-VASc score, all patients older than 75 years of age and all females older than 65 years of age are automatically considered at high risk, so they do not need further formal risk assessment other than consideration of bleeding risk.

Assessment of Bleeding Risk

- Before starting anticoagulation, an assessment of bleeding risk should be undertaken. Major bleeding, especially

TABLE 6.3 CHA$_2$DS$_2$-VASc Score[a]

	Risk Factor	Score
C	Congestive heart failure	1
H	Hypertension	1
A$_2$	Age 75 years or older	2
D	Diabetes	1
S$_2$	CVA or TIA	2
V	Vascular disease	1
A	Age 65 years or older	1
Sc	Sex category (i.e., female)	1

[a]Total score:
0 = low risk (0.8% annual stroke rate).
1 = moderate risk (1.75% annual stroke rate).
≥2 = high risk (>2.7% annual stroke rate).
3 = 3.2%; 5 = 6.7%; 7 = 9.6%.
CVA, Cardiovascular accident; *TIA*, transient ischaemic attack.

TABLE 6.4 The HAS-BLED Bleeding Risk Score (Pisters et al, 2010)

Letter	Clinical Characteristic	Points
H	Hypertension[a]	1
A	Abnormal renal and liver function (1 point each)[b,c]	1 or 2
S	Stroke	1
B	Bleeding[d]	1
L	Labile INRs[e]	1
E	Older (older than 65 years of age)	1
D	Drugs or alcohol use (1 point each)[f]	1 or 2
TOTAL		

[a]*Hypertension* is defined as systolic blood pressure greater than 160 mm Hg.
[b]*Abnormal kidney function* is defined as the presence of chronic dialysis or renal transplantation or serum creatinine of 200 mmol/L or greater.
[c]*Abnormal liver function* is defined as chronic hepatic disease (e.g., cirrhosis) or biochemical evidence of significant hepatic derangement (e.g., bilirubin greater than two times the upper limit of normal, in association with aspartate aminotransferase, alanine aminotransferase, or alkaline phosphatase greater than three times the upper limit normal.).
[d]*Bleeding* refers to previous bleeding history or predisposition to bleeding (e.g., bleeding diathesis, anaemia).
[e]*Labile international normalized ratios (INRs)* refers to unstable or high INRs or poor time in therapeutic range (e.g., <60%).
[f]*Drugs or alcohol use* refers to concomitant use of drugs, such as antiplatelet agents, nonsteroidal antiinflammatory drugs, alcohol abuse, and so on.

intracranial haemorrhage (ICH), is the most feared complication of anticoagulation therapy and confers a high risk of death and disability (Connolly et al, 2011).

- Several different guidelines recommend the use of the HAS-BLED score, which has been validated in many cohort studies and correlates well with ICH risk (Cairns et al, 2011; Lip et al, 2011; Camm et al, 2010) (Table 6.4).
- A HAS-BLED score of 3 or more indicates a bleeding risk (ICH or requiring admission) on anticoagulation over the next year sufficient to justify caution with anticoagulation.
- A score of 3 or more does not exclude patients from receiving anticoagulation but does require extra caution to control bleeding risks (e.g., closer monitoring of renal function and international normalised ratio [INR], better management of hypertension).

Anticoagulation

- For more than half a century, warfarin has been the primary medication used to reduce the risk of thromboembolic events in patients with AF (Mega, 2011).
- Research has confirmed that warfarin is superior to antiplatelet therapy (e.g., aspirin) in the management of AF in the community even in older people (Mant et al, 2007). Aspirin should no longer be used for stroke prevention in AF; such patients should be reviewed.
- Despite its clinical efficacy, warfarin has several limitations, including drug interactions and the need for regular blood monitoring (INR should be controlled to between 2 and 3) and dose adjustments. See in Box 6.6 for contraindications to warfarin.
- As a result, alternative anticoagulants that are at least as efficacious but easier to administer have been developed and widely promoted.

- Four novel oral anticoagulant agents (NOACs) have been approved by NICE as alternatives to warfarin in patients with nonvalvular AF. These are dabigatran, rivaroxaban, apixaban, and edoxaban.
- The main advantages of these agents are that they are fixed dose, are less susceptible to interactions, and do not require monitoring.
- The main disadvantages are that there is no antidote, and it is not possible to monitor concordance in the same way as it is with warfarin.
- A number of studies have concluded that the NOACs compare favourably to warfarin in terms of both efficacy (reducing overall mortality risk and strokes) and safety profile (less intracranial bleeding) (Dentali et al, 2012; Rasmussen et al, 2012).
- For patients switching from warfarin to a NOAC, warfarin should be stopped and the NOAC started as soon as the INR is below 2.

Dabigatran

- Dabigatran is recommended by NICE as an option for the prevention of stroke in nonvalvular AF in patients with one or more of the following risk factors (NICE, 2012):
  - Heart failure: left ventricular ejection fraction below 40% or symptomatic with NYHA class II or above
  - Previous cardiovascular accident (CVA), transient ischaemic attack (TIA), or embolism

• BOX 6.6 Contraindications to Warfarin in Patients With Atrial Fibrillation (Man-Son-Hing & Laupacis, 2003)

Absolute Contraindications

- Pregnancy
- Active peptic ulcer or other active source of GI bleeding
- Current major trauma or surgery
- Uncontrolled hypertension
- A bleeding diathesis
- Bacterial endocarditis
- Alcoholism.
- Inability to control the INR

Factors Which Increase the Risk of Bleeding Slightly but Only Enough to Alter the Decision in Cases in Which the Benefit Is Already Borderline

- Current NSAID use (add gastroprotection or change to a COX-2 inhibitor)
- Activities that involve a high risk of injury

Factors Often Erroneously Thought to Contraindicate Warfarin

- Old age. The INR is no harder to control in older adults than in younger patients. There is a slight increase in bleeding risk in older patients but with increasing age the benefit from warfarin rises more than the risk
- Past history of peptic ulcer or GI bleeding, now resolved
- Hypertension controlled (blood pressure <160/90 mm Hg)
- Patients at risk of falling
- Previous stroke
- Alcohol intake of one to two drinks a day

COX, Cyclooxygenase; *GI,* gastrointestinal; *INR,* international normalised ratio; *NSAID,* nonsteroidal antiinflammatory drug.

- Age 75 years or older
- Age 65 years or older and with diabetes, CHD, or high blood pressure
- The recommended daily dose is 300 mg taken as one 150-mg capsule twice daily. Therapy is continued long term.
- Patients 80 years of age or older and those with renal impairment (eGFR 30–49 percentages) should be treated with a daily dose of 220 mg taken as one 110-mg capsule twice daily because of the increased risk of bleeding in this population.
- It is contraindicated in people with severe renal impairment (eGFR <30%) and those at increased risk of bleeding, including previous GI ulceration, recent surgery, hepatic impairment, or liver disease. Concomitant use of dronedarone is also contraindicated.
- Check renal function before starting. Do not start in any patient with severe renal impairment (eGFR <30%).

Rivaroxaban, Apixaban, and Edoxaban

- NICE has approved rivaroxaban, apixaban, and edoxaban as alternatives to warfarin in people with nonvalvular AF and one or more of the following risk factors (NICE, 2012, 2013):
  - Heart failure

- Previous CVA or TIA
- Hypertension
- Age older than 75 years
- Diabetes
- The recommended daily dose of rivaroxaban is 20 AP mg/day, reduced to 15 mg/day in people with renal impairment (eGFR 30–49 percentages). It should be taken after food.
- The dose of apixaban is 5 mg bd, reduced to 2.5 mg bd in those with renal impairment AP.
- Edoxaban is administered once a day, 60 mg for those weighing more than 60 kg and 30 mg od (Once a day) for those weighing less than 60 kg AP.

Left Atrial Appendage Closure

- The left atrial appendage (LAA) is considered the main (though not the only) site of thrombus formation leading to ischaemic stroke in people with AF (ESC, 2012). 2012 focused update of the ESC Guidelines for the management of atrial fibrillation: An update of the 2010 ESC Guidelines for the management of atrial fibrillation
- Minimally invasive techniques have been developed to occlude the LAA orifice and thereby reduce stroke risk, with results equivalent to those of warfarin (Holmes, 2009).
- At present, this procedure is only considered for patients in whom oral anticoagulation is contraindicated.

Paroxysmal Atrial Fibrillation

- Paroxysmal atrial fibrillation (PAF) is defined as recurrent (two or more) episodes of AF that terminate spontaneously in less than 7 days and usually less than 24 hours.
- Tailor the treatment to the severity.
- For patients with infrequent attacks and no serious symptoms or attacks that can be averted by avoiding a precipitating cause (e.g., alcohol or caffeine), give one of the following:
  - No drug treatment
  - A 'pill in the pocket' to be taken at the onset of an attack if the patient is suitable (Box 6.7)
- For patients with more frequent attacks or more severe symptoms:
  - Give a standard beta-blocker.
  - If the standard beta-blocker is ineffective or not tolerated, refer for specialist assessment. Other medications

• BOX 6.7 NICE Recommendations for the Suitability of a Patient for a 'Pill in the Pocket'

a. Infrequent episodes (e.g., between once per month and once per year)
b. Sufficiently reliable to use the treatment correctly
c. No structural heart disease, CHD, or left ventricular dysfunction
d. Satisfactory baseline state: systolic blood pressure >100 mm Hg and resting heart rate >70 beats/min.

CHD, Coronary heart disease; *NICE,* National Institute for Health and Clinical Excellence.

such as sotalol, flecainide, propafenone, or amiodarone may be considered. Dronedarone, which is structurally related to amiodarone, has been approved for the treatment of PAF or persistent AF but only under specialist initiation and supervision. It should not be given to patients with moderate or severe heart failure and should be avoided in patients with less severe heart failure if appropriate alternatives exist.

- NICE warns of the danger of initiating drugs other than standard beta-blockers for PAF in general practice without specialist advice because of the risk that the drug will itself cause ventricular arrhythmias. This is most likely in those with underlying heart disease. In practice, the patient will often have been assessed already by a cardiologist and had previous experience of an antiarrhythmic drug without adverse effects, obviating the need for rereferral.
- If a paroxysm becomes persistent (arbitrarily defined as lasting ≥7 days), refer for consideration of cardioversion. Refer immediately if the patient develops heart failure or hypotension.

Catheter Ablation

- The ESC guidelines recommend that catheter ablation (by pulmonary vein isolation) be considered as a first-line therapy for AF rhythm control in selected patients (i.e., those with PAF with a preference for interventional treatment and a low-risk profile for procedural complications).
- Studies have shown promising results (Nielsen et al, 2012), but the procedure carries the risk of invasive complications. In one study, complication rates were 0.6% for stroke, 1.3% for tamponade, 1.3% for peripheral vascular complications, and around 2% for pericarditis (Arbelo et al, 2012).

Anticoagulation

A patient with PAF should be considered for antithrombotic treatment according to the presence of risk factors (e.g., as assessed by CHA_2DS_2-VASc score). The risk of stroke, although less well defined in PAF, is considered to be the same as in persistent or permanent AF regardless of the number and severity of paroxysms (Friberg et al, 2010).

Atrial Flutter

- Atrial flutter should be approached in a similar way to AF, with a focus on:
  a. Rate control
  b. Rhythm control
  c. Prevention of thromboembolic complications
- It is much less common than AF and usually less well tolerated, often presenting with palpitations.
- Episodes of atrial flutter and AF can occur in the same person.
- Refer all suspected cases for specialist assessment.
- Radiofrequency catheter ablation is first-line treatment (Sawhney & Feld, 2008).

Paroxysmal Supraventricular Tachycardia

If the patient is seen during the attack:
- Get the patient to perform a Valsalva manoeuvre. This can be described to the patient as trying to breathe out forcefully while keeping the mouth closed and nose pinched or simulating straining on the toilet (Whinnett et al, 2012).
- Apply carotid sinus massage except when the patient has any of the following:
  a. Is an older adult
  b. Has IHD
  c. Is likely to be digoxin toxic
  d. Has a carotid bruit
  e. Has a history of TIAs
  Note: The BNF (British National Formulary) recommends ECG monitoring during carotid sinus massage.
- Admit if the attack continues and there is no clear history of previous attacks which have terminated themselves. Even if there is such a history, keep the patient at the surgery until the attack terminates.
- Record an ECG and give the patient a copy.
- If supraventricular tachycardia (SVT) is diagnosed from the patient's history or if the attack has terminated before admission was needed:
  - Refer for specialist confirmation and initiation of treatment. Referral should be urgent if attacks are associated with chest pain, dizziness, or breathlessness.
  - Catheter ablation is the first-line definitive management option for SVT.
  - Drug treatment is reserved for minimising symptoms while awaiting catheter ablation or for those who decline catheter ablation or in whom the procedure carries an unacceptably high risk.
  - Discuss with a cardiologist before starting an antiarrhythmic drug (e.g., sotalol, flecainide, verapamil) while awaiting the cardiology appointment.
  - A baseline ECG, with a further ECG before each dose increase, is recommended to look for prolongation of the QT interval, an indicator that there is a risk of drug-induced *torsades de pointes*. A final decision on the most appropriate drug will depend on the electropathology in the individual patient.
  - Instruct the patient in the use of the Valsalva manoeuvre and check that he or she is not smoking or misusing alcohol or caffeine.

Ventricular Tachycardia

- Ventricular tachycardia associated with loss of consciousness or hypotension is a medical emergency requiring immediate cardioversion.
- Call 999 emergency ambulance.
- Remember the ABCs (airway, breathing, circulation), oxygen, and ECG monitoring.
- If the patient is conscious but in extremis, consider IV lidocaine 100 mg if available while waiting for the ambulance.

- After discharge, prophylaxis will be needed. If amiodarone is chosen, thyroid function tests and liver function tests every 6 months are necessary.

Sick Sinus Syndrome

This requires admission for pacing. Drugs are likely to make symptoms worse because of the variability of the rhythms.

Bradycardia

- Refer all patients with bradycardia, other than sinus bradycardia, even if they are asymptomatic. A pacemaker might be needed and may be lifesaving. Untreated second-degree and complete AV block have a mortality rate of 25% to 50% in the first year after diagnosis. For this reason, even asymptomatic patients with a rate of 40 beats/min or below should be paced.
- Admit a patient in acute AV block with hypotension caused by the bradycardia. Give IV atropine if available while waiting for the ambulance.

PATIENT SUPPORT GROUPS

Arrhythmia Alliance. http://www.heartrhythmcharity.org.uk
    Atrial Fibrillation Association. https://www.facebook.com/atrialfibrillation/
    Sudden Adult Death Trust. http://www.sadsuk.org
    Cardiac Risk in the Young. http://www.c-r-y.org.uk

Prophylaxis of Infective Endocarditis

GUIDELINE

National Institute for Health and Clinical Excellence. (2016). *Prophylaxis against infective endocarditis. NICE clinical guideline 64.* Retrieved from https://www.nice.org.uk/guidance/cg64.

- Antibiotic prophylaxis aims to reduce the incidence of infective endocarditis (IE).
- The NICE guidance represented a major shift in advice on antibiotic prophylaxis.
- Do not offer antibiotics to prevent IE for any of the following procedures:
  - Any dental procedure
  - An obstetric or gynaecologic procedure or childbirth
  - A procedure on the bladder or urinary tract
  - A procedure on the oesophagus, stomach, or intestines
  - A procedure on the airways (including ear, nose, and throat and bronchoscopy)
- People with the following cardiac conditions should be regarded as being at risk of developing IE:
  - Acquired valvular heart disease with stenosis or regurgitation
  - Valve replacement

- Structural congenital heart disease, including surgically corrected or palliated structural conditions but excluding isolated atrial septal defect, fully repaired ventricular septal defect, or fully repaired patent ductus arteriosus and closure devices that are judged to be endothelialised
  - Hypertrophic cardiomyopathy
  - Previous IE
- People at risk of IE should be offered clear and consistent information about prevention, including:
  - The benefits and risks of antibiotic prophylaxis and an explanation of why antibiotic prophylaxis is no longer routinely recommended
  - The importance of maintaining good oral health
  - Symptoms that may indicate IE and when to seek expert advice
  - The risks of undergoing invasive procedures, including nonmedical procedures such as body piercing or tattooing
- In people at risk for IE, it is important to investigate and treat promptly all episodes of infection to reduce the risk of the development of endocarditis.
- If a person at risk of IE is receiving antimicrobial therapy because they are undergoing a GI or genitourinary procedure at a site where there is a suspected infection, offer an antibiotic that covers organisms that cause IE.

PATIENT INFORMATION

A range of resources are available through the British Heart Foundation's website at http://www.bhf.org.uk. Their helpline (0300 330 3311) is open Monday to Friday, 9 a.m. to 5 p.m.

Prevention of Cardiovascular Disease

GUIDELINE

National Institute for Health and Clinical Excellence. (2023). *Cardiovascular disease: Risk assessment and reduction, including lipid modification. NICE clinical guideline 181.* Retrieved from https://www.nice.org.uk/guidance/cg181.

- CVD predominantly affects people older than 50 years, and age is the main determinant of risk (NICE, 2014). There are significant gender differences in cardiovascular risk, including biological differences associated with pregnancy and menopause (Parikh, 2011), as well as differences in behavioural risk factors (Huxley & Woodward, 2011).
- Worldwide, the two most important modifiable cardiovascular risk factors are smoking and abnormal lipids (SIGN, 2017).
- The next most important modifiable cardiovascular risk factors are hypertension, diabetes, psychosocial factors (including deprivation), and abdominal obesity, but their relative effects vary in different regions of the world.

- Risk factors tend to cluster, and their effects are multiplicative, not additive. The presence of one or more of the following increases the chance that other risk factors will also be present: hypertension, increased cholesterol, inactivity, obesity, smoking, and glucose intolerance (Perry et al, 1995).
- Strategies for the prevention of CVD can be divided into primary and secondary prevention. Primary prevention is concerned with preventing the occurrence of CVD in those who are currently unaffected. Secondary prevention relates to delaying or reversing the progression of disease in those already affected. Although targeting those at highest risk is known to be most cost-effective, most countries recognise the importance of a multifaceted approach, adopting both population-based and more targeted interventions (Rose, 1981).

Primary Prevention

- For the primary prevention of CVD in primary care, a systematic strategy should be used to identify people aged older than 40 years who are likely to be at high risk, now considered to be a 10% 10-year risk after lifestyle modification. This should be done at least every 5 years.
- The following groups of people should be assumed to be at high risk based on clinical history alone and do not require risk assessment with a scoring system:
  - People who have had a previous cardiovascular event (angina, MI, stroke, TIA, or peripheral arterial disease)
  - People with diabetes (type 1 or 2) older than the age of 40 years
  - People with familial hypercholesterolaemia (FH)
- CVD risk should be estimated using information already contained in the patient's records and using a chart or computer programme based on epidemiological data such as the US Framingham Heart Study data (Anderson et al, 1991), according to:
  - Age
  - Sex
  - Lifetime smoking habit
  - Blood pressure (If treated, use pretreatment level.)
  - Serum lipids if known. (If treated, use pretreatment level.)
- A number of different validated resources are available to calculate the 10-year risk of CVD, but NICE now recommends the use of the QRISK2 assessment tool.
- Asymptomatic individuals should be considered at high risk if they are assessed as having 10% or more risk of a first cardiovascular event over 10 years. Such individuals warrant intervention with lifestyle changes and consideration for drug therapy to reduce their absolute risk.
- NICE now recommends that the QRISK2 tool be used up to and including age 84 years.
  Consider people aged 85 years and older to be at increased risk of CVD because of their age alone.
  A further consideration when assessing someone's CVD risk is the presence of xanthelasmata. A 2011 study found that xanthelasmata predicts an increased risk of cardiovascular

events, particularly in females, even if their serum lipid levels are normal (Christoffersen et al, 2011). The authors suggest that xanthelasmata may be a sign of an increased propensity to deposit lipid in soft tissues and is therefore a cutaneous marker of atheroma. There is no such increased risk with arcus corneae.

Lifestyle Changes

- *Stop smoking.* A person who smokes 20 cigarettes a day or less and stops has a risk of CHD 10 years later almost the same as in one who has never smoked. Recovery is, however, less the longer the person has smoked (Doll et al, 2004). Nicotine replacement therapy increases the rate of quitting by 50% to 70%, regardless of the setting and independent of whether support, other than brief advice, is offered (Stead et al, 2008).
- *Alcohol.* Keep alcohol intake within safe limits. Current UK recommendations are 14 units of alcohol or less per week for both males and females.
- *Take exercise.* Encourage patients to incorporate exercise into their daily lives rather than rely on visiting a gym or playing football at the weekend. Simple advice from GPs is unlikely to change behaviour; a more supportive programme is needed.
- *Manage social isolation.* Depression and lack of social support are associated with an increased risk of CVD (Bunker et al, 2003), as is the combination of high workload and low autonomy at work (Aboa-Eboule et al, 2007).
- *Control weight.* Central obesity, rather than an increased BMI, carries the greater cardiovascular risk and can be assessed by measuring the waist circumference, with a single cutoff point for each sex. Males with a waist circumference greater than 94 cm and females with a waist circumference greater than 80 cm are likely to have other risk factors for CVD. Males with a waist circumference over 102 cm (females >88 cm) are 2.5 to 4.5 times as likely to have other major cardiovascular risk factors (Han et al, 1995). Small losses of weight are possible in primary care if advice on diet and exercise is accompanied by a behavioural programme.
- *Diet.* Encourage patients to:
  - Reduce their meat and fat intake.
  - Eat oily fish at least twice a week.
  - Eat bread, pasta, and potatoes as sources of carbohydrate.
  - Eat at least five portions a day of fruit or vegetables.
  - Use olive oil and rape seed margarine instead of butter.

Intensive Management When a 10-Year Cardiovascular Risk of At Least 20% Is Detected

Lipid Lowering

- Check thyroid function tests, creatinine, liver function tests, and fasting glucose level. Note that elevated liver enzymes are not a contraindication to the use of a statin. They are not associated with subsequent statin-induced toxicity (Chalasani et al, 2004).
- Check baseline lipids. NICE no longer recommends a fasting test.

- NICE now recommends offering atorvastatin 20 mg for the primary prevention of CVD to people who have a 10% or greater 10-year risk of developing CVD. The reduction in major coronary events is likely to be 30%. How useful this is depends on the patient's baseline risk.
- NICE recommends annual medication reviews for patients and consideration of an annual, nonfasting, non-HDL cholesterol blood test to inform the discussion. Aim for a reduction of greater than 40% in non-HDL cholesterol in both primary and secondary prevention.
- Strongly encourage physical activity in all those taking statins. In combination, the mortality risk is greatly reduced in those with dyslipidaemia (Kokkinos et al, 2013).
- Warn the patient to report muscle pain or weakness; if present, check creatine kinase (CK) and thyroid-stimulating hormone (Lasker & Chowdhury, 2012).
  - If CK is 10 or more times the upper limit of normal, *stop* immediately. This is a risk of rhabdomyolysis.
  - If CK is 5 or less times normal, it is rarely clinically significant and is often related to exercise.
  - If CK is not significantly increased, suggest rechallenging with a statin at a lower dose or switching the statin (e.g., 10 mg of atorvastatin is equivalent to 40 mg of simvastatin). If myalgia recurs, try a nonstatin treatment (i.e., ezetimibe 10 mg AP).
- Continue indefinitely unless adverse effects occur.
- Be aware of interactions:
  - When macrolides (e.g., erythromycin and clarithromycin) must be prescribed, stop the statin and restart 1 week after the macrolide is finished.
  - Avoid itraconazole and ketoconazole (contraindicated with simvastatin)
  - Reduce statin dose (maximum, 20 mg of simvastatin) with amlodipine, diltiazem, verapamil, and amiodarone.
- On subsequent visits, check that the patient is taking the statin. A study from Liverpool found that a quarter of patients took their statin less than 80% of the time and had a higher mortality rate (Howell et al, 2004).

Blood Pressure Control
- Check blood pressure annually.
- Treat if levels are sustained at 140/90 mm Hg or above.
- Aim for a level of less than 140/90 mm Hg or less than 140/80 mm Hg in those with type 2 diabetes (and 130/80 mm Hg if microalbuminuria or proteinuria is present).

Talking to the Patient About Absolute Risks When Taking A Statin (Tables 6.5 and 6.6)

Secondary Prevention

Consider the following measures in those with CVD, diabetes, CKD, or primary hyperlipidaemia.
- Recommend *lifestyle changes* as for primary prevention.
- *Lipid lowering*
  - Order the tests recommended under primary prevention and give the same warnings.

TABLE 6.5 Benefits (Based on Simvastatin 40 mg/day)

Patient Characteristics	NNT Over 5 Years[a]
MI	10
Angina	13
Stroke, PVD, or diabetes	15
No CVD but a 30% 10-year CVD risk	32
No CVD but a 20% 10-year CVD risk	48

[a]Heart Protection Study Collaborative Group, 2002; Cholesterol Treatment Trialists' Collaborators, 2005.
CVD, Cardiovascular disease; MI, myocardial infarction; NNT, number needed to treat; PVD, peripheral vascular disease.

TABLE 6.6 Harms of Statins (Law & Rudnicka, 2006)

Harm[a]	NNH Over 5 Years
Rhabdomyolysis	0.00017 or 1 per 30,000 patient-years
Statin-related myopathy	0.0005 or 1 per 10,000 patient-years
Statin-related peripheral myopathy	0.0006 or 1 per 8000 patient-years

[a]Of these, only rhabdomyolysis may be irreversible, with a mortality rate of 10%. The chance of dying of rhabdomyolysis may be expressed as being 15 times less likely than being killed in a car accident. Other adverse effects are documented (depression, sleep disturbance, memory loss, sexual dysfunction, diarrhoea) but their frequency is less clear. NNH, number needed to harm.

- Offer a statin regardless of baseline cholesterol level.
- Start atorvastatin 80 mg in patients with CVD. Use a lower dose if there are potential drug interactions, a high risk of adverse effects, or patient preference.
- Recheck the serum lipids after 3 months. If TC is 4 mmol/L or greater or low-density lipoprotein (LDL) cholesterol level is 2 mmol/L or greater, consider intensifying treatment. If targets are still not reached, add ezetimibe. Other options are a fibrate (but with a warning about the increased risk of rhabdomyolysis), nicotinic acid, or an omega-3 fatty acid.
- If adverse effects occur, consider reducing the statin dose; changing to another statin; or using ezetimibe, a fibrate, or nicotinic acid.
- *Blood pressure.* Treat if levels are sustained at 140/90 mm Hg or above. Aim for a level below 140/90 or below 130/80 mm Hg in those with diabetes.
- *Antiplatelet therapy.* Recommendations for antiplatelet therapy vary in different scenarios. These are now largely specialist-led decisions:
  - Stable angina and history of MI: aspirin 75 mg/day ap for life

- ACSs
  - Unstable angina (non–ST-segment elevation MI) medically managed: aspirin 75 mg indefinitely and clopidogrel 75 mg ap/day for 12 months
  - Unstable angina with acute primary PCI: aspirin 75 mg indefinitely plus ticagrelor 90 mg bd ap for 12 months (NICE, 2011)
- ST-segment elevation MI
  - Immediate PCI followed by aspirin 75 mg indefinitely plus ticagrelor *or* prasugrel for 12 months (NICE, 2009)
  - If no PCI, use aspirin and clopidogrel for at least 1 month; then aspirin thereafter
- Elective PCI with stenting
  - Drug-eluting stents: aspirin plus clopidogrel for at least 12 months; then aspirin thereafter
  - Bare-metal stents: aspirin plus clopidogrel for a period of between 1 to 12 months; then aspirin thereafter
  - Gastroprotection (e.g., PPI) should be used with dual antiplatelet therapy.
- *ACE inhibition.* Prescribe an ACE inhibitor to all patients with CHD. Titrate to the maximum tolerated doses and continue long term.
- Prescribe a beta-blocker to all those who have had an MI. Start them in patients whose MI was in the previous 5 years and who therefore missed the opportunity to have them started in the acute stage. Patients at the highest risk benefit most from beta-blockade (e.g., those who are older than 50 years with angina, hypertension, or heart failure).
- *Eplerenone.* This aldosterone antagonist is now preferred to spironolactone in patients who have left ventricular dysfunction after MI.

Annual Workup at a Coronary Heart Disease Prevention Clinic

- *Check:*
  a. Fasting sugar, HbA1c, or both
  b. Lipid profile
  c. Urine protein
  d. Blood pressure
  e. Weight, height, and BMI
- *Proteinuria.* If 1+ or more, repeat after 1 week on the first morning specimen. If still 1+ or more, check the midstream specimen of urine, serum creatinine and electrolytes, and an ACR on a single urine sample. If the urine ACR is greater than 30, there is haematuria, or the creatinine is increased, this is significant proteinuria. (Different thresholds apply in patients with diabetes.)

Familial Hypercholesterolaemia

GUIDELINE

National Institute for Health and Clinical Excellence. (2019). *Familial hypercholesterolaemia. NICE clinical guideline 71.* Retrieved from https://www.nice.org.uk/guidance/cg71.

- FH is important because it carries a very high risk of premature cardiovascular morbidity and mortality. It is generally asymptomatic, so it is easily missed in general practice (Gill et al, 2012).
- It is present in about 1 in 500 of the population in the United Kingdom and for males carries a 50% risk of a major coronary event by the age of 50 years. In females, the risk is 30% by the age of 60 years. This risk is far higher than would be predicted from the cholesterol level alone and requires intensive therapy (high-dose statins and ezetimibe).
- The possibility of FH is raised in two situations:
  a. Opportunistic case finding
    - Ask about family history in every patient with an increased cholesterol level, especially if the TC is greater than 7.5 mmol/L or the LDL cholesterol is 5 mmol/L or greater. These cutoffs should be lowered in younger patients and in females. For instance, for a female up to 24 years, an LDL cholesterol level of 3.9 mmol/L or greater suggests FH. See the charts in the NICE guideline (NICE, 2008).
  b. Screening because of an affected relative
    - Screen children with an affected parent by the age of 10 years or by the age of 5 years if both parents are affected or if the child has clinical signs (e.g., skin lipid deposits).
    - Screen adults with a diagnosis of FH in a relative as remote as third degree or with a family history of premature CHD.
- If suspicion of FH is raised:
  - Recheck the serum lipids with a fasting specimen.
  - Check for other causes of raised cholesterol (e.g., hypothyroidism, excess alcohol consumption).
  - Ask about the family history across three generations. Accept that the patient may need to return with these details after consultation with the family.
  - Ask about symptoms of CVD.
  - Examine for evidence of CVD or skin or tendon manifestations of hyperlipidaemia.
- Make a clinical diagnosis of FH according to the Simon Broome criteria:
  - *FH exists* if the TC is greater than 7.5 mmol/L or the LDL cholesterol is greater than 4.9 mmol/L *and* tendon xanthomas are present (in the patient or a first- or second-degree relative).
  - FH is possible if one of the following is present:
    a. The TC is greater than 7.5 mmol/L or the LDL cholesterol is greater than 4.9 mmol/L *and* there is a first-degree relative with an MI before the age of 60 years or a second-degree relative with an MI before the age of 50 years.
    b. The TC is greater than 7.5 mmol/L or the LDL cholesterol is greater than 4.9 mmol/L in the patient *and* in a first- or second-degree relative (or >6.7 mmol/L or >4.0 mmol/L, respectively, in a brother or sister younger than 16 years old).

c. There is a personal or family history of premature CHD (younger than 60 years old in the individual or first-degree relative).
- NICE now recommends searching primary care records for patients who are younger than 30 years of age with a TC greater than 7.5 mmol/L and those older than their 30s with TC greater than 9 mmol/L.
- Referral is needed:
  a. *To a specialist with expertise in FH* for all with a definite or possible clinical diagnosis. Further investigation will include DNA testing for relevant mutations and family screening.
  b. *To a cardiologist* if there are symptoms of CHD. Consider referral if the patient has no symptoms but there is a family history of CHD in early adult life or the patient has two or more other risk factors for CHD.
- Cholesterol lowering in a patient with a confirmed diagnosis of FH
  - Give a high-intensity statin (e.g., atorvastatin 40 mg/day).
  - Aim for an LDL cholesterol more than 50% below the pretreated level.
  - If the target is not met, increase the statin to the maximum licensed dose, provided it is tolerated, or add ezetimibe.
  - Re-refer if the target is not met.
  - Review annually when stable. Stress that lifestyle changes are even more important in someone with FH than in the general population.

References

Aboa-Eboule, C., Brisson, C., Maunsell, E., Mâsse, B., Bourbonnais, R., Vézina, M., Milot, A., Théroux, P., & Dagenais, G. R. (2007). Job strain and risk of acute recurrent coronary heart disease events. *JAMA, 298,* 1652–1660.

Aguilar, M. I., & Hart, R. (2005). Oral anticoagulants for preventing stroke in patients with non-valvular atrial fibrillation and no previous history of stroke or transient ischemic attacks. *Cochrane Database of Systematic Reviews, 3,* CD001927.

Al-Mohammad, A., Mant, J., Laramee, P., Swain, S., & Chronic Heart Failure Guideline Development Group. (2010). Diagnosis and management of adults with chronic heart failure: Summary of updated NICE guidance. *BMJ (Clinical research ed.), 341,* c4130.

Anderson, K. M., Odell, P. M., Wilson, P. W., & Kannel, W. B. (1991). Cardiovascular disease risk profiles. *American Heart Journal, 121*(1 Pt 2), 293–298.

Appel, L. J., Moore, T. J., Obarzanek, E., Vollmer, W. M., Svetkey, L. P., Sacks, F. M., Bray, G. A., Vogt, T. M., Cutler, J. A., Windhauser, M. M., Lin, P. H., & Karanja, N. (1997). The effect of dietary patterns on blood pressure: Results from the Dietary Approaches to Stop Hypertension trial. *New England Journal of Medicine, 336,* 1117–1124.

Arbelo, E., Brugada, J., Hindricks, G., Maggioni, A., Tavazzi, L., Vardas, P., Anselme, F., Inama, G., Jais, P., Kalarus, Z., Kautzner, J., Lewalter, T., Mairesse, G., Perez-Villacastin, J., Riahi, S., Taborsky, M., Theodorakis, G., Trines, S., & Atrial Fibrillation Ablation Pilot Study Investigators. (2012). ESC-EURObservational research programme: The atrial fibrillation ablation pilot study, conducted by the European Heart Rhythm Association. *Europace, 14,* 1094–1103.

Arroll, B., Doughty, R., & Andersen, V. (2010). Investigation and management of congestive heart failure. *BMJ (Clinical research ed.), 341,* c3657.

Atrial Fibrillation Follow-up Investigation of Rhythm Management (AFFIRM) Investigators. (2002). A comparison of rate control and rhythm control in patients with atrial fibrillation. *New England Journal of Medicine, 347,* 1825–1833.

Baigent, C., Keech, A., Kearney, P. M., Blackwell, L., Buck, G., Pollicino, C., Kirby, A., Sourjina, T., Peto, R., Collins, R., Simes, R., & Cholesterol Treatment Trialists' (CTT) Collaborators. (2005). Efficacy and safety of cholesterol-lowering treatment: prospective meta-analysis of data from 90,056 participants in 14 randomised trials of statins. *Lancet (London, England), 366*(9493), 1267–1278.

Barnett, H., Burrill, P., & Iheanacho, I. (2010). Don't use aspirin for primary prevention of cardiovascular disease. *BMJ (Clinical research ed.), 340,* c1805.

Barnett, K., Mercer, S. W., Norbury, M., Watt, G., Wyke, S., & Guthrie, B. (2012). Epidemiology of multimorbidity and implications for health care, research, and medical education: A cross-sectional study. *Lancet (London, England), 380*(9836), 37–43.

Bass, C., & Mayou, R. (2002). Chest pain. *BMJ (Clinical research ed.), 325,* 588–591.

Beckett, N., Peters, R., Tuomilehto, J., Swift, C., Sever, P., Potter, J., McCormack, T., Forette, F., Gil-Extremera, B., Dumitrascu, D., Staessen, J. A., Thijs, L., Fletcher, A., Bulpitt, C., & HYVET Study Group. (2011). Immediate and late benefits of treating very elderly people with hypertension: Results from active treatment extension to Hypertension in the Very Elderly randomised controlled trial. *BMJ (Clinical research ed.), 344,* d7541.

Beckett, N. S., Peters, R., Fletcher, A. E., Staessen, J. A., Liu, L., Dumitrascu, D., Stoyanovsky, V., Antikainen, R. L., Nikitin, Y., Anderson, C., Belhani, A., Forette, F., Rajkumar, C., Thijs, L., Banya, W., Bulpitt, C. J., & HYVET Study Group. (2008). Treatment of hypertension in patients 80 years of age or older. *New England Journal of Medicine, 358,* 1887–1898.

Benson, J., & Britten, N. (2002). Patients' decisions about whether or not to take antihypertensive drugs: Qualitative study. *BMJ (Clinical research ed.), 325,* 873–876.

Brown, M. J., Cruickshank, J. K., Dominiczak, A. F., MacGregor, G. A., Poulter, N. R., Russell, G. I., Thom, S., Williams, B., & Executive Committee, British Hypertension Society. (2003). Better blood pressure control: How to combine drugs. *Journal of Human Hypertension, 17,* 81–86.

Bunker, S. J., Colquhoun, D. M., Esler, M. D., Hickie, I. B., Hunt, D., Jelinek, V. M., Oldenburg, B. F., Peach, H. G., Ruth, D., Tennant, C. C., & Tonkin, A. M. (2003). "Stress" and coronary heart disease: Psychosocial risk factors. *Medical Journal of Australia, 178,* 272–276.

Cairns, J. A., Connolly, S., McMurtry, S., Stephenson, M., & Talajic, M. (2011). Canadian Cardiovascular Society atrial fibrillation guidelines 2010: Prevention of stroke and systemic thromboembolism in atrial fibrillation and flutter. *Canadian Journal of Cardiology, 27,* 74–90.

Camm, A. J., Kirchhof, P., Lip, G. Y., Schotten, U., Savelieva, I., Ernst, S., Van Gelder, I. C., Al-Attar, N., Hindricks, G., Prendergast, B., Heidbuchel, H., Alfieri, O., Angelini, A., Atar, D., Colonna, P., De Caterina, R., De Sutter, J., Goette, A., ... Rutten, F. H. (2010). Guidelines for the management of atrial fibrillation: The Task Force for the Management of Atrial Fibrillation of the European Society of Cardiology (ESC). *Europace, 12,* 1360–1420.

Camm, A. J., Lip, G. Y., De Caterina, R., Savelieva, I., Atar, D., Hohnloser, S. H., Hindricks, G., & Kirchhof, P., (2012). 2012 focused update of the ESC Guidelines for the management of atrial fibrillation: An update of the 2010 ESC Guidelines for the management of atrial fibrillation. Developed with the special contribution of the European Heart Rhythm Association. *Europace, 14,* 1385–1413.

Chalasani, N., Aljadhey, H., Kesterson, J., Murray, M. D., & Hall, S. D. (2004). Patients with elevated liver enzymes are not at higher risk for statin hepatotoxicity. *Gastroenterology, 126,* 1287–1292.

Chen, L. Y., Sotoodehnia, N., & Bůžková, P. (2013). Atrial fibrillation and the risk of sudden cardiac death. *JAMA Internal Medicine, 173*(1), 29–35.

Chobanian, A. V., Bakris, G. L., Black, H. R., Cushman, W. C., Green, L. A., Izzo, J. L., Jr, Jones, D. W., Materson, B. J., Oparil, S., Wright, J. T., Jr, & Roccella, E. J., (2003). The seventh report of the Joint National Committee on Prevention, Detection, Evaluation, and Treatment of High Blood Pressure: The JNC 7 report. *JAMA, 289,* 2560–2571.

Christoffersen, M., Frikke-Schmidt, R., Schnohr, P., Jenson, G. B., Nordestgaard, B. G., & Tybjærg-Hansen, A. (2011). Xanthelasmata, arcus corneae, and ischaemic vascular disease and death in general population: Prospective cohort study. BM*J, 343,* d5497.

Clark, C. E., Taylor, R. S., Shore, A. C., & Campbell, J. L. (2012). The difference in blood pressure readings between arms and survival: Primary care cohort study. *BMJ (Clinical research ed.), 344,* e1327.

Clark, C. E., Taylor, R. S., Shore, A. C., Ukoumunne, O. C., & Campbell, J. L. (2012). Association of a difference in systolic blood pressure between arms with vascular disease and mortality: A systematic review and meta-analysis. *Lancet, 379,* 905–914.

Connell, P., McKevitt, C., & Wolfe, C. (2005). Strategies to manage hypertension: A qualitative study with black Caribbean patients. *British Journal of General Practice, 55,* 357–361.

Connolly, S. J., Eikelboom, J. W., Ng, J., Hirsh, J., Yusuf, S., Pogue, J., de Caterina, R., Hohnloser, S., Hart, R. G., & ACTIVE (Atrial Fibrillation Clopidogrel Trial with Irbesartan for Prevention of Vascular Events) Steering Committee and Investigators. (2011). Net clinical benefit of adding clopidogrel to aspirin therapy in patients with atrial fibrillation for whom vitamin K antagonists are unsuitable. *Annals of Internal Medicine, 155,* 579–586.

Cooper, A., Timmis, A., Skinner, J., & Guideline Development Group. (2010). Assessment of recent onset chest pain or discomfort of suspected cardiac origin: Summary of NICE guidance. *BMJ (Clinical research ed.), 340,* c1118.

Cox, K. L., Puddey, I. B., Morton, A. R., Burke, V., Beilin, L. J., & McAleer, M. (1996). Exercise and weight control in sedentary overweight men: Effects on clinic and ambulatory blood pressure. *Journal of Hypertension, 14,* 779–790.

Czernichow, S., Zanchetti, A., Turnbull, F., Barzi, F., Ninomiya, T., Kengne, A. P., Lambers Heerspink, H. J., Perkovic, V., Huxley, R., Arima, H., Patel, A., Chalmers, J., Woodward, M., MacMahon, S., Neal, B., & Blood Pressure Lowering Treatment Trialists' Collaboration. (2011). The effects of BP reduction and of different blood pressure-lowering regimens on major cardiovascular events according to baseline blood pressure: Meta-analysis of randomized trials. *Journal of Hypertension, 29,* 4–16.

Dargie, H., & McMurray, J. (1994). Diagnosis and management of heart failure. *BMJ (Clinical research ed.), 308,* 321–328.

Dentali, F., Riva, N., & Crowther, M., Turpie, A. G., Lip, G. Y., & Ageno, W. (2012). Efficacy and safety of the novel oral anticoagulants in atrial fibrillation: A systematic review and meta-analysis of the literature. *Circulation, 126,* 2381–2391.

Diao, D., Wright, J. M., Cundiff, D. K., & Gueyffier, F. (2012). Pharmacotherapy for mild hypertension. *Cochrane Database of Systematic Reviews, 8,* CD006742.

Doll, R., Peto, R., Boreham, J., & Sutherland, I. (2004). Mortality in relation to smoking: 50 years' observations on male British doctors. *BMJ (Clinical research ed.), 328,* 1519–1528.

Elliott, A. M., McAteer, A., & Hannaford, P. C. (2011). Revisiting the symptom iceberg in today's primary care: Results from a UK population survey. *BMC Family Practice. 12,* 16.

European Society of Cardiology. (2012).

Fitzmaurice, D. A., Hobbs, F. D. R., Jowett, S., Mant, J., Murray, E. T., Holder, R., Raftery, J. P., Bryan, S., Davies, M., Lip, G. Y., & Allan, T. F. (2007). Screening versus routine practice in detection of atrial fibrillation in peoples aged 65 or over: Cluster randomised controlled trial. *BMJ (Clinical research ed.), 335,* 383–386.

Friberg, L., Hammar, N., & Rosenqvist, M. (2010). Stroke in paroxysmal atrial fibrillation: Report from the Stockholm Cohort of Atrial Fibrillation. *European Heart Journal, 31,* 967–975.

Gage, B. F., Waterman, A. D., Shannon, W., Boechler, M., Rich, M. W., & Radford, M. J. (2001). Validation of clinical classification schemes for predicting stroke. *JAMA, 285,* 2864–2870.

Gill, P. J., Harnden, A., & Karpe, F. (2012). Familial hypercholesterolaemia. *BMJ (Clinical research ed.), 344,* e3228.

Goodacre, S., Cross, E., Arnold, J., Angelini, K., Capewell, S., & Nicholl, J. (2005). The health care burden of acute chest pain. *Heart (British Cardiac Society), 91,* 229–230.

Gordon, S, Hickman, M., & Pentney, V. (2012). Screening for asymptomatic atrial fibrillation at seasonal influenza vaccination. *Primary Care Cardiovascular Journal, 5,* 161–164.

Grasko, J. M., Nguyen, H. H., & Glendenning, P. (2010). Delayed diagnosis of primary hyperaldosteronism. *BMJ (Clinical research ed.), 340,* c2461.

Haasenritter, J., Bösner, S., Vaucher, P., Herzig, L., Heinzel-Gutenbrunner, M., Baum, E., & Donner-Banzhoff, N. (2012). Ruling out coronary heart disease in primary care: External validation of a clinical prediction rule. *British Journal of General Practice, 62*(599), e415–e421.

Hagens, V., Vermeulen, K., & TenVergert, E. (2004). Rate control is more cost-effective than rhythm control for patients with persistent atrial fibrillation - results from the RAte Control versus Electrical cardioversion (RACE) study. *European Heart Journal, 25,* 1542–1549.

Han, T. S., van Leer, E. M., Seidell, J. C., & Lean, M. E. (1995). Waist circumference action levels in the identification of cardiovascular risk factors: Prevalence study in a random sample. BMJ (Clinical research ed.), *311,* 1401–1405.

He, F. J., & MacGregor, G. A. (2011). Comment: Salt reduction lowers cardiovascular risk: Meta-analysis of outcome trials. *Lancet, 378,* 380–382.

Health and Social Care Information Centre. (2011). *Health Survey for England – 2011,* Chapter 3: Hypertension. Retrieved from http://www.hscic.gov.uk/

Heart Protection Study Collaborative Group. (2002). MRC/BHF Heart Protection Study of cholesterol lowering with simvastatin in 20,536 high-risk individuals: a randomised placebo-controlled trial. *Lancet (London, England),* 360(9326), 7–22. doi:10.1016/S0140-6736(02)09327-3.

Hobbs, F. D., Fitzmaurice, D. A., Mant, J., Murray, E., Jowett, S., Bryan, S., Raftery, J., Davies, M., & Lip, G. (2005). A randomised controlled trial and cost-effectiveness study of systematic screening (targeted and total population screening) versus routine practice for the detection of atrial fibrillation in people aged 65 and over. The

SAFE study. *Health Technology Assessment (Winchester, England)*. *9*(40), iii–iv, ix–x, 1–74

Hobbs, F. D., Roalfe, A. K., Lip, G. Y., Fletcher, K., Fitzmaurice, D. A., Mant, J., & Birmingham Atrial Fibrillation in the Aged Investigators and Midland Research Practices Consortium Network. (2011). Performance of stroke risk scores in older people with atrial fibrillation not taking warfarin: Comparative cohort study from BAFTA trial. *BMJ (Clinical research ed.)*, *342*, d3653.

Hodgkinson, J., Mant, J., Martin, U., Guo, B., Hobbs, F. D., Deeks, J. J., Heneghan, C., Roberts, N., & McManus, R. J. (2011). Relative effectiveness of clinic and home blood pressure monitoring compared with ambulatory blood pressure monitoring in diagnosis of hypertension: Systematic review. *BMJ (Clinical research ed.)*, *342*, d3621.

Hoefman, E., Boer, K. R., van Weert, H. C., Reitsma, J. B., Koster, R. W., & Bindels, P. J. (2007). Predictive value of history taking and physical examination in diagnosing arrhythmias in general practice. *Family Practice*, *24*(6), 636–641.

Holmes, D. R., Reddy, V. Y., Turi, Z. G., Doshi, S. K., Sievert, H., Buchbinder, M., Mullin, C. M., Sick, P., & PROTECT AF Investigators. (2009). Percutaneous closure of the left atrial appendage versus warfarin therapy for prevention of stroke in patients with atrial fibrillation: A randomised non-inferiority trial. *Lancet*, *374*(9689), 534–542.

Holt, T. A., Hunter, T. D., Gunnarsson, C., Khan, N., Cload, P., & Lip, G. Y. (2012). Risk of stroke and oral anticoagulant use in atrial fibrillation: A cross-sectional survey. *British Journal of General Practice*, *62*(603), e710–e717.

Howell, N., Trotter, R., Mottram, D., & Rowe, P. (2004). Compliance with statins in primary care. *Pharmaceutical Journal*, *272*, 23–26.

Hughes, J. W., Fresco, D. M., Myerscough, R., van Dulmen, M. H., Carlson, L. E., & Josephson, R. (2013). Randomized controlled trial of mindfulness-based stress reduction for prehypertension. *Psychosomatic Medicine*, *75*(8), 721.

Huxley, R. R., & Woodward, M. (2011). Cigarette smoking as a risk factor for coronary heart disease in women compared with men: A systematic review and meta-analysis of prospective cohort studies. *Lancet*, *378*(9799), 1297–1305.

James, M. A., & Campbell, J. L. (2012). Better prevention of stroke through screening for atrial fibrillation. *British Journal of General Practice*, *62*(598), 234–235.

Jong, P., McKelvie, R., & Yusuf, S. (2010). Should treatment for heart failure with preserved ejection fraction differ from that for heart failure with reduced ejection fraction? *BMJ (Clinical research ed.)*, *341*, c4202.

Kokkinos, P. F., Faselis, C., Myers, J., Panagiotakos, D., & Doumas, M. (2013). Interactive effects of fitness and statin treatment on mortality risk in veterans with dyslipidaemia: A cohort study. *Lancet*, *381*, 394–399.

Kostis, J. B., Wilson, A. C., Freudenberger, R. S., Cosgrove, N. M., Pressel, S. L., Davis, B. R., & SHEP Collaborative Research Group. (2005). Long-term effect of diuretic-based therapy on fatal outcomes in subjects with isolated systolic hypertension with and without diabetes. *American Journal of Cardiology*, *95*, 29–35.

Krause, T., Lovibond, K., Caulfield, M., McCormack, T., Williams, B., & Guideline Development Group. (2011). Management of hypertension: Summary of NICE guidance. *BMJ (Clinical research ed.)*, *343*, d4891.

Lasker, S. S., & Chowdhury, T. A. (2012). Myalgia while taking statins. *BMJ*, *345*, e5348.

Law, M., Wald, N., Morris, J., & Jordan, R. (2003). Value of low dose combination treatment with blood pressure lowering drugs: Analysis of 354 randomised trials. *BMJ (Clinical research ed.)*, *326*, 1427–1434.

Law, M., & Rudnicka, A. R. (2006). Statin safety: a systematic review. *The American journal of Cardiology*, *97*(8A), 52C–60C. doi:10.1016/j.amjcard.2005.12.010.

Lip, G., Chin, B., & Prasad, N. (2002). Antithrombotic therapy in myocardial infarction and stable angina. *BMJ (Clinical research ed.)*, *325*, 1287–1289.

Lip, G. Y., Andreotti, F., Fauchier, L., Huber, K., Hylek, E., Knight, E., Lane, D., Levi, M., Marín, F., Palareti, G., Kirchhof, P., & European Heart Rhythm Association. (2011). Bleeding risk assessment and management in atrial fibrillation patients. Executive Summary of a Position Document from the European Heart Rhythm Association [EHRA], endorsed by the European Society of Cardiology [ESC] Working Group on Thrombosis. *Thrombosis and Haemostasis*, *106*(6), 997–1011.

Little, P., Barnett, J., Barnsley, L., Marjoram, J., Fitzgerald-Barron, A., & Mant, D. (2002). Comparison of agreement between different measures of blood pressure in primary care and daytime ambulatory blood pressure. *BMJ (Clinical research ed.)*, *325*, 254–257.

Mackenzie, I. S., Rogers, A., Poulter, N. R., Williams, B., Brown, M. J., Webb, D. J., Ford, I., Rorie, D. A., Guthrie, G., Grieve, J. W. K., Pigazzani, F., Rothwell, P. M., Young, R., McConnachie, A., Struthers, A. D., Lang, C. C., MacDonald, T. M., TIME Study Group. (2022). Cardiovascular outcomes in adults with hypertension with evening versus morning dosing of usual antihypertensives in the UK (TIME study): a prospective, randomised, open-label, blinded-endpoint clinical trial. *Lancet*, *400*(10361), 1417–1425. doi:10.1016/S0140-6736(22)01786-X.

Man-Son-Hing, M., & Laupacis, A. (2003). Anticoagulant-related bleeding in older persons with atrial fibrillation. *Archives of Internal Medicine*, *163*, 1580–1586.

Mant, D., Hobbs, F. R., Glasziou, P., Wright, L., Hare, R., Perera, R., Price, C., & Cowie, M. (2008). Identification and guided treatment of ventricular dysfunction in general practice using blood B-type natriuretic peptide. *British Journal of General Practice*, *58*, 393–399.

Mant, J., Hobbs, F. D., Fletcher, K., Roalfe, A., Fitzmaurice, D., Lip, G. Y., Murray, E., BAFTA investigators, & Midland Research Practices Network (MidReC). (2007). Warfarin versus aspirin for stroke prevention in an elderly community population with atrial fibrillation (the Birmingham Atrial Fibrillation Treatment of the Aged Study, BAFTA): a randomised controlled trial. *Lancet (London, England)*, *370*, 493–503.

Martin, U., & Coleman, J. J. (2006). Monitoring renal function in hypertension. *BMJ (Clinical research ed.)*, *333*, 896–899.

Mayou, R., Sprigings, D., Birkhead, J., & Price, J. (2002). A randomized controlled trial of a brief educational and psychological intervention for patients presenting to a cardiac clinic with palpitation. *Psychological Medicine*, *32*: 699–706.

Mayou, R., Sprigings, D., Birkhead, J., & Price, J. (2003). Characteristics of patients presenting to a cardiac clinic with palpitations. *Quarterly Journal of Medicine*, *96*, 115–123.

Mega, J. L. (2011). A new era for anticoagulation in atrial fibrillation. *New England Journal of Medicine*, *365*(11), 1052–1054.

Myat, A., Redwood, S. R., Qureshi, A. C., Spertus, J. A., & Williams, B. (2012). Resistant hypertension. *BMJ (Clinical research ed.)*, *345*, e7473.

Nash, I. S. (2007). Reassessing normal blood pressure. *BMJ (Clinical research ed.)*, *335*, 408–409.

National Institute for Health and Clinical Excellence. (2011, August). *Hypertension: Clinical management of primary hypertension in adults (update). (Clinical guideline 127)*. Retrieved from http://guidance.nice.org.uk/CG127.

National Institute for Health and Clinical Excellence. (2013, February). *Apixaban for preventing stroke and systemic embolism in people with non-valvular atrial fibrillation. NICE TA275.* Retrieved from https://www.nice.org.uk/guidance/ta275.

National Institute for Health and Clinical Excellence. (2010, March). *Chest pain of recent onset. NICE Clinical Guideline 95.* Retrieved from https://www.nice.org.uk/guidance/cg95.

National Institute for Health and Clinical Excellence. (2010, August). *Chronic heart failure:Management of chronic heart failure in adults in primary and secondary care. NICE CG 108.* Retrieved from https://www.nice.org.uk/guidance/ng106.

National Institute for Health and Clinical Excellence. (2008, September). *Chronic kidney disease: Early identification and management of chronic kidney disease in adults in primary and secondary care. NICE CG 73.* Retrieved from http://guidance.nice.org.uk/CG73.

National Institute for Health and Clinical Excellence. (2012, March). *Dabigatran etexilate for the prevention of stroke and systemic embolism in atrial fibrillation. NICE TA249.* Retrieved from https://www.nice.org.uk/guidance/ta275.

National Institute for Health and Clinical Excellence. (2012, November). *Ivabradine for treating chronic heart failure. NICE Technology Appraisal Guidance, TA267.*

National Institute for Health and Clinical Excellence. (2010, Reissued March). *Lipid modification: Cardiovascular risk assessment and the modification of blood lipids for the primary and secondary prevention of cardiovascular disease. NICE CG 67, May 2008.* Retrieved from http://guidance.nice.org.uk/CG67.

National Institute for Health and Clinical Excellence. (2012, December). *Management of stable angina. NICE Clinical Guideline 126.* Retrieved from https://www.nice.org.uk/guidance/cg126.

National Institute for Health and Clinical Excellence. (2009, October). *Prasugrel for the treatment of acute coronary syndromes with percutaneous coronary intervention. NICE TA182.* Retrieved from https://www.nice.org.uk/guidance/ta182.

National Institute for Health and Clinical Excellence. (2012, May). *Rivaroxaban for the prevention of stroke and systemic embolism in people with atrial fibrillation. NICE TA256.* Retrieved from https://www.nice.org.uk/guidance/ta256.

National Institute for Health and Clinical Excellence. (2011, October). *Ticagrelor for the treatment of acute coronary syndromes. NICE TA236.* Retrieved from https://www.nice.org.uk/guidance/ta236.

NICE. (2007). *Secondary prevention in primary and secondary care for patients following a myocardial infarction. NICE clinical guideline 48.* Retrieved from https://www.nice.org.uk/guidance/cg48.

Nielsen, J. C., Johannessen, A., Raatikainen, P., Hindricks, G., Walfridsson, H., Kongstad, O., Pehrson, S., Englund, A., Hartikainen, J., Mortensen, L. S., & Hansen, P. S. (2012). Radiofrequency ablation as initial therapy in paroxysmal atrial fibrillation. *New England Journal of Medicine, 367,* 1587–1595.

O'Flynn, N., Timmis, A., Henderson, R., Rajesh, S., Fenu, E., & Guideline Development Group. (2011). Management of stable angina: Summary of NICE guidance. *BMJ (Clinical research ed.), 343,* d4147.

Olesen, J. B., Lip, G. Y., Hansen, M. L., Hansen, P. R., Tolstrup, J. S., Lindhardsen, J., Selmer, C., Ahlehoff, O., Olsen, A. M., Gislason, G. H., & Torp-Pedersen, C. (2011). Validation of risk stratification schemes for predicting stroke and thromboembolism in patients with atrial fibrillation: Nationwide cohort study. *BMJ (Clinical research ed.), 342,* d124.

Owan, T. E., Hodge, D. O., Herges, R. M., et al. (2006). Trends in prevalence and outcome of heart failure with preserved ejection fraction. *New England Journal of Medicine, 355,* 251–259.

Parikh, N. I. (2011). Sex differences in the risk of cardiovascular disease. *BMJ (Clinical research ed.), 343,* d5526.

Perry, I., Wannamethee, S., & Walker, M. (1995). Prospective study of risk factors for development of non-insulin dependent diabetes in middle-aged British men. *BMJ (Clinical research ed.), 310,* 560–564.

Pisters, R., Lane, D. A., Nieuwlaat, R., de Vos, C. B., Crijns, H. J., & Lip, G. Y. (2010). A novel user-friendly score (HAS-BLED) to assess 1-year risk of major bleeding in patients with atrial fibrillation: The Euro Heart Survey. *Chest, 138*(5), 1093–1100.

Rasmussen, L. H., Larsen, T. B., Graungaard, T., Skjøth, F., & Lip, G. Y. H. (2012). Primary and secondary prevention with new oral anticoagulant drugs for stroke prevention in atrial fibrillation: Indirect comparison analysis. *BMJ (Clinical research ed.), 345,* e7097.

Raviele, A., Giada, F., Bergfeldt, L., Blanc, J. J., Blomstrom-Lundqvist, C., Mont, L., Morgan, J. M., Raatikainen, M. J., Steinbeck, G., Viskin, S., Kirchhof, P., Braunschweig, F., Borggrefe, M., Hocini, M., Della Bella, P., Shah, D. C., & European Heart Rhythm Association. (2011). Management of patients with palpitations: A position paper from the European Heart Rhythm Association. *Europace, 13,* 920–934.

Rhys, G. C., Azhar, M. F., & Foster, A. (2013). Screening for atrial fibrillation in patients aged 65 years or over attending annual flu vaccination clinics at a single general practice. *Quality in Primary Care, 21*(2), 131–140.

Ritchie, L. D., Campbell, N. C., & Murchie, P. (2011). New NICE guidelines for hypertension. *BMJ (Clinical research ed.), 343,* d5644.

Rose, G. (1981). Strategy of prevention: Lessons from cardiovascular disease. *BMJ (Clinical research ed.), 282*(6279), 1847–1851.

Sacks, F. M., & Campos, H. (2010). Dietary therapy in hypertension. *New England Journal of Medicine, 362,* 2102–2112.

Salpeter, S., Ormiston, T., & Salpeter, E. (2005). Cardioselective beta-blockers for chronic obstructive pulmonary disease. *Cochrane Database of Systematic Reviews,* (4), CD003566. doi:10.1002/14651858.CD003566.pub2.

Sawhney, N. S., & Feld, G. K. (2008). Diagnosis and management of typical atrial flutter. *Medical Clinics of North America, 92*(1), 65–85.

Scottish Intercollegiate Guidelines Network. (2013, February). *Acute coronary syndromes.* Edinburgh: SIGN; 2013. (SIGN publication no.93). Retrieved from http://www.sign.ac.uk.

Scottish Intercollegiate Guidelines Network. (2010, March). *Management of diabetes: A national clinical guideline.* Retrieved from http://www.sign.ac.uk/pdf/sign116.pdf.

Sharma, A. M., Wittchen, H. U., Kirch, W., Pittrow, D., Ritz, E., Göke, B., Lehnert, H., Tschöpe, D., Krause, P., Höfler, M., Pfister, H., Bramlage, P., Unger, T., & HYDRA Study Group. (2004). High prevalence and poor control of hypertension in primary care: Cross-sectional study. *Journal of Hypertension, 22,* 479–486.

Stead, L. F., Perera, R., Bullen, C., Mant, D., & Lancaster, T. (2008). Nicotine replacement therapy for smoking cessation. *Cochrane Database of Systematic Reviews,* (1), CD000146.

Steffen, M., Kuhle, C., Hensrud, D., Erwin, P. J., & Murad, M. H. (2012). The effect of coffee consumption on blood pressure and the development of hypertension: A systematic review and meta-analysis. *Journal of Hypertension, 30*(12), 2245–2254.

Stevens, V., Obarzanek, E., & Cook, N. (2001). Long-term weight loss and changes in blood pressure: Results of the Trials of Hypertension Prevention, phase 2. *Annals of Internal Medicine, 134,* 1–11.

Taylor, C. J., Roalfe, A. K., Iles, R., & Hobbs, F. D. R. (2012). Ten-year prognosis of heart failure in the community: Follow-up data from the Echocardiographic Heart of England Screening (ECHOES) study. *European Journal of Heart Failure, 14*(2), 176–184.

Taylor, R. S., Ashton, K. E., Moxham, T., Hooper, L., & Ebrahim, S. (2011). Reduced dietary salt for the prevention of cardiovascular disease. *Cochrane Database of Systematic Reviews,* (7), CD009217.

van den Born, B. J. H., Hulsman, C. A. A., Hoekstra, J. B. L., Schlingemann, R. O., & van Montfrans, G. A. (2005). Value of routine funduscopy in patients with hypertension: Systematic review. *BMJ (Clinical research ed.), 331,* 73–76.

Wald, D. S., Law, M., Morris, J. K., Bestwick, J. P., & Wald, N. J. (2009). Combination therapy versus monotherapy in reducing blood pressure: Meta-analysis on 11,000 participants from 42 trials. *American Journal of Medicine, 122,* 290–300.

Whelton, S., Chin, A. V., Xin, X., & He, J. (2002). Effect of aerobic exercise on blood pressure: A meta-analysis for randomised controlled trials. *Annals of Internal Medicine, 136,* 493–503.

Whinnett, Z. I., Sohaib, S. M., & Davies, D. W. (2012). Diagnosis and management of supraventricular tachycardia. *BMJ (Clinical research ed.), 345,* e7769.

Wilber, J., & Barrow, J. (1972). Hypertension: Community problem. *American Journal of Medicine, 52,* 653–663.

Wolff, A., & Cowan, C. (2009). 10 steps before your refer for palpitations. *British Journal of Cardiology, 16,* 182–186.

World Health Organization. *Global Health Observatory. Raised blood pressure.* Retrieved from https://www.who.int/data/gho/indicator-metadata-registry/imr-details/3155

World Health Organisation (2023). Fact Sheets: Hypertension. https://www.who.int/news-room/fact-sheets/detail/hypertension

Writing Group of the PREMIER Collaborative Research Group. (2003). Effects of comprehensive lifestyle modification on blood pressure control. *JAMA, 289,* 2083–2093.

Xin, X., He, J., Frontini, M. G., Ogden, L. G., Motsami, O. I., & Whelton, P. K. (2001). Effects of alcohol reduction on blood pressure: A meta-analysis of randomized controlled trial. *Hypertension, 38,* 1112–1117.

7

Respiratory Problems

Kristian Brooks

CHAPTER CONTENTS

> ### PROFESSIONAL RESOURCES
>
> National Institute for Health and Care Excellence. This is a public body under the Department of Health and Social Care that generates evidence-based guidelines for use in the NHS in England and Wales. (Services in Scotland and Northern Ireland often use similar recommendations.) Available at http://www.nice.org.uk.
>
> Primary Care Respiratory Society UK. A group of primary care professionals with an interest in respiratory disease. They are active in lobbying, research, and education and publish the *Primary Care Respiratory Journal.* Their website provides online access to the journal, opinion sheets, and resources for primary care practitioners. Available at http://www.pcrs-uk.org.
>
> British Thoracic Society. The multidisciplinary society for all professionals with an interest in respiratory disease. Guidelines, quality standards, and clinical statements are available on their website, and they also publish novel research in the journal *Thorax.* Available at http://www.brit-thoracic.org.uk.

Asthma

> ### GUIDELINES
>
> National Institute for Health and Care Excellence. (2017; updated March 2021). *Asthma: Diagnosis, monitoring and*
>
> *chronic asthma management. NICE clinical guideline 80.* Retrieved from https://www.nice.org.uk/guidance/ng80.
> British Thoracic Society, Scottish Intercollegiate Guidelines Network. (2019). *British guideline on the management of asthma*. Retrieved from https://www.brit-thoracic.org.uk/quality-improvement/guidelines/asthma.

Diagnosis

Adults (17 Years of Age and Older)

- There is no single test to diagnose asthma. The diagnosis is based on the presence of typical symptoms combined with objective measures of variable airflow obstruction.
- It is important to document the basis upon which the diagnosis has been made so it is clear to future users of the clinical record.
- If the patient's symptoms change or they fail to respond to asthma treatment, then the diagnosis of asthma should be revisited. Clinical history and investigations have poor individual sensitivity and specificity for asthma, and other conditions may produce similar results.

History and Examination

- There are six key points to elicit, which may require a review of a patient's records:

a. Episodic symptoms of cough, wheeze, chest tightness, or dyspnoea. There may be clear exacerbators (e.g., exercise, cold weather, viral infections or known allergens), but there should be periods of reduced symptoms in between.

b. Variability of symptoms throughout the day. Symptoms are often worse at night, but this is not universal.

c. Wheeze, heard by a healthcare professional on auscultation

d. Personal or family history of atopy (e.g., hay fever, allergic rhinitis, or eczema)

e. Record of variable peak flow or forced expiratory volume in 1 second (FEV_1)

f. No features to suggest an alternative diagnosis (see Differential Diagnosis)

Objective Testing

- The goal of testing is to demonstrate variable airflow obstruction; therefore, it may be necessary to repeat investigations when a patient is both symptomatic and asymptomatic.

- Lung function testing does not generate aerosols, and provision of lung function testing in primary care should have resumed after the COVID-19 pandemic (Sheikh, Hamilton, & Nava, 2022).

- Investigations should be performed in the following order:

  1. *Simple spirometry.* An FEV_1/forced vital capacity (FEV_1/FVC) ratio below 0.7 is the definition of airflow obstruction. The FEV_1/FVC ratio changes with age; therefore, if the lower limit of normal (LLN) is available, then this can be used as a more accurate cutoff for airflow obstruction

  2. *Bronchodilator reversibility.* If the patient has airflow obstruction, give 400 mcg of salbutamol by metered-dose inhaler (MDI) via a spacer and repeat spirometry after 10 to 15 minutes. An improvement in FEV_1 12% or greater (and 200 mL or greater) is a positive test result.

  3. *Peak flow diary.* This can be used in patients with normal spirometry, although variable patient effort means the results are less reliable than observed testing. To increase accuracy, two or more readings per day (but ideally four or more) are required for 2 to 4 weeks; electronic meters and diaries increase compliance. Variability greater than 20%, with a typical 'sawtooth' pattern, indicates possible variable airflow obstruction.

  4. *Tests of eosinophilic inflammation.* If available, fractional exhaled nitric oxide (FeNO) is a simple test that can be performed at the same time as spirometry. Levels of 40 ppb or greater suggest eosinophilic airway inflammation, but false-positive results can be seen in allergic rhinitis, nasal polyposis, and tall people. Smokers and those on inhaled corticosteroids (ICSs) lower levels (Murugesan et al, 2023). FeNO can be supplemented by checking blood eosinophil count and immunoglobulin (Ig) E levels (total IgE and specific IgE to common aeroallergens). It should be noted that 25% of patients with asthma have 'noneosinophilic' asthma and therefore have minimal evidence of eosinophilic inflammation on testing (Carr, Zeki, & Kraft, 2018).

Making a Diagnosis

- If there is a high probability of asthma based on the initial assessment, then a 6-week trial of treatment can be started (see Management). If the patient shows a subjective and objective response to treatment, then the diagnosis of asthma is confirmed.

- If a patient does not have a typical asthma presentation, then further primary care investigations should be arranged (see Objective Testing). A treatment trial can be performed if this testing provides evidence supporting a diagnosis of asthma.

- If the patient has a poor response to a trial of treatment or there is a low probability of asthma on the initial assessment, consider investigating for other diagnoses.

- If asthma remains a possibility or the diagnosis is unclear, consider referring the patient to secondary care for a specialist opinion. Always include the results of previous investigations and treatment trials in all referrals.

Differential Diagnosis

- *Chronic obstructive pulmonary disease (COPD).* Patients usually have a greater than 20-pack-year smoking history and minimal wheeze. COPD causes obstructive spirometry with minimal reversibility and FeNO is typically negative.

- *Bronchiectasis.* This is suggested by chronic productive cough, recurrent chest infections, and positive sputum bacterial culture results (especially *Pseudomonas*). Variable airflow obstruction is caused by mucus plugging and is dependent on the effectiveness of chest clearance.

- *Occupational asthma.* Suspect in adult-onset asthma or patients with recently deteriorating asthma control. Always ask patients whether symptoms improve on days away from work. When suspected, it requires referral to specialist occupational lung disease services for further assessment.

- *Inducible laryngeal obstruction (ILO)* or *vocal cord dysfunction.* This is inappropriate partial closure of the vocal cords causing symptoms that mimic asthma but do not respond to asthma management. 'Wheezing' is often inspiratory, and ILO can also cause hypersensitivity to strong smells or aerosols, a change in voice, and a sensation of tightness or persistent mucus in the throat.

- *Dysfunctional breathing.* Breathlessness is the predominant symptom with dizziness, lightheadedness, and peripheral paraesthesia.

- *Eosinophilic granulomatosis with polyangiitis (formerly Churg-Strauss syndrome).* This is vasculitis that begins with asthma but proceeds to systemic disease with a very high serum eosinophil count. It requires specialist respiratory management.

Children (16 Years of Age and Younger)

- The typical asthma symptoms of episodic wheeze, cough, and exercise limitation are much more sensitive in children than in adults. Asthma is very unlikely when these symptoms are absent (Galant et al, 2004).
- It is important to clarify the exact nature of parent-reported 'wheeze' because this term is often used indiscriminately to refer to any abnormal respiratory sound made by a child.
- The diagnosis remains a combination of typical symptomology supported by objective measures of respiratory function (when possible).
- Testing of respiratory function is not possible in preschool children; therefore, it is pragmatic to manage patients based on symptoms and overall clinical assessment. Regular review is required in this age group to assess response to treatment.
- When a child reaches 5 years of age, objective testing should be attempted. If they are unable to reliably perform the tests, the tests should be repeated every 6 to 12 months.
- Children of school age are usually able to perform the same measures of respiratory function that are used in adults, although they may require additional training to obtain usable results.
- All children with typical symptoms and reversible airflow obstruction should be managed as having asthma. An FEV_1 improvement of 12% or greater is a positive test result in children.
- FeNO can be used when there is diagnostic uncertainty; a reading of 35 ppb or greater is positive in children. If spirometry and FeNO are inconclusive, then consider measuring peak flow readings for at least 2 weeks; 20% or greater variability is a positive test result.
- A child with obstructive spirometry but no bronchodilator reversibility and negative FeNO must be referred to secondary paediatric services for further assessment.
- Referral could also be considered in a child with typical asthma symptoms who has either failed to respond to treatment (any age) or has normal objective test results (aged 5–16 years).

Differential Diagnosis

- *Bronchiolitis.* This is seen in infants younger than 12 months. Cough, wheeze, and feeding difficulty occur over days and then plateau. These infants do not respond to bronchodilators and may require hospital review if there are any clinical concerns.
- *Viral-associated wheeze.* This is uncommon after age 5 years. It includes a short history of wheeze that gets progressively worse. Wheeze is caused by bronchospasm and tends to respond to bronchodilators.
- *Croup.* This is inflammation of the upper airway causing coryzal symptoms, stridor (inspiratory, high-pitched squeal), and a harsh barking cough. Patients require steroids, not bronchodilators.
- *Tracheal stenosis.* This can be congenital but more commonly occurs after infection, injury, or inhalation of a foreign body. Stridor is audible, and children may develop sudden and severe breathing problems if stenosis is associated with an acute event.
- *Cystic fibrosis.* Symptoms are often present from birth and include a productive cough, failure to thrive, and recurrent chest infections.
- *Primary ciliary dyskinesia.* This is associated with recurrent ear, nose, and throat symptoms, including otitis media and sinusitis.
- *Gastro-oesophageal reflux.* Children may have recurrent vomiting and may have features of aspiration, including recurrent respiratory infections and failure to thrive.
- *Congenital heart disease.* This includes persistent (rather than episodic) wheeze, failure to thrive, increased respiratory effort, excessive tachycardia, and an audible murmur.

Management

- Treatment should be started at a stage appropriate to the severity of the patient's initial presentation and escalated in a stepwise manner (summarised in Tables 7.1 and 7.2).
- Inhaler technique should always be checked before starting treatment or escalating asthma therapy.
- Any changes to a treatment regimen should be made sequentially. After a change is made, the patient should be reviewed in 4 to 8 weeks to assess response before further additions are contemplated.
- Control should be achieved by continuing on the lowest dose of treatment required to maintain adequate asthma control. This includes reducing treatment doses when

TABLE 7.1	Asthma Management in Adults
Step 1	Regular preventer: low-dose ICS
Step 2	Initial add-on therapy: inhaled LABA
Step 3	Additional control: medium-dose ICS or LTRA
Step 4	Specialist therapies: refer to specialist respiratory services

All symptomatic patients should be prescribed a SABA as reliever therapy.

ICS, Inhaled corticosteroid; *LABA*, long-acting beta-agonist; *LTRA*, leukotriene receptor antagonist; *SABA*, short-acting beta-agonist.

TABLE 7.2	Asthma Management in Children

Step 1	Regular preventer: very low-dose ICS
Step 2	Initial add-on therapy: • Younger than 5 years: LTRA • 5 years or older: LABA or LTRA
Step 3	Additional control: low-dose ICS or LTRA
Step 4	Specialist therapies: refer to specialist paediatric respiratory services

All symptomatic patients should be prescribed a SABA as reliever therapy.

ICS, Inhaled corticosteroid; *LABA,* long-acting beta agonist; *LTRA,* leukotriene receptor antagonist; *SABA,* short-acting beta-agonist.

possible and stopping all treatments that have not produced a demonstrable benefit.
• Uncontrolled asthma is more likely to be secondary to external factors rather than underdosing of asthma-specific pharmacologic therapies (see Monitoring) (Chapman et al, 2008).

Nonpharmacologic Management
• *Smoking cessation* should be considered a priority in all current smokers diagnosed with asthma. It is the most important modifiable risk factor for symptom management and the reduction of exacerbations (Polosa & Thomson, 2013).
• *Reducing secondhand smoke exposure* is also of importance, especially in children. Parents and other household members should be offered support to stop smoking.
• *Aeroallergen avoidance* can help patients with known triggers, and they should be provided with appropriate advice (see Patient Information). Chemical and physical measures for reducing house dust mite levels are of no benefit and should not be routinely recommended for asthma management (Gøtzsche & Johansen, 2008).
• *Weight loss* can lead to improvement in asthma control in both adults and children, although more than 10% weight loss may be required to obtain benefit (Ma et al, 2015). Dietary interventions and exercise programmes should be considered in overweight patients.
• *Annual influenza vaccination* is recommended for all patients with asthma who are taking regular inhaled or oral corticosteroids. The pneumococcal vaccine is only recommended for use in patients older than 65 years or taking regular oral prednisolone ($\geq$ 20 mg/day).
• *Breathing exercise programmes* led by specialist physiotherapists can be used in those with features of dysfunctional breathing patterns. They have been shown to improve asthma symptoms and overall quality of life in adults (Freitas et al, 2013).

Pharmacologic Management in Adults
Intermittent Reliever Therapy
• All patients with asthma should be provided with an inhaled short-acting beta-agonist (SABA) as reliever therapy to be used in the event of acute symptoms.
• Salbutamol is preferred to terbutaline because it has greater initial bronchodilation, although both can cause side effects such as tremor, palpitations, anxiety, and headache (Hartnett & Marlin, 1977).
• A SABA alone may be sufficient for patients with infrequent symptoms and normal spirometry results. Those with severe symptoms (especially nighttime symptoms) or using a SABA three or more times per week should be offered maintenance therapy.
• Any patient who has had an asthma attack requiring oral corticosteroids in the past 2 years should also be offered regular treatment.

Regular Preventer Therapy
• ICSs are the most effective means of improving lung function, symptoms, and frequency of asthma attacks. As such, they are the preferred option for patients requiring regular preventive treatment.
• Regular treatment improves lung function, reduces symptoms, reduces use of rescue bronchodilation, and reduces the risk of exacerbations (Adams et al, 2005a, 2005b; Adams, Bestall, & Jones, 1999).
• Most adults should be started on a low-dose ICS. There is no benefit of starting patients on higher doses, and there is a significant plateau to the treatment effect of ICS dosages beyond this initial low dose (Gaddie et al, 1973).
• Examples of low-dose ICSs are beclomethasone 200 mcg, budesonide 200 mcg, fluticasone 100 mcg, and mometasone 200 mcg. All are given twice daily. Various inhaler forms are available and should be chosen to suit the patient's needs (see Inhaler Devices).
• Although fluticasone is more potent than beclomethasone or budesonide, there is no strong evidence to suggest any particular ICS has fewer side effects.
• At low doses, the main side effects of ICS are oral candidiasis and hoarseness, both of which can be reduced by using spacer devices or rinsing the mouth with water after use. Bone density reduction and other adverse steroid outcomes are minimal at low doses, and patients should be actively reassured about their safety (Tattersfield et al, 2001).

Initial Add-On Therapy
• Many patients obtain greater benefit from adding a different agent rather than increasing the dose of ICS. This avoids exposing the patient to the increased frequency of side effects at higher ICS doses.
• If there is insufficient control on low-dose ICS, then a long-acting beta-agonist (LABA) should be added; examples include formoterol, salmeterol, and vilanterol. LABAs improve symptoms and reduce the risk of asthma

attacks but should not be used as monotherapy without ICS (Chauhan & Ducharme, 2014).

- For simplicity and to improve adherence, treatment is given in the form of a combined ICS and LABA inhaler. Again, various forms are available, and the choice mostly depends on patient preference (see Routine Review).
- The National Institute for Health and Care Excellence (NICE) suggest the use of leukotriene receptor antagonists (LTRAs) as the initial add-on therapy to ICSs in asthma. This recommendation is based on cost-effectiveness rather than clinical effectiveness; it is not recommended by the British Thoracic Society (BTS)/Scottish Intercollegiate Guidelines Network (SIGN) guidelines and is not followed by most asthma practitioners.

Maintenance and Reliever Therapy

- Maintenance and reliever therapy (MART) should be considered in patients who have recurrent asthma attacks despite low-dose ICS–LABA. It uses combined inhalers that contain formoterol (a fast-acting LABA), which is used as both regular maintenance therapy and a symptomatic reliever.
- When symptoms worsen and the patient requires increasing reliever usage, they also receive increasing doses of the preventive ICS. This can reduce the number of asthma attacks and the need for courses of oral steroids (Cates & Karner, 2013).
- Appropriate patient selection for MART is important because it requires a good understanding of how the regimen is intended to be used. Ideally, a self-management plan should be made with the patient (see Monitoring).
- Not all ICS–LABA combinations are licensed for MART regimens; therefore, the chosen product should be prescribed by the specific trade name.
- Patients should not be prescribed a SABA alongside their MART inhaler as this negates the intended benefit of increased ICS dosage with reliever use.

Additional Control

- If asthma control remains suboptimal, then the next options are either increasing the dose of ICS or adding an LTRA. If the addition of LABA has produced no subjective or objective improvement, then it should be stopped.
- Medium-dose ICSs are approximately double the low-dose ICS values: beclomethasone 400 mcg, budesonide 400 mcg, fluticasone 250 mcg, and mometasone 400 mcg (all given twice daily). When appropriate, MART can still be used with medium-dose ICS–LABA combinations inhalers.
- Although LTRAs improve lung function, symptoms, and rate of asthma attacks, they are less effective than LABAs (Chauhan & Ducharme, 2014). However, some patients may derive additional benefit from the inclusion of an LTRA to their current regimen. Montelukast (10mg, at nigh) is the most commonly used LTRA in the United Kingdom.

Specialist Therapies

- If a patient remains symptomatic despite medium-dose ICS ± LABA ± LTRA, they should be referred to secondary respiratory services for further review.
- Options at this stage include high-dose ICSs, long-acting muscarinic antagonists (LAMAs), and theophylline. Primary care clinicians may be asked to continue these treatments on a patient's regular prescription.
- Patients may also be considered for novel biologic agents, which include monoclonal antibodies to various mediators of airway inflammation. These treatments require regular specialist input and are prescribed separately by tertiary referral centres. General practitioner (GP) practices should not be asked to prescribe or monitor these treatments.
- With the advent of these further treatment options, regular oral steroid use is now avoided other than in exceptional circumstances. All patients who are unable to wean off their oral steroid dose after an acute exacerbation should be referred for specialist review.

Pharmacologic Management in Children

- Treatment options available for use in children are similar to those in adults, but it should be noted that not all preparations of SABAs, ICS,s LABAs, and LTRAs have marketing authority to be used in children. Local formularies should be checked before prescribing any branded product.
- Patients and their families may raise concerns about the use of ICSs in children. At low doses, the risks are minimal, but medium- or high-dose ICSs may be associated with systemic side effects, including reduced bone mineral density and adrenal suppression (Gray et al, 2018). Despite causing an initial reduction in growth velocity, final height is not affected by ICS use (Agertoft & Pedersen, 2000). Patients younger than 16 years of age should have their growth monitored annually.
- It is important to provide reassurance that ICSs reduce the frequency of asthma attacks and result in fewer courses of oral steroids, which pose a greater danger than regular ICS use.

Children 5 to 16 Years of Age

- All patients should be offered a SABA as reliever therapy; this may be sufficient for those with minimal symptoms and normal lung function.
- The indications for maintenance therapy are the same as in adults (i.e., uncontrolled symptoms on SABA alone, symptoms three or more times per week, nocturnal symptoms, or an asthma attack requiring oral steroids in the past 2 years).
- First-line treatment is very low-dose ICS: beclomethasone 100 mcg, budesonide 100 mcg, or fluticasone 50 mcg. (Mometasone is not available at very low doses.) All are given twice daily.
- Initial add-on therapy to very low-dose ICSs can be either an LABA or LTRA. Both have evidence to support

their use in this age group, but neither has been shown to be superior (Chauhan & Ducharme, 2014). They should be trialled sequentially (not simultaneously) and stopped if there has been no benefit.

- MART is only licensed for use in children 12 years of age or older, although the only available ICS–LABA combination are Symbicort Turbohaler (100/6 and 200/6 forms) and DuoResp Spiromax (160/4.5 form).
- If further treatment escalation is warranted, then low-dose ICS can be used: beclomethasone 200 mcg, budesonide 200 mcg, fluticasone 100 mcg, or mometasone 200 mcg (all taken twice daily).
- If there is an inadequate response to low-dose ICSs, the patient should be referred to specialist paediatric services for review and consideration of more intensive treatments.
- Medium-dose ICSs and theophylline should not be started in primary care; these patients should be under the supervision of specialist paediatric services.

Children Younger Than 5 Years of Age

- A SABA should be given as reliever therapy to all patients.
- Because of the difficulty of confirming asthma in very young children, a trial of low-dose ICS (e.g., beclomethasone 200 mcg twice a day) may be used as a diagnostic tool in patients with suspected asthma.
- After 8 weeks of low-dose ICS, it is important to stop treatment and observe the child for up to 4 weeks amended for clarity to see if symptoms recur. This is to exclude coincidental improvement because of an alternative diagnosis (e.g., bronchiolitis or viral-associated wheeze).
- If symptoms improve with the treatment trial, then the child can be started on regular very-low dose ICS (as per management of patients 5–16 years of age).
- In children who are unable to take ICSs or when ICSs have not sufficiently controlled their symptoms, an LTRA can be added (Knorr et al, 2001). LABAs are not licensed for patients in this age category.
- If the use of very low-dose ICSs or LTRAs has been unsuccessful, then referral to specialist paediatric services is appropriate.

Inhaler Devices

- The effectiveness of inhaled therapy depends heavily on the patient's inhaler technique. This should be checked before an inhaler is prescribed, when considering treatment escalation, and during every routine asthma review.
- Inhalers should always be prescribed by brand name to ensure patients receive the inhaler devices they are used to. If patients are prescribed separate preventer and reliever inhalers, the same device type should be used for each inhaler to reduce the risk of user error.

Types of Devices

- Inhalers are either MDIs or dry powder inhalers (DPIs). MDI can be pressurised (pMDI) or breath actuated; all DPIs are breath actuated.

- pMDIs require the patient to synchronise pressing the inhaler canister and breathing in at the same time. This can be somewhat overcome by using a spacer.
- Breath-actuated devices avoid the need to coordinate these two actions; the dose is instead triggered by taking a deep breath from the mouthpiece. A critical flow rate is required to activate the inhaler, which may be a limiting factor for some patients.
- All types of inhaler device are used incorrectly by up to three-quarters of patients, although pMDIs without spacers are particularly prone to this. With effective training, correct usage of all inhaler types can improve to approximately 80% (Brocklebank et al, 2001).
- The RightBreathe website and app contains videos demonstrating correct technique for all inhalers available in the United Kingdom (see Patient Information).

Choosing a Device

- Choice of inhaler device should be individualised to the patient. Factors to be considered include:
  a. *Patient preference.* Choice of inhaler device may be affected by any number of subjective factors that are relevant to the individual patient. These may include device size and portability, the patient's lifestyle, ease of use, and side effects. Ultimately, the correct device is the one which the patient accepts for regular use.
  b. *Treatment regimen.* The choice of device may be limited by the intended asthma treatment. Local formularies should be checked to see which devices are available.
  c. *Device effectiveness.* In adults, there is no significant difference in the effectiveness of drug delivery between pMDI and DPI regardless of whether a spacer is used (Brocklebank et al, 2001).
     In children 5 years of age or older, pMDI is as effective as DPI, provided a spacer is used (Brocklebank et al, 2001; Ram et al, 2001). In children younger than 5 years, there is no evidence to compare effectiveness of different devices; in practice, a pMDI with a spacer and a face mask is normally used.
  d. *pMDI coordination.* The coordination required for pMDI inhalers may not be possible for some patients. Additionally, those with significant arthritis may lack the dexterity required to activate pMDI devices.
  e. *Spacers.* Spacers improve pMDI effectiveness in younger patients and remove the need to coordinate the delivery action in all patients. However, many patients are not willing to carry a spacer device with them at all times
  f. *Peak inspiratory flow rate (PIFR).* Breath-actuated devices require significant breath strength to be used correctly. PIFR can be determined by using inspiratory flow meters such as the In-Check DIAL device. PIFR greater than 30 L/min (and ideally >60 L/min) is required for optimal use of breath-actuated inhalers.

g. *Environmental impact.* MDI devices use compressed gas, which has high global warming potential and contributes 3.5% of the total NHS carbon footprint (House of Commons Environmental Audit Committee, 2018). All prescribers should consider using DPI when they are likely to equally effective.

Monitoring

- Patients receiving asthma treatment should be reviewed regularly by a GP or trained asthma nurse. This should be at least annually but may be more frequent in patients with suboptimal control. This allows care to be targeted to patients at higher risk of further deterioration or future asthma attacks (Royal College of Physicians, 2014).
- Inadequate monitoring, failure to escalate treatment appropriately, and underuse of written management plans are all associated with increased risk of fatal asthma attacks.
- Face-to-face consultations are often preferred by patients, but telephone reviews are equally effective, more cost-effective, and may suit some patients (Pinnock et al, 2007).
- Routine review should include three key components (Pinnock et al, 2010):
  1. Assess overall asthma control.
  2. Identify and address any reasons for poor control.
  3. Facilitate supported self-management strategies to maintain control.

Assessing Overall Asthma Control

- *Initial screening questions.* Underreporting of symptoms is common in asthma (Haughney et al, 2004). Using the Royal College of Physicians' 'three questions' (Table 7.3) allows for a standardised approach to screening during routine review (Thomas et al, 2009). A negative response to all three questions suggests good control, whereas having two or three positive answers indicates poor control (Pinnock et al, 2012).
- *Patient-reported outcomes.* The Asthma Control Questionnaire and Asthma Control Test are well-validated methods for obtaining a subjective measure of a patient's asthma control (Juniper et al, 2006; Nathan et al, 2004). They should be completed without the assistance of the clinician and can be given to the patient in the waiting area before the start of a consultation.
- *Use of relief medications.* Good asthma control is associated with minimal need for reliever therapy. Patients

TABLE 7.3	Royal College of Physicians 'Three Questions' for Asthma

In the past month:

1. Have you had difficulty sleeping because of your asthma symptoms (including cough)?
2. Have you had your usual asthma symptoms during the day (cough, wheeze, tight chest, or breathlessness)?
3. Has your asthma interfered with your usual activities (housework, work or school, and so on.)?

prescribed two or more SABA inhaler devices per month or using SABA three or more times per week are at high risk for asthma attacks and require urgent assessment of the reasons for their poor asthma control.

- *Frequency of asthma attacks.* Acute attacks requiring courses of oral steroids are markers of uncontrolled asthma. All patients requiring three or more courses of steroids in 12 months (despite optimisation of their asthma treatment) should be offered referral to specialist respiratory services.
- *De-escalating treatment.* A reduction in the patient's maintenance therapy should be contemplated when a patient has achieved acceptable asthma control for 3 months or more. The risks and benefits of reducing treatment should be discussed with the patient and a plan made for monitoring the response (this may include self-monitoring of symptoms or peak flow measurements). Stopping ICSs completely is often not advisable.

Identifying and Addressing Any Reasons for Poor Control

- If assessment indicates poor asthma control, systematically consider the possible causes:
  a. *Inhaler technique.* Inhaler technique should be checked with every patient at every asthma review. If required, the patient should receive training on the correct use of their inhaler devices. Placebo devices are widely available and are particularly helpful in assessing technique. If the patient is unable to use an inhaler, then consider switching to an alternative device or using a spacer (see Inhaler Devices).
  b. *Treatment adherence.* Patients may not be a reliable source for assessing their overall treatment compliance. Adherence can be objectively assessed by comparing the number of pharmacy-collected prescriptions with the expected number of prescriptions.
  c. *Smoking.* Current smokers have worse asthma control, an increased number of asthma attacks, and worse lung function than nonsmokers (Tiotiu et al, 2021). Smoking also reduces the effectiveness of ICSs, and smokers subsequently need higher ICS doses (Lazarus et al, 2007). Smoking cessation advice should be given to current smokers at every review, and nicotine replacement therapy should be actively encouraged.
  d. *Comorbidities.* Any pulmonary, cardiac, or systemic comorbidities that may be contributing to respiratory symptoms should be addressed. In appropriate patients, this may include referral to pulmonary rehabilitation. Rhinitis is present in more than 80% of people with asthma, and symptomatic patients should be managed with intranasal corticosteroids. This has not been shown to improve asthma control, but it may improve quality of life (Simons, 1999).
  e. *Medications.* Beta-blockers (oral and ocular) are contraindicated in people with asthma. Nonsteroidal antiinflammatory drugs (NSAIDs) and aspirin may also cause deterioration in asthma control.

f. *Occupation.* Ask about any recent change in job or whether the patient's duties have changed in their current position. The patient may notice their symptoms improve on days away from work or when on holiday. The patient should be referred to an occupational lung disease clinic if there is a possibility of occupational asthma or work-aggravated asthma.

g. *Psychosocial factors.* Deteriorating asthma control may be caused by mental health disorders, alcohol and drug abuse, learning difficulties, financial troubles, social isolation, or severe domestic stress. These elements should be recognised and their impact on asthma control discussed with the patient.

- *Review the diagnosis.* Failure to respond to treatment may imply that the diagnosis of asthma is incorrect. Review the evidence for which the diagnosis was made and repeat any equivocal objective investigations. If there is suspicion that an alternative diagnosis may be present, referral to specialist respiratory services should be considered (see Differential Diagnosis).

- *Increase asthma therapy.* If no other causes for poor control are identified, then asthma-specific treatment can be escalated as per published evidence-based guidelines (see Pharmacologic Management).

Facilitating Supported Self-Management Strategies to Maintain Control

- Asthma is a chronic condition with variable symptoms. Self-management strategies allow patients to cope with the impact of their disease and help them maintain long-term control, particularly by identifying the signs and symptoms of both acute and chronic deterioration.

- Every asthma consultation is an opportunity to review, reinforce, and extend asthma knowledge and skills. Education should aim to empower patients to be in control of their asthma and should include the provision of written Personal Asthma Action Plans (PAAPs), which have been shown to reduce hospitalisations, emergency consultations, days off work or school, and nocturnal symptoms (Gibson et al, 2003; Wolf et al, 2003).

- All patients with asthma should be offered a PAAP, which should be tailored to the individual patient, and include (Kouri et al, 2017):
  a. A description of their regular medications and when to take them
  b. How to monitor their condition, based on symptoms or peak flow measurements, and who to contact on a nonurgent basis if their asthma worsens
  c. How to recognise an asthma attack and information on increasing ICSs or starting oral steroids. It should also include when to call 999 or seek urgent medical assistance (see Acute Asthma).

- In general, adult PAAPs should advise patients to quadruple their ICS dose at the start of an asthma attack and continue this for 14 days to reduce the risk of requiring oral steroids (McKeever et al, 2018). Those using combined ICS–LABA inhaler devices may require a separate ICS inhaler to achieve this. It is important to be aware that patients who are more than 90% adherent with their regular medications may gain no benefit from this increase in their ICS dose.

- Rescue packs of oral steroids may be given to patients with a history of frequent or severe exacerbations. The indications for using these packs should be clearly documented in the patient's PAAP and the patient reviewed before further rescue packs are dispensed.

- *Exercise-induced asthma* may need to be specifically addressed for some patients. In most cases, it represents poorly controlled asthma, and treatment should be escalated as per standard recommendations (see Pharmacologic Management).

- The patient's PAAP should advise on the use of SABAs immediately before exercise (Raissy et al, 2008).

- Examples and further guidance on PAAPs can be found on the Asthma + Lung UK website at https://www.asthmaandlung.org.uk/conditions/asthma/your-asthma-action-plan.

Acute Asthma

- Delays in recognition of an asthma attack and seeking further medical attention are the commonest contributors to asthma deaths.

- Most deaths occur in those with chronic severe asthma, although fatal asthma attacks have also occurred in patients with mild to moderate disease (Harrison et al, 2000). Severe asthma includes patients on multiple asthma therapies, those with previous hospitalisation for asthma exacerbations, and those using excessive amounts of SABAs (Suissa, Blais, & Ernst, 1994).

- Adults and children with adverse psychosocial factors are also at risk of severe asthma attacks, and these patients should be highlighted during regular asthma review (SIGN, 2019) (Box 7.1).

- Severe asthma attacks usually progress slowly over at least 6 hours; in 80% of cases, they develop over more than 48 hours (Turner et al, 1998). Therefore, in most cases,

---

• BOX 7.1 Adverse Behavioural and Psychosocial Features Associated with Increased Risk of Developing Near-Fatal or Fatal Asthma (SIGN, 2019)

Nonadherence with treatment or monitoring	Alcohol or drug abuse
Failure to attend appointments	Obesity
Fewer general practitioner contacts	Learning difficulties
Frequent home visits	Employment problems
Self-discharge from hospital	Income problems
Psychiatric illness or self-harm	Social isolation
Current or recent major tranquiliser use	Childhood abuse
Denial	Severe domestic, marital, or legal stress

there is an opportunity to intervene to reduce the number of attacks that require hospitalisation.

- All patients with asthma should have their own peak flow meters and a PAAP with clear instructions for self-treatment in the event of an asthma attack.
- The routine prescribing of antibiotics for asthma attacks is not required unless there are specific features of possible bacterial infection (e.g., purulent sputum).

Acute Asthma in Adults

Assessment

- The initial assessment includes key parameters that allow for immediate stratification of acute asthma severity (Table 7.4):
  a. Clinical features: severity of dyspnoea, auscultation of the chest, use of accessory muscles, level of consciousness
  b. Peak expiratory flow (PEF): compared with the patient's best (or their predicted if best PEF within 2 years is unknown)
  c. Heart rate and respiratory rate
  d. Peripheral oxygen saturations
  e. Blood pressure
- Any features of life-threatening asthma should trigger urgent admission to hospital. Whilst awaiting transfer, initial treatment can be administered in the GP practice.
- All patients who have previously had a near-fatal asthma attack are at significantly higher risk and should always be admitted to hospital even if their presentation is moderate.

Initial Treatment

1. *Oxygen.* To maintain oxygen saturation (SpO_2) at 94 to 98%.
2. *Bronchodilators.* In moderate asthma attacks, salbutamol should be given via MDI and spacer: 1 puff every minute, up to a maximum of 10 puffs
   In acute-severe or life-threatening asthma, oxygen-driven nebulised salbutamol 5 mg is preferred (if available).

   Nebulised ipratropium 0.5 mg should be added in life-threatening asthma.
3. *Steroids.* Prednisolone 40 to 50 mg or intravenous (IV) hydrocortisone 100 mg if the oral route is unavailable.
4. *Reassess.* If there are any features of acute severe asthma after the initial management, the patient must be admitted to hospital and continued on oxygen-driven nebulisers whilst awaiting transfer.

   If symptoms, respiratory rate, and heart rate improve and PEF is greater than 50% best or predicted, then continue the patient's usual asthma treatment and give prednisolone 40 mg for minimum 5 days.
5. *Review.* Arrange for a review of asthma treatment and revision of PAAP after the patent has returned to baseline. All patients admitted to hospital should have GP review within 2 working days of discharge, but should also remain under specialist follow-up for at least 12 months.

Acute Asthma in Children

Assessment

- Assessing children younger than 5 years of age is difficult, especially because of the common alternative causes of acute wheeze in this age group (e.g., bronchiolitis and viral-associated wheeze).
- The initial priority is determining the severity of the patient's presentation (Table 7.5). Assess the child's heart rate, respiratory rate, and degree of breathlessness and whether they are agitated or confused. Oxygen saturations should be checked if pulse oximetry is available.
- PEF can be helpful in children who are able to use the device. However, PEF measurements in children during an asthma attack may be significantly more unreliable than when they are well, and these measurements must not be the sole indicator for treatment decisions.

TABLE 7.4	Assessing Level of Asthma Attack Severity in Adults in General Practice
Moderate	Peak flow 50%–75% of best or predicted
	No features of acute-severe or life-threatening asthma
Acute-severe	Peak flow 33%–50% of best or predicted
	Respiratory rate ≥25 breaths/min
	Heart rate ≥110 beats/min
	Unable to complete sentences in one breath
Life threatening	Peak flow <33% of best or predicted
	SpO_2 <92%
	Silent chest, cyanosis, or poor respiratory effort
	Arrhythmia or hypotension
	Exhaustion or altered consciousness

SpO_2, Oxygen saturation.

TABLE 7.5	Assessing Level of Asthma Attack Severity in Children in General Practice
Moderate	SpO_2 ≥92%
	No features of acute-severe or life-threatening asthma
Acute-severe	SpO_2 <92%
	Respiratory rate >30 breaths/min (aged older than 5 years), >40 breaths/min (aged 2–5 years)
	Heart rate ≥125 beats/min (aged older than 5 years), >140 beats/min (aged 2–5 years)
	Too breathless to talk or feed
	Use of accessory neck muscles
Life-threatening	SpO_2 <92% plus ≥1 of: • Confusion • Agitation
	• Silent chest
	• Cyanosis
	• Poor respiratory effort

SpO_2, Oxygen saturation.

- All children with life-threatening asthma should be immediately referred to hospital for emergency management. Treatment can be started and continued whilst this is being arranged.

Initial Treatment

Treatment follows the same principles as in adults, although the treatment doses are different:

1. *Oxygen.* This is given via facemask to maintain SpO_2 at 94% to 98%.
2. *Bronchodilators.* In moderate asthma attacks, children of all ages can be given salbutamol via MDI and spacer. Give 1 puff every minute according to response (maximum 10 puffs).

   In acute severe or life-threatening asthma, it is preferable to give salbutamol by oxygen-driven nebuliser (2.5 mg if 2–5 years of age; 5 mg if older than 5 years of age). Nebulised ipratropium 0.25 mg should be added in life-threatening asthma (same dose in all ages).
3. *Steroids.* 2 to 5 years of age: prednisolone 20 mg or IV hydrocortisone 50 mg

   Older than 5 years of age: prednisolone 30 to 40 mg or IV hydrocortisone 100 mg
4. *Reassess.* If there is a poor response to treatment, regardless of the initial severity assessment, then the patient should be admitted to hospital.

   There should be a lower threshold for admission in patients who present later in the day, have had previous severe attacks, or when there is concern about their social circumstances.

   If there is a good response to treatment, then SABA can be used up to every 4 hours. If symptoms recur within 4 hours, then repeat medical review should be sought. Prednisolone should be continued for 3 minimum to 5 days.
5. *Review.* If admission is not required, a primary care review should take place within 48 hours. Maintenance asthma treatment and the patient's PAAP should be reconsidered at this point.

   If the patient has had a previous asthma attack within the past 12 months, referral to a specialist paediatric asthma clinic should be made.

PATIENT INFORMATION

Asthma + Lung UK (previously known separately as 'Asthma UK' and 'British Lung Foundation'). Provides patient information leaflets about asthma. Resources such as Personalised Asthma Action Plans can be ordered or downloaded from their website. They also run support groups and the 'Breathe Easy' programme. Telephone helpline: 0300 222 5800. Available at http://www.asthmaandlung.org.uk.

Allergy UK. Charity that runs a dedicated helpline, support network, and online forum for those with allergy and intolerance. Also contains advice on allergen avoidance. Telephone helpline: 01322 619 898. Available at http://www.allergyuk.org.

Right Breathe. Online resource containing dosing information, safety advice, and instructional videos for all inhalers available in the United Kingdom. Available at https://www.rightbreathe.com.

Chronic Obstructive Pulmonary Disease

GUIDELINES

Global Initiative for Chronic Obstructive Lung Disease (GOLD). (2023).
Global strategy for prevention, diagnosis and management of COPD: 2023 report. https://goldcopd.org/2023-gold-report-2/

National Institute for Health and Care Excellence. (2018; updated 2019). *Chronic obstructive pulmonary disease in over 16s: Diagnosis and management. NICE guideline 115.* Retrieved from https://www.nice.org.uk/guidance/ng115.

National Institute for Health and Care Excellence. (2021; updated 2023). *Tobacco: preventing uptake, promoting quitting and treating dependence. NICE guideline 209.* Retrieved from https://www.nice.org.uk/guidance/ng209.

Clinical Assessment

- Approximately 1.4 million people in the United Kingdom have COPD, but it is estimated there are up to 2 million undiagnosed patients. Almost 25% of those diagnosed wait 5 years or more for their diagnosis (Nacul et al, 2011).
- The signs and symptoms of COPD are nonspecific, but the diagnosis requires:
  a. Progressive shortness of breath
  b. A significant smoking history (or exposure to other smoke or dusts)
  c. Evidence of fixed airflow obstruction on spirometry
- COPD is a particularly heterogenous disease, with a highly variable set of symptoms and complications and no set disease path for every patient.
- Assessment should centre on identifying particular 'treatable traits'. This subsequently helps provide effective patient-focussed management rather than applying a one-size-fits-all model (Cardoso et al, 2021).

History Taking

- Shortness of breath is the principal symptom of COPD, but it can be difficult to quantify objectively. Asking the patient to estimate their exercise tolerance (how long they can walk before having to stop) is useful but is affected by nonrespiratory factors.
- Chronic cough, regular sputum production, and wheeze are other symptoms which may raise suspicion about the presence of COPD.
- COPD increases the risk of respiratory tract infections, especially over the winter months. Any previous hospitalisations or antibiotic courses required for chest infections should be documented. (This may require review of the patient's records.)
- Direct questioning can be used to identify symptoms of relevant associated conditions and complications of COPD:
  a. *Asthma.* Variable wheeze and cough, with relative normality in between. Clear triggers for symptoms, often worse at night.
  b. *Bronchiectasis.* Large-volume sputum production and repeated chest infections.

c. *Cor pulmonale.* Right-sided heart failure can cause peripheral oedema, cyanosis, lightheadedness, and syncope.

d. *Lung cancer.* Weight loss is common in both cancer and COPD, but haemoptysis and pain are unusual in COPD and should raise suspicion.

e. *Respiratory failure.* Raised CO_2 from nocturnal hypoventilation can cause morning headaches, increasing fatigue and poor cognition.

- Smoking causes 95% of COPD in the United Kingdom, with smoking duration being of more importance than pack years (Chang et al, 2021). A smoking history is crucial and includes whether household members smoke as well.
- Occupations such as mining and construction that inherently surround workers with smoke and dust carry an additional risk of COPD. Check whether personal protective equipment was worn whilst working.
- The patient's social circumstances should be established. COPD can drastically affect a person's ability to provide self-care; even if they do not have care needs at the time of initial consultation, they may arise over time. Understanding the patient's support network will allow appropriate intervention if required in the future.

Examination

- Document the patient's weight and body mass index (BMI) at every routine appointment; a low BMI is associated with a poor prognosis in COPD (Eriksson et al, 2017). Weight loss and anorexia may also be signs of underlying malignancy or chronic infection.
- Peripheral oxygen saturations must also be measured at every routine review.
- Examination of the chest is often entirely normal in early COPD. Hyperexpansion of the chest, widespread reduced air entry, and basal crackles may develop as the disease progresses.
- Focal chest signs are unusual in COPD and may be a presenting feature of lung cancer. Finger clubbing, cervical or supraclavicular lymphadenopathy, and unilateral basal dullness to percussion (suggesting pleural effusion) are all uncommon in patients with COPD but are potential signs of lung cancer.
- Cardiac examination may reveal signs of cor pulmonale, including a systolic murmur (tricuspid regurgitation), bounding pulse, peripheral oedema, raised jugular venous pressure, and plethoric conjunctivae.

Investigations

- *Spirometry* is essential to make a diagnosis of COPD and should be performed during a period of clinical stability, at least 6 weeks after an exacerbation. Irreversible airflow obstruction must be demonstrated: defined as a FEV_1/FVC ratio less than 0.7.
- The FEV_1/FVC ratio naturally declines with age, so using 0.7 as a cutoff can lead to overdiagnosis of COPD in older adult patients. The LLN should be used instead if available (van Dijk et al, 2015).

- *Bronchodilator reversibility testing* should always be performed after airflow obstruction is proven. A dose of 400 mcg of salbutamol is given via a spacer and spirometry repeated after 15 minutes; if the FEV_1/FVC ratio remains below 0.7, this supports the diagnosis of COPD.
- Even if the FEV_1/FVC ratio remains below 0.7, bronchodilator use may lead to an improvement in airflow obstruction. If FEV_1 improves by 12% or greater (and ≥ 200 mL), then the patient may have combined COPD and asthma.
- *Chest radiography* is not required for diagnosis but should be considered in every patient diagnosed with COPD. The purposes of radiography are to establish a baseline in case of future deterioration and to screen for alternative diagnoses and comorbidities (e.g., pulmonary fibrosis, bronchiectasis, lung cancer).
- A *full blood count* should be performed to check the eosinophil count and look for polycythaemia (haematocrit >0.55).
- *Sputum culture and sensitivity* should be performed in all patients with a productive cough to look for evidence of bacterial colonisation.
- Detailed pulmonary function testing, further imaging (e.g., computed tomography of the chest), echocardiography, and serum alpha-1-antitrypsin testing should not be performed routinely in primary care unless other indications are present.

Severity Assessment

Airflow Obstruction

- Postbronchodilator FEV_1 is used to classify the severity of airflow obstruction:
  a. Mild: FEV_1 greater than 80% of predicted
  b. Moderate: FEV_1 50% to 80% of predicted
  c. Severe FEV_1 30% to 50% of predicted
  d. Very severe: FEV_1 less than 30% of predicted
- The degree of airflow obstruction is linked to overall prognosis and can be used for monitoring disease progression. However, it correlates poorly with symptoms and response to bronchodilator therapy, so it should not be used to inform management decisions (Albert et al, 2012; Han, 2013).

Patient-Reported Symptoms

- The modified Medical Research Council Dyspnoea Scale (mMRCD) relates breathlessness to functional disability and predicts future mortality risk (American Thoracic Society, 1982; Nishimura et al, 2002) (Table 7.6).
- A multidimensional model, the COPD Assessment Tool (CAT), can be used to gauge a more comprehensive view of the symptomatic burden of COPD (Jones et al, 2009). It is available at www.catestonline.org.
- Patients with mMRCD of 2 or greater or CAT score of 10 or greater should be considered for more aggressive COPD management.

Grade	Degree of Breathlessness Related to Activities
TABLE 7.6 — Modified Medical Research Council Dyspnoea Scale Dyspnoea Scale (American Thoracic Society, 1982)	
0	I only get breathless with strenuous exercise.
1	I get short of breath when hurrying on the level or walking up a slight hill.
2	I walk slower than people of the same age on the level because of breathlessness, or I have to stop for breath when walking at my own pace on the level.
3	I stop for breath after walking about 100 m or after a few minutes on the level.
4	I am too breathless to leave the house, or I am breathless when dressing and undressing.

Exacerbation Risk

- The frequency and severity of COPD exacerbations should be documented, making particular note of how many hospital admissions have been required.
- The best predictor of future exacerbation risk is a history of previous exacerbations, but increasing airflow obstruction and an increased eosinophil count are also associated with increased exacerbation rate.

Comorbidities

- Other chronic diseases represent an additional component of severity in COPD and can affect mortality and hospitalisation rates, irrespective of the degree of airflow obstruction (Mannino et al, 2008).
- Cardiovascular disease, metabolic syndrome, osteoporosis, and mental health disorders are regularly seen in patients with COPD and require separate management (Soriano et al, 2005).

Management

- There are no therapies currently available that can reverse the underlying pathology of COPD. Indeed, the only treatment that can affect disease progression is smoking cessation, which should be encouraged at every opportunity (Kohansal et al, 2009).
- All other management options aim to improve symptoms and quality of life; the treatment goals are individual to each patient. Management includes pharmacologic, behavioural, and social interventions tailored to the patient's needs and wishes. This is the 'treatable traits' model of COPD, which relies on a thorough patient assessment, which will be an evolving process throughout the patient's lifetime (Agusti et al, 2016).
- Lung function should not be used on its own when assessing the response to any pharmacologic or non-pharmacologic treatment. Consider symptoms, ability to complete activities of daily living, exercise tolerance, and exacerbation frequency as additional measures of effectiveness.
- All patients with COPD should have at least annual review in primary care. This should increase to every 6 months in those with very severe disease so that palliative care can be instigated at the correct time.

Pharmacologic Management

- It is essential that inhaler technique is checked by a trained professional before starting any inhaled therapy. It should be rechecked at every routine review and before starting any new pharmacologic therapy.
- Further information on the types of inhaler device available and choosing specific devices can be found in the Asthma, Inhaler Devices section.

Bronchodilators

- All patients should be trialled initially on a SABA or short-acting muscarinic antagonist (SAMA). These can be used to relieve breathlessness or for use before exertion expected to cause dyspnoea; they have approximately equal efficacy (Appleton et al, 2006).
- For patients that remain breathless or are having recurrent exacerbations, a fixed-dose combination LAMA–LABA inhaler can be started. Combination inhalers are simpler for patients, improve adherence, and are more cost-effective.
- Both LAMAs and LABAs improve breathlessness, overall quality of life, and exacerbation rates (Chong, Karner, & Poole, 2012). The different mechanisms of action result in a cumulative effect, and the current NICE recommendation is to start them simultaneously rather than sequentially.
- Increasing the LAMA–LABA dose has minimal additional bronchodilator effect, although toxicity does increase. The starting LAMA–LABA dose should be maintained and given on a regular basis to have the greatest impact.

Inhaled Corticosteroids

- ICSs must be used judiciously as they are associated with an increased rate of pneumonia, *Pseudomonas* colonisation, and nontuberculous mycobacteria (NTM) infection in COPD (Andréjak et al, 2013; Crim et al, 2017; Eklöf et al, 2022). This is addition to the increased risk of systemic side effects such as diabetes, cataracts, and reduced bone mineral density.
- In patients with moderate to severe COPD and a history of exacerbations, ICSs improve lung function and exacerbation rates (Nannini et al, 2013). There is also a strong relationship between higher blood eosinophil count and ICS response (Singh et al, 2022). As a result, ICSs should only be considered when there is any of:
  a. A history of hospitalisation for COPD exacerbation
  b. Two or more exacerbations of COPD requiring oral steroids per year
  c. Blood eosinophil count of 0.3×10^9/L or greater
  d. Evidence of concomitant asthma

- Unless there is associated asthma, patients should be started on a fixed-dose combination LAMA–LABA–ICS inhaler device. This should be trialled for 3 months and switched back to LAMA–LABA if there has been no significant improvement. A longer trial period may be required if ICS was started primarily to reduce exacerbation frequency.

Additional Pharmacologic Treatments

- *Mucolytic therapies* (e.g., carbocisteine) can be used to aid chest clearance in patients with a chronic productive cough. They can improve symptoms and reduce exacerbations (Poole, Black, & Cates, 2012).
- *Nebulised bronchodilators* are not recommended for regular unsupervised home use because they may inappropriately delay patients from seeking medical attention during acute exacerbations.
- *Theophylline* has a modest bronchodilator effect compared with placebo, but it has no effect on exacerbation frequency (Ram et al, 2002). It should only be used after other treatment trials have failed. There has been a move away from using theophylline in patients with COPD because of frequent side effects in older people; these include severe gastrointestinal upset, insomnia, arrhythmias, and seizures.
- *Diuretics* are used to treat cor pulmonale that is causing significant peripheral oedema. They should be started at low doses and titrated according to response and renal function. Alpha-blockers, angiotensin-converting enzyme inhibitors, calcium channel blockers, and digoxin are of no benefit.
- *Long-term antibiotics*, commonly azithromycin, can be used in nonsmokers with frequent or prolonged exacerbations. They should only be started after review in a specialist respiratory clinic.
- *Roflumilast* is an oral phosphodiesterase-4 inhibitor used to reduce exacerbation frequency in patients with COPD and severe airflow obstruction. It should also only be started after review in a specialist respiratory clinic.
- *Oral prednisolone* has no role in the long-term management of COPD. Any perceived benefits are substantially outweighed by the significant side effects of long-term oral steroids (Renkema et al, 1996).

Nonpharmacologic Management

Smoking Cessation

- Smoking cessation should be offered to all patients with COPD who continue to smoke and to other household members. Stopping smoking confers ongoing benefits to prognosis, disease progression, and symptoms, even in those with severe disease (Montes de Oca, 2020).
- The combination of pharmacotherapy and appropriate support can achieve long-term quit rates of up to 25% (van Eerd et al, 2016). Many NHS trusts and city councils have dedicated 'stop smoking' services which accept primary care referrals, but local variances exist.
- Despite the withdrawal of Varenicline (Champix) from the UK market, multiple forms of nicotine replacement therapy are still available.
- The long-term safety of electronic cigarettes and vaping is uncertain, but there is some evidence they can be an effective means to stopping smoking (Hajek et al, 2019). It should be noted they are not licensed medications and cannot be prescribed.

Oxygen Therapy

- Any patient with a resting SpO_2 of 92% or less should be referred for an oxygen assessment and consideration of LTOT. This has been shown to increase life expectancy in appropriate patients (Pavlov et al, 2018).
- LTOT must be worn for 15 or more hours per day to obtain the mortality benefit and requires regular reassessment by an oxygen team. Patients should be made aware that an oxygen concentrator will need to be fitted in their house, although they will also be given portable cylinders as per their individual needs.
- Ambulatory oxygen is a separate option that may be offered to patients who demonstrate both exertional desaturation and improved exercise tolerance with oxygen.
- NICE and BTS do not make smoking cessation mandatory for the provision of home oxygen, but local services may have different restrictions. In patients who continue to smoke, a safety assessment needs to be made, and oxygen therapy may be refused based on the results.
- Some patients on LTOT benefit from the addition of HMV. This is limited to those with persistent hypercapnia after a COPD exacerbation that required noninvasive ventilation. HMV is managed by specialist services.

Additional Nonpharmacologic Management

- *Education.* Patients should be offered written information about their conditions at every routine appointment. This can include additional details on smoking cessation, inhaler technique, symptom and exacerbation management, and support networks.
- *Pulmonary rehabilitation.* Physiotherapist-led structured exercise programmes improve exercise capacity, quality of life, and mortality rates (Garvey et al, 2016). They are tailored to the individual needs of the patient and are usually held in community facilities to improve accessibility. Pulmonary rehabilitation should be offered to all patients with an MRCD of 2 or greater.
- *Vaccinations.* All patients with COPD are eligible for annual influenza and COVID-19 vaccination and should be actively invited during seasonal campaigns. They should also receive a one-off pneumococcal vaccination (UK Health Security Agency, 2021).
- *Lung cancer screening.* Targeted lung health checks are currently only available in certain parts of the United Kingdom but will likely become more widespread in the near future. If available locally, patients should be referred if they are aged 55 to 74 years with 10-pack-year smoking history or longer.
- *Nutrition.* Low BMI is associated with worse respiratory function, lower exercise capacity, and increased mortality

rates. All underweight patients should be offered dietetic referral and nutritional supplements (Ferreira et al, 2005). Obese patients should be advised to lose weight to reduce their respiratory muscle load.

- *Mood.* Anxiety and depression are common in patients with COPD. Psychological or lifestyle interventions that include an exercise component significantly improve symptoms (Coventry et al, 2013). Some patients may require antidepressant medications.
- *Social support.* Walking aids, stair lifts, and bath aids may all help patients maintain independence. A wheelchair and a disabled parking permit may prevent patients with COPD from becoming housebound and improve their social contact. Day centres can provide short respite periods for both the patient and their family. As care needs increase, patients may need a social worker to help arrange care assistance.
- *Financial support.* Patients with COPD may qualify for state benefits with different options available for working-age and retired individuals. Further advice may be obtained from the Asthma + Lung website (see Patient Information).

Exacerbations

- Acute episodes of worsened COPD symptoms have significant associated morbidity and mortality. Recurrent exacerbations lead to more rapid FEV_1 decline and earlier death (Soler-Cataluña et al, 2005).
- Increased symptoms typically last 7 to 10 days, but 20% of patients have not returned to their premorbid state by 8 weeks (Seemungal et al, 2000).
- Infections, usually viral, are the commonest cause of exacerbations, but environmental pollution and temperature changes are increasingly being recognised as triggers (Li et al, 2022).
- Pulmonary embolism, pneumothorax, acute coronary syndrome, arrhythmias, and decompensated heart failure all have increased prevalence in patients with COPD and may present in a similar manner to an exacerbation.

Assessment

- Any patient describing a less than 14-day history of increased breathlessness or cough should be assessed for a possible exacerbation. In primary care, the severity of dyspnoea can be quickly assessed using a 0 to 10 visual analogue scale (Prins et al, 2021).
- Wheeze, purulent sputum, and increased sputum volume are other potential features of a COPD exacerbation but are not universal. Specific attention should be made to ask about more concerning symptoms such as new confusion, reduced conscious level, or cyanosis.
- Clarifying the patient's social circumstances and support network is also essential for deciding whether exacerbation management can continue safely at home.
- Examination should identify all features of increased respiratory effort such as accessory muscle use, paradoxical abdominal movement, and evidence of exhaustion. Auscultation of the chest is primarily to identify wheeze (suggesting acute airway inflammation and narrowing) or focal crackles (signifying possible pneumonia).

- Baseline observations can isolate any physiological features of sepsis (e.g., hypotension, tachycardia, pyrexia). Pulse oximetry can screen for hypoxia: SpO_2 less than 92% (or a decrease $\geq$3% in a patient with low baseline SpO_2).
- Sputum culture and chest radiography are not routinely required for COPD exacerbations.
- Assessment should allow an exacerbation to be classified as mild, moderate, or severe (Table 7.7) (Celli et al, 2021). C-reactive protein (CRP) and arterial blood gas measurement are typically unavailable in primary care, so erring on the side of caution is advised.
- It should be emphasised that some severe exacerbations may fall outside of this classification; it should not be the sole determinant for management decision making.

Management

- About 80% of patients present with 'mild' exacerbations and can be managed in the community with appropriate therapy. Hospital admission should be offered for 'moderate' exacerbations and should also be considered if there are other concerning symptoms or the patient's care needs are unlikely to be met at home.
- *Bronchodilators.* Increased SABA or SAMA usage is the initial management for a COPD exacerbation. An MDI (with or without a spacer) is as effective as a nebuliser, and 1 or 2 puffs can be given every hour according to the patient's response (van Geffen et al, 2016). If a patient is too breathless to use an inhaler, they are likely to require hospital review.

 TABLE 7.7 Classification of the Severity of Chronic Obstructive Pulmonary Disease Exacerbations (Celli et al, 2021)

Severity	Criteria
Mild	Dyspnoea VAS <5 Respiratory rate <24 breaths/minute Heart rate <95 beats/min Resting SpO_2 ≥92% on air or usual LTOT and ≤3% change from baseline CRP <10 mg/L (if available)
Moderate (requires three of five)	Dyspnoea VAS ≥5 Respiratory rate ≥24 breaths/min Heart rate ≥95 beats/min Resting SpO_2 <92% on air or usual LTOT and/or ≤3% change from baseline CRP ≥10 mg/L (if available)
Severe	Same criteria as moderate exacerbation Plus hypercapnia ($PaCO_2$ >6 kPa) and acidosis (pH <7.35)

CRP, C-reactive protein; *LTOT,* long-term oxygen therapy; *SpO₂,* Oxygen saturation; *VAS,* visual analogue scale.

- *Steroids.* Oral steroids shorten recovery time from an exacerbation, improve lung function, and reduce the risk of treatment failure and early relapse (Alía et al, 2011). Prednisolone 30 mg for 5 days should be given to anyone with an exacerbation and breathlessness causing increased functional limitation.
- *Antibiotics.* Not every patient requires antibiotics; they should only be prescribed if there is a change in sputum colour, volume, or viscosity. Amoxicillin (500mg, three times a day) is first-line treatment, with doxycycline and clarithromycin as options in penicillin allergy. A 5-day course is sufficient (NICE, 2018).
- *Hospital-at-home.* This multidisciplinary service provides an alternative method of managing patients who otherwise may require hospital admission. Nebulised bronchodilators can be given and patients monitored closely. Selection criteria vary, so local referral guidelines should be followed and patient preference taken into account.
- *Review.* Patients should be advised to seek repeat consultation or attend an emergency department if their condition fails to improve or deteriorates despite the recommended measures. After an exacerbation, a review should be arranged to optimise the patient's regular treatment, encourage smoking cessation, and provide other lifestyle advice.

Referring to Secondary Care

- The majority of patients with COPD are managed entirely in primary care, where there is greater continuity and patients have easier access to healthcare professionals. Nevertheless, there are scenarios when referral to specialist services is required:
  a. When the diagnosis of COPD is unclear or when important differential diagnoses cannot be excluded
  b. Rapid deterioration in symptoms or lung function
  c. Symptoms that are disproportionate to the severity of airflow obstruction
  d. Aged younger than 40 years or if there is a family history of alpha-1-antitrypsin deficiency
  e. To assess suitability for lung transplantation or lung volume reduction surgery (LVRS)
  f. Frequent infective exacerbations or to consider suitability for long-term antibiotic therapy
  g. Haemoptysis or abnormal chest radiography findings when lung cancer needs to be excluded (2-week-wait referral)
  h. When there is a possibility of an occupational cause or concomitant industrial disease (e.g., pneumoconiosis); refer to a specialist occupational lung disease clinic
  i. Onset of cor pulmonale or suspected pulmonary hypertension
  j. Assessment for long-term oxygen therapy (LTOT), home mechanical ventilation (HMV), or regular nebuliser use
  k. Assessment for pulmonary rehabilitation (refer to respiratory physiotherapy directly)
  l. When the patient requests a second opinion

Palliative Care

- COPD is a progressive disease and is ultimately the cause of death for many patients. When a patient is nearing the end of their life, the decision to add someone to a palliative care register can be useful as it denotes that treatment priorities have changed.
- Identifying this moment is difficult, but regular reviews can help monitor disease progress. Indicators of advancing disease include progression of symptoms, increasing functional limitation, chronic hypoxia, and repeated hospital admissions (Pinnock et al, 2011).
- Despite this, only 17% of patients with COPD receive palliative care support compared with 57% of patients with lung cancer (Bloom et al, 2018).
- Breathlessness is often the most troublesome symptom for patients with COPD at the end of their lives. Morphine, palliative oxygen, and fans can all provide some relief.
- If the patient begins to become agitated, then benzodiazepines are a useful adjunct, often given as oral lorazepam or subcutaneous midazolam. Further support and advice regarding symptomatic management can be obtained from local palliative care services
- Palliative care for patients with COPD should always include conversations with the patient and their family about resuscitation, advanced directives, and the preferred place of death (Seamark et al, 2007). Advanced care planning can reduce anxiety and reassure the patient that the care they will receive is in keeping with their stated wishes.
- Patients may find it useful to document these discussions in an Advanced Health Care Plan. Community palliative care services and Macmillan teams can help with this process and with arranging hospice care or increased home support when the patient is nearing the end of their life.

PATIENT INFORMATION

Asthma + Lung UK (including the charity previously known as the British Lung Foundation). This provides patient information leaflets about COPD and resources such as COPD self-management plans and Patient Passports. They also run support groups and the 'Breathe Easy' programme. Telephone helpline: 0300 222 5800. Available at http://www. asthmaandlung.org.uk.

    RightBreathe. Online resource containing dosing information, safety advice, and instructional videos for all inhalers available in the United Kingdom. Available athttps://www. rightbreathe.com.

Lower Respiratory Tract Infection

GUIDELINES

British Thoracic Society. (2009). *Guidelines for the management of community acquired pneumonia in adults*. Retrieved from http://www.brit-thoracic.org.uk/quality-improvement/guidelines/pneumonia-adults.

National Institute for Health and Care Excellence. (2014; updated 2022). *Pneumonia in adults: Diagnosis and management. NICE clinical guideline 191*. Retrieved from http://www.nice.org.uk/guidance/cg191.

National Institute for Health and Care Excellence. (2019). *Pneumonia (community-acquired): Antimicrobial prescribing. NICE clinical guideline 138*. Retrieved from https://www.nice.org.uk/guidance/ng138.

• BOX 7.2 Risk Factors for Increased Mortality Rate in Lower Respiratory Tract Infections (Torres et al, 2013)

COPD and asthma	Age 65 years or older
Previous pneumonia	Nursing home residents
Heart failure	High alcohol intake
Chronic kidney disease	Smoking
Chronic liver disease	Low BMI or malnutrition
Cerebrovascular disease	Immunosuppressive therapy
Dementia	Long-term steroid use
Cancer	Social deprivation
Diabetes mellitus	Poor dental health

BMI, Body mass index; *COPD*, chronic obstructive pulmonary disease.

Clinical Assessment

- Lower respiratory tract infection (LRTI) can be diagnosed in any patient presenting with an otherwise unexplained acute illness (<21 days) including cough with one or more other symptom: fever, sputum production, dyspnoea, wheeze, or chest discomfort.
- 'Pneumonia' refers to an LRTI with new radiologic changes. Only 12% of patients with LRTI have community-acquired pneumonia (CAP), but the risk is two to four times greater in people older than 60 years (Macfarlane et al, 1993).
- Most patients presenting with an LRTI to primary care have a self-limiting illness that does not require antibiotics (Macfarlane et al, 2001). Therefore, the role of the GP is to:
  a. Identify patients with severe LRTI that require active treatment.
  b. Identify patients at high risk for progression to severe infection.
  c. Reassure patients about the natural disease process of uncomplicated LRTI.
  d. Ensure selected patients receive appropriate follow-up after LRTI.

History Taking and Examination

- History taking primarily focuses on making the diagnosis of respiratory infection because there are no sensitive or specific symptoms for pneumonia (Metlay, Kapoor, & Fine, 1997).
- Establishing the degree of breathlessness by comparing it with the patient's baseline can be useful to establish the impact of the acute illness, a factor that may influence the decision to treat at home or arrange admission to hospital.
- If infection is suspected, specific attention should be made to exclude systemic symptoms that may suggest early sepsis, including (but not limited to) fever, rigors, confusion, slurred speech, lightheadedness, dizziness, reduced urine output, and diarrhoea.

- Direct questioning and review of the patient's records should take place to determine whether the patient has any important comorbidities that put them at high-risk for death from LRTI (Box 7.2) (Torres et al, 2013). The clinician needs to have a lower threshold for starting antibiotics or admitting to hospital in these circumstances.
- Chest examination may detect focal chest signs, which are positively correlated with pneumonia; their absence does not exclude the diagnosis (Metlay et al, 1997).
- It should be possible to measure basic physical observations in the GP practice. Significant pyrexia (>40°C), tachypnoea (>30 breaths/min), and hypotension (blood pressure ≤90/60 mm Hg) indicate severe infection and possible sepsis.
- SpO_2 less than 92% on pulse oximetry indicates significant hypoxia and should trigger hospital referral even without other signs of sepsis. In patients with chronic lung disease, a SpO_2 drop of 3% or less from a previously recorded baseline can be used.

CRB65 Score

- The CRB65 score stratifies adult patients in primary care with CAP according to their mortality risk. It can aid decision making regarding admission to hospital but should be used in conjunction with other components of the clinical assessment.
- Score 1 point for the following prognostic factors:
  a. Confusion: abbreviated mental test score of 8 or less or new disorientation
  b. Respiratory rate of 30 breaths/min or greater
  c. Blood pressure less than 90 mm Hg systolic or less than 60 mm Hg diastolic
  d. Age 65 years or older
- Patients with a score of 0 have less than a 1% mortality risk, and treatment at home is recommended. Review in hospital should be considered for all other patients as the mortality risk rapidly increases (McNally et al, 2010).

Investigations

- *Serum CRP* may help with antibiotic decision making as increased levels correlate with pneumonia (Verbakel et al,

2019). Antibiotics should not be routinely offered when CRP is below 20 mg/L, but there is a strong recommendation that antibiotics should be given if CRP is greater than 100 mg/L. If CRP is 20 to 100 mg/L, an antibiotic prescription can be given to the patient for use only if symptoms worsen.

- Other blood tests should only be performed when there are features of severe infection (not requiring hospital admission) or if the patient has not responded to initial treatment.
- *Chest radiography* is rarely indicated in primary care but may be requested if there are focal chest signs or unusual symptoms (e.g., haemoptysis) or in high-risk patients even in the absence of chest signs.
- *Sputum samples* should be sent for culture in any patient for whom antibiotics are being considered. If the patient has COPD or bronchiectasis, this should be included on all request forms as additional microbiological tests may need to be performed.

Differential Diagnosis

- The signs and symptoms of LRTI are nonspecific; the primary care clinician should bear in mind other potential diagnoses which can present in a similar manner.
- *Noninfective exacerbation of chronic lung disease.* Asthma and COPD can present with acute worsening causing shortness of breath, cough, and wheeze.
- *Pulmonary embolism.* Sudden-onset shortness of breath and chest pain should raise the suspicion of PE, especially in those with risk factors (e.g., recent immobility, cancer, signs of deep vein thrombosis, previous blood clots).
- *Heart failure.* Decompensation of heart failure can present with shortness of breath, which usually has a more insidious onset than infection. New arrhythmias or ischemic events can cause acute presentations with pulmonary oedema.
- *Lung cancer.* This should always be suspected in patients with a smoking history and new respiratory symptoms. Even if antibiotics are prescribed, appropriate follow-up is required (see Follow-up).

Management

- In patients without severe infection or significant co-morbidities, LRTI can be managed with self-management and without antibiotics. In this population, antibiotics do not improve the patient's symptoms and only reduce the symptom duration by half a day (Bent et al, 1999).
- Antibiotics commonly cause side effects, including nausea and diarrhoea, and inappropriate prescribing contributes to the development of antibiotic resistance.
- Steroids should not be routinely offered unless the patient has another condition for which they are required. This includes exacerbations of asthma or COPD.
- Simple symptomatic treatment, including paracetamol, increased fluid intake, and bed rest, should be recommended.

Patients may wish to use other self-care treatments such as honey, herbal medicines, and over-the-counter cough medicines. There is limited evidence that these may improve cough symptoms.

- Antihistamines, NSAIDs, decongestants, and codeine linctus have been shown to have no effect on cough symptoms (Chang, Cheng, & Chang, 2014).
- Repeat consultation rates can be reduced by providing written information on the nature of cough and the expected duration (≤4 weeks) (Macfarlane, Holmes, & Macfarlane, 1997).

Antibiotics

- When an antibiotic prescription is deemed necessary, all previous microbiology results should be reviewed to guide the choice of antibiotic.
- Initial antibiotic prescriptions should be for 5 days. Failure to improve as expected, deterioration, or development of new symptoms should prompt the patient to seek further medical advice.
- The antibiotics options in primary care are summarised in Table 7.8. All the listed antibiotics have similar efficacy in low-severity CAP (Pakhale, 2014). Amoxicillin is the first-line treatment for all age groups unless the patient has a penicillin allergy or atypical organisms are suspected.
- Doxycycline should be used with caution in children and pregnant females due to its potential effects on the growth of teeth and bones.

TABLE 7.8 Antibiotic Options for Lower Respiratory Tract Infections in Primary Care

Age (years)	First Choice	Penicillin Allergy
18 and older	Amoxicillin 500 mg tds	Doxycycline 200 mg stat; then 100 mg od; Clarithromycin 500 mg bd; Erythromycin 500 mg qds
12–17	Amoxicillin 500 mg tds	Clarithromycin 250–500 mg bd; Erythromycin 250–500 mg qds; Doxycycline 200 mg stat; then 100 mg od
5–11	Amoxicillin 500 mg tds	Clarithromycin, dose weight dependant (see BNF for children)
1–4	Amoxicillin 250 mg tds	Clarithromycin, dose weight dependant (see BNF for children)
<1	Amoxicillin 125 mg tds	Clarithromycin, dose weight dependant (see BNF for children)

Bd, Twice a day; *BNF,* British National Formulary; *od,* once a day; *qds,* four times a day; *tds,* three times a day.

Follow-up

- A noticeable improvement should be observed within days of treatment being started. Those who fail to respond should have a further review, and there should be strong consideration for performing blood tests and chest radiography.
- If there is a significant clinical deterioration despite home-based treatment, then the patient should be referred to hospital for further assessment.
- Patients with LRTI or CAP should gradually improve along a predictable tautology trajectory, although this may take longer than some patients expect (Hounkpatin et al, 2023):
  - 1 week: resolution of fever
  - 4 weeks: chest pain and sputum production significantly improved
  - 6 weeks: cough and dyspnoea largely settled
  - 3 months: most symptoms fully resolved; some fatigue may remain
  - 6 months: complete resolution back to baseline
- On occasion, CAP represents the initial presentation of an underlying malignancy. Primary lung cancer or metastatic lymph node spread can cause airway obstruction, mucus impaction, bacterial growth, and lobar collapse.
- If there has been an identified chest X-ray abnormality, then repeat imaging is required after 6 weeks if the patient has any one of:
  a. Persisting symptoms or signs
  b. A significant smoking history
  c. Is 50 years of age or older
- Any persisting radiologic changes should immediately elicit a 2-week-wait referral to specialist respiratory services. Do not request further imaging because this can lead to unnecessary delays; the specialist centre will have more ready access to further scans.
- If there has been chest radiography resolution, then use the opportunity to provide smoking cessation advice and ensure influenza, COVID-19, and pneumococcal vaccinations are up to date.

Tuberculosis

GUIDELINES

National Institute for Health and Care Excellence. (2016; updated 2019). *Tuberculosis. NICE clinical guideline 33*. Retrieved from https://www.nice.org.uk/guidance/ng33.

UK Health Security Agency. (2013; updated 2018). Tuberculosis. In *Immunisation Against Infectious Disease, 'The Green Book'*. Retrieved from https://www.gov.uk/government/publications/tuberculosis-the-green-book-chapter-32.

Role of Primary Care in Tuberculosis Management

Be Alert to the Possibility of Tuberculosis

- Although a quarter of tuberculosis (TB) cases in this country occur in people born in the United Kingdom, the incidence rates for those born in South Asia, China, and sub-Saharan Africa are up to 14 times greater than UK-born individuals. There are also considerable geographic differences, with rates highest in major cities and especially in London, where one-third of all UK cases are identified (UK Health Security Agency, 2023).
- New patient medicals are an opportunity to screen recent entrants to the United Kingdom, but only 14% develop TB infection within 2 years of entry, and in some populations, the median latency is more than 10 years (UK Health Security Agency, 2023).
- Other high-risk groups include patients with impaired immunity (e.g., people living with human immunodeficiency virus [HIV] or long-term corticosteroid use), homeless people, those with alcohol or drug misuse, prisoners, patients with high socioeconomic deprivation, and people with medical comorbidities (including diabetes, renal failure, use of anti–tumor necrosis factor-α medications, and cancer).

Consider the Diagnosis

- Most patients present with nonspecific respiratory symptoms such as productive cough, shortness of breath, or haemoptysis.
- Further investigations should be prompted by the presence of TB risk factors or when there are associated systemic symptoms such as fever, night sweats, or weight loss.
- TB is an insidious disease and can present in almost any way and affect any body system. Primary care clinicians should be alert to the wide range of nonspecific symptoms which can occur in people with TB (Metcalf et al, 2007).

Request Appropriate Tests

- Chest radiography should be arranged in all cases.
- If the patient has a productive cough, three sputum samples should be sent for TB microscopy and culture. These should be from different days and ideally be early-morning samples.

Refer Promptly to Secondary Care

- Management of all patients with TB should be supervised by specialist hospital teams, which will include infectious diseases or respiratory physicians supported by TB nurse specialists and health visitors.
- The long antibiotic course and relatively high likelihood of adverse drug reactions mean that treatment compliance can be difficult to maintain. Given the important public health significance of TB, specialist teams can provide increased patient support and organise appropriate contact tracing.

- Most patients can be managed in the community. Inpatient care is sometimes required in severe cases, in those with resistant TB, or when medication compliance needs additional monitoring (e.g., because of drug side effects or uncertain social circumstances).
- All TB treatment is free in the United Kingdom regardless of a patient's eligibility for other NHS care.

Be Aware of the Side Effects of Tuberculosis Treatment

- If a patient presents with potential side effects of TB treatment, they should always be discussed with the local TB specialist team. Liver function tests should be checked because most antituberculous antibiotics can cause hepatotoxicity.
- Rifampicin and isoniazid are frequently used in TB treatment and are potent enzyme inducers and inhibitors. All prospective new medications should be checked for possible drug interactions; common examples include oral contraception, warfarin, and antiepileptic drugs.

Provide Advice to Contacts of Patients Diagnosed With Tuberculosis

- Contact tracing is undertaken by TB specialist nurses and is only required for close contacts (i.e., people from the same household or frequent visitors to the household).
- Other contacts, including most work colleagues, are 'casual contacts' and are at considerably lower risk of infection. Casual contacts are not screened unless the index patient is particularly infectious or if the contact person is at high risk for infection.

Latent Tuberculosis Infection (LTBI) Testing

- LTBI represents dormant infection, which can become active during periods of immunosuppression (which includes increasing age).

BOX 7.3	**Indications for Latent Tuberculosis Infection Testing in New UK Entrants**

Born or spent >6 months in a country with TB incidence >150 per 100,000 or sub-Saharan Africa
Entered the United Kingdom within the past 5 years
Aged 16–35 years
No previous history of TB or latent TB
Not previously screened in the United Kingdom

TB, Tuberculosis.

- Interferon-gamma release assays (IGRA; QuantiFERON-TB GOLD, T-SPOT) are more readily available than Mantoux tuberculin skin tests (TSTs) and are as effective at identifying LTBI (Auguste et al, 2017).
- New UK entrants should be offered LTBI testing in primary care if they are meet criteria set out by NICE (Box 7.3).
- LTBI testing of immunocompromised patients, close contacts of TB cases, and new NHS workers should be performed by secondary care services.

Bacillus Calmette-Guérin (BCG) Vaccination

- The bacillus Calmette-Guérin (BCG) vaccine is up to 80% effective against TB meningitis in children but is less effective against pulmonary disease. Protection lasts at least 15 years (Colditz et al, 1994).
- Newborn vaccination programmes include BCG, but other eligible patients should be identified when registering with primary care providers (Table 7.9).
- As a live attenuated vaccine, it should not be given to any HIV-positive, pregnant, or significantly immunosuppressed patients. BCG should also never be given to patients who have been previously vaccinated.

TABLE 7.9 **Bacillus Calmette-Guérin Vaccination Eligibility Criteria**

Category	Criteria for Vaccination
Infants (0–12 months)	All newborns in an area of the United Kingdom with TB incidence >40 per 100,000 ≥1 parent or grandparent born in a country with TB incidence >40 per 100,000
Children (1–16 years)	Born in or lived for ≥3 months in a country with TB incidence >40 per 100,000 ≥1 parent or grandparent born in a country with TB incidence >40 per 100,000 (TST or IGRA not required if ≤5 years)
New entrants	Younger than 16 years of age from a country with TB incidence >40 per 100,000 16–35 years of age from sub-Saharan Africa or a country with TB incidence >500 per 100,000
TB contact	35 years of age or younger, close contact only Healthcare worker or contact with patients or clinical materials (any age)
Occupational exposure	Healthcare workers with direct contact with TB patients or infectious materials (any age) 35 years of age or younger: workers in prisons, care homes with older patients, or hostels for homeless, refugees, or asylum-seekers; vets and other handlers of animals susceptible to TB
Travellers	35 years of age or younger living or working with local people for >3 months in a country with TB incidence >40 per 100,000

IGRA, Interferon-gamma release assay; *TB,* tuberculosis; *TST,* tuberculin skin test.

- In patients older than 12 months of age, LTBI should be excluded with a negative IGRA or TST result before administering BCG vaccination.

PATIENT INFORMATION

British Lung Foundation. Patient information on tuberculosis (TB), treatment, and TB in children. Telephone helpline: 0300 222 5800. Available at http://www.blf.org.uk/conditions/tuberculosis.

TB Alert. Specialist UK TB charity that provides patient support groups and a patient support fund. Contains multiple TB Patient Information leaflets. Available at http://www.tbalert.org.

References

Adams, N., Bestall, J., & Jones, P. W. (2001). Budesonide for chronic asthma in children and adults. *Cochrane Database of Systematic Reviews, 1999*(4), CD003274.

Adams, N. P., Bestall, J. B., Malouf, R., Lasserson, T. J., & Jones, P. W. (2005a). Inhaled beclomethasone versus placebo for chronic asthma. *Cochrane Database of Systematic Reviews, 2005*(1), CD002738.

Adams, N. P., Bestall, J. C., Lasserson, T. J., Jones, P. W., & Cates, C. (2005b). Fluticasone versus placebo for chronic asthma in adults and children. *Cochrane Database of Systematic Reviews*, (4), CD003135.

Agertoft, L., & Pedersen, S. (2000). Effect of long-term treatment with inhaled budesonide on adult height in children with asthma. *New England Journal of Medicine, 343*(15), 1064–1069.

Agusti, A., Bel, E., Thomas, M., Vogelmeier, C., Brusselle, G., Holgate, S., Humbert, M., Jones, P., Gibson, P. G., Vestbo, J., Beasley, R., & Pavord, I. D. (2016). Treatable traits: Toward precision medicine of chronic airway diseases. *European Respiratory Journal, 47*(2), 410–419.

Albert, P., Agusti, A., Edwards, L., Tal-Singer, R., Yates, J., Bakke, P., Celli, B. R., Coxson, H. O., Crim, C., Lomas, D. A., Macnee, W., Miller, B., Rennard, S., Silverman, E. K., Vestbo, J., Wouters, E., & Calverley, P. (2012). Bronchodilator responsiveness as a phenotypic characteristic of established chronic obstructive pulmonary disease. *Thorax, 67*(8), 701–708.

Alía, I., de la Cal, M. A., Esteban, A., Abella, A., Ferrer, R., Molina, F. J., Torres, A., Gordo, F., Elizalde, J. J., de Pablo, R., Huete, A., & Anzueto, A. (2011). Efficacy of corticosteroid therapy in patients with an acute exacerbation of chronic obstructive pulmonary disease receiving ventilatory support. *Archives of Internal Medicine, 171*(21), 1939–1946.

Andréjak, C., Nielsen, R., Thomsen, V. Ø., Duhaut, P., Sørensen, H. T., & Thomsen, R. W. (2013). Chronic respiratory disease, inhaled corticosteroids and risk of non-tuberculous mycobacteriosis. *Thorax, 68*(3), 256–262.

Appleton, S., Jones, T., Poole, P., Pilotto, L., Adams, R., Lasserson, T. J., Smith, B., & Muhammad, J. (2006). Ipratropium bromide versus short acting beta-2 agonists for stable chronic obstructive pulmonary disease. *Cochrane Database of Systematic Reviews, 2006*(2), CD001387.

Auguste, P., Tsertsvadze, A., Pink, J., Court, R., McCarthy, N., Sutcliffe, P., & Clarke, A. (2017). Comparing interferon-gamma release assays with tuberculin skin test for identifying latent tuberculosis infection that progresses to active tuberculosis: Systematic review and meta-analysis. *BMC Infectious Diseases, 17*(1), 200.

Bent, S., Saint, S., Vittinghoff, E., & Grady, D. (1999). Antibiotics in acute bronchitis: A meta-analysis. *American Journal of Medicine, 107*(1), 62–67.

Bloom, C. I., Slaich, B., Morales, D. R., Smeeth, L., Stone, P., & Quint, J. K. (2018). Low uptake of palliative care for COPD patients within primary care in the UK. *European Respiratory Journal, 51*(2), 1701879.

Brocklebank, D., Ram, F., Wright, J., Barry, P., Cates, C., Davies, L., Douglas, G., Muers, M., Smith, D., & White, J. (2001). Comparison of the effectiveness of inhaler devices in asthma and chronic obstructive airways disease: A systematic review of the literature. *Health Technology Assessment (Winchester, England), 5*(26), 1–149.

Cardoso, J., Ferreira, A. J., Guimarães, M., Oliveira, A. S., Simão, P., & Sucena, M. (2021). Treatable traits in COPD - a proposed approach. *International Journal of Chronic Obstructive Pulmonary Disease, 16*, 3167–3182.

Carr, T. F., Zeki, A. A., & Kraft, M. Eosinophilic and noneosinophilic asthma. *American Journal of Respiratory and Critical Care Medicine, 197*(1), 22–37.

Cates, C. J., & Karner, C. (2013). Combination formoterol and budesonide as maintenance and reliever therapy versus current best practice (including inhaled steroid maintenance), for chronic asthma in adults and children. *Cochrane Database of Systematic Reviews, 2013*(4), CD007313.

Celli, B. R., Fabbri, L. M., Aaron, S. D., Agusti, A., Brook, R., Criner, G. J., Franssen, F. M. E., Humbert, M., Hurst, J. R., O'Donnell, D., Pantoni, L., Papi, A., Rodriguez-Roisin, R., Sethi, S., Torres, A., Vogelmeier, C. F., & Wedzicha, J. A. (2021). An updated definition and severity classification of chronic obstructive pulmonary disease exacerbations: The Rome proposal. *American Journal of Respiratory and Critical Care Medicine, 204*(11), 1251–1258.

Chang, C. C., Cheng, A. C., & Chang, A. B. (2014). Over-the-counter (OTC) medications to reduce cough as an adjunct to antibiotics for acute pneumonia in children and adults. *Cochrane Database of Systematic Reviews*, (3), CD006088.

Chang, J. T., Meza, R., Levy, D. T., Arenberg, D., & Jeon, J. (2021). Prediction of COPD risk accounting for time-varying smoking exposures. *PLoS One, 16*(3), e0248535.

Chapman, K. R., Boulet, L. P., Rea, R. M., & Franssen, E. (2008). Suboptimal asthma control: Prevalence, detection and consequences in general practice. *European Respiratory Journal, 31*(2), 320–325.

Chauhan, B. F., & Ducharme, F. M. (2014). Addition to inhaled corticosteroids of long-acting beta2-agonists versus anti-leukotrienes for chronic asthma. *Cochrane Database of Systematic Reviews, 2014*(1), CD003137.

Chong, J., Karner, C., & Poole, P. (2012). Tiotropium versus long-acting beta-agonists for stable chronic obstructive pulmonary disease. *Cochrane Database of Systematic Reviews, 2012*(9), CD009157.

Colditz, G. A., Brewer, T. F., Berkey, C. S., Wilson, M. E., Burdick, E., Fineberg, H. V., & Mosteller, F. (1994). Efficacy of BCG vaccine in the prevention of tuberculosis. Meta-analysis of the published literature. *JAMA, 271*(9), 698–702.

Coventry, P. A., Bower, P., Keyworth, C., Kenning, C., Knopp, J., Garrett, C., Hind, D., Malpass, A., & Dickens, C. (2013). The effect of complex interventions on depression and anxiety in chronic obstructive pulmonary disease: Systematic review and meta-analysis. *PLoS One, 8*(4), e60532.

Crim, C., Calverley, P. M. A., Anderson, J. A., Holmes, A. P., Kilbride, S., Martinez, F. J., Brook, R. D., Newby, D. E., Yates, J. C., Celli, B. R., Vestbo, J., & SUMMIT investigators. (2017). Pneumonia risk with inhaled fluticasone furoate and vilanterol in COPD patients with moderate airflow limitation: The SUMMIT trial. *Respiratory Medicine, 131*, 27–34.

Eklöf, J., Ingebrigtsen, T. S., Sørensen, R., Saeed, M. I., Alispahic, I. A., Sivapalan, P., Boel, J. B., Bangsborg, J., Ostergaard, C., Dessau, R. B., Jensen, U. S., Hansen, E. F., Lapperre, T. S., Meteran, H., Wilcke, T., Seersholm, N., & Jensen, J. S. (2022). Use of inhaled corticosteroids and risk of acquiring *Pseudomonas aeruginosa* in patients with chronic obstructive pulmonary disease. *Thorax, 77*(6), 573–580.

Eriksson, B., Backman, H., Bossios, A., Bjerg, A., Hedman, L., Lindberg, A., Rönmark, E., & Lundbäck, B. (2016). Only severe COPD is associated with being underweight: Results from a population survey. *ERJ Open Research, 2*(3), 00051-2015.

Ferreira, I. M., Brooks, D., Lacasse, Y., Goldstein, R. S., & White, J. (2005). Nutritional supplementation for stable chronic obstructive pulmonary disease. *Cochrane Database of Systematic Reviews*, (2), CD000998.

Freitas, D. A., Holloway, E. A., Bruno, S. S., Chaves, G. S., Fregonezi, G. A., & Mendonça, K. P. (2013). Breathing exercises for adults with asthma. *Cochrane Database of Systematic Reviews*, (10), CD001277.

Gaddie, J., Petrie, G. R., Reid, I. W., Skinner, C., Sinclair, D. J., & Palmer, K. N. (1973). Aerosol beclomethasone dipropionate: A dose-response study in chronic bronchial asthma. *Lancet (London, England), 2*(7824), 280–281.

Galant, S. P., Crawford, L. J., Morphew, T., Jones, C. A., & Bassin, S. (2004). Predictive value of a cross-cultural asthma case-detection tool in an elementary school population. *Pediatrics, 114*(3), e307–e316.

Garvey, C., Bayles, M. P., Hamm, L. F., Hill, K., Holland, A., Limberg, T. M., & Spruit, M. A. (2016). Pulmonary rehabilitation exercise prescription in chronic obstructive pulmonary disease: Review of selected guidelines: an official statement from the American Association of Cardiovascular and Pulmonary Rehabilitation. *Journal of Cardiopulmonary Rehabilitation and Prevention, 36*(2), 75–83.

Gibson, P. G., Powell, H., Coughlan, J., Wilson, A. J., Abramson, M., Haywood, P., Bauman, A., Hensley, M. J., & Walters, E. H. (2003). Self-management education and regular practitioner review for adults with asthma. *Cochrane Database of Systematic Reviews*, (1), CD001117.

Gøtzsche, P. C., & Johansen, H. K. (2008). House dust mite control measures for asthma. *Cochrane Database of Systematic Reviews, 2008*(2), CD001187.

Gray, N., Howard, A., Zhu, J., Feldman, L. Y., & To, T. (2018). Association between inhaled corticosteroid use and bone fracture in children with asthma. *JAMA Pediatrics, 172*(1), 57–64.

Hajek, P., Phillips-Waller, A., Przulj, D., Pesola, F., Myers Smith, K., Bisal, N., Li, J., Parrott, S., Sasieni, P., Dawkins, L., Ross, L., Goniewicz, M., Wu, Q., & McRobbie, H. J. (2019). A randomized trial of e-cigarettes versus nicotine-replacement therapy. *New England Journal of Medicine, 380*(7), 629–637.

Han, M. K., Muellerova, H., Curran-Everett, D., Dransfield, M. T., Washko, G. R., Regan, E. A., Bowler, R. P., Beaty, T. H., Hokanson, J. E., Lynch, D. A., Jones, P. W., Anzueto, A., Martinez, F. J., Crapo, J. D., Silverman, E. K., & Make, B. J. (2013). GOLD 2011 disease severity classification in COPDGene: A prospective cohort study. *Lancet Respiratory Medicine, 1*(1), 43–50.

Harrison, B., Slack, R., Berrill, W. T., & Bur, M. L. (2000). Results of a national confidential enquiry into asthma deaths. *Asthma Journal, 5*(4), 180–186.

Hartnett, B. J., & Marlin, G. E. (1977). Comparison of terbutaline and salbutamol aerosols. *Australian and New Zealand Journal of Medicine, 7*(1), 13–15.

Haughney, J., Barnes, G., Partridge, M., & Cleland, J. (2004). The Living & Breathing Study: A study of patients' views of asthma and its treatment. *Primary Care Respiratory Journal, 13*(1), 28–35.

Hounkpatin, H., Stuart, B., Zhu, S., Yao, G., Moore, M., Löffler, C., Little, P., Kenealy, T., Gillespie, D., Francis, N. A., Bostock, J., Becque, T., Arroll, B., Altiner, A., Alonso-Coello, P., & Hay, A. D. (2023). Post-consultation acute respiratory tract infection recovery: A latent class-informed analysis of individual patient data. *British Journal of General Practice, 73*(728), e196–e203.

House of Commons Environmental Audit Committee. (2018). *UK progress on reducing F-Gas emissions inquiry. Fifth Report of Session 2017-19.* Retrieved from https://publications.parliament.uk/pa/cm201719/cmselect/cmenvaud/469/469.pdf. Accessed May 30, 2024.

Jones, P. W., Harding, G., Berry, P., Wiklund, I., Chen, W. H., & Kline Leidy, N. (2009). Development and first validation of the COPD Assessment Test. *European Respiratory Journal, 34*(3), 648–654.

Juniper, E. F., Bousquet, J., Abetz, L., Bateman, E. D., & GOAL Committee. (2006). Identifying 'well-controlled' and 'not well-controlled' asthma using the Asthma Control Questionnaire. *Respiratory Medicine, 100*(4), 616–621.

Knorr, B., Franchi, L. M., Bisgaard, H., Vermeulen, J. H., LeSouef, P., Santanello, N., Michele, T. M., Reiss, T. F., Nguyen, H. H., & Bratton, D. L. (2001). Montelukast, a leukotriene receptor antagonist, for the treatment of persistent asthma in children aged 2 to 5 years. *Pediatrics, 108*(3), E48.

Kohansal, R., Martinez-Camblor, P., Agustí, A., Buist, A. S., Mannino, D. M., & Soriano, J. B. (2009). The natural history of chronic airflow obstruction revisited: An analysis of the Framingham offspring cohort. *American Journal of Respiratory and Critical Care Medicine, 180*(1), 3–10.

Kouri, A., Boulet, L. P., Kaplan, A., & Gupta, S. (2017). An evidence-based, point-of-care tool to guide completion of asthma action plans in practice. *European Respiratory Journal, 49*(5), 1602238.

Lazarus, S. C., Chinchilli, V. M., Rollings, N. J., Boushey, H. A., Cherniack, R., Craig, T. J., Deykin, A., DiMango, E., Fish, J. E., Ford, J. G., Israel, E., Kiley, J., Kraft, M., Lemanske, R. F., Jr, Leone, F. T., Martin, R. J., Pesola, G. R., Peters, S. P., Sorkness, C. A., Szefler, S. J., ... National Heart Lung and Blood Institute's Asthma Clinical Research Network. (2007). Smoking affects response to inhaled corticosteroids or leukotriene receptor antagonists in asthma. *American Journal of Respiratory and Critical Care Medicine, 175*(8), 783–790.

Li, N., Ma, J., Ji, K., & Wang, L. (2022). Association of PM2.5 and PM10 with acute exacerbation of chronic obstructive pulmonary disease at lag0 to lag7: A systematic review and meta-analysis. *COPD, 19*(1), 243–254.

Ma, J., Strub, P., Xiao, L., Lavori, P. W., Camargo, C. A., Jr, Wilson, S. R., Gardner, C. D., Buist, A. S., Haskell, W. L., & Lv, N. (2015). Behavioral weight loss and physical activity intervention in obese adults with asthma. A randomized trial. *Annals of the American Thoracic Society, 12*(1), 1–11.

Macfarlane, J., Holmes, W., Gard, P., Macfarlane, R., Rose, D., Weston, V., Leinonen, M., Saikku, P., & Myint, S. (2001). Prospective study of the incidence, aetiology and outcome of adult lower respiratory tract illness in the community. *Thorax*, *56*(2), 109–114.

Macfarlane, J. T., Colville, A., Guion, A., Macfarlane, R. M., & Rose, D. H. (1993). Prospective study of aetiology and outcome of adult lower-respiratory-tract infections in the community. *Lancet (London, England)*, *341*(8844), 511–514.

Macfarlane, J. T., Holmes, W. F., & Macfarlane, R. M. (1997). Reducing reconsultations for acute lower respiratory tract illness with an information leaflet: A randomized controlled study of patients in primary care. *British Journal of General Practice*, *47*(424), 719–722.

Mannino, D. M., Thorn, D., Swensen, A., & Holguin, F. (2008). Prevalence and outcomes of diabetes, hypertension and cardiovascular disease in COPD. *European Respiratory Journal*, *32*(4), 962–969.

McKeever, T., Mortimer, K., Wilson, A., Walker, S., Brightling, C., Skeggs, A., Pavord, I., Price, D., Duley, L., Thomas, M., Bradshaw, L., Higgins, B., Haydock, R., Mitchell, E., Devereux, G., & Harrison, T. (2018). Quadrupling inhaled glucocorticoid dose to abort asthma exacerbations. *New England Journal of Medicine*, *378*(10), 902–910.

McNally, M., Curtain, J., O'Brien, K. K., Dimitrov, B. D., & Fahey, T. (2010). Validity of British Thoracic Society guidance (the CRB-65 rule) for predicting the severity of pneumonia in general practice: Systematic review and meta-analysis. *British Journal of General Practice*, *60*(579), e423–e433.

Metcalf, E. P., Davies, J. C., Wood, F., & Butler, C. C. (2007). Unwrapping the diagnosis of tuberculosis in primary care: A qualitative study. *British Journal of General Practice*, *57*(535), 116–122.

Metlay, J. P., Kapoor, W. N., & Fine, M. J. (1997). Does this patient have community-acquired pneumonia? Diagnosing pneumonia by history and physical examination. *JAMA*, *278*(17), 1440–1445.

Montes de Oca, M. (2020). Smoking cessation/vaccinations. *Clinics in Chest Medicine*, *41*(3), 495–512.

Murugesan, N., Saxena, D., Dileep, A., Adrish, M., & Hanania, N. A. (2023). Update on the role of FeNO in asthma management. *Diagnostics (Basel, Switzerland)*, *13*(8), 1428.

Nacul, L., Soljak, M., Samarasundera, E., Hopkinson, N. S., Lacerda, E., Indulkar, T., Flowers, J., Walford, H., & Majeed, A. (2011). COPD in England: A comparison of expected, model-based prevalence and observed prevalence from general practice data. *Journal of Public Health (Oxford, England)*, *33*(1), 108–116.

Nannini, L. J., Poole, P., Milan, S. J., & Kesterton, A. (2013). Combined corticosteroid and long-acting beta(2)-agonist in one inhaler versus inhaled corticosteroids alone for chronic obstructive pulmonary disease. *Cochrane Database of Systematic Reviews*, *2013*(8), CD006826.

Nathan, R. A., Sorkness, C. A., Kosinski, M., Schatz, M., Li, J. T., Marcus, P., Murray, J. J., & Pendergraft, T. B. (2004). Development of the asthma control test: A survey for assessing asthma control. *Journal of Allergy and Clinical Immunology*, *113*(1), 59–65.

National Institute for Health and Clinical Excellence. (2018). *Chronic obstructive pulmonary disease (acute exacerbation): Antimicrobial prescribing*. NICE guideline [NG114]. Retrieved from https://www.nice.org.uk/guidance/ng114. Accessed May 30, 2024.

Nishimura, K., Izumi, T., Tsukino, M., & Oga, T. (2002). Dyspnea is a better predictor of 5-year survival than airway obstruction in patients with COPD. *Chest*, *121*(5), 1434–1440.

Pakhale, S., Mulpuru, S., Verheij, T. J., Kochen, M. M., Rohde, G. G., & Bjerre, L. M. (2014). Antibiotics for community-acquired pneumonia in adult outpatients. *Cochrane Database of Systematic Reviews*, *2014*(10), CD002109.

Pavlov, N., Haynes, A. G., Stucki, A., Jüni, P., & Ott, S. R. (2018). Long-term oxygen therapy in COPD patients: Population-based cohort study on mortality. *International Journal of Chronic Obstructive Pulmonary Disease*, *13*, 979–988.

Pinnock, H., Adlem, L., Gaskin, S., Harris, J., Snellgrove, C., & Sheikh, A. (2007). Accessibility, clinical effectiveness, and practice costs of providing a telephone option for routine asthma reviews: Phase IV controlled implementation study. *British Journal of General Practice*, *57*(542), 714–722.

Pinnock, H., Burton, C., Campbell, S., Gruffydd-Jones, K., Hannon, K., Hoskins, G., Lester, H., & Price, D. (2012). Clinical implications of the Royal College of Physicians three questions in routine asthma care: A real-life validation study. *Primary Care Respiratory Journal*, *21*(3), 288–294.

Pinnock, H., Fletcher, M., Holmes, S., Keeley, D., Leyshon, J., Price, D., Russell, R., Versnel, J., & Wagstaff, B. (2010). Setting the standard for routine asthma consultations: A discussion of the aims, process and outcomes of reviewing people with asthma in primary care. *Primary Care Respiratory Journal*, *19*(1), 75–83.

Pinnock, H., Kendall, M., Murray, S. A., Worth, A., Levack, P., Porter, M., MacNee, W., & Sheikh, A. (2011). Living and dying with severe chronic obstructive pulmonary disease: Multi-perspective longitudinal qualitative study. *BMJ (Clinical research ed.)*, *342*, d142.

Polosa, R., & Thomson, N. C. (2013). Smoking and asthma: Dangerous liaisons. *European Respiratory Journal*, *41*(3), 716–726.

Poole, P., Black, P. N., & Cates, C. J. (2012). Mucolytic agents for chronic bronchitis or chronic obstructive pulmonary disease. *Cochrane Database of Systematic Reviews*, (8), CD001287.

Prins, H. J., Duijkers, R., Daniels, J. M. A., van der Molen, T., van der Werf, T. S., & Boersma, W. (2021). COPD-Lower Respiratory Tract Infection Visual Analogue Score (c-LRTI-VAS) validation in stable and exacerbated patients with COPD. *BMJ Open Respiratory Research*, *8*(1), e000761.

Raissy, H. H., Harkins, M., Kelly, F., & Kelly, H. W. (2008). Pretreatment with albuterol versus montelukast for exercise-induced bronchospasm in children. *Pharmacotherapy*, *28*(3), 287–294.

Ram, F. S., Jones, P. W., Castro, A. A., De Brito, J. A., Atallah, A. N., Lacasse, Y., Mazzini, R., Goldstein, R., & Cendon, S. (2002). Oral theophylline for chronic obstructive pulmonary disease. *Cochrane Database of Systematic Reviews*, *2002*(4), CD003902.

Ram, F. S., Wright, J., Brocklebank, D., & White, J. E. (2001). Systematic review of clinical effectiveness of pressurised metered dose inhalers versus other hand held inhaler devices for delivering beta (2) agonists bronchodilators in asthma. *BMJ (Clinical research ed.)*, *323*(7318), 901–905.

Renkema, T. E., Schouten, J. P., Ko°ter, G. H., & Postma, D. S. (1996). Effects of long-term treatment with corticosteroids in COPD. *Chest*, *109*(5), 1156–1162.

Royal College of Physicians. (2014, May). *Why asthma still kills: The National Review of Asthma Deaths (NRAD)*. Confidential Enquiry Report. https://www.rcp.ac.uk/media/i2jjkbmc/why-asthma-still-kills-full-report.pdf. Accessed May 30, 2024.

Scottish Intercollegiate Guidelines Network. (2019, July). *British guideline on the management of asthma. A national clinical guideline* (Revised ed.). Retrieved from https://www.sign.ac.uk/our-guidelines/british-guideline-on-the-management-of-asthma/. Accessed May 30, 2024.

Seamark, D. A., Seamark, C. J., & Halpin, D. M. (2007). Palliative care in chronic obstructive pulmonary disease: A review for clinicians. *Journal of the Royal Society of Medicine*, *100*(5), 225–233.

Seemungal, T. A., Donaldson, G. C., Bhowmik, A., Jeffries, D. J., & Wedzicha, J. A. (2000). Time course and recovery of exacerbations in patients with chronic obstructive pulmonary disease. *American Journal of Respiratory and Critical Care Medicine*, *161*(5), 1608–1613.

Sheikh, S., Hamilton, F. W., Nava, G. W., Gregson, F. K. A., Arnold, D. T., Riley, C., Brown, J., AERATOR Group, Reid, J. P., Bzdek, B. R., Maskell, N. A., & Dodd, J. W. (2022). Are aerosols generated during lung function testing in patients and healthy volunteers? Results from the AERATOR study. *Thorax*, *77*(3), 292–294.

Simons, F. E. (1999). Allergic rhinobronchitis: The asthma-allergic rhinitis link. *Journal of Allergy and Clinical Immunology*, *104*(3 Pt 1), 534–540.

Singh, D., Agusti, A., Martinez, F. J., Papi, A., Pavord, I. D., Wedzicha, J. A., Vogelmeier, C. F., & Halpin, D. M. G. (2022). Blood eosinophils and chronic obstructive pulmonary disease: A Global Initiative for Chronic Obstructive Lung Disease Science Committee 2022 Review. *American Journal of Respiratory and Critical Care Medicine*, *206*(1), 17–24.

Soler-Cataluña, J. J., Martínez-García, M. A., Román Sánchez, P., Salcedo, E., Navarro, M., & Ochando, R. (2005). Severe acute exacerbations and mortality in patients with chronic obstructive pulmonary disease. *Thorax*, *60*(11), 925–931.

Soriano, J. B., Visick, G. T., Muellerova, H., Payvandi, N., & Hansell, A. L. (2005). Patterns of comorbidities in newly diagnosed COPD and asthma in primary care. *Chest*, *128*(4), 2099–2107.

Suissa, S., Blais, L., & Ernst, P. (1994). Patterns of increasing beta-agonist use and the risk of fatal or near-fatal asthma. *European Respiratory Journal*, *7*(9), 1602–1609.

Surveillance for respiratory hazards in the occupational setting [American Thoracic Society]. (1982). *American Review of Respiratory Disease*, *126*(5), 952–956.

Tattersfield, A. E., Town, G. I., Johnell, O., Picado, C., Aubier, M., Braillon, P., & Karlström, R. (2001). Bone mineral density in subjects with mild asthma randomised to treatment with inhaled corticosteroids or non-corticosteroid treatment for two years. *Thorax*, *56*(4), 272–278.

Thomas, M., Gruffydd-Jones, K., Stonham, C., Ward, S., & Macfarlane, T. V. (2009). Assessing asthma control in routine clinical practice: Use of the Royal College of Physicians '3 questions'. *Primary Care Respiratory Journal*, *18*(2), 83–88.

Tiotiu, A., Ioan, I., Wirth, N., Romero-Fernandez, R., & González-Barcala, F. J. (2021). The impact of tobacco smoking on adult asthma outcomes. *International Journal of Environmental Research and Public Health*, *18*(3), 992.

Torres, A., Peetermans, W. E., Viegi, G., & Blasi, F. (2013). Risk factors for community-acquired pneumonia in adults in Europe: A literature review. *Thorax*, *68*(11), 1057–1065.

Turner, M. O., Noertjojo, K., Vedal, S., Bai, T., Crump, S., & Fitzgerald, J. M. (1998). Risk factors for near-fatal asthma. A case-control study in hospitalized patients with asthma. *American Journal of Respiratory and Critical Care Medicine*, *157*(6 Pt 1), 1804–1809.

UK Health Security Agency. (2021, January). *Department of Health & Social Care. Immunisation against infectious disease*. Retrieved from https://www.gov.uk/government/collections/immunisation-against-infectious-disease-the-green-book. Accessed May 30, 2024.

UK Health Security Agency. (2023, March). *Tuberculosis in England, 2022 report*. Retrieved from https://www.gov.uk/government/publications/tuberculosis-in-england-2022-report-data-up-to-end-of-2021. Accessed May 30, 2024.

van Dijk, W., Tan, W., Li, P., Guo, B., Li, S., Benedetti, A., Bourbeau, J., & CanCOLD Study Group. (2015). Clinical relevance of fixed ratio vs lower limit of normal of FEV1/FVC in COPD: Patient-reported outcomes from the CanCOLD cohort. *Annals of Family Medicine*, *13*(1), 41–48.

van Eerd, E. A., van der Meer, R. M., van Schayck, O. C., & Kotz, D. (2016). Smoking cessation for people with chronic obstructive pulmonary disease. *Cochrane Database of Systematic Reviews*, *2016*(8), CD010744.

van Geffen, W. H., Douma, W. R., Slebos, D. J., & Kerstjens, H. A. (2016). Bronchodilators delivered by nebuliser versus pMDI with spacer or DPI for exacerbations of COPD. *Cochrane Database of Systematic Reviews*, *2016*(8), CD011826.

Verbakel, J. Y., Lee, J. J., Goyder, C., Tan, P. S., Ananthakumar, T., Turner, P. J., Hayward, G., & Van den Bruel, A. (2019). Impact of point-of-care C reactive protein in ambulatory care: A systematic review and meta-analysis. *BMJ Open*, *9*(1), e025036.

Wolf, F. M., Guevara, J. P., Grum, C. M., Clark, N. M., & Cates, C. J. (2003). Educational interventions for asthma in children. *Cochrane Database of Systematic Reviews*, (1), CD000326.

8

Gastroenterologic Problems

Vincent Cheung & Lulia Al-Hillawi

CHAPTER CONTENTS

Disorders of the Upper Gastrointestinal Tract

GUIDELINES

National Institute for Health and Clinical Excellence. (2019). *Gastro-oesophageal reflux disease and dyspepsia in adults: Investigation and management. NICE clinical guideline 184.* Retrieved from http://www.nice.org.uk/guidance/cg184.

National Institute for Health and Clinical Excellence. (2021). *Suspected cancer: Recognition and referral. NICE clinical guideline 12.* Retrieved from http://www.nice.org.uk/guidance/ng12.

- Upper gastrointestinal (GI) symptoms are extremely common in the general population, and the vast majority of patients have benign disease (Maconi et al., 2008).
- Broadly speaking, symptoms are combined under the umbrella term of 'dyspepsia' and may include upper abdominal or epigastric pain, nausea, vomiting, belching, bloating, and borborygmi (National Institute for Health and Clinical Excellence [NICE], 2014c). Reflux symptoms of heartburn, reflux, or regurgitation should be *initially* managed/investigated in the same way.
- Although benign disease predominates, the possibility of cancer is often a significant concern for patients, families, and treating clinicians.

Initial Management in Primary Care

- If a previous diagnosis has been made at endoscopy with no new alarm symptoms, then manage as previously advised.
- Encourage lifestyle modification with avoidance of food triggers, alcohol reduction, smoking cessation, and weight loss.
- Check that the patient is not taking a drug that can cause dyspepsia (e.g., aspirin or a nonsteroidal antiinflammatory drug (NSAID), a calcium antagonist, a nitrate, a theophylline, a bisphosphonate, or a steroid).
- Offer to 'test and treat' *Helicobacter pylori* infection.
- Consider a 4-week empirical trial of a proton pump inhibitor (PPI) (e.g., omeprazole 20 mg once daily to increase to 40 mg once daily if refractory symptoms) in *Helicobacter*-negative patients. If symptoms recur after initial treatment, step down the PPI to the lowest dose required to control symptoms. Encourage self-management and discuss using treatment on an 'as required' basis.
- Offer histamine-2-antagonists, (e.g., famotidine 20 mg once daily) in patients with inadequate response to a PPI.

Alarm Symptoms

- 'Alarm features' have been shown to be sensitive, but not specific, in screening for upper GI carcinoma. In a UK study of 1852 patients referred to a rapid access upper GI cancer service, only dysphagia, weight loss, and age older than 55 years were independent significant predictors of cancer. Furthermore, older than 55 years was only a significant predictor if at least one other alarm feature was present (anaemia, anorexia, vomiting, dysphagia, weight loss, or 'high-risk features'). Simple dyspepsia, even if new or continuous, was *inversely* correlated with the finding of cancer in these older patients (Kapoor et al, 2005).

Investigation and Referral

- Patients presenting with UGI symptomology (dyspepsia, heartburn, epigastric pain) and significant acute GI bleeding require immediate (same-day) referral for assessment with or without endoscopy.
- Consider referral to exclude upper GI cancer in the following circumstances:
  a. Consider a suspected cancer pathway referral (for an appointment within 2 weeks) for people with an upper abdominal mass consistent with gastric cancer.
  b. Offer urgent direct access upper GI endoscopy (to be performed within 2 weeks) to assess for oesophago-gastric cancer in people with dysphagia or aged 55 years or older with weight loss and upper abdominal pain, reflux, or dyspepsia.
  c. Consider nonurgent direct access upper GI endoscopy to assess for oesophagogastric cancer in people with haematemesis.
  d. Consider nonurgent direct access upper GI endoscopy to assess for oesophagogastric cancer in people with any of the following:
     - Treatment-resistant dyspepsia
     - Upper abdominal pain with low haemoglobin levels
     - Raised platelet count with nausea, vomiting, weight loss, reflux, dyspepsia, or upper abdominal pain
     - Nausea or vomiting with weight loss, reflux, dyspepsia, or upper abdominal pain
- Consider referral to a specialist service for patients:
  - Of any age with upper GI symptoms that are nonresponsive to treatment or unexplained
  - With suspected gastro-oesophageal reflux disease (GORD) who are considering surgery
  - With *H. pylori* infection that has not responded to second-line therapy
  - For consideration of surveillance in patients with Barrett oesophagus (taking into account it's ≥10 mm,

presence of dysplasia, person's risk factors, and patient preference).

Dyspepsia

- Dyspepsia is not a diagnosis but rather describes a range of symptoms that should prompt doctors to consider underlying disease of the upper GI tract. These symptoms may include upper abdominal or epigastric pain, nausea, vomiting, belching, bloating and borborygmi (NICE, 2014c).
- In Western countries, one-third of the population have symptoms of dyspepsia, but of them, only 25% seek medical attention. Ten percent are investigated by endoscopy with only 2% of patients undergoing endoscopy being diagnosed with gastric cancer (NICE, 2004).
- In 90% of patients (including 75% of patients with *H. pylori* infection), the final diagnosis is functional dyspepsia (FD), and most disease is managed symptomatically (Briggs et al, 1996).

Helicobacter pylori

- *H. pylori* is a gram-negative bacterium identified in 1982 by Australian scientists Barry Marshall and Robin Warren (Marshall & Warren, 1984) and recognised to affect at least 50% of the population worldwide.
- Infection usually occurs in the first few years of life and tends to persist indefinitely unless treated.
- *H. pylori* infection is recognised as a risk factor for peptic ulcer disease (reported to develop in 1%–10% of infected patients) and gastric cancer (occurring in 0.1%–3%) (McColl, 2010).

Testing for H. pylori

- *H. pylori* serology testing is inexpensive, convenient, and widely available. However, a meta-analysis of commercially available antibody assays demonstrates a sensitivity and specificity of only 85% and 79%, respectively (Loy et al, 1996). A further limitation is that this test has little value in confirming eradication of the infection because the antibodies persist for many months, if not longer, after eradication.
- The urea breath test (UBT) involves drinking 13C- or 14C-labelled urea, which is converted to labelled carbon dioxide by the urease in *H. pylori*. The infection can also be detected by identifying *H. pylori*–specific antigens in a stool sample. These tests have much better sensitivity (95%) and specificity (95%) than serologic testing (Gisbert & Pajares, 2004; Vaira & Vakil, 2001).
- For both the UBT and the faecal antigen test, the patient should stop taking PPIs 2 weeks before testing, should stop taking H$_2$ receptor antagonists for 24 hours before testing, and should avoid taking antimicrobial agents for 4 weeks before testing because these

medications may suppress the infection and reduce the sensitivity of testing.

Test and Treat

- The rationale for 'test and treat' is that *H. pylori* eradication can effectively treat undiagnosed peptic ulcer disease in uninvestigated dyspepsia without alarm symptoms. A large randomised control study found this to be cost effective because of the reduction in unnecessary endoscopy despite having a number needed to treat (NNT) of seven patients (Ford et al, 2005).
- *H. pylori* eradication is likely to be helpful in patients with duodenal ulceration (DU); gastric ulceration (GU); gastritis; duodenitis; and, marginally, in functional dyspepsia (FD) (NNT = 15) (McColl, 2010).

Eradicating H. pylori

- NICE recommends a 1-week triple therapy regimen as first-line eradication therapy. The optimum regimen consists of a full-dose PPI, with amoxicillin 1 g and either clarithromycin 500 mg or in the case of penicillin hypersensitivity, metronidazole 400 mg and clarithromycin 500 mg, all given twice daily.
- Eradication is effective in 80% to 85% of patients on triple therapy using either antibiotic combination.
- Prescribing amoxicillin and tetracycline rarely results in *H. pylori* resistance, whereas resistance occurs after limited exposure to clarithromycin and quinolones. Exposure to metronidazole also results in *H. pylori* resistance, but this has less of an impact on the effectiveness of treatment regimens.
- *First-line therapy.* Choose the treatment regimen with the lowest acquisition cost and consider previous exposure to clarithromycin or metronidazole. (It is not necessary to consider previous metronidazole exposure in patients with penicillin allergy.)
- *Second-line therapy* should use different antibiotics to first-line therapy.
- Seek advice from a gastroenterologist if eradication of *H. pylori* is not successful with second-line therapy.
- Before prescribing further therapy with quadruple or sequential therapy, it is important to confirm that the infection is still present and to consider whether additional antimicrobial treatment is appropriate (e.g., patients with confirmed peptic ulcer disease). This is likely to require endoscopy with rapid-urease testing or gastric histology used to confirm persistent infection. It may also allow tissue to be sent for culture and sensitivity to guide antibiotic prescribing when appropriate (McColl, 2010).
- However, patients with no endoscopic evidence of significant *Helicobacter*-related pathology are likely to have functional dyspepsia, and given the marginal benefit of *Helicobacter* eradication in this group (NNT =15), symptomatic management with long-term acid suppression may be more appropriate (McColl, 2010).

Confirmation of Successful Eradication

- It is good practice to confirm successful eradication. Confirmation should definitely be performed in the following circumstances:
  a. Ongoing or recurrent symptoms after eradication therapy
  b. Partial resection for gastric cancer
  c. Mucosa associated lymphoid tissue (MALT) lymphoma
  d. Complicated peptic ulcer disease (e.g., after perforation or ulcer bleed)
- Wait 4 weeks after eradication before repeating UBT or faecal antigen.

Other Considerations and Controversies

- *H. pylori and reflux.* Chronic *Helicobacter* infection may result in atrophic gastritis and reduced acid secretion, which is protective against significant reflux disease. Most epidemiologic studies have demonstrated a negative association between *H. pylori* infection and GORD or its complications with the prevalence of *H. pylori* infection being lower in reflux patients than in control participants. Numerous studies have now reported a strong negative association between *H. pylori* infection and risk of adenocarcinoma of the oesophagus or gastro-oesophageal junction.
- *Population screening.* Despite being identified as a carcinogen, there is no consensus that population screening and eradication of asymptomatic individuals is beneficial. Given the negative association of *Helicobacter* with oesophageal adenocarcinoma, it has been postulated that eradication might increase the risk of oesophageal adenocarcinoma because of increased acid secretion and reflux, thus potentially trading one cancer risk for another (Islami & Kamangar, 2008).
- *Other people to test and treat.* European guidelines recommend eradicating *H. pylori* infection in first-degree relatives of patients with gastric cancer and in patients with atrophic gastritis, unexplained iron-deficiency anemia, or chronic idiopathic thrombocytopenic purpura (Malfertheiner et al, 2007).
- *Reinfection.* This rarely occurs, and many reported cases may simply represent recrudescence (i.e., failure of initial eradication) (van der et al, 1997).

Peptic Ulcer Disease

- The vast majority of peptic ulcer disease cases are caused by *H. pylori* infection or use of NSAIDs.
- *H. pylori*–positive patients should receive eradication therapy.
- Offer *H. pylori*–negative patients who are not taking NSAIDs a full-dose PPI (e.g., omeprazole 20 mg/day) or H_2RA for 4 to 8 weeks.
- Patients taking NSAIDs should stop where possible and be offered full-dose PPI (e.g., omeprazole 20 mg/day) or H_2RA for 8 weeks.

- Patients continuing NSAIDs should be coprescribed a PPI, counselled regarding the risk with the need for treatment reviewed regularly, and a switch to cyclooxygenase-2 selective NSAID considered.
- Patients with gastric ulcer should undergo repeat endoscopy after 6 to 8 weeks with or without biopsy to ensure healing and exclude malignancy.
- Consider repeat testing to confirm successful eradication in *H. pylori*–positive patients with complicated peptic ulcer disease (e.g., perforation or bleeding) and depending on the size and extent of ulceration.

Functional Dyspepsia

- FD is defined as the presence of symptoms thought to originate in the gastroduodenal region in the absence of any organic, systemic, or metabolic disease that is likely to explain the symptoms (Tack et al, 2006).
- FD is diagnosed in approximately 80% of patients referred for endoscopy to investigate dyspepsia (Ford et al, 2010).
  - The Rome IV criteria for FD should be used to make a diagnosis (criteria fulfilled for the past 3 months with symptom onset at least 6 months before diagnosis) and must include:
    1. *One or more of:*
       a. Bothersome epigastric pain
       b. Bothersome epigastric burning
       c. Bothersome postprandial fullness
       d. Bothersome early satiation
    (in which 'bothersome' is used to describe symptoms severe enough to interfere with daily activities)
    and
    2. No evidence of structural disease (including at upper endoscopy) that is likely to explain the symptoms
- The Rome IV criteria have further been classified into two distinct subtypes: postprandial distress syndrome (PDS), in which symptoms are mainly triggered by meals and occur at least 3 days a week, and epigastric pain syndrome (EPS), in which symptoms are often present regardless of meals and occur at least 1 day a week, though patients with FD can have overlapping features of both subtypes. To have a diagnosis of FD, one must fulfil criteria for PDS or EPS.

Management of Functional Dyspepsia

- Reassurance and explanation regarding the diagnosis should be provided.
- The evidence base in FD is limited by high placebo response rates (20%–60%) and many small, heterogenous studies, but acid suppression remains the first-line management. Meta-analyses have shown PPIs and H_2 antagonists to be effective with NNTs of 7 and 8, respectively (Moayyedi et al, 2003b). However, some of the benefit with these drugs may be from treating undiagnosed reflux.
- *Helicobacter* spp. eradication provides only marginal benefit (NNT = 17) (Moayyedi et al, 2003a).

- Prokinetics (e.g., domperidone and metoclopramide) appear efficacious but are limited by risk of cardiac arrhythmia and extrapyramidal side effects such that they are largely restricted to use for short-term symptomatic relief (Moayyedi et al, 2003b).
- Regular aerobic exercise is also recommended first-line treatment for FD in national guidance (Black et al, 2022).
- Referral of patients with FD to gastroenterology in secondary care is appropriate when there is diagnostic doubt, when symptoms are severe or refractory to first-line treatments, or when the individual requests a specialist opinion.

Gastroesophageal Reflux Disease

- GORD is defined as excessive reflux of gastric contents into the oesophagus that causes symptoms or complications.
- GORD typically presents with heartburn and regurgitation, but extra-oesophageal symptoms do occur (Vakil et al, 2006).
- It is the most common chronic disease in Western countries with 25% experiencing monthly symptoms and 5% having reflux daily (Moayyedi & Talley, 2006).
- A positive diagnosis of reflux cannot necessarily be established endoscopically because up to 60% of endoscopies show normal results in patients with GORD. Further oesophageal studies may be required if symptoms are refractory to treatment in endoscopy-negative reflux disease.
- Patients with an insufficient therapeutic response to the standard dose of one PPI may benefit from one of the other PPIs, an increased dose of the same PPI, or a twice-a-day PPI regimen (Boeckxstaens et al, 2014).
- In patients with functional heartburn, there is evidence for selective serotonin reuptake inhibitors (SSRIs) and tricyclic antidepressants (TCAs) (Viazis et al, 2012).
- Complications of reflux include oesophagitis, peptic stricture formation, columnar metaplasia (Barrett oesophagus), and oesophageal adenocarcinoma.
- Screening for Barrett oesophagus with endoscopy is not feasible or justified for an unselected population with reflux symptoms but can be considered in patients with chronic GORD symptoms and multiple risk factors (at least three of age 50 years or older, White race, male sex, and obesity). The threshold should be lowered if there is a family history of Barrett or oesophageal adenocarcinoma in one or more first-degree relative (Fitzgerald et al, 2014).
- Because of the increased risk of oesophageal adenocarcinoma in patients with Barrett oesophagus, surveillance endoscopy is recommended (Fitzgerald et al, 2014). High-grade and persistent low-grade dysplasia may now be treated endoscopically with radiofrequency ablation, often avoiding the need for oesophagectomy (NICE, 2014a).

Dysphagia

- Urgent direct-access endoscopy should be considered in all patients presenting with dysphagia. However, many will subsequently have a normal examination or be found to have benign disease, so an approach to further investigation is required (Abdel Jalil et al, 2015).
- Patients with peptic oesophageal strictures may require balloon dilatation (perforation risk of ~1%) and should be maintained on long-term PPI to prevent recurrence.
- Eosinophilic oesophagitis typically presents as food bolus obstruction in young males with a history of atopy. Characteristic endoscopic appearances have been described (concentric ringlike oesophagus called trachealisation, furrowing, white exudates, strictures), but it should be considered particularly in young patients presenting with dysphagia. Proximal and distal oesophageal biopsies (showing >15 eosinophils per high-power field) may help to confirm or refute the diagnosis. Many patients respond to acid suppression, but in others, elimination diets, topical steroids, or both may be required. There is a new oral budesonide tablet for eosinophilic oesophagitis that should be specialist initiated.
- Chest radiography should be considered in smokers to exclude extrinsic compression from a bronchial neoplasm with or without mediastinal mass.
- Barium swallow may identify the presence of a pharyngeal pouch or oesophageal dysmotility in patients with persistent dysphagia.
- Oesophageal manometry (with or without pH monitoring to exclude significant reflux) helps to diagnose motility disorders of the oesophagus (e.g., diffuse oesophageal spasm or achalasia).
- Oesophageal spasm often presents with chest pain, and achalasia is characterised by weight loss and frequent regurgitation. Heller myotomy, pneumohydraulic balloon dilatation, and Botox injection to the lower oesophageal sphincter are therapeutic options that may be considered in those with confirmed achalasia.
- Functional dysphagia is less common than FD but is similarly a diagnosis of exclusion. Empirical trials of antireflux therapy are appropriate but not always effective (Clouse et al, 1999).
- Patients with 'high' dysphagia (i.e., above the level of the suprasternal notch) should be considered for otolaryngology referral and nasendoscopy, particularly if current or ex-smokers.

Gallstone Disease

GUIDELINES

National Institute for Health and Clinical Excellence. (2014). *Gallstone disease: Diagnosis and management. NICE clinical guideline 188.* Retrieved from https://www.nice.org.uk/guidance/cg188.
National Institute for Health and Clinical Excellence. (2015). *Suspected cancer: Recognition and referral. NICE clinical guideline 12.* Retrieved from https://www.nice.org.uk/guidance/ng12.

- If endoscopy is negative and symptoms do not respond to *H. pylori* eradication or acid suppression, consider alternative investigations such as abdominal ultrasonography, amylase, and liver function tests (LFT), which may point to biliary or pancreatic disease.
- Gallstone disease affects up to 15% of the adult population, but the majority experience no symptoms (NICE, 2014).
- Cholecystitis typically presents with persistent pain (lasting >6 hours) and fever. In contrast, the pain from biliary colic is intermittent and lasts from a few minutes up to 1 hour before subsiding after less than 4 to 6 hours. In both cases, pain classically occurs postprandially.
- Ultrasound examination is effective in detecting cholecystitis and gallstones (sensitivity, >95%) (Shea et al, 1994) but is inferior to magnetic resonance cholangiopancreatography (MRCP) for identifying biliary obstruction (e.g., common bile duct stones) (Singh et al, 2014).
- Biliary colic can often be controlled in primary care with appropriate analgesia, with advice for a low-fat diet to prevent further episodes (successful in 30% of patients).
- Patients with suspicion of acute cholecystitis, cholangitis, or acute pancreatitis should be referred to hospital as an emergency (Association of Upper Gastrointestinal Surgeons of Great Britian and Ireland, 2016).
- In patients with recurrent biliary colic, chronic cholecystitis, or previous gallstone pancreatitis, surgical referral for cholecystectomy should be considered.
- Endoscopic retrograde cholangiopancreatography (ERCP) with or without sphincterotomy is required for bile duct stones. Cholecystectomy should subsequently be performed.
- Functional disorders can also affect the gallbladder (e.g., biliary dyskinesia) and biliary tree (biliary sphincter disorders formerly known as sphincter of Oddi dysfunction). Pharmacologic therapy seems to be ineffective, and ERCP with sphincterotomy is sometimes considered for certain cases, usually when there is derangement in LFTs with or without abnormal imaging (Sgouros & Pereira, 2006).

Pancreatic Disease

GUIDELINES

National Institute for Health and Clinical Excellence. (2015). *Suspected cancer: Recognition and referral. NICE clinical guideline 12*. Retrieved from http://www.nice.org.uk/guidance/ng12.
National Institute for Health and Clinical Excellence. (2018). *Pancreatitis. NICE clinical guideline 104*. Retrieved from http://www.nice. org.uk/guidance/ng104.

Pancreatic cancer remains in the top 5 most common cause of cancer death in the UK. Survival rates are poor due to late diagnosis, with an average life expectancy of 3-6 months. 70% of tumours occur in the head of the pancreas. Symptoms commonly include jaundice, weight loss, nausea and non-specific abdominal pain. Late-onset diabetes can also occur.

Consider an urgent direct-access computed tomography (CT) scan (to be performed within 2 weeks) to assess for pancreatic cancer in people aged 60 years and older with weight loss and diarrhoea, back pain, abdominal pain, nausea, vomiting, constipation, or new-onset diabetes.

Acute pancreatitis presents with typical, acute, upper abdominal pain. It can carry significant morbidity and mortality. Urgent A&E assessment is warranted if suspected.

Risk factors include gallstones, alcohol excess and certain medications (e.g. thiopurines, tetracyclines, thiazides, sulfonamides, metronidazole, sodium valproate).

Chronic pancreatitis can occur with ongoing inflammation of the pancreas. Chronic pain can become an issue. Whilst alcohol excess and ongoing consumption account for a large proportion of these patients, other long-term conditions can be associated (e.g. cystic fibrosis, autoimmune pancreatitis).

Pancreatic pseudocysts are cysts of pancreatic enzymes which can occur as a consequence of pancreatitis. Often self-limiting, they can however cause long-term issues in a small subset of patients requiring specialist hepatobiliary input with repeated drainage +/− antibiotics.

Irritable Bowel Syndrome

GUIDELINES

National Institute for Health and Clinical Excellence. (2017). *Irritable bowel syndrome in adults: Diagnosis and management. NICE clinical guideline 61*. Retrieved from http://www.nice.org.uk/guidance/cg61.
Vasant, D. H., Paine, P. A., Black, C. J., Houghton, L. A., Everitt, H. A., Corsetti, M., Agrawal, A., Aziz, I., Farmer, A. D., Eugenicos, M. P., Moss-Morris, R., Yiannakou, Y., & Ford, A. C. (2021). British Society of Gastroenterology guidelines on the management of irritable bowel syndrome. *Gut, 70*, 1214–1240.

- Irritable bowel syndrome (IBS) is a common, chronic GI condition of unknown cause (Vasant et al, 2021).
- About 10% to 20% of the UK population is estimated to be affected with the condition. It is twice as common in females, and the peak incidence between the ages of 20 and 30 years (NICE, 2008).
- It is characterised by abdominal pain or discomfort associated with defaecation, abdominal bloating, and bowel dysfunction (constipation, diarrhoea, or both).
- IBS can also affect sleep and cause stress, anxiety, and lethargy. It is associated with reduced work productivity and quality of life.

Diagnosis and Referral

- Consider IBS in patients presenting with ≥6 months of **a**bdominal pain or discomfort, **b**loating, or **c**hange in bowel habit (think 'ABC').
- It is defined by the Rome III diagnostic criteria as recurrent abdominal pain or discomfort at least 3 days per month in the previous 3 months associated with two or more of the following:
    a. Improvement with defecation
    b. Onset associated with a change in frequency of stool
    c. Onset associated with a change in form (appearance) of stool
- Symptom onset should be at least 6 months before diagnosis. Refer to secondary care patients with any of the following 'red flags':
    a. Unintentional and unexplained weight loss
    b. Rectal bleeding
    c. Family history of bowel or ovarian cancer
    d. Change in bowel habit in patients older than 60 years
    e. Anaemia
    f. Abdominal or rectal masses
    g. Increased inflammatory markers

Investigation

- Full blood count (FBC), erythrocyte sedimentation rate, C-reactive protein (CRP), and antibody testing for coeliac disease (tissue transglutaminase [tTG] or endomysial antibodies) should be performed in all patients with suspected IBS (NICE, 2008).
- Faecal immunochemical testing should be used when appropriate to triage referral to secondary care for those patients with 'red flag' symptoms concerning for lower gastrointestinal (LGI) cancer (Monahan et al, 2022).
- Although not necessary to confirm the diagnosis in those meeting diagnostic criteria, consider testing thyroid function.
- In females with bloating symptoms, consider ruling out gynaecologic causes.
- Faecal calprotectin (FCP) has been shown to be a useful screening test to differentiate between inflammatory bowel disease (IBD) and IBS. It is a calcium and zinc-binding protein within the cytosol of neutrophils and a sensitive but nonspecific marker of inflammation within the GI tract.
- NICE recommend using FCP to support the diagnosis of IBS when cancer is not suspected (NICE, 2013a).
- Some studies suggest the manufacturer's FCP cut-off values are too low for use in clinical practice with levels less than 200 µg/g rarely associated with any organic disease (Seenan et al, 2014).

Irritable Bowel Syndrome Subtypes

- IBS can be classified based on the predominant symptoms into:
    - Constipation-predominant IBS (IBS-C)
    - Diarrhoea-predominant IBS (IBS-D)
    - Mixed-type IBS (IBS-M)

- This allows treatment to be tailored to the most troublesome symptom (Longstreth et al, 2006).

Treatment

- A diagnosis of IBS should be made with emphasis on reassurance and explanation.
- Patient self-management should be encouraged. This should include information on general lifestyle, physical activity, and diet (including limiting intake of insoluble fibre) (NICE, 2008).
- More detailed dietary advice is provided in the British Dietetic Association's Food Facts for IBS Factsheet (www.bda.uk.com/foodfacts/IBSfoodfacts.pdf).
- If further dietary management is required, such as trialling a low-FODMAP (fermentable oligosaccharides, disaccharides, monosaccharides, and polyols) diet, it should be led by a healthcare professional with relevant expertise (i.e., Registered Dietician).
- The evidence for probiotics is weak but they may help bloating and flatulence in some patients (Didari et al, 2015; DuPont, 2014; Zhang et al, 2016).
- Consider prescribing antispasmodic agents (e.g., peppermint oil) for patients with IBS (Ruepert et al, 2011).
- Laxatives should be considered for constipated patients but lactulose avoided because it may exacerbate bloating and discomfort (NICE, 2008).
- Loperamide should be the first-choice antimotility agent for patients with IBS-D.
- Consider TCAs as second-line treatment for patients with IBS if laxatives, loperamide, or antispasmodics have not helped. Start at a low dose (e.g., amitriptyline 10 mg nocte) to minimise sedation. Increase the dose if necessary and tolerated (maximum 30 mg). TCAs are effective (NNT = 3) and primarily reduce pain but also have an antimotility effect with a suggestion that patients with IBS-D obtain the greatest benefit (Ruepert et al, 2011).
- Consider SSRIs (e.g., fluoxetine 20mg/day) only if TCAs are ineffective (Ruepert et al, 2011).
- Linaclotide (290 µg once daily) is a guanylate cyclase C agonist that elevates cyclic guanosine monophosphate, accelerating transit in the GI tract through increased fluid transit and reducing visceral hypersensitivity. It improves pain, bloating, and constipation in IBS-C and should be considered if optimal or maximum tolerated doses of laxatives from different classes have not helped in patients with constipation for 12 months or more (Chey et al, 2012; Quigley et al, 2013).
- Prucalopride (1–2mg/day) is a highly selective serotonin 5-HT4 agonist that stimulates gut motility. It has been shown to be effective in patients (85% females) with chronic constipation with an expected onset of effect within 4 weeks (Camilleri et al, 2008, 2010, 2016).

Inflammatory Bowel Disease

GUIDELINES

Lamb, C. A., Kennedy, N. A., Raine, T., Hendy, P. A., Smith, P. J., Limdi, J. K., Hayee, B., Lomer, M. C. E., Parkes, G. C., Selinger, C., Barrett, K. J., Davies, R. J., Bennett, C., Gittens, S., Dunlop, M. G., Faiz, O., Fraser, A., Garrick, V., Johnston, P. D., Parkes, M., … Hawthorne, A. B. (2019). British Society of Gastroenterology consensus guidelines on the management of inflammatory bowel disease in adults. *Gut, 68,* S1–S106.
National Institute for Health and Clinical Excellence. (2019). *Crohn's disease: Management.. NICE clinical guideline 129.* Retrieved from http://www.nice.org.uk/guidance/ng129.
National Institute for Health and Clinical Excellence. (2019). *Ulcerative colitis: Management. NICE clinical guideline 1302.* Retrieved from https://www.nice.org.uk/guidance/ng130.

Ulcerative Colitis

- Ulcerative colitis (UC) is the commoner form of IBD with an incidence of 10 per 100,00 and prevalence of 240 per 100,000. This means there are an estimated 146,000 patients with UC across the United Kingdom.
- Presentation peaks between the ages of 15 and 25 years with a smaller peak later in life from 55 to 65 years.
- UC typically affects the colon continuously from the rectum to a variable distance proximally. The extent is therefore described as proctitis (limited to the rectum), distal or left sided, extensive or pancolitis.
- It usually presents with bloody diarrhoea, urgency, and abdominal pain. Weight loss and extraintestinal symptoms can also occur (NICE, 2019a).
- 1 in 10 patients will require a colectomy within the first 10 years of diagnosis.

Crohn's Disease

- Crohn's disease affects an estimated 115,000 people in the United Kingdom.
- One-third of cases present before the age of 21 years.
- Unlike UC, it causes transmural inflammation and can affect anywhere in the GI tract from the mouth to the anus.
- Crohn's disease is described by location in the GI tract (e.g., small bowel, ileocolonic, colonic, or perianal) and phenotype (inflammatory, structuring, penetrating/fistulising).
- Historically, 50% to 80% of patients require surgery because of complications such as perforation, obstruction caused by stricture formation, or fistulisation.
- Crohn's disease is multifactorial thought to be due to a combination of genetic and environmental factors such as smoking, which in combination lead to immune dysfunction (NICE, 2019b).

General Points

- Patients with IBD should be under a specialist service to oversee care.

- There is a multidisciplinary approach to IBD care, and most centres have dedicated specialist nurse teams for support (Lamb et al, 2019).
- Cigarette smoking has a negative impact on the clinical course of Crohn's disease, and those that continue to smoke are more likely to have recurrence of disease after resection. Given the risk of widespread harm to health for all patients, efforts should be made to help patients with IBD quit smoking.
- The Crohn's and Colitis UK Charity is an excellent resource for patients and healthcare professionals (https://crohnsandcolitis.org.uk).

Pharmacologic Treatment

Topical Therapy

- *Indication,* Induction and maintenance of remission in patients with UC and Crohn's colitis.
- Particularly effective in distal disease. Consider using suppositories in proctitis and enemas in patients with distal or left-sided colitis. Various enema preparations are available, including liquid, foam, and retention enemas. Choice of preparation depends on patient preference.
- Topical therapy can also provide additional benefit to oral therapy in patients with extensive colitis (inflammation that extends beyond splenic flexure).
- Studies suggest aminosalicylate preparations are more effective than steroid suppositories or enemas (Marshall & Irvine, 1997; Munkholm et al, 2010).
- Topical therapy may be used to treat acute exacerbations, as 'as required therapy' in patients with limited disease (proctitis), or as regular maintenance therapy.
- *Typical doses.* Mesalazine suppositories usual dose 1 g/day, mesalazine enemas 1 to 2 g/day, prednisolone rectal foam 20 to 40mg/day (for ≤4 weeks).
- *Monitoring.* Not required.

Oral Aminosalicylates

- *Indications.* Induction and maintenance of remission in patients with mild to moderate or moderate to severe (high-dose) UC.
- Sulfasalazine and oral aminosalicylates are effective therapy for both inducing and maintaining remission in UC.
- Oral aminosalicylates are preferred because of their improved side effect profile. Diarrhoea (3%), headache (2%), nausea (2%), and rash (1%) are reported, but a systematic review has shown that adverse events are similar to placebo for mesalazine.
- All aminosalicylates have been associated with nephrotoxicity (including interstitial nephritis and nephrotic syndrome). Patients receiving oral aminosalicylates should have their renal function monitored at commencement and then annually (Mowat et al, 2011).
- Studies suggest that doses greater than 2 g are more effective at inducing remission in patients with moderate to severe disease (Ford et al, 2011). Higher doses (4.8 g vs 2.4 g/day) are associated with increased rates of

response and earlier mucosal healing (Hanauer et al, 2005; Hanauer et al, 2007; Lichtenstein et al, 2011).

- Oral therapy can be combined with topical aminosalicylates if required.
- Except in patients with proctitis, treatment is continued indefinitely to reduce the risk of relapse (Feagan & MacDonald 2012) and mitigate colorectal cancer (CRC) risk (van Staa et al, 2005). The threshold dose to reduce CRC risk appears to be 1.2 g/day (Rubin et al, 2006). Modified-release preparations should be used to reduce the pill burden, minimise dosing, and improve patient compliance.
- There is limited evidence to support the use of aminosalicylates in active Crohn's disease. However, they may have a role in reducing the risk of colorectal neoplasia in Crohn's colitis (van Staa et al, 2005) and the prevention of postoperative recurrence (Gordon et al, 2011).
- *Typical doses.* Mesalazine 2.4 to 4.8 g/day (active disease) and 1.2 to 2.4 g (maintenance).
- *Recommended monitoring.* Renal function annually.

Oral Steroids

- *Indication.* Induction of remission in patients with both UC and Crohn's disease.
- Effective in inducing remission but maintenance therapy is avoided because of the side effects of long-term use (e.g., hypertension, diabetes, osteoporosis, cataracts, glaucoma).
- Patients receiving systemic steroids should be coprescribed calcium and vitamin D as bone protection.
- Budesonide can be used in both UC (Cortiment, Ferring, Budesonide MMX, colonic release) and mild to moderate ileocaecal Crohn's disease (Entocort, Tillotts, or Budenofalk, Dr Falk, terminal ileal release). It may be preferred because of its high first-pass metabolism, low systemic absorption, and better side effect profile.
- Consider prescribing steroids in patient unresponsive or intolerant to aminosalicylates.
- *Typical doses*
  - Prednisolone 40mg/day reducing by 5 mg per week over 8 weeks to stop
  - Budesonide MMX (Cortiment) 9 mg for 8 weeks; then stop
  - Budesonide (Entocort, Budenofalk) 9 mg for 8 weeks; then 6 mg for 2 weeks and 3 mg for further 2 weeks
- *Monitoring.* Consider the risk of diabetes in symptomatic patients and screening for osteoporosis, hypertension, cataracts, and glaucoma with high cumulative doses.

Thiopurines

- *Indication.* Maintenance of remission in moderate-severe UC and Crohn's disease.
- Thiopurines have demonstrated efficacy in maintaining remission for both UC (Gisbert et al, 2009) and Crohn's disease (Chande et al, 2013). They may also have a role in the preventing postoperative recurrence in Crohn's disease (Gordon et al, 2014).
- Check thiopurine methyltransferase (TPMT) activity before staring. One in 300 will have absent TPMT

activity putting, them at risk for life-threatening myelosuppression (Mowat et al, 2011).

- Other side effects (e.g., pancreatitis, hepatitis, myalgia, nausea, vomiting) appear to be independent of TPMT activity. Patients should also be advised regarding the increased relative risk (approximately two- to threefold) of nonmelanoma skin cancer (NMSC) and lymphoma. Advice to reduce the risk of NMSC by avoiding excessive sun exposure should be offered (see www.bad.org.uk).
- Mercaptopurine may be used in patients with normal TPMT activity who are intolerant of azathioprine without pancreatitis (Hindorf et al, 2009; Lees et al, 2008).
- Thiopurine metabolite monitoring can identify noncompliance and patients in whom coprescription of allopurinol to low-dose azathioprine may be beneficial to improve efficacy and prevent drug-induced hepatitis (Smith et al, 2012).
- Given the potential side effects of long-term use, cessation may be an option for those in long-term (≥5–10 years) clinical, endoscopic, and histologic remission, with the benefits and risks of continuing azathioprine discussed with individual patients. Those stopping maintenance therapy with thiopurine should be receiving aminosalicylate therapy if tolerated (Lamb et al, 2019).
- Typical doses
  - Azathioprine 2 to 2.5 mg/kg daily
  - Mercaptopurine 1 to 1.5 mg/kg daily
- *Monitoring.* Please refer to the local 'shared-care protocol' but typically requires FBC, urea and electrolytes (U&Es), and LFTs weekly for 4 weeks then monthly for 3 months and 3-monthly thereafter.

Methotrexate

- *Indication.:* Induction and maintenance therapy in patients with Crohn's disease.
- Methotrexate been shown to be effective as both induction (Alfadhli et al, 2003; McDonald et al, 2014) and maintenance therapy for Crohn's disease (Feagan et al, 2000).
- It is often used in patients who are intolerant to thiopurines.
- Coprescription of folic acid 5 mg (once a week taken 3 days after methotrexate) limits GI side effects of nausea, vomiting, diarrhoea, and stomatitis. Long-term concerns are hepatotoxicity, pneumonitis, and opportunistic infections.
- Methotrexate is teratogenic and should not be used in females or males considering conception. It may persist in tissues for long periods; therefore, conception should be avoided for 3 to 6 months after withdrawal of therapy (Mowat et al, 2011).
- *Monitoring.* Please refer to the local 'shared-care protocol'. Measurement of FBC and LFTs are generally advisable before and within 4 weeks of starting therapy, then monthly.

Biologics

- *Indication.* Induction and maintenance therapy in patients with moderate to severe UC and Crohn's disease who are unresponsive to, intolerant of, or unsuitable for conventional therapy.

- Infliximab, adalimumab (anti–tumour necrosis factor [TNF]-α), vedolizumab (anti-integrin), and ustekinumab (anti-interleukin [IL]-12 and IL-23) are now approved for use in both UC and Crohn's disease in the United Kingdom. Golimumab (anti–TNF-α) is only approved for use in UC.
- Before initiation, patients are screened for tuberculosis (TB) based on history, chest radiography, and blood testing (interferon-γ release assays (e.g., T-spot or QuantiFERON-TB Gold). Human immunodeficiency virus (HIV), hepatitis B, and hepatitis C serology should also be performed. It is good practice to check varicella zoster virus status if there is no confirmed history of chicken pox, with vaccination in those not previously exposed.
- Anti-TNFs are avoided in patients with history of confirmed or suspected demyelination.
- *Monitoring.* Please refer to the local 'shared-care protocol'.

Small Molecules

- Janus kinase (JAK) inhibitors are small molecules that target the JAK–STAT signalling pathway in lymphocytes. There are currently three used for patients with IBD: tofacitinib, filgotinib, and upadacitinib.
  - *Indication.* Induction and maintenance therapy in patients with moderate to severe UC who are unresponsive to, intolerant of, or unsuitable for conventional therapy.
  - Upadacitinib has recently been licensed for use in moderate to severe Crohn's disease by the Medicines and Healthcare Products Regulatory Agency (MHRA), and a decision is awaited from NICE about whether it will be recommended for use on the NHS (NICE, 2023).
  - A higher rate of venous thromboembolism and major adverse cardiovascular events has been seen in patients on the higher induction dose of tofacitinib. All JAK inhibitors carry increased risk of shingles, and treatment is associated with a dose-dependent increase in lipid parameters.
  - *Monitoring.* Please refer to the local 'shared-care protocol'. Of note, for JAK-inhibitors such as upadacitinib, lipid profile should form part of blood monitoring.
- The sphingosine-1-phosphate receptor (S1PR) modulator ozanimod
  - *Indication.* Induction and maintenance therapy in patients with moderate to severe UC who are unresponsive to, intolerant of, or unsuitable for conventional therapy.
  - Ozanimod may cause transient bradycardia and cardiac rhythm disturbance. It is not recommended in patients with significant cardiac history, uncontrolled hypertension, or cerebrovascular disease. There is an increased risk of macular oedema in those with preexisting retinal disease.
  - *Before treatment*: Patients require electrocardiography and blood pressure checks before starting treatment. Patients with certain preexisting cardiac conditions or

bradycardia require cardiac monitoring for 6 hours after the first dose. Eye examination is recommended in patients with diabetes, uveitis, or retinal disease.
  - *Monitoring.* Please refer to the local 'shared-care protocol'. Patients require intermittent blood pressure monitoring; FBC and LFT blood monitoring; and periodic eye examination in those with a history of diabetes, uveitis, or retinal disease.

Surgery

Ulcerative Colitis

- *Indications*
  - Severe colitis refractory to medical therapy; may be an emergency or semielective procedure
  - Dysplasia or cancer
- Acutely patients usually undergo subtotal colectomy. In some cases, an ileoanal pouch anastomosis (IPAA) will be considered at a later stage (e.g., 6 months after initial surgery).
- In UC, surgery can generally be considered 'curative' and removes both the risk of CRC and need for colonoscopic surveillance. Laparoscopic surgery with enhanced recovery and early discharge is increasingly available.
- However, there are morbidity and mortality risks attached to surgery. Furthermore, IPAA is not always possible, and some patients may require a permanent stoma. Pouch function may be variable, and increased stool frequency and volume is expected.
- After proctocolectomy with IPAA, the median stool frequency is four to eight motions per day with a volume of around 700 mL (compared with 200 mL in healthy subjects).
- Pouchitis (nonspecific inflammation of the pouch) occurs in up to 50% of patients after 10 years. After being confirmed (endoscopically and histologically), antibiotics (metronidazole, ciprofloxacin, or both) often induce remission. This can be maintained with the probiotic VSL#3 (Singh et al, 2015). Other treatments for refractory pouchitis include infliximab (IFX), vedolizumab, steroids (e.g., budesonide), and removal of the pouch (van Assche et al, 2013).

Crohn's Disease

- *Indications*
  - Severe colitis refractory to medical therapy: subtotal colectomy or panproctocolectomy without IPAA
  - Stricturing disease causing obstruction
  - Crohn's mass or abscess
  - Fistulising disease (including perianal disease with associated sepsis)
  - Colonic dysplasia or cancer
- Patients with perianal sepsis associated with Crohn's should undergo an examination under anaesthesia, ideally by a colorectal surgeon experienced in managing IBD. This often involves drainage of any abscess or collection and laying open of fistula tracts with or without insertion of a noncutting Seton suture to allow drainage and prevent recurrent sepsis.

TABLE 8.1 Truelove and Witts' (1955) Criteria for Acute Severe Colitis

Criterion	Description
Bowel movements (number per day)	Six or more plus at least one of the features of systemic upset (marked with * below)
Blood in stools	Visible blood
Pyrexia (temperature >37.8°C)*	Yes
Pulse rate greater than 90 beats/min*	Yes
Anaemia*	Yes
Erythrocyte sedimentation rate (mm/h)*	>30

- Perianal disease may also be treated with antibiotics (e.g., metronidazole or ciprofloxacin). However long-term use of these drugs is limited by concerns regarding antibiotic resistance, antibiotic-associated diarrhoea, and other side effects (e.g., neuropathy with metronidazole and seizures with ciprofloxacin). When sepsis is controlled, patients with perianal disease are treated with biologic agents, such as infliximab and ustekinumab.

Indications for Admission

- Patients with acute severe colitis require hospital admission for intravenous steroids with or without rescue medical therapy with infliximab (or, in cases when this is contraindicated, cyclosporin). The rate of colectomy (nonelective) for inpatients with UC remains relatively high at 10% to 15% (Royal College of Physicians, 2014). Acute severe colitis is defined according to Truelove and Witts' (1955) criteria as shown in Table 8.1.
- Other indications for admission include:
  - Acute obstruction
  - Suspected intrabdominal or perianal sepsis
  - Significant GI bleeding

Cancer Surveillance

- Patients with UC and Crohn's disease are considered to have an equivalent increased risk of CRC provided there is a similar extent and duration of colonic inflammation.
- Risk factors for CRC in patients with IBD include:
  - Duration and extent of disease
  - Family history of CRC (Patients with an affected first-degree relative have a twofold increased risk.)
  - Primary sclerosing cholangitis (PSC)
  - Young age at diagnosis
  - Evidence also suggests that persistent inflammation increases the risk of CRC and is now considered when

determining surveillance intervals. This emphasises the importance of compliance to treatment and good disease control
- All patients should undergo a repeat colonoscopy at 8 to 10 years from initial diagnosis or at diagnosis if there is concurrent PSC. This should ideally be performed as a dye-spray chromoendoscopy with the patient in clinical remission and will guide the need for further surveillance, which may be at 1, 3, or 5 years depending on the estimated risk.

Fertility and Pregnancy

- Patients with inactive IBD can be expected to have normal fertility levels, but they are reduced by active disease.
- Both male and female patients undergoing surgery are at risk of resultant infertility (via impotence or ejaculatory problems and impaired tubular function respectively). This is of particular concern when pouch formation or rectal excision is performed. Sulfasalazine (but not other aminosalicylates or thiopurines) cause a reversible and dose-dependent decrease in sperm motility and count.
- Methotrexate is teratogenic, therefore should not be used in females wishing to conceive (van Assche et al, 2010).
- There is concern from animal studies regarding teratogenicity in higher doses of tofacitinib. There is not enough data regarding the safety of other small molecules; therefore, small molecules (JAK inhibitors, S1PR modulators) should not be used or started in females wishing to conceive.
- Patients should be in clinical remission before conception because it is associated with better pregnancy outcomes.
- Folate supplementation is important to prevent neural tube defects. This is particularly important when Sulfasalazine is used because it may interfere with folate absorption. Some patients with IBD will therefore be advised to take high-dose folic acid of 5 mg/day rather than standard 400 mcg/day dosing. Pre-conception counselling should therefore be offered, and if not possible, advice sought as soon as pregnancy is determined in IBD patients.
- IBD is a risk for preterm birth and low birth weight but not stillbirth or congenital malformations.
- If conception occurs when disease is quiescent, the risk of relapse during pregnancy is the same as in nonpregnant females. However, in patients who conceive when the disease is active, the majority will continue to have active disease during pregnancy (e.g., in Crohn's disease, two-thirds of those with active disease at conception continue to have active disease with the majority deteriorating clinically during their pregnancies).
- Medical treatment (except for methotrexate, JAK inhibitors, and S1PR modulators) should generally be continued throughout pregnancy because the benefits of good disease control outweigh the risks of therapy.
- Specific guidance
  - Metronidazole should be used with caution and only of there is no alternative because of the risk of prematurity.

Ciprofloxacin or co-amoxiclav is preferable, but to minimise risk, the shortest possible course should always be used.

- Suppositories and enemas are safe until the third trimester.
- Despite having a US Food and Drug Administration rating of D, which is extrapolated from animal studies, human studies suggest that azathioprine and mercaptopurine are safe and well tolerated (Alstead et al, 1990; Francella et al, 2003; Norgard et al, 2003; Zlatanic et al, 2003).
- Anti-TNF drugs are recognised to cross the placenta in the late second and third trimesters. To minimise foetal exposure and subsequent immunosuppression, consideration may be given to discontinuing these drugs at 24 weeks' gestation if patients are in remission. However, it is now common practice to continue throughout the pregnancy. If continued in pregnancy, a neonatologist should be consulted and live vaccines avoided in the foetus until they are 12 months old (Lamb et al, 2019).
- Flares should be treated aggressively and similar to in nonpregnant patients. Endoscopic investigation and some imaging modalities can be undertaken safely when needed.
- Patients with uncomplicated IBD can deliver vaginally. Caesarean section should be preferred in perianal Crohn's disease, active rectal disease, or when an IPAA is present. Colectomy or ileostomy patients can deliver vaginally.
- Close collaboration between gastroenterologists and obstetricians is encouraged, and in complex cases, consideration should be given to early referral via pregnancy planning or medical obstetric clinics (van Assche et al, 2010).

Breastfeeding

- Sulfasalazine, other aminosalicylates, thiopurines, and anti-TNF therapy are all considered safe in breastfeeding.
- Ustekinumab and vedolizumab are generally considered to be safe in breastfeeding, though there are limited data.
- Metronidazole and ciprofloxacin should be avoided.
- Methotrexate is contraindicated.
- Small molecules (JAK inhibitors, S1PR modulators) should be avoided.
- Steroids appear in low concentrations in breast milk. To minimise exposure, a 4-hour delay after oral dosing may be considered (van Assche et al, 2010).

Vaccinations

- A vaccine and infection history, including TB exposure, chickenpox history, and risk of hepatitis B, should be obtained at diagnosis in patients with IBD.

- Varicella zoster serology should be checked if there is no history of infection and immunisation considered before initiation of steroids or immunosuppressants.
- Hepatitis B serology should be checked in high-risk patients (please refer to 'Immunisation against Infectious Diseases: The Green Book', Department of Health, United Kingdom) and vaccination considered before initiation of steroids, immunosuppressants, or anti-TNF monoclonal antibody therapy in nonimmune patients.
- Influenza, pneumococcal, and human papillomavirus (females) vaccination is recommended for immunosuppressed adults and is best considered for all patients with IBD, given the frequent need for steroid and immunosuppressive therapy. Booster vaccinations are appropriate for influenza (annually) and pneumococcus (after 3 years).
- Live vaccines should be avoided in patients on immunosuppression or steroids (measles, mumps, and rubella; oral polio; yellow fever; live typhoid; varicella; bacillus Calmette–Guérin).
- Immunoglobulin postexposure prophylaxis of non-immune individuals on high-dose steroid or immunosuppression should be considered after exposure to varicella or measles. Acyclovir prophylaxis may also be used for varicella (van Assche et al, 2010).

Chronic Diarrhoea

> ### GUIDELINES
>
> Arasaradnam, R. P., Brown, S., Forbes, A., Fox, M. R., Hungin, P., Kelman, L., Major, G., O'Connor, M., Sanders, D. S., Sinha, R., Smith, S. C., Thomas, P., & Walters, J. R. F. (2018). Guidelines for the investigation of chronic diarrhoea in adults: British Society of Gastroenterology, 3rd edition. *Gut; 67(8)*, 1380–1399.
> National Institute for Health and Clinical Excellence. (2015). *Suspected cancer: Recognition and referral. NICE clinical guideline 12*. Retrieved from https://www.nice.org.uk/guidance/ng12.

- Chronic diarrhoea may be defined as the abnormal passage of three or more loose or liquid stools per day for more than 4 weeks or a daily stool weight greater than 200 g/day.

Further Investigation

- Refer to secondary care for further investigation patients older than 60 years with a change in bowel habit to looser or more frequent stools.
- Stool culture (including analysis for ova, cysts, and parasites) should always be considered.
- Coeliac disease occurs in approximately 1 in 100 patients in the United Kingdom. Therefore, serologic testing for coeliac disease should be performed in all patients

presenting with diarrhoea (see subsection on coeliac disease).

- Microscopic colitis (lymphocytic or collagenous colitis) is increasingly recognised as a cause of chronic watery diarrhoea. The aetiology is unclear, and it may occur as a postinfectious phenomenon but is often drug induced. Commonly implicated drugs include lansoprazole, NSAIDs, and SSRIs and should be withdrawn if possible. Budesonide (9 mg/day for 6 weeks) is effective at controlling diarrhoea in approximately 80%, but symptoms often recur on discontinuation, so patients may need several courses. Other therapeutic options include antidiarrhoeals, bismuth, prednisolone, and aminosalicylates with or without bile acid sequestrants. However, microscopic colitis is distinct from conventional IBD and, importantly, is not associated with any long-term complication, so it should be managed symptomatically (Nguyen et al, 2016).
- Malabsorption is often accompanied by steatorrhoea and the passage of bulky, malodorous, pale stools. It may be associated with biochemical or haematological abnormalities suggesting nutritional deficiency (e.g., electrolyte deficiencies, hypocalcaemia, low vitamin D, elevated prothrombin time suggesting vitamin K deficiency, macrocytosis, or haematinic deficiencies).
- In patients in whom history or investigations are suggestive of malabsorption, consider the following:
  a. Faecal elastase (normal >500, low if pancreatic exocrine failure) with or without CT of the pancreas
  b. Hydrogen breath test or empirical trial of antibiotics for small bowel bacterial overgrowth, particularly in patients with increased risk of this such as those with gut dysmotility or altered anatomy (e.g., blind loop) because of previous surgery
  c. Small bowel imaging (e.g., CT enterography or magnetic resonance imaging of the small bowel) to exclude small bowel Crohn's disease (Headstrom & Surawicz, 2005; Schiller, 2004)
- Bile salt malabsorption may occur after terminal ileal resection but has also been described after cholecystectomy and in postinfectious or idiopathic diarrhoea. A ^{75}Se homotaurocholate (75Se-HCAT) scan demonstrating poor retention (<5% at 7 days) or an elevated serum 7-alpha cholestenone level suggests the diagnosis. However, a therapeutic trial of bile acid sequestrant (e.g., cholestyramine 4 g twice daily (bd) or colesevelam 3.75 g daily) is often preferred.
- Other rare causes of diarrhoea include:
  a. Carcinoid syndrome: may be associated with flushing and diagnosed by demonstrating elevated urinary 5-hydroxyidolacetic acid
  b. Gastrointestinal neurointestinal tumours (Consider gut hormone analysis)
  c. Factitious diarrhoea e.g., laxative abuse (Arasaradnam et al, 2018)

Coeliac Disease

GUIDELINES

Ludvigsson, J. F., Bai, J. C., Biagi, F., Card, T. R., Ciacci, C., Ciclitira, P. J., Green, P. H., Hadjivassiliou, M., Holdoway, A., van Heel, D. A., Kaukinen, K., Leffler, D. A., Leonard, J. N., Lundin, K. E., McGough, N., Davidson, M., Murray, J. A., Swift, G. L., Walker, M. M., Zingone, F., ... British Society of Gastroenterology. (2014). Diagnosis and management of adult coeliac disease: Guidelines from the British Society of Gastroenterology. *Gut, 63*(8),1210–1228.

National Institute for Health and Clinical Excellence. (2015). *Coeliac disease: Recognition, assessment and management. NICE clinical guideline 20.* Retrieved from http://www.nice.org.uk/guidance/ng20.

- Coeliac disease is an autoimmune condition causing inflammation of the proximal small bowel induced by the ingestion of gluten.
- It affects around 1% of the world's population, but the incidence varies geographically.
- The prevalence of coeliac disease has increased in the past 50 years, but most patients are undiagnosed.
- Human leukocyte antigen (HLA) types DQ2 (95%) or DQ8 is present in more than 99% of individuals affected by coeliac disease.
- Histologic features on duodenal biopsy are subtotal villous atrophy associated with crypt hyperplasia and increase in intraepithelial lymphocytes.
- Coeliac disease is associated with an increased risk of non-Hodgkin lymphoma and small bowel adenocarcinoma but not an overall increase in malignant conditions (Mooney et al, 2014).
- The interest in gluten as a factor in other conditions has increased, and many individuals without coeliac disease may identify themselves as gluten sensitive. The mechanism for gluten sensitivity is unclear (Aziz et al, 2014; Lebwohl et al, 2015).

Initial Testing and Referral

- Many individuals with coeliac disease are asymptomatic, but presenting symptoms that should prompt testing for coeliac disease include:
  - In children
    a. Recurrent abdominal pain
    b. Failure to thrive or short stature
    c. Diarrhoea: only in 10%
  - In adults
    a. Diarrhoea: fewer than 50% of patients
    b. Nonspecific abdominal symptoms often mimicking IBS
    c. Anaemia: around 50% of patients at diagnosis may be iron deficient, but vitamin B_{12} and folate may also be low
    d. Elevated liver enzymes
    e. Osteoporosis

f. Dermatitis herpetiformis: itchy blistering rash on the trunk; may precede clinical evidence of intestinal involvement, but duodenal biopsies are abnormal

g. Aphthous stomatitis

h. Unexplained neurologic symptoms: may relate to micronutrient deficiency

i. Subfertility and low-birthweight offspring

- In addition to the above, in patients with a clinical picture suggesting possible coeliac disease, testing is recommended in the following groups:
  - First-degree relatives of patients with coeliac disease: risk is 10%
  - Patients with type 1 diabetes: risk is 4% to 7%
  - Patients with other autoimmune disease with unexplained symptoms
  - Individuals with Down syndrome or Turner syndrome
- Immunoglobulin A (IgA) tTG antibody has 98% specificity and 95% sensitivity and is the initial investigation of choice.
- When IgA deficiency is present (2%–3% of patients with coeliac disease), IgG antiendomysial antibody should be tested.
- Adult patients with positive antibody screening should be referred for oesophagogastroscopy (OGD) and duodenal biopsy.
- Patients referred for biopsy should be told to continue to take gluten in at least one meal per day in the interim.
- In symptomatic children, an IgA tTG titre more than 10 times the upper limit of normal may be sufficient for diagnosis without biopsy (Murch et al, 2013).
- HLA typing should only be carried out in specialist settings to exclude coeliac disease:
  - In patients who exclude gluten before biopsy and are not willing to reintroduce it
  - To minimise future testing in high-risk individuals such as first-degree relatives (NICE, 2015a)

Further Management

- When coeliac disease is confirmed by duodenal biopsy, patients should be advised on lifelong exclusion of gluten from their diet.
- Patients diagnosed with coeliac disease should be referred to a dietitian.
- Patients should be advised to avoid all wheat, rye, and barley.
- Guidance on prescription of gluten-free products can be found in the document 'Gluten Free Foods: a Revised Prescribing Guide' online (http://www.coeliac.org.uk). Prescribing of gluten-free products may be restricted according to local integrated care board policy in the United Kingdom.
- Oats should be avoided initially, but certified gluten-free oats may be introduced after 6 to 12 months with follow-up assessment and serologic testing to assess tolerance (NICE, 2015a).

- Patients should have repeat biopsy if tTG titre has not fallen to normal range after 12 months on a gluten-free diet (Ludvigsson et al, 2014).
- Patients should be encouraged to join national coeliac support group (e.g., Coeliac UK).
- Patients with coeliac disease should be vaccinated against:
  - Pneumococcus
  - Meningitis C
  - Haemophilus influenza B
  - Influenza annually

Ongoing Management

- Patients should be seen on an annual basis to:
  - Measure weight and height.
  - Assess symptoms.
  - Assess diet and adherence to a gluten-free diet and consider need for specialist dietetic advice.
- Suggested investigations:
  - Measure tTG titre.
  - Measure FBC, ferritin, folate, and vitamin B_{12}.
  - Check calcium levels, alkaline phosphatase, and vitamin D levels (Ludvigsson et al, 2014).
- Bone densitometry scan should be offered to patients with two or more of body mass index (BMI) less than 20, weight loss greater than 10%, age older 70 years, or persisting symptoms or poor adherence to a gluten-free diet (Scott et al, 2000).
  - If osteopenia, repeat after 3 years on a gluten-free diet.
  - Repeat at age 55 years for males or at menopause for females if normal at baseline.
  - Patients with osteoporosis should be treated according to current guidance.
  - All patients should be encouraged to assure adequate calcium intake, taking supplements, if necessary, to achieve this.
- Other autoimmune conditions are common in individuals with coeliac disease, and these should be tested for when there are symptoms.

Refractory or Recurrent Symptoms

- Patients with refractory symptoms or recurrence of symptoms should be referred to gastroenterology for assessment.
- Causes of ongoing diarrhoea include:
  - Noncompliance with a gluten-free diet or inadvertent gluten ingestion
  - Lymphocytic colitis
  - Small bowel bacterial overgrowth
  - Lactose intolerance
  - Hyperthyroidism
  - Pancreatic insufficiency
  - Refractory coeliac disease
  - Small bowel lymphoma or adenocarcinoma (Mooney et al, 2014)

Refractory Coeliac Disease

- Refractory coeliac disease (RCD) is diagnosed when clinical and histologic features of coeliac disease persist despite strict gluten exclusion for at least 6 to 12 months.
- The incidence is uncertain but rare.
- *Type 1 RCD.* Small bowel lymphocytes are polyclonal and express typical CD3/CD8 positivity. Response to treatment with steroids and immunosuppression is good, and the 5-year survival is greater than 90%.
- *Type 2 RCD* has aberrant or clonal T-cell lines with loss of CD3/CD8 positivity.
  - Response to treatment is poor, and progression to lymphoma is common. The 5-year survival rate is 40% to 60% (Al Toma et al, 2007; Rubio-Tapia & Murray, 2010).
  - There are no guidelines for treatment of patients with this condition, so patients should be referred to a tertiary centre.

Lymphoma and Cancer Risk

- Individuals with coeliac disease should be reassured that that life expectancy is not reduced.
- Patients with coeliac disease have around a two- to four-fold increased risk of non-Hodgkin lymphoma, equating to about 1 in 2000 per year (Mooney et al, 2014).
- Enteropathy-associated T-cell lymphoma (type 1)
  - This is a rare form of lymphoma associated with coeliac disease, particularly type 2 RCD.
  - The prognosis is poor with a 2-year survival rate of less than 20% (Al Toma et al, 2007).
  - The highest rate of diagnosis is in the first year after diagnosis, and the risk reduces with compliance with a gluten-free diet.
- The risk of small bowel adenocarcinoma is more than 30 times higher in patients with coeliac disease, although it is still rare (Howdle et al, 2003; Mooney et al, 2014).
- A gluten-free diet is thought to reduce the risk of lymphoma and small bowel cancer.

Noncoeliac Gluten Sensitivity

- Many people without coeliac disease perceive that there are health benefits to excluding gluten from the diet (Lebwohl et al, 2015).
- In a population study of 1002 people in the United Kingdom, 13% reported gluten sensitivity, and 3.7% avoid eating gluten (Aziz et al, 2014).
- Some patients with IBS improve when gluten is restricted.
- Some of these patients will have IBS and be sensitive to FODMAPs.
- The biologic basis for noncoeliac gluten sensitivity is not established; therefore, a frank discussion with patients regarding the risks and benefits of dietary restriction is recommended.

Iron-Deficiency Anaemia

GUIDELINES

National Institute for Health and Clinical Excellence. (2021). *Suspected cancer: Recognition and referral. NICE clinical guideline 12.* Retrieved from http://www.nice.org.uk/guidance/ng12.
Snook, J., Bhala, N., Beales, I. L. P., Cannings, D., Kightley, C., Logan, R. P., Pritchard, D. M., Sidhu, R., Surgenor, S., Thomas, W., Verma, A. M., & Goddard, A. F. (2021). British Society of Gastroenterology guidelines for the management of iron deficiency anaemia in adults. *Gut, 70,* 2030–2051.

- Iron deficiency is common, affecting up to 2% to 5% of males and postmenopausal females in developed countries (Snook et al, 2021).
- Causes of iron deficiency include dietary deficiency, lack of absorption from the diet, and chronic loss of blood.
- Endoscopic investigation of iron deficiency in the absence of anaemia rarely yields a diagnosis of malignancy. Risks and benefits of investigation should be discussed with the individual patient and should only be considered in patients aged older than 50 years or with GI symptoms (Snook et al, 2021).

Causes

- Coeliac disease is the commonest cause of iron deficiency from malabsorption (prevalence, 4%–6%). Other causes, including postgastrectomy, *Helicobacter* colonisation, gut resection, and small bowel bacterial overgrowth, are less common.
- Benign sources of GI blood loss, including aspirin and NSAID use, account for 10% to 20% of patients.
- Prevalence of GI tract cancers are in the region of:
  - Colonic: 5% to 10%
  - Gastric: 5%
  - Oesophageal: 2%
  - Small bowel tumours: 1% to 2%
  - Ampullary carcinoma: less than 1% (NICE, 2021)

  Non-GI sources of blood loss include menstruation (20%–30%), blood donation (5%), and haematuria (1%). If the latter is present, urology referral is warranted (Snook et al, 2021).

History

- The history should include a dietary review and a careful history for any source of blood loss or associated symptoms (e.g., dyspepsia, altered bowel habits, weight loss).
- Ask about previous history of anaemia and investigation.
- Ask about family or personal history of haemoglobinopathies, telangiectasia, and other bleeding disorders.
- Enquire about family history of GI tract cancer, IBD, and coeliac disease.
- Check drug history (e.g., anticoagulants, antiplatelets, NSAIDs).
- Ask about previous surgical history (e.g., gastrectomy).

TABLE 8.2	Interpretation of Iron Studies	
Test	Iron-Deficiency Anaemia	Anaemia of Chronic Disease
Mean corpuscular volume and mean corpuscular haemoglobin	Low	Low to normal
Ferritin	Low	Normal to high
Iron	Low	Low
Transferrin	High	Low
Transferrin saturation	Low	Normal

Examination

- Clinical signs of iron deficiency are unusual, but patients should be examined to exclude an abdominal mass, and those with rectal bleeding or tenesmus should have a digital rectal examination (Snook et al, 2021).

Initial Investigation

- FBC with mean cell volume, blood film, and ferritin level.
  - Low serum ferritin is recognised as the best indicator of iron deficiency.
  - Ferritin is elevated in inflammatory states, so iron deficiency can exist in the presence of normal ferritin.
  - Iron studies may help to clarify iron deficiency but can be difficult to interpret. Table 8.2 may help interpretation.
- IgA tTG antibody for coeliac disease
- Urinalysis in all patients (Snook et al, 2021)
- The 2015 NICE guidelines for recognition of lower GI cancers, revised in 2023, suggest offering testing with quantitative faecal immunochemical tests in any adult patient with iron-deficiency anaemia, and in those over 60 years old with anaemia even in the absence of iron deficiency (Table 8.2).

Further Investigation

- Menstruating females with no GI symptoms should be screened for coeliac disease with IgA tTG antibody.
- More invasive GI investigation is only warranted when there are GI symptoms or other high-risk factors (i.e., age older than 50 years or strong family history of GI tract malignancy) (Snook et al, 2021).
- Females who are not menstruating and not pregnant and males of any age should have both upper and lower GI investigations (Snook et al, 2021).
- Endoscopy is the best test for investigation of the upper GI tract.
- Distal duodenal biopsies should be taken to exclude coeliac disease.
- Colonoscopy is the optimal lower GI investigation because of its high sensitivity and ability to biopsy or provide therapy (e.g., polypectomy).
- CT virtual colonoscopy is up to 90% sensitive for lesions larger than 1 cm but does not allow for biopsy and histologic diagnosis. This investigation usually still involves full bowel preparation but can be performed with minimal preparation or without contrast on request (Spada et al, 2014).
- After CT colonoscopy, flexible sigmoidoscopy may be required for completion because views of the rectum can be suboptimal.
- Small bowel investigation is not indicated in every patient with iron-deficiency anaemia but should be considered in those who become anaemic again after iron replacement, particularly if the patient is young or transfusion dependent despite iron supplementation (Snook et al, 2021; Sidhu et al, 2008).
- In such cases:
  - Capsule endoscopy has a high diagnostic yield but is not a therapeutic modality, so it may need to be followed up by push or balloon enteroscopy.
  - Magnetic resonance or CT enterography is sensitive for diagnosing inflammation and mucosal thickening but may not show up small vascular abnormalities or flat lesions.

Treatment

- Initial treatment of iron-deficiency anaemia should be with one tablet per day of ferrous sulphate, fumarate, or gluconate (Snook et al, 2021).
- Patients should be monitored in the first 4 weeks for a haemoglobin response, and treatment should be continued for a period of around 3 months after normalisation of the haemoglobin level to ensure adequate repletion of the marrow iron stores (Snook et al, 2021).
- Lack of response should prompt assessment of compliance or consideration of ongoing blood loss or problems with absorption.
- Parenteral iron can be used when oral preparations are not tolerated or not absorbed adequately (Snook et al, 2021).

Weight Loss

GUIDELINES

National Institute for Health and Clinical Excellence. (2017). *Nutrition support for adults: oral nutrition support, enteral tube feeding and parenteral nutrition 32. ICE clinical guideline.* Retrieved from http://www.nice.org.uk/guidance/cg32.
National Institute for Health and Clinical Excellence. (2021). *Suspected cancer: Recognition and referral. ICE clinical guideline 12.* Retrieved from http://www.nice.org.uk/guidance/ng12.

- Unintentional weight loss is common, particularly in older adult patients with 15% to 20% of those aged older than 65 years but as many as 50% to 60% of those residing in nursing homes affected (McMinn et al, 2011; NICE, 2006).
- Weight loss of 5% of body weight over 6 to 12 months is generally accepted as significant, but smaller losses in frailer patients may also be important.
- Weight loss may be caused by reduced calorie intake and conditions causing malabsorption, but in other conditions such as weight loss in malignancy, the mechanism is less well understood.
- Weight loss is not exclusively a symptom of GI disease, which is the cause in about one-third of cases, so a holistic approach to the patient is important.
- Exclusion of malignancy is often the primary concern for both the patient and doctor. Referral via urgent suspicion of cancer pathway for assessment or investigation should be offered (NICE, 2015b).
- No cause may be found in up to 25% of older adults. Malignancy may be the cause in a similar proportion. Data for younger adults are lacking (Gaddey & Holder, 2014; McMinn et al, 2011).
- The incidence of eating disorders in increasing. Both genders can be affected, as can people from a wide range of ages from childhood upwards (Micali et al, 2013). Patients with eating disorders have significantly increased mortality rates (Arcelus et al, 2011); therefore, it is important to have a high index of suspicion.

History and Examination

- Many conditions and medications can lead to reduced appetite. Careful history of what the patient eats as well as factors associated with their ability to access, prepare, and consume food is important (Gaddey & Holder, 2014).
- Medication side effects, including nausea and altered sense of taste, may be important (Alibhai et al, 2005).
- A thorough systematic review is key to elicit other symptoms, which can guide referral pathway.
- It is *essential* to document the patient's weight because self-reporting of weight is often not reliable.
- Full examination of all systems and examination for lymphadenopathy is indicated.

Investigation

- There are no guidelines specifically for the investigation of weight loss in all patients, but there are many recommendations for investigation of suspected cancer. Patients' symptoms should guide the initial investigation.
- Laboratory investigation
  - tTG antibody
  - FBC
  - Thyroid function tests
  - CRP
  - Glucose

- There is some evidence that in older patients, elevated serum lactate dehydrogenase is predictive of an organic cause (McMinn et al, 2011).
- Tumour markers are generally unhelpful ,but CA-125 should be tested in females with weight loss, loss of appetite, or early satiety (NICE, 2015b).
- HIV test should be performed (British HIV Association, 2008).
- Faecal elastase should be performed if the patient has diarrhoea or risk factors for pancreatic disease.
- FCP should be performed if diarrhoea is suspicious for IBD.

Endoscopy

- OGD should be done in all patients with unintentional weight loss. Patients aged older than 55 years with abdominal pain, dyspepsia, reflux, or nausea and vomiting with weight loss should be referred for urgent direct-access OGD.
- Patients with weight loss associated with altered bowel habits, rectal bleeding, or iron-deficiency anaemia should be referred for urgent assessment or direct-access colonoscopy (NICE, 2015b).

Imaging

- Ultrasound (USS) pelvis females older than 40 years, especially if they have bloating
- Chest radiography for all 'ever' smokers or any respiratory symptom
- CT of the abdomen as urgent direct access in patients aged 60 or older with diarrhoea, constipation, nausea and vomiting, or abdominal or back pain or new-onset diabetes (NICE, 2015b)

Further Management

- In older adult patients who have been investigated along the lines above with negative results, malignant diagnosis is uncommon.
- The yield from further blind investigation is low, and an approach of watchful waiting over 3 to 6 months may be appropriate at this stage, particularly in older adult patients (Alibhai et al, 2005; McMinn et al, 2011).
- In younger patients and those in whom malignancy is still strongly suspected, CT of the thorax, abdomen, and pelvis may be the next investigation of choice.

Treatment

- Nutrition support is advised in patients with a BMI below 18.5 kg/m^2, loss of 10% body weight in 3 to 6 months, or BMI below 20 and loss of more than 5% body weight in 3 to 6 months.
- Dietetic input is essential to ensure micronutrient needs as well as energy and protein needs are met (NICE, 2006).
- Social support, aids, and equipment may be just as important for some patients, so a full multidisciplinary approach is required.

- No pharmacologic treatments have a proven benefit in improving weight gain. In patients with depression, mirtazapine may be appropriate. Megestrol is sometimes used in patients with poor appetite, but the evidence base for this is poor, and side effects may limit its use (Alibhai et al, 2005; McMinn et al, 2011).

Jaundice and Abnormal Liver Function Test Results

GUIDELINES AND REVIEWS

Dyson, J. K., Anstee, Q. M., & McPherson, S. (2014). Non-alcoholic fatty liver disease: A practical approach to treatment. *Frontline Gastroenterology, 5*(4), 277–286.

European Association for the Study of the Liver. (2018). EASL Clinical Practice Guidelines. Management of alcohol-related liver disease. *Journal of Hepatology,* 69(1):154–181.

Lilford, R., J., Bentham, L. M., Armstrong, M. J., Neuberger, J., & Girling, A. J. (2013). What is the best strategy for investigating abnormal LFTs in primary care? *BMJ Open,* 3(6), e003099.

National Institute for Health and Clinical Excellence. (2016). *Assessment and management of cirrhosis. NICE clinical guideline 50.* Retrieved from http://www.nice.org.uk/guidance/ng50.

National Institute for Health and Clinical Excellence. (2021). *Suspected cancer: Recognition and referral. NICE clinical guideline 12.* Retrieved from http://www.nice.org.uk/guidance/ng12.

Williams, R., Aspinall, R., Bellis, M., Camps-Walsh, G., Cramp, M., Dhawan, A., Ferguson, J., Forton, D., Foster, G., Gilmore, I., Hickman, M., Hudson, M., Kelly, D., Langford, A., Lombard, M., Longworth, L., Martin, N., Moriarty, K., Newsome, P., O'Grady, J., … Smith, T. (2014). Addressing liver disease in the United Kingdom: A blueprint for attaining excellence in health care and reducing premature mortality from lifestyle issues of excess consumption of alcohol, obesity, and viral hepatitis. *Lancet, 29, 384*(9958),1953–1997.

- Liver disease is increasing in prevalence, and general oractitioners (GPs) will see many patients with abnormal LFT results.
- About 600,000 people in England and Wales have some form of liver disease with around 60,000 with cirrhosis (Williams et al, 2014).
- Death from liver disease is increasing and is the third most common cause of premature death in the United Kingdom.
- GPs are best placed to identify patients at risk of liver disease and intervene to modify risk factors.
- Fewer than 5% of people with abnormal LFT results have a specific liver disease, and fewer require treatment (Lilford et al, 2013a, 2013b).
- Conversely, many individuals will be developing liver fibrosis with normal LFT results (Williams et al 2014).

Special Situations

- Patients with jaundice and fever with right upper quadrant pain may have ascending cholangitis and require urgent admission for antibiotics and definitive management with ERCP.
- All patients aged over 40 years with jaundice should be referred as urgent to be seen within 2 weeks by a specialist (NICE, 2015b).
- Patients with evidence of impending liver failure such as altered mental status or in whom paracetamol overdose is suspected should be admitted as an emergency (Bernal et al, 2010).
- Jaundice or abnormal LFT results in pregnant patients, particularly in the third trimester, may indicate acute fatty liver of pregnancy, preeclampsia, or HELLP (hemolysis, elevated liver enzymes, low platelet count) syndrome and requires urgent admission to an obstetric unit (Hay, 2008).
- Patients with decompensation of chronic liver disease with jaundice, encephalopathy, tense ascites, or evidence of bleeding are likely to require emergency admission.
- Patients with isolated elevation of bilirubin are likely to have Gilbert syndrome and should have levels of conjugated and unconjugated bilirubin measured and be screened for evidence of haemolysis.

History

History of the Presenting Complaint

- History of the presenting complaint may give the diagnosis, for example, when right upper quadrant pain is associated with dark urine and pale stools in choledocholithiasis.
- Hepatitis may present with general malaise and nonspecific symptoms.
- Many patients with abnormal LFT results are entirely asymptomatic and are picked up incidentally.

Drug history

- The incidence of drug-induced liver injury (DILI) is in the region of 20 per 100000 per year (Bjornsson et al, 2013).
- A careful drug history should go back at least 6 months before the abnormality.
- Ask about nonprescribed drugs; Chinese, herbal, and other complementary therapies; and dietary supplements.
- Common causes of DILI
  a. Antibiotics: co-amoxiclav, nitrofurantoin.
  b. NSAID: diclofenac.
  c. Immunomodulators: azathioprine, infliximab.
  d. Diet and weight loss supplements are increasingly common causes of DILI (Bjornsson et al, 2013).
  e. Immunotherapy-related hepatitis occurs in approximately 10% of patients receiving immune checkpoint inhibitors as part of metastatic cancer treatment (e.g., melanoma, lung cancer, renal cell carcinoma). Management is distinct from other forms of DILI and often includes use of steroids. We suggest contacting

the treating oncology team with or without a specialist hepatologist as appropriate for advice (Cheung et al, 2019).

For more information on DILI, see www.livertox.nih.gov.

Social History

- Alcohol history (units per day or week)
  a. The department of health recommends that to reduce the risk of harm from alcohol, all adults drink no more than 14 units of alcohol per week spread evenly over 3 days of the week (UK Department of Health advice, January 2016).
  b. Daily alcohol of less than 20 g for a female or less than 30 g for a male is unlikely to be the cause of liver disease.
  c. Patients with harmful drinking should be offered interventions to reduce this (NICE, 2016a).
- Risk factors for bloodborne and sexually transmitted infections
- Travel history
- Family history (e.g., haemochromatosis, Gilbert syndrome)

Past Medical History

- Comorbidities: diabetes and metabolic syndrome, autoimmune diseases

Examination

- This may reveal evidence of underlying chronic liver disease, tender hepatomegaly in acute hepatitis, right upper quadrant tenderness, and Murphy sign in cholecystitis.
- It is useful to document the patient's weight and BMI.

Initial Investigations

- Blood tests
  - Initial LFT panel: Alanine transaminase (ALT) and alkaline phosphatase (ALP) are the most useful to guide whether it is a hepatitis or cholestatic picture (Lilford et al, 2013b).
  - Coagulation: Prolongation of prothrombin time may indicate liver failure or vitamin K deficiency in cholestasis.
  - FBC: Thrombocytopaenia may indicate chronic liver disease and portal hypertension.
- Initial liver screen
  - A prospective cohort study has shown that repeating abnormal LFT results after a period of time is an inefficient use of resource and suggests that individuals are instead tested for significant liver diagnoses directly (Lilford et al, 2013b).
  - The following panel is suggested:
    a. Hepatitis B and C serology (hepatitis A, hepatitis E, Epstein–Barr virus, and cytomegalovirus in an acute hepatitis)
    b. Immunoglobulin levels
    c. Antinuclear antibody, antimitochondrial antibody, anti–smooth muscle antibody, antinucleolar cytoplasmic antibody, liver kidney microsomal antibody, and soluble liver antigen
    d. Ferritin and (if elevated) transferrin saturation and *HFE* gene
    e. Caeruloplasmin
    f. Alpha-1 antitrypsin level
    g. tTG antibody
    h. HIV test (particularly when risk factors are identified)
- Imaging
  - Ultrasound scan of the liver and biliary system is often a useful first-line investigation, especially when biliary obstruction is suspected. MRCP is indicated for abnormal biliary dilatation or persistent cholestatic LFT results.
  - ERCP is reserved for patients in whom intervention is planned and is no longer regarded as a diagnostic procedure.
  - Ultrasound examination may also be useful as a screening tool to identify steatosis.
- Transient elastography ('FibroScan')
  - Transient elastography (TE) gives a measurement of liver stiffness that correlates with severity of liver fibrosis and can be a useful tool in staging liver disease and prognosticating. It is particularly well validated for viral hepatitis. It may be less accurate in patients with high BMIs (Castera, 2010a, 2010b; Czul & Bhamidimarri, 2016).
  - NICE recommend the use of TE to screen for cirrhosis in high-risk groups, including individuals with hepatitis B or hepatitis C and those who drink in excess of 50 units of alcohol per week.
- Serum biomarkers of fibrosis
  - These include direct markers such as hyaluronic acid or PIIINP, proprietary panels of tests such as ELF or FibroTest, or scoring systems based on a range of laboratory results (e.g., APRI score or FIB-4). Again, these are validated against biopsy scores and can help to stage liver disease without the need for biopsy (Castera et al, 2013; Czul & Bhamidimarri, 2016)
  - NICE has recommended ELF for identifying advanced fibrosis in patients with nonalcoholic fatty liver disease (NICE, 2016b).
- Liver biopsy
  - This is mainly required when there is diagnostic uncertainty rather than for staging of liver disease; however, it may be carried out when surrogate markers for fibrosis are borderline. Liver biopsy carries significant risks of haemorrhage (0.05%–0.1%) and death (0.1%–0.01%). In patients with coagulopathy or ascites, a transjugular approach may be undertaken that reduces risk but gives smaller samples.

Specific Liver Diseases

Viral Hepatitis

- Chronic viral hepatitis B and C are important long-term conditions with significant morbidity and mortality and highly effective available treatments. Patients at risk should be encouraged to have testing (Williams et al, 2014; NICE 2013b, NICE 2013c).

Hepatitis B

- Hepatitis B has a prevalence of 0.1% to 0.5% in the United Kingdom, but this varies between individual communities. It is estimated that 350 million people are infected worldwide. Transmission is predominantly vertical in developing countries. The majority of patients diagnosed in the United Kingdom have migrated from endemic areas.
- All pregnant females in the United Kingdom should be screened antenatally and referred to a specialist within 6 weeks to allow treatment in the third trimester.
- Arrange the following tests in primary care for patients who are hepatitis B surface antigen (HBsAg) positive, and refer to a specialist with the results:
  a. Hepatitis B e antigen (HBeAg) or antibody (anti-HBe) status
  b. HBV DNA level
  c. IgM antibody to hepatitis B core antigen (anti-HBc IgM)
  d. Hepatitis C virus antibody (anti-HCV)
  e. Hepatitis delta virus antibody (anti-HDV)
  f. HIV antibody
  g. IgG antibody to hepatitis A virus (anti-HAV)
  h. LFTs (albumin, bilirubin, ALP, ALT, aspartate aminotransferase [AST], gamma-glutamyl transferase), total globulins, FBC, and prothrombin time
  i. Tests for hepatocellular carcinoma (HCC), including ultrasound and alpha-fetoprotein testing
- Not all patients require treatment at diagnosis but should have monitoring by a specialist to determine if and when treatment should be started.
- Treatment, when required, is with a finite course of 48 weeks of pegylated interferon monotherapy or with (usually indefinite) treatment with antivirals, now usually tenofovir or entecavir (NICE, 2013b).
- Patients should be given advice on prevention of transmission of the virus and testing and vaccination should be offered to sexual partners and the patients' children.
- Hepatitis B is associated with increased risk of HCC in certain groups even in the absence of cirrhosis, and surveillance will be offered (European Association for the Study of the Liver [EASL], 2012).

Hepatitis C

- The number of people in the United Kingdom with chronic HCV is approximately 215,000.
- Injecting drug use is the main risk factor, but migration from endemic areas and receipt of blood products before 1991 are also important risk factors.
- HCV rarely causes acute hepatitis, and 75% to 85% of patients develop chronic active hepatitis.
- All patients with chronic HCV infection should be considered for treatment of the virus and should be referred to specialist care.

- Treatment of HCV has advanced rapidly in recent years with the advent of a range of direct-acting antivirals (DAAs). These used in combination, either with or without pegylated interferon, offer higher cure rates with shorter, better tolerated treatment.
- DAAs are usually taken for 8 to 12 weeks and clear the infection in more than 90% of patients.
  - Risk of reinfection after successful treatment and education to reduce this risk should be stressed, especially in high-risk groups.

Hepatitis A

- This virus transmitted via the faecal–oral route is a cause of acute hepatitis, often in returning travellers.
- Vaccination with two doses 6 months apart is effective for prevention in high-risk groups, including travellers to endemic areas, those in high-risk occupations, and males who have sex with males with high-risk sexual behaviours. Intravenous drug users and their close contacts should also be considered as being at high risk.
- The illness is usually self-limiting with mild symptoms occasionally lasting up to 6 months. In a minority (<1%) of cases, fulminant hepatitis may occur (Rezende et al, 2003).

Hepatitis E

- Also transmitted through the faecal–oral route, it usually causes a mild self-limiting acute hepatitis or subclinical infection.
- It can present with fulminant hepatic failure in pregnant females.
- It has been linked to outbreaks in places with contaminated water supply in the developing world. In the United Kingdom more recently, the incidence is rising and may be linked to a reservoir of infection among animal populations, including pigs with ingestion of undercooked or cured meats or seafood being particular culprits.
- Chronic infection with rapid progression to cirrhosis has been documented in immunosuppressed groups (e.g., after liver transplant), and in these groups, treatment using ribavirin may be indicated.
- The virus has been detected in donated blood from asymptomatic donors; however, the risk of transmission to immunocompetent individuals is unclear, and the role for screening of blood products has not been established.
- Patients may present with extrahepatic features, including up to 5% with neurologic syndromes, including a Guillain–Barré syndrome (Dalton et al, 2013).

Autoimmune Hepatitis

- Presentation of this condition can range from a minor elevation of transaminases with or without symptoms of general malaise through acute hepatitis to subacute liver failure, though the latter is rare. A relapsing remitting course may mean LFT results fluctuate with repeat testing.

- One-third of patients have cirrhosis at diagnosis.
- There is a female preponderance (female: male ratio, 2:1), and there may be a history of other associated autoimmune conditions, including rheumatoid arthritis, Graves disease, and coeliac disease.
- The diagnosis is usually based on typical biochemistry along with positive autoantibodies and elevated IgG.
- Liver biopsy is regarded as a prerequisite to confirm the diagnosis and for staging and prognosis. The validity of noninvasive fibrosis markers is not well established (EASL, 2015).
- Treatment is with steroids initially, which may be in the form of prednisolone or budesonide, before introducing a steroid-sparing agent, usually a thiopurine.
- Occasionally, second-line immunosuppressive agents are required, including mycophenolate mofetil or tacrolimus.
- Withdrawal of treatment should be undertaken with caution because up to 50% to 90% of patients relapse. Treatment should be for at least 3 years and at least 24 months from normalisation of LFT results. Biopsy should be repeated before treatment withdrawal to exclude disease activity (EASL, 2015).

Primary Sclerosing Cholangitis

- PSC has a male predominance and strong association with IBD (in 80% of cases). All patients with PSC should have a screening colonoscopy for IBD.
- The diagnosis is usually made by MRCP with characteristic appearances of stricturing and dilatation with a typical beading appearance.
- No specific treatment has been shown to prevent progression. Some studies report improvement in biochemistry with certain doses of ursodeoxycholic acid, but evidence is insufficient to recommend it universally, and US guidelines state this treatment should not be used because of an excess mortality rate in study of higher doses (Chapman et al, 2010; EASL, 2009).
- Patients with PSC carry a significant increased risk of cholangiocarcinoma (which can be difficult to diagnose), colon cancer, and gallbladder cancer.
- Surveillance is recommended with:
  - Annual colonoscopy (chromoendoscopy when possible) with biopsies.
  - Annual abdominal ultrasound examination of the gallbladder (cholecystectomy if there is any abnormality). Some clinicians may perform interval MRCP, but the evidence base for this is lacking.
  - If a dominant stricture is identified, then ERCP with brushings with or without intervention may be required.

Primary Biliary Cholangitis

- Primary biliary cholangitis (PBC) has a female preponderance (female:male ratio, 3:1) and association with other autoimmune conditions.
- Symptoms of itch and fatigue are typical.
- Cholestatic LFT results, IgM is elevated, and positive antimitochondrial antibody are found.
- The typical phenotype associated with positive serology is sufficient for the diagnosis, and biopsy is not always necessary (EASL, 2009; Lindor et al, 2009).
- Treatment with ursodeoxycholic acid at a dosage of 13 to 15 mg/kg per day has been shown to improve the long-term prognosis in patients with PBC who respond biochemically (Hirschfield et al, 2018).
- Treatment of itch initially is with antihistamines. Bile sequestrants can be used (patients must be advised not to take ursodeoxycholic acid with 2–4 hours of taking these) and in some cases rifaximin or naltrexone (Lindor et al, 2009).
- Hyperlipidaemia occurs but may not reflect increased cardiovascular risk.
- The risk of osteoporosis is increased and should be screened for by dual x-ray absorptiometry (Lindor et al, 2009).

Overlap Syndromes

- Patients may have features of two or more of the conditions discussed. Treatment often follows the predominant condition, or patients may receive a combination of immunosuppression and ursodeoxycholic acid.

Nonalcoholic Fatty Liver Disease

- This is the commonest liver disease in the Western world, and with increasing prevalence, is possibly the biggest challenge in liver disease in the developed world in the next decades. About 17% to 40% of adults have some degree of nonalcoholic fatty liver disease.
- The disease is on a spectrum from steatosis to steatohepatitis to fibrosis and cirrhosis.
- Death in these patients is mostly from cardiovascular disease and cancer, but there is significant risk of progression to liver cirrhosis (Angulo et al, 2015).
- Fibrosis on biopsy is still the best predictor of prognosis, but in practice, noninvasive tests are usually preferred (Angulo et al, 2015; EASL, 2016).
- No specific treatments are available, but patients should be counselled on lifestyle and risk factors.
- Weight loss of 7% to 10% of body weight has been shown to improve fibrosis, but the optimum method has not been proven.
- There is some evidence of benefit from pioglitazone, vitamin E, or obeticholic acid; however, these should only be used within specialist settings (NICE, 2016b; Rinella, 2015).
- Statins are generally safe in this patient group and may be beneficial; therefore, they should not be discontinued.

Alcoholic Hepatitis

- Alcoholic hepatitis presents with recent-onset jaundice and carries a very high mortality rate when severe. The diagnosis is usually based on the history of excessive alcohol consumption within 4 weeks before presentation and typical biochemistry with bilirubin greater than 80 μmol/L, AST or ALT typically below 500 units U/L and an AST-to-ALT ratio greater than 1.5 to 2.0 units U/L (EASL, 2018).
- It can present with or without other signs of liver decompensation. Jaundice is often associated with fever, malaise, weight loss, and malnutrition. (Clinical features of the syndrome can also result from sepsis, DILI, gallstone migration, and so on.)
- The Maddrey discriminant function was the first score that reliably defined individuals at the highest risk of death in the short term and is still widely used in practice. A cutoff of 32 identifies patients with severe alcoholic hepatitis.
- These patients should be typically managed in the acute hospital setting. Alcohol abstinence, supplementation with B-complex vitamins, and management of sepsis and nutrition are key.
- Treatment with corticosteroids may be considered under specialist supervision in the absence of sepsis (Thursz et al, 2015).

Hereditary Haemochromatosis

- This is an autosomal recessive inherited condition with homozygosity of *C282Y* mutation most common.
  - *H63D/C282Y* 'compound' heterozygote is associated with some risk of iron overload.
- Associated with iron overload from the third or fourth decade of life. It occurs later in females because of menstrual blood loss.
- Patients may present with joint pains or fatigue (van Bokhoven et al, 2011).
- Genetic testing is not recommended as a screening test because of low penetrance of the condition (EASL, 2010).
- A ferritin level below 1000 ug/L with normal LFT results has a good negative predictive value for cirrhosis.
- Treatment is with venesection until iron stores (ferritin) are depleted (<50 ug/L) and as required venesection thereafter (target ferritin, 50–100 ug/L).
- In patients in whom cirrhosis is suspected, biopsy should be performed.

Wilson Disease

- Wilson disease is a rare genetic condition with associated neuropsychiatric features.
- It can present as fulminant hepatic failure typically associated with haemolytic anaemia.
- Caeruloplasmin measurement is useful screening test (levels will be low), but the diagnosis requires liver biopsy and urinary copper.
- Treatment is with chelating agents (i.e., penicillamine or trientine) (Ferenci, 2004).

Chronic Liver Disease

- Cirrhosis results from injury (caused by a variety of mechanisms or disease processes), leading to necroinflammation and fibrinogenesis within the liver. Histologic features of liver cirrhosis include diffuse nodular regeneration, fibrous septa, collapse of the normal liver architecture, and distortion of vascular structures.
- Clinical examination findings in advanced liver disease may include:
  - Palmar erythema, spider naevi (more than five is considered abnormal)
  - Caput medusae
  - Loss of body hair in males
  - Gynaecomastia
  - Testicular atrophy
  - All or none of these signs may be present.
- Patients at risk of cirrhosis include individuals with BMIs greater than 30, those who misuse alcohol, patients with type 2 diabetes, and patients with hepatitis B or C infection, as well as patients with other forms of liver disease as previously discussed.
- NICE recommend testing for cirrhosis with FibroScan in all males drinking more than 50 units alcohol per week (females >35 units) or anyone diagnosed with alcohol-related liver disease.

Staging of Advanced Liver Disease

- Liver cirrhosis or advanced liver disease can be thought of as a spectrum of clinical states from early disease with compensated disease and absence of oesophageal varices, through the development of portal hypertension, to decompensated liver disease with complications of varices and ascites.
- The prognosis varies between these stages with a 1-year mortality rate of 1% per year for early stage to more than 50% for decompensated disease (Tsochatzis et al, 2014).
- Child–Pugh classification can be used to describe the stage or severity of liver cirrhosis. The The Model for End-stage Liver Disease (MELD) and UK Model for End-stage Liver Disease (UKELD) scores are used in the transplant assessment process to risk stratify patients and select those in whom risk of transplant is outweighed by risk of death without transplant (Table 8.3).

TABLE 8.3	Child–Pugh Classification of Chronic Liver Disease		
Measure	1 Point	2 Points	3 Points
Total bilirubin (μmol/L)	<34	34–50	>50
Prothrombin time prolongation (s)	<4.0	4.0–6.0	>6.0
Ascites	None	Mild	Moderate to severe
Hepatic encephalopathy	None	Grade I or II (or suppressed with medication)	Grade III or IV (or refractory)
Serum albumin (g/L)	<28	28–35	>35

Management of Patients With Cirrhosis

- Patients with stable compensated cirrhosis are usually seen at liver clinics every 6 to 12 months for monitoring and to arrange surveillance for HCC:
  - Ultrasound examination of the liver every 6 months is currently recommended as HCC surveillance (Bruix & Sherman, 2011).
  - Patients should receive appropriate treatment depending on the underlying cause of their liver disease (e.g., antiviral therapy or venesection in haemochromatosis).
  - Patients should be advised on lifestyle factors, including weight reduction in obesity, management of type 2 diabetes, smoking cessation, and abstinence from alcohol.

Ascites

- Half of patients with compensated cirrhosis develop ascites within a 10-year period.
- The development of ascites marks progression of liver disease and an associated 2-year mortality rate of up to 50%. The development of ascites should prompt consideration of assessment for transplantation.
- Treatment is with a low-sodium diet (<2000 mg/day) and an aldosterone antagonist (e.g., spironolactone 100 mg, increasing in increments of 100 mg to a maximum of 300 mg) with the addition of loop diuretic (e.g., furosemide 40–120 mg) in some cases.
- Fluid restriction is not indicated unless the patient has hyponatraemia.
- Hyponatraemia is common and may limit diuretic use. Diuretics should be reduced or stopped if serum sodium is below 125 mmol/L (Moore & Aithal, 2006).
- NSAID should be avoided in patients with ascites caused by cirrhosis.
- Angiotensin-converting enzyme inhibitors and angiotensin receptor blockers may be harmful in patients with ascites and should be stopped.
- Rapid accumulation of ascites may be caused by the development of portal vein thrombosis or HCC and should prompt referral and consideration of imaging.

- Spontaneous bacterial peritonitis (SBP) may present with decompensation without specific symptoms and should prompt urgent admission. Signs of peritonism are usually absent. The in-hospital mortality rate from SBP is around 20%.
- After one episode of SBP, patients should receive long-term antibiotic prophylaxis. Antibiotic choice is usually a quinolone or cotrimoxazole but should be guided by local protocols and sensitivities.

Hepatic Encephalopathy

- Hepatic encephalopathy (HE) will affect 30% to 40% of patients with cirrhosis at some time in their clinical course.
- HE can be classified according to the West Haven criteria. Minimal encephalopathy may be apparent only on psychometric testing, but it may still lead to a reduction in quality of life for patients.
- Overt hepatic encephalopathy (OHE) classically presents with deficit in attention, reduced visuospatial awareness, disorientation, alteration of the sleep–wake cycle, change in personality, and reduced a consciousness level in the later stages. OHE usually has a precipitant such as variceal bleeding or infection.
- It is important in acute confusion to consider other causes and to be aware that patients with advanced liver disease are at risk of intracranial bleeding. There should be a low threshold for referral for urgent assessment and imaging in patients with new confusion (EASL & American Association for the Study of Liver Diseases [AASLD], 2014).
- Lactulose is usually given to treat and prevent encephalopathy, and rifaximin is added in as a second-line treatment. Both treatments are usually continued indefinitely.

Varices

- All patients at risk of varices should have a screening endoscopy. Until recently, this included all patients with cirrhosis, but evidence now suggests that those with lower fibrosis scores (i.e., TE with stiffness <20 kPA with platelet count $>150 \times 10^9$/L) may not require screening (Bosch & Sauerbruch, 2016; Tripathi et al, 2015).

- Patients with grade 1 varices without red spots do not require primary prophylaxis but should have further endoscopy after 1 year.
- Patients with grade 2 or 3 varices a receive nonselective beta-blocker (NSBB) as primary prophylaxis (e.g., carvedilol 6.25 mg/day increasing to 12.5mg/day after 1 week if tolerated or propranolol 40 mg twice daily increased to the maximum tolerated dose). Patients on NSBB for primary prophylaxis do not require routine endoscopy.
- When NSBB is contraindicated, patients should have primary prophylaxis by endoscopic band ligation (EBL).
- Patients who have had a variceal bleed should undergo a programme of EBL every 2 to 4 weeks until varices are obliterated. They should also receive NSBB unless there is a contraindication.
- Transjugular intrahepatic portosystemic shunt (TIPSS) may be required as a recue therapy in patients with acute variceal bleeding.
- Bleeding from gastric varices can be more difficult to manage endoscopically and more commonly requires TIPSS.
- There is controversy regarding the treatment with NSBB in advanced decompensated liver disease with some studies indicating loss of benefit or harm from NSBB in more advanced disease but others showing benefit. More research is needed in this area, and the decision to stop or restart NSBB should be made by a specialist (Krag & Madsen 2015).

Transjugular Intrahepatic Portosystemic Shunt

- TIPSS is indicated as a rescue therapy in acute variceal haemorrhage or for high-risk gastric varices.
- It may be indicated for refractory ascites in appropriate patients.
- The main adverse effect is encephalopathy, which occurs in up to 10% to 50% of patients; therefore, careful patient selection is very important (EASL & AASLD, 2014).

Hepatocellular Carcinoma

- HCC is diagnosed by characteristic contrast-enhanced imaging on one or two modalities. Biopsy not usually required.
- Treatment options depend on the stage of liver disease as well as the number, size, and site of tumours by the Barcelona Clinic Liver Cancer staging.
- Resection is reserved for those with Child–Pugh with one small (<2 cm) lesion.
- Transplant is considered for those with three or fewer lesions, all less than 3 cm in size, who are otherwise candidates for transplantation.

- Transarterial chemoembolisation and radiofrequency ablation are effective palliative treatment but are not suitable for patients with Child–Pugh or cirrhosis and good performance status.
- Sorafenib is an oral kinase inhibitor used as a palliative treatment, which has recently been approved by NICE for use in selected patients.

Liver Transplant

- Liver transplant should be considered in all patients with advanced liver disease.
- Many patients will not be suitable because of comorbidity or risk of recidivism.
- After transplant, the vast majority of patients will remain on lifelong immunosuppression.
- They will be seen at least every 6 months by a specialist who will review immunosuppression and aim to minimise toxicity. Changes to immunosuppression should not be made by nonspecialists (AASLD & American Society of Transplantation [AST], 2012).
- In the first year, complications of surgery, rejection, and infections are the greatest causes of morbidity and mortality.
- In patients who survive after 1 year from transplant, renal disease and cardiovascular disease are the main cause of morbidity and malignancy, and cardiovascular disease accounts for most deaths. Many patients undergoing transplant have multiple risk factors, including obesity, metabolic syndrome, and type 2 diabetes (AASLD & AST, 2012).
- Patients should be given the following lifestyle advice:
  - Diet: Avoid unpasteurised dairy products and raw or undercooked meat or eggs.
  - Avoid smoking.
  - Use high-factor sun protection and stay out of strong sunlight. Patients should also be counselled to self-examine their skin for suspicious lesions (AASLD & AST, 2012).
- Cardiovascular risk factors should be addressed, including weight management, hypertension, and diabetes.
- Bone density should be considered and appropriately managed according to protocols.

References

American Association for the Study of Liver Diseases, & American Society of Transplantation. (2012). *Long-term management of the successful adult liver transplant: 2012 practice guideline by AASLD and the American Society of Transplantation*. Retrieved from: https://www.aasld.org/sites/default/files/2022-07/Long-Term%20Management%20of%20the%20Successful%20Adult%20Liver%20Transplant.pdf

Abdel Jalil, A. A., Katzka, D. A., & Castell, D. O. (2015). Approach to the patient with dysphagia. *American Journal of Medicine*, *128*(10), 1138–1123.

Alfadhli, A. A., McDonald, J. W., & Feagan, B. G. (2003). Methotrexate for induction of remission in refractory Crohn's disease. *Cochrane Database of Systematic Reviews*, (1), CD003459.

Alibhai, S. M., Greenwood, C., & Payette, H. (2005). An approach to the management of unintentional weight loss in elderly people. *CMAJ, 172*(6), 773–780.

Alstead, E. M., Ritchie, J. K., Lennard-Jones, J. E., Farthing, M. J., & Clark, M. L. (1990). Safety of azathioprine in pregnancy in inflammatory bowel disease. *Gastroenterology*, 99(2), 443–446.

Al Toma, A., Verbeek, W. H., Hadithi, M., von Blomberg, B. M., & Mulder, C. J. (2007). Survival in refractory coeliac disease and enteropathy-associated T-cell lymphoma: Retrospective evaluation of single-centre experience. *Gut, 56*(10), 1373–1378.

Angulo, P., Kleiner, D. E., Dam-Larsen, S., Adams, L. A., Bjornsson, E. S., Charatcharoenwitthaya, P., Mills, P. R., Keach, J. C., Lafferty, H. D., Stahler, A., Haflidadottir, S., & Bendtsen, F. (2015). Liver fibrosis, but no other histologic features, is associated with long-term outcomes of patients with nonalcoholic fatty liver disease. *Gastroenterology, 149*(2), 389–397.

Arcelus, J., Mitchell, A. J., Wales, J., & Nielsen, S. (2011). Mortality rates in patients with anorexia nervosa and other eating disorders. A meta-analysis of 36 studies. *Archives of General Psychiatry, 68*(7), 724–731.

Arasaradnam, R. P., Brown, S., Forbes, A., Fox, M. R., Hungin, P., Kelman, L., Major, G., O'Connor, M., Sanders, D. S., Sinha, R., Smith, S. C., Thomas, P., & Walters, J. R. F. (2018). Guidelines for the investigation of chronic diarrhoea in adults: British Society of Gastroenterology, 3rd Edition. *Gut, 67*(8), 1380–1399.

Association of Upper Gastrointestinal Surgeons of Great Britian and Ireland. (2016). *Commissioning Guide: Gallstone disease*. Retrieved from http://www.rcseng.ac.uk; https://www.rcseng.ac.uk/-/media/files/rcs/standards-and-research/commissioning/gallstone-disease-commissioning-guide-for-republication.pdf. Accessed April 18th, 2023.

Aziz, I., Lewis, N. R., Hadjivassiliou, M., Winfield, S. N., Rugg, N., Kelsall, A., Newrick, L., & Sanders, D. S. (2014). A UK study assessing the population prevalence of self-reported gluten sensitivity and referral characteristics to secondary care. *European Journal of Gastroenterology & Hepatology, 26*(1), 33–39.

Bernal, W., Auzinger, G., Dhawan, A., & Wendon, J. (2010). Acute liver failure. *Lancet, 376*(9736), 190–201.

Bjornsson, E. S., Bergmann, O. M., Bjornsson, H. K., Kvaran, R. B., & Olafsson, S. (2013). Incidence, presentation, and outcomes in patients with drug-induced liver injury in the general population of Iceland. *Gastroenterology, 144*(7), 1419–1425.

Black, C. J., Paine, P. A., Agrawal, A., Aziz, I., Eugenicos, M. P., Houghton, L. A., Hungin, P., Overshott, R., Vasant, D. H., Rudd, S., Winning, R. C., Corsetti, M., & Ford, A. C. (2022). British Society of Gastroenterology guidelines on the management of functional dyspepsia. *Gut, 71*, 1697–1723.

Boeckxstaens, G., El Serag, H. B., Smout, A. J., & Kahrilas, P. J. (2014). Symptomatic reflux disease: The present, the past and the future. *Gut, 63*(7), 1185–1193.

Bosch, J., & Sauerbruch, T. (2016). Esophageal varices: Stage-dependent treatment algorithm. *Journal of Hepatology, 64*(3), 746–748.

Briggs, A. H., Sculpher, M. J., Logan, R. P., Aldous, J., Ramsay, M. E., & Baron, J. H. (1996). Cost effectiveness of screening for and eradication of Helicobacter pylori in management of dyspeptic patients under 45 years of age. *BMJ, 312*(7042), 1321–1325.

British HIV Association. *UK National Guidelines for HIV Testing 2008*. 2008. Retrieved from: https://www.bhiva.org/file/RHNUJgIseDaML/GlinesHIVTest08.pdf

Bruix, J., & Sherman, M. (2011). Management of hepatocellular carcinoma: An update. *Hepatology, 53*(3), 1020–1022.

Camilleri, M., Kerstens, R., Rykx, A., & Vandeplassche, L. (2008). A placebo-controlled trial of prucalopride for severe chronic constipation. *New England Journal of Medicine, 358*(22), 2344–2354.

Camilleri, M., Piessevaux, H., Yiannakou, Y., Tack, J., Kerstens, R., Quigley, E. M., Ke, M., Da Silva, S., & Levine, A. (2016). Efficacy and safety of prucalopride in chronic constipation: An integrated analysis of six randomized. Controlled Clinical Trials. *Digestive Diseases and Sciences, 61*(8), 2357–2372.

Camilleri, M., Van Outryve, M. J., Beyens, G., Kerstens, R., Robinson, P., & Vandeplassche, L. (2010). Clinical trial: The efficacy of open-label prucalopride treatment in patients with chronic constipation - follow-up of patients from the pivotal studies. *Alimentary Pharmacology & Therapeutics, 32*(9), 1113–1123.

Castera, L. (2010a). Diagnosing cirrhosis non-invasively: Sense the stiffness but don't forget the nodules!. *Journal of Hepatology, 52*(6), 786–787.

Castera, L., Sebastiani, G., Le Bail, B., de, L., V, Couzigou, P., & Alberti, A. (2010b). Prospective comparison of two algorithms combining non-invasive methods for staging liver fibrosis in chronic hepatitis C. *Journal of Hepatology, 52*(2), 191–198.

Castera, L., Vilgrain, V., & Angulo, P. (2013). Noninvasive evaluation of NAFLD. *Nature Reviews Gastroenterology & Hepatology, 10*(11), 666–675.

Chande, N., Tsoulis, D. J., & MacDonald, J. K. (2013). Azathioprine or 6-mercaptopurine for induction of remission in Crohn's disease. *Cochrane Database of Systematic Reviews*, (4), CD000545.

Chapman, R., Fevery, J., Kalloo, A., Nagorney, D. M., Boberg, K. M., Shneider, B., & Gores, G. J. (2010). Diagnosis and management of primary sclerosing cholangitis. *Hepatology, 51*(2), 660–678.

Cheung, V., Gupta, T., Payne, M., Middleton, M. R., Collier, J. D., Simmons, A., Klenerman, P., Brain, O., & Cobbold, J. F. (2019). Immunotherapy-related hepatitis: Real-world experience from a tertiary centre. *Frontline Gastroenterol, 10*(4), 364–371.

Chey, W. D., Lembo, A. J., Lavins, B. J., Shiff, S. J., Kurtz, C. B., Currie, M. G., MacDougall, J. E., Jia, X. D., Shao, J. Z., Fitch, D. A., Baird, M. J., Schneier, H. A., & Johnston, J. M. (2012). Linaclotide for irritable bowel syndrome with constipation: A 26-week, randomized, double-blind, placebo-controlled trial to evaluate efficacy and safety. *American Journal of Gastroenterology, 107*(11), 1702–1712.

Clouse, R. E., Richter, J. E., Heading, R. C., Janssens, J., & Wilson, J. A. (1999). Functional esophageal disorders. *Gut, 45*(2), 1131–1136.

Czul, F., & Bhamidimarri, K. R. (2016). Noninvasive markers to assess liver fibrosis. *Journal of Clinical Gastroenterology, 50*(6), 445–457.

Dalton, H. R., Hunter, J. G., & Bendall, R. P. (2013). Hepatitis E. *Current Opinion in Infectious Diseases, 26*(5), 471–478.

Didari, T., Mozaffari, S., Nikfar, S., & Abdollahi, M. (2015). Effectiveness of probiotics in irritable bowel syndrome: Updated systematic review with meta-analysis. *World Journal of Gastroenterology, 21*(10), 3072–3084.

DuPont, H. L. (2014). Review article: Evidence for the role of gut microbiota in irritable bowel syndrome and its potential influence on therapeutic targets. *Alimentary Pharmacology & Therapeutics, 39*(10), 1033–1042.

European Association for the Study of the Liver. (2009). EASL Clinical Practice Guidelines: Management of cholestatic liver diseases. *Journal of Hepatology, 51*(2), 237–267.

European Association for The Study of The Liver. (2010). EASL clinical practice guidelines for HFE hemochromatosis. *Journal of Hepatology, 53*(1), 3–22.

European Association for The Study of The Liver, & European Organisation for Research and Treatment of Cancer. (2012). EASL-

EORTC clinical practice guidelines: Management of hepatocellular carcinoma. *Journal of Hepatology, 56*(4), 908–943.

European Association for the Study of the Liver. (2015). EASL Clinical Practice Guidelines: Autoimmune hepatitis. *Journal of Hepatology, 63*(4), 971–1004.

EASL, EASD, & EASO. (2016). EASL-EASD-EASO Clinical Practice Guidelines for the management of non-alcoholic fatty liver disease. *Journal of Hepatology, 64*(6), 1388–1402.

European Association for the Study of the Liver. (2018). EASL Clinical Practice Guidelines: Management of alcohol-related liver disease. *Journal of Hepatology, 69*(1), 154–181.

EASL & AASLD. Hepatic Encephalopathy in Chronic Liver Disease: 2014 Practice Guideline by the European Association for the Study of the Liver and the American Association for the Study of Liver Diseases. 2014. Retrieved from: https://www.aasld.org/sites/default/files/2022-07/Hepatic%20Encephalopathy%20in%20Chronic%20Liver%20Disease%202014.pdf

Feagan, B. G., Fedorak, R. N., Irvine, E. J., Wild, G., Sutherland, L., Steinhart, A. H., Greenberg, G. R., Koval, J., Wong, C. J., Hopkins, M., Hanauer, S. B., & McDonald, J. W. (2000). A comparison of methotrexate with placebo for the maintenance of remission in Crohn's disease. North American Crohn's Study Group Investigators. *New England Journal of Medicine, 342*(22), 1627–1632.

Feagan, B. G., & MacDonald, J. K. (2012). Oral 5-aminosalicylic acid for maintenance of remission in ulcerative colitis. *Cochrane Database of Systematic Reviews, 10*, CD000544.

Ferenci, P. (2004). Review article: Diagnosis and current therapy of Wilson's disease. *Alimentary Pharmacology & Therapeutics, 19*(2), 157–165.

Fitzgerald, R. C., di Pietro, M., Ragunath, K., Ang, Y., Kang, J. Y., Watson, P., Trudgill, N., Patel, P., Kaye, P. V., Sanders, S., O'Donovan, M., Bird-Lieberman, E., Bhandari, P., Jankowski, J. A., Attwood, S., Parsons, S. L., Loft, D., Lagergren, J., Moayyedi, P., Lyratzopoulos, G., & de Caestecker, J. (2014). British Society of Gastroenterology guidelines on the diagnosis and management of Barrett's oesophagus. *Gut, 63*(1), 7–42.

Ford, A. C., Achkar, J. P., Khan, K. J., Kane, S. V., Talley, N. J., Marshall, J. K., & Moayyedi, P. (2011). Efficacy of 5-aminosalicylates in ulcerative colitis: Systematic review and meta-analysis. *American Journal of Gastroenterology, 106*(4), 601–616.

Ford, A. C., Marwaha, A., Lim, A., & Moayyedi, P. (2010). What is the prevalence of clinically significant endoscopic findings in subjects with dyspepsia? Systematic review and meta-analysis. *Clinical Gastroenterology and Hepatology, 8*, 830–837, 837.e1-2.

Ford, A. C., Qume, M., Moayyedi, P., Arents, N. L., Lassen, A. T., Logan, R. F., McColl, K. E., Myres, P., & Delaney, B. C. (2005). Helicobacter pylori 'test and treat' or endoscopy for managing dyspepsia: An individual patient data meta-analysis. *Gastroenterology, 128*(7), 1838–1844.

Francella, A., Dyan, A., Bodian, C., Rubin, P., Chapman, M., & Present, D. H. (2003). The safety of 6-mercaptopurine for childbearing patients with inflammatory bowel disease: A retrospective cohort study. *Gastroenterology, 124*(1), 9–17.

Gaddey, H. L., & Holder, K. (2014). Unintentional weight loss in older adults. *American Family Physician, 89*(9), 718–722.

Gisbert, J. P., Linares, P. M., McNicholl, A. G., Mate, J., & Gomollon, F. (2009). Meta-analysis: The efficacy of azathioprine and mercaptopurine in ulcerative colitis. *Alimentary Pharmacology & Therapeutics, 30*(2), 126–137.

Gisbert, J. P., & Pajares, J. M. (2004). Stool antigen test for the diagnosis of Helicobacter pylori infection: A systematic review. *Helicobacter, 9*(4), 347–368.

Gordon, M., Naidoo, K., Thomas, A. G., & Akobeng, A. K. (2011). Oral 5-aminosalicylic acid for maintenance of surgically-induced remission in Crohn's disease. *Cochrane Database of Systematic Reviews, (1),* CD008414.

Gordon, M., Taylor, K., Akobeng, A. K., & Thomas, A. G. (2014). Azathioprine and 6-mercaptopurine for maintenance of surgically-induced remission in Crohn's disease. *Cochrane Database of Systematic Reviews, (8),* CD010233.

Hanauer, S. B., Sandborn, W. J., Dallaire, C., Archambault, A., Yacyshyn, B., Yeh, C., & Smith-Hall, N. (2007). Delayed-release oral mesalamine 4.8 g/day (800 mg tablets) compared to 2.4 g/day (400 mg tablets) for the treatment of mildly to moderately active ulcerative colitis: The ASCEND I trial. *Canadian Journal of Gastroenterology, 21*(12), 827–834.

Hanauer, S. B., Sandborn, W. J., Kornbluth, A., Katz, S., Safdi, M., Woogen, S., Regalli, G., Yeh, C., Smith-Hall, N., & Ajayi, F. (2005). Delayed-release oral mesalamine at 4.8 g/day (800 mg tablet) for the treatment of moderately active ulcerative colitis: The ASCEND II trial. *American Journal of Gastroenterology, 100*(11), 2478–2485.

Hay, J. E. (2008). Liver disease in pregnancy. *Hepatology, 47*(3), 1067–1076.

Headstrom, P. D., & Surawicz, C. M. (2005). Chronic diarrhea. *Clinical Gastroenterology and Hepatology, 3*(8), 734–737.

Hindorf, U., Johansson, M., Eriksson, A., Kvifors, E., & Almer, S. H. (2009). Mercaptopurine treatment should be considered in azathioprine intolerant patients with inflammatory bowel disease. *Alimentary Pharmacology & Therapeutics, 29*(6), 654–661.

Hirschfield, G. M., Dyson, J. K., Alexander, G. J. M. et al. (2018). The British Society of Gastroenterology/UK-PBC primary biliary cholangitis treatment and management guidelines. *Gut, 67*(9): 1568–1594.

Howdle, P. D., Jalal, P. K., Holmes, G. K., & Houlston, R. S. (2003). Primary small-bowel malignancy in the UK and its association with coeliac disease. *QJM, 96*(5), 345–353.

Immunisation against Infectious Diseases: The Green Book, Department of Health, United Kingdom.

Islami, F., & Kamangar, F. (2008). Helicobacter pylori and esophageal cancer risk: A meta-analysis. *Cancer Prevention Research (Philadelphia, Pa.), 1*(5), 329–338.

Kapoor, N., Bassi, A., Sturgess, R., & Bodger, K. (2005). Predictive value of alarm features in a rapid access upper gastrointestinal cancer service. *Gut, 54*(1), 40–45.

Krag, A., & Madsen, B. S. (2015). To block, or not to block in advanced cirrhosis and ascites: That is the question. *Gut, 64*(7), 1015–1017.

Lamb, C. A., Kennedy, N. A., Raine, T., Hendy, P. A., Smith, P. J., Limdi, J. K., Hayee, B., Lomer, M. C. E., Parkes, G. C., Selinger, C., Barrett, K. J., Davies, R. J., Bennett, C., Gittens, S., Dunlop, M. G., Faiz, O., Fraser, A., Garrick, V., Johnston, P. D., Parkes, M., Sanderson, J., Terry, H., IBD guidelines eDelphi consensus group, Gaya, D .R., Iqbal, T. H., Taylor, S. A., Smith, M,, Brookes, M., Hansen, R., & Hawthorne, A. B. (2019). British Society of Gastroenterology consensus guidelines on the management of inflammatory bowel disease in adults. *Gut, 68*(3), s1–s106.

Lebwohl, B., Ludvigsson, J. F., & Green, P. H. (2015). Celiac disease and non-celiac gluten sensitivity. *BMJ, 351*, h4347.

Lees, C. W., Maan, A. K., Hansoti, B., Satsangi, J., & Arnott, I. D. (2008). Tolerability and safety of mercaptopurine in azathioprine-intolerant patients with inflammatory bowel disease. *Alimentary Pharmacology & Therapeutics, 27*(3), 220–227.

Lichtenstein, G. R., Ramsey, D., & Rubin, D. T. (2011). Randomised clinical trial: Delayed-release oral mesalazine 4.8 g/day vs.

2.4 g/day in endoscopic mucosal healing—ASCEND I and II combined analysis. *Alimentary Pharmacology & Therapeutics*, *33*(6), 672–678.

Lilford, R. J., Bentham, L., Girling, A., Litchfield, I., Lancashire, R., Armstrong, D., Jones, R., Marteau, T., Neuberger, J., Gill, P., Cramb, R., Olliff, S., Arnold, D., Khan, K., Armstrong, M. J., Houlihan, D. D., Newsome, P. N., Chilton, P. J., Moons, K., & Altman, D. (2013a). Birmingham and Lambeth Liver Evaluation Testing Strategies (BALLETS): A prospective cohort study. *Health Technology Assessment*, *17*(28), i–xiv, 1–307.

Lilford, R. J., Bentham, L. M., Armstrong, M. J., Neuberger, J., & Girling, A. J. (2013b). What is the best strategy for investigating abnormal liver function tests in primary care? Implications from a prospective study. *BMJ Open*, *3*(6), e003099.

Lindor, K. D., Gershwin, M. E., Poupon, R., Kaplan, M., Bergasa, N. V., & Heathcote, E. J. (2009). Primary biliary cirrhosis. *Hepatology*, *50*(1), 291–308.

Longstreth, G. F., Thompson, W. G., Chey, W. D., Houghton, L. A., Mearin, F., & Spiller, R. C. (2006). Functional bowel disorders. *Gastroenterology*, *130*(5), 1480–1491.

Loy, C. T., Irwig, L. M., Katelaris, P. H., & Talley, N. J. (1996). Do commercial serological kits for Helicobacter pylori infection differ in accuracy? A meta-analysis. *American Journal of Gastroenterology*, *91*(6), 1138–1144.

Ludvigsson, J. F., Bai, J. C., Biagi, F., Card, T. R., Ciacci, C., Ciclitira, P. J., Green, P. H., Hadjivassiliou, M., Holdoway, A., van Heel, D. A., Kaukinen, K., Leffler, D. A., Leonard, J. N., Lundin, K. E., McGough, N., Davidson, M., Murray, J. A., Swift, G. L., Walker, M. M., Zingone, F., & Sanders, D. S. (2014). Diagnosis and management of adult coeliac disease: Guidelines from the British Society of Gastroenterology. *Gut*, *63*(8), 1210–1228.

Maconi, G., Manes, G., & Porro, G. B. (2008). Role of symptoms in diagnosis and outcome of gastric cancer. *World Journal of Gastroenterology*, *14*(8), 1149–1155.

Malfertheiner, P., Megraud, F., O'Morain, C., Bazzoli, F., El Omar, E., Graham, D., Hunt, R., Rokkas, T., Vakil, N., & Kuipers, E. J. (2007). Current concepts in the management of Helicobacter pylori infection: The Maastricht III Consensus Report. *Gut*, *56*(6), 772–781.

Marshall, B. J., & Warren, J. R. (1984). Unidentified curved bacilli in the stomach of patients with gastritis and peptic ulceration. *Lancet*, *1*(8390), 1311–1315.

Marshall, J. K., & Irvine, E. J. (1997). Rectal corticosteroids versus alternative treatments in ulcerative colitis: A meta-analysis. *Gut*, *40*(6), 775–781.

McColl, K. E. (2010). Clinical practice. Helicobacter pylori infection. *New England Journal of Medicine*, *362*(17), 1597–1604.

McDonald, J. W., Wang, Y., Tsoulis, D. J., MacDonald, J. K., & Feagan, B. G. (2014). Methotrexate for induction of remission in refractory Crohn's disease. *Cochrane Database of Systematic Reviews*, (8), CD003459.

McMinn, J., Steel, C., & Bowman, A. (2011). Investigation and management of unintentional weight loss in older adults. *BMJ*, *342*, d1732.

Micali, N., Hagberg, K. W., Petersen, I., & Treasure, J. L. (2013). The incidence of eating disorders in the UK in 2000-2009: Findings from the General Practice Research Database. *BMJ Open*, *3*(5), e002646.

Moayyedi, P., Soo, S., Deeks, J., Delaney, B., Harris, A., Innes, M., Oakes, R., Wilson, S., Roalfe, A., Bennett, C., & Forman, D. (2003a). Eradication of Helicobacter pylori for non-ulcer dyspepsia. *Cochrane Database of Systematic Reviews*, (1), CD002096.

Moayyedi, P., Soo, S., Deeks, J., Delaney, B., Innes, M., & Forman, D. (2003b). Pharmacological interventions for non-ulcer dyspepsia. *Cochrane Database of Systematic Reviews*, (1), CD001960.

Moayyedi, P., & Talley, N. J. (2006). Gastro-oesophageal reflux disease. *Lancet*, *367*(9528), 2086–2100.

Monahan, K. J., Davies, M. M., Abulafi, M., Banerjea, A., Nicholson, B. D., Arasaradnam, R., Barker, N., Benton, S., Booth, R., Burling, D., Carten, R. V., D'Souza, N., East, J. E., Kleijnen, J., Machesney, M., Pettman, M., Pipe, J., Saker, L., Sharp, L., Stephenson, J., Steele, R. J. C. (2022). Faecal immunochemical testing (FIT) in patients with signs or symptoms of suspected colorectal cancer (CRC): A joint guideline from the Association of Coloproctology of Great Britain and Ireland (ACPGBI) and the British Society of Gastroenterology (BSG). *Gut*, *71*, 1939–1962.

Mooney, P. D., Hadjivassiliou, M., & Sanders, D. S. (2014). Coeliac disease. *BMJ*, *348*, g1561.

Moore, K. P., & Aithal, G. P. (2006). Guidelines on the management of ascites in cirrhosis. *Gut*, *55*(Suppl. 6), vi1–vi12.

Mowat, C., Cole, A., Windsor, A., Ahmad, T., Arnott, I., Driscoll, R., Mitton, S., Orchard, T., Rutter, M., Younge, L., Lees, C., Ho, G. T., Satsangi, J., & Bloom, S. (2011). Guidelines for the management of inflammatory bowel disease in adults. *Gut*, *60*(5), 571–607.

Munkholm, P., Michetti, P., Probert, C. S., Elkjaer, M., & Marteau, P. (2010). Best practice in the management of mild-to-moderately active ulcerative colitis and achieving maintenance of remission using mesalazine. *European Journal of Gastroenterology & Hepatology*, *22*(8), 912–916.

Murch, S., Jenkins, H., Auth, M., Bremner, R., Butt, A., France, S., Furman, M., Gillett, P., Kiparissi, F., Lawson, M., McLain, B., Morris, M. A., Sleet, S., & Thorpe, M. (2013). Joint BSPGHAN and Coeliac UK guidelines for the diagnosis and management of coeliac disease in children. *Archives of Disease in Childhood*, *98*(10), 806–811.

National Institute for Health and Clinical Excellence. (2004). *Dyspepsia: Managing dyspepsia in adults in primary care*. https://www.nice.org.uk/guidance/cg184

National Institute for Health and Clinical Excellence. (2006). *Nutrition support for adults: Oral nutrition support, enteral tube feeding and parenteral nutrition*. https://www.nice.org.uk/guidance/cg32

National Institute for Health and Clinical Excellence. (2008). *Irritable bowel syndrome in adults: Diagnosis and management*. https://www.nice.org.uk/guidance/cg61

National Institute for Health and Clinical Excellence. (2013a). *Faecal calprotectin diagnostic tests for inflammatory diseases of the bowel*. https://www.nice.org.uk/guidance/dg11

National Institute for Health and Clinical Excellence. (2013b). *Hepatitis B (chronic): Diagnosis and management (CG165)*. https://www.nice.org.uk/guidance/cg165

National Institute for Health and Clinical Excellence. (2013c). *Hepatitis B and C testing: people at risk of infection*. https://www.nice.org.uk/guidance/ph43

National Institute for Health and Clinical Excellence. (2014a). *Endoscopic radiofrequency ablation for Barrett's oesophagus with low-grade dysplasia or no dysplasia*. https://www.nice.org.uk/guidance/ipg496

National Institute for Health and Clinical Excellence. (2014b). *Gallstone disease: Diagnosis and management*. https://www.nice.org.uk/guidance/cg188

National Institute for Health and Clinical Excellence. (2014c). *Gastro-oesophageal reflux disease and dyspepsia in adults: Investigation and management*. https://www.nice.org.uk/guidance/cg184

National Institute for Health and Clinical Excellence. (2015). *Suspected cancer: Recognition and referral. NICE clinical guideline 12.* Retrieved from http://www.nice. org.uk/guidance/ng12.

National Institute for Health and Clinical Excellence. (2015a). *Coeliac disease: Recognition, assessment and management (NG29).* https://www.nice.org.uk/guidance/ng20

National Institute for Health and Clinical Excellence. (2015b). *Suspected cancer: Recognition and referral.* https://www.nice.org.uk/guidance/ng12

National Institute for Health and Clinical Excellence. (2016a). *Assessment and management of cirrhosis.* https://www.nice.org.uk/guidance/ng50

National Institute for Health and Clinical Excellence. (2016b). *Non-alcoholic fatty liver disease (NAFLD): Assessment and management.* https://www.nice.org.uk/guidance/ng49

National Institute for Health and Clinical Excellence. (2018). *Pancreatitis. NICE clinical guideline 104.* Retrieved from http://www. nice. org.uk/guidance/ng104.

National Institute for Health and Clinical Excellence. (2019a). *Ulcerative colitis: Management.* https://www.nice.org.uk/guidance/ng130

National Institute for Health and Clinical Excellence. (2019b). *Crohn's disease: Management.* https://www.nice.org.uk/guidance/ng129

National Institute for Health and Clinical Excellence. (2023). *Updacitinib for previously treated moderately to severely active Crohn's disease (ID4027) NICE medical technologies guidance.* Retrieved from https://www.nice.org.uk/guidance/indevelopment/gid-ta10997.

Nguyen, G. C., Smalley, W. E., Vege, S. S., & Carrasco-Labra, A. (2016). American Gastroenterological Association Institute Guideline on the Medical Management of Microscopic Colitis. *Gastroenterology, 150*(1), 242–246.

Norgard, B., Pedersen, L., Fonager, K., Rasmussen, S. N., & Sorensen, H. T. (2003). Azathioprine, mercaptopurine and birth outcome: A population-based cohort study. *Alimentary Pharmacology & Therapeutics, 17*(6), 827–834.

Quigley, E. M., Tack, J., Chey, W. D., Rao, S. S., Fortea, J., Falques, M., Diaz, C., Shiff, S. J., Currie, M. G., & Johnston, J. M. (2013). Randomised clinical trials: Linaclotide phase 3 studies in IBS-C - a prespecified further analysis based on European Medicines Agency-specified endpoints. *Alimentary Pharmacology & Therapeutics, 37*(1), 49–61.

Rezende, G., Roque-Afonso, A. M., Samuel, D., Gigou, M., Nicand, E., Ferre, V., Dussaix, E., Bismuth, H., & Feray, C. (2003). Viral and clinical factors associated with the fulminant course of hepatitis A infection. *Hepatology, 38*(3), 613–618.

Rinella, M. E. (2015). Nonalcoholic fatty liver disease: A systematic review. *JAMA, 313*(22), 2263–2273.

Royal College of Physicians (2014). National audit of inflammatory bowel disease (IBD) service provision. *UK IBD audit.* Retrieved from: https://www.rcp.ac.uk/improving-care/resources/ibd-organisational-audit-adult-report-round-four-2014/

Rubin, D. T., LoSavio, A., Yadron, N., Huo, D., & Hanauer, S. B. (2006). Aminosalicylate therapy in the prevention of dysplasia and colorectal cancer in ulcerative colitis. *Clinical Gastroenterology and Hepatology, 4*(11), 1346–1350.

Rubio-Tapia, A., & Murray, J. A. (2010). Classification and management of refractory coeliac disease. *Gut, 59*(4), 547–557.

Ruepert, L., Quartero, A. O., de Wit, N. J., van der Heijden, G. J., Rubin, G., & Muris, J. W. (2011). Bulking agents, antispasmodics and antidepressants for the treatment of irritable bowel syndrome. *Cochrane Database of Systematic Reviews, (8),* CD003460.

Schiller, L. R. (2004). Chronic diarrhea. *Gastroenterology, 127*(1), 287–293.

Scott, E. M., Gaywood, I., Scott, B. B. (2000). Guidelines for osteoporosis in coeliac disease and inflammatory bowel disease. British Society of Gastroenterology. *Gut; 46*(1): i1–8.

Seenan, J. P., Thomson, F., Rankin, K., Smith, K., & Gaya, D. R. (2015). Are we exposing patients with a mildly elevated faecal calprotectin to unnecessary investigations? *Frontline Gastroenterology; 6*(3); 156–160.

Sgouros, S. N., & Pereira, S. P. (2006). Systematic review: Sphincter of Oddi dysfunction—non-invasive diagnostic methods and long-term outcome after endoscopic sphincterotomy. *Alimentary Pharmacology & Therapeutics, 24*(2), 237–246.

Shea, J. A., Berlin, J. A., Escarce, J. J., Clarke, J. R., Kinosian, B. P., Cabana, M. D., Tsai, W. W., Horangic, N., Malet, P. F., & Schwartz, J. S. (1994). Revised estimates of diagnostic test sensitivity and specificity in suspected biliary tract disease. *Archives of Internal Medicine, 154*(22), 2573–2581.

Sidhu, R., Sanders, D. S., Morris, A. J., & McAlindon, M. E. (2008). Guidelines on small bowel enteroscopy and capsule endoscopy in adults. *Gut, 57*(1), 125–136.

Singh, A., Mann, H. S., Thukral, C. L., & Singh, N. R. (2014). Diagnostic accuracy of MRCP as compared to ultrasound/CT in patients with obstructive jaundice. *Journal of Clinical and Diagnostic Research, 8*(3), 103–107.

Singh, S., Stroud, A. M., Holubar, S. D., Sandborn, W. J., & Pardi, D. S. (2015). Treatment and prevention of pouchitis after ileal pouch-anal anastomosis for chronic ulcerative colitis. *Cochrane Database of Systematic Reviews, (11),* CD001176.

Smith, M. A., Blaker, P., Marinaki, A. M., Anderson, S. H., Irving, P. M., & Sanderson, J. D. (2012). Optimising outcome on thiopurines in inflammatory bowel disease by co-prescription of allopurinol. *Journal of Crohn's & Colitis, 6*(9), 905–912.

Snook, J., Bhala, N., Beales, I. L. P., Cannings, D., Kightley, C., Logan, R. P. H., Pritchard, D. M., Sidhu, R., Surgenor, S., Thomas, W., Verma, A. M., & Goddard, A. (2021). British Society of Gastroenterology guidelines for the management of iron deficiency anaemia in adults. *Gut, 70,* 2030–2051.

Spada, C., Stoker, J., Alarcon, O., Barbaro, F., Bellini, D., Bretthauer, M., De Haan, M. C., Dumonceau, J. M., Ferlitsch, M., Halligan, S., Helbren, E., Hellstrom, M., Kuipers, E. J., Lefere, P., Mang, T., Neri, E., Petruzziello, L., Plumb, A., Regge, D., Taylor, S. A., Hassan, C., & Laghi, A. (2014). Clinical indications for computed tomographic colonography: European Society of Gastrointestinal Endoscopy (ESGE) and European Society of Gastrointestinal and Abdominal Radiology (ESGAR) Guideline. *Endoscopy, 46*(10), 897–915.

Spiller, R., Aziz, Q., Creed, F., Emmanuel, A., Houghton, L., Hungin, P., Jones, R., Kumar, D., Rubin, G., Trudgill, N., & Whorwell, P. (2007). Guidelines on the irritable bowel syndrome: Mechanisms and practical management. *Gut, 56*(12), 1770–1798.

Tack, J., Talley, N. J., Camilleri, M., Holtmann, G., Hu, P., Malagelada, J. R., & Stanghellini, V. (2006). Functional gastroduodenal disorders. *Gastroenterology, 130*(5), 1466–1479.

Thursz, M. R., Richardson, P., Allison, M., Austin, A., Bowers, M., Day, C. P., Downs, N., Gleeson, D., MacGilchrist, A., Grant, A., Hood, S., Masson, S., McCune, A., Mellor, J., O'Grady, J., Patch, D., Ratcliffe, I., Roderick, P., Stanton, L., Vergis, N., Wright, M., Ryder, S., & Forrest, E. H. (2015). Prednisolone or pentoxifylline for alcoholic hepatitis. *New England Journal of Medicine, 372*(17), 1619–1628.

Tripathi, D., Stanley, A. J., Hayes, P. C., Patch, D., Millson, C., Mehrzad, H., Austin, A., Ferguson, J. W., Olliff, S. P., Hudson, M., & Christie, J. M. (2015). U.K. guidelines on the management of variceal haemorrhage in cirrhotic patients., *Gut*, *64*(11), 1680–1704.

Truelove, S. C., & Witts, L. J. (1955). Cortisone in ulcerative colitis; final report on a therapeutic trial. *British Medical Journal*, *2*(4947), 1041–1048.

Tsochatzis, E. A., Bosch, J., & Burroughs, A. K. (2014). Liver cirrhosis. *Lancet*, *383*(9930), 1749–1761.

UK Department of Health. (2016). *UK Chief Medical Officers' Low Risk Drinking Guidelines*. Retrieved from: https://assets.publishing.service.gov.uk/media/5a80b7ed40f0b623026951db/UK_CMOs__report.pdf

Vaira, D., & Vakil, N. (2001). Blood, urine, stool, breath, money, and Helicobacter pylori. *Gut*, *48*(3), 287–289.

Vakil, N., van Zanten, S. V., Kahrilas, P., Dent, J., & Jones, R. (2006). The Montreal definition and classification of gastroesophageal reflux disease: A global evidence-based consensus. *American Journal of Gastroenterology*, *101*, 1900–1920.

van Assche, G., Dignass, A., Bokemeyer, B., Danese, S., Gionchetti, P., Moser, G., Beaugerie, L., Gomollon, F., Hauser, W., Herrlinger, K., Oldenburg, B., Panes, J., Portela, F., Rogler, G., Stein, J., Tilg, H., Travis, S., & Lindsay, J. O. (2013). Second European evidence-based consensus on the diagnosis and management of ulcerative colitis part 3: Special situations. *Journal of Crohn's & Colitis*, *7*(1), 1–33.

van Assche, G., Dignass, A., Reinisch, W., van der Woude, C. J., Sturm, A., De Vos, M., Guslandi, M., Oldenburg, B., Dotan, I., Marteau, P., Ardizzone, A., Baumgart, D. C., d'Haens, G., Gionchetti, P., Portela, F., Vucelic, B., Soderholm, J., Escher, J., Koletzko, S., Kolho, K. L., Lukas, M., Mottet, C., Tilg, H., Vermeire, S., Carbonnel, F., Cole, A., Novacek, G., Reinshagen, M., Tsianos, E., Herrlinger, K., Oldenburg, B., Bouhnik, Y., Kiesslich, R., Stange, E., Travis, S., & Lindsay, J. (2010). The second European evidence-based Consensus on the diagnosis and management of Crohn's disease: Special situations. *Journal of Crohn's & Colitis*, *4*(1), 63–101.

van Bokhoven, M. A., van Deursen, C. T., & Swinkels, D. W. (2011). Diagnosis and management of hereditary haemochromatosis. *BMJ*, *342*, c7251.

van der, E. A., van der Hulst, R. W., Dankert, J., & Tytgat, G. N. (1997). Reinfection versus recrudescence in Helicobacter pylori infection. *Alimentary Pharmacology & Therapeutics*, *11*(Suppl. 1), 55–61.

van Staa, T. P., Card, T., Logan, R. F., & Leufkens, H. G. (2005). 5-Aminosalicylate use and colorectal cancer risk in inflammatory bowel disease: A large epidemiological study. *Gut*, *54*(11), 1573–1578.

Vasant, D. H., Paine, P. A., Black, C. J., Houghton, L. A., Everitt, H. A., Corsetti, M., Agrawal, A., Aziz, I., Farmer, A. D., Eugenicos, M. P., Moss-Morris, R., Yiannakou, Y., & Ford, A. C. (2021). British Society of Gastroenterology guidelines on the management of irritable bowel syndrome. *Gut*, *70*, 1214–1240.

Viazis, N., Keyoglou, A., Kanellopoulos, A. K., Karamanolis, G., Vlachogiannakos, J., Triantafyllou, K., Ladas, S. D., & Karamanolis, D. G. (2012). Selective serotonin reuptake inhibitors for the treatment of hypersensitive esophagus: A randomized, double-blind, placebo-controlled study. *American Journal of Gastroenterology*, *107*, 1662–1667.

Williams, R., Aspinall, R., Bellis, M., Camps-Walsh, G., Cramp, M., Dhawan, A., Ferguson, J., Forton, D., Foster, G., Gilmore, I., Hickman, M., Hudson, M., Kelly, D., Langford, A., Lombard, M., Longworth, L., Martin, N., Moriarty, K., Newsome, P., O'Grady, J., Pryke, R., Rutter, H., Ryder, S., Sheron, N., & Smith, T. (2014). Addressing liver disease in the UK: A blueprint for attaining excellence in health care and reducing premature mortality from lifestyle issues of excess consumption of alcohol, obesity, and viral hepatitis. *Lancet*, *384*(9958), 1953–1997.

Zhang, Y., Li, L., Guo, C., Mu, D., Feng, B., Zuo, X., & Li, Y. (2016). Effects of probiotic type, dose and treatment duration on irritable bowel syndrome diagnosed by Rome III criteria: A meta-analysis. *BMC Gastroenterology*, *16*(1), 62.

Zlatanic, J., Korelitz, B. I., Rajapakse, R., Kim, P. S., Rubin, S. D., Baiocco, P. J., & Panagopoulos, G. (2003). Complications of pregnancy and child development after cessation of treatment with 6-mercaptopurine for inflammatory bowel disease. *Journal of Clinical Gastroenterology*, *36*(4), 303–309.

9

Surgical Problems

Iain Wilson & Jennifer Stevens

CHAPTER CONTENTS

Gallstones and Gallbladder Disease

GUIDELINE

National Institute for Health and Clinical Excellence. (2014). *Gallstone disease and management. NICE clinical guideline 188.* Available at https://www.nice.org.uk/guidance/cg188.

PATIENT INFORMATION

National Health Service. *Gallbladder removal.* Available at https://www.nhs.uk/conditions/gallbladder-removal.
Royal College of Surgeons of England. *Get well soon. Helping you to make a speedy recovery after gallbladder removal.* Available at http://www.rcseng.ac.uk/library-and-publications/rcs-publications/docs/gall-bladder-removal.

- Gallstones are common; they are present in 10% to 15% of the population.
- Most gallstones are asymptomatic; 80% of people with gallstones have no symptoms.
- About 2% to 4% of people with gallstones will develop symptoms or complications each year (Gurusamy & Davidson, 2014).
- Complications of gallstones include biliary colic, cholecystitis, pancreatitis, choledocholithiasis, cholangitis, obstructive jaundice, and gallbladder cancer.

Biliary Colic

Diagnosis

- Classically, patients report colicky pain (pain that comes and goes, like a contraction) in the right upper quadrant that radiates to the back or shoulder.
- Pain commonly occurs one hour after eating (usually rich or fatty foods). This is usally in the evening or at night
- Patinets with biliary colic will have gallstones in a thin walled gallbladder on ultrasound.

Management

- Patients with biliary colic require analgesia as per the World Health Organization's pain ladder.
- Refer to secondary care for laparoscopic cholecystectomy.
- It can be difficult to differentiate between biliary colic and other acute biliary problems both clinically and radiologically. Patients whose symptoms cannot be managed with simple analgesia require emergency referral to secondary care.

Cholecystitis

GUIDELINES

National Institute for Health and Clinical Excellence. (2014). *Gallstone disease and management. NICE clinical guideline 188.* Available at https://www.nice.org.uk/guidance/cg188.
World Society of Emergency Surgery Guideline. (2020). *World Society of Emergency Surgery updated guidelines for the diagnosis and treatment of acute calculous cholecystitis.* Available at https://pubmed.ncbi.nlm.nih.gov/33153472/.

Diagnosis

- Symptoms include right upper quadrant pain, fever, nausea, and vomiting.
- On examination, there may be tenderness in the right upper quadrant. Patients may have a positive Murphy sign (severe pain in the right upper quadrant on deep inspiration)
- Bloods are likely to show raised WCC (white blood cell count) and C-reactive protein.
- Signs of cholecysttis on ultrasound include a thickened gallbladder and pericholecystic fluid

Management

- Antibiotics should be commenced if there is evidence of sepsis, cholangitis, abscess, or perforation.
- Patients with suspected cholecysttis require emergency referral to secondary care
- Laparoscopic cholecystectomy is the first-line treatment for patients with acute cholecystitis (WSES, 2020).
- Patients with acute cholecystitis should be offered early laparoscopic cholecystectomy (to be carried out within 1 week of diagnosis) (NICE, 2014).
- When early laparoscopic cholecystectomy is not possible, surgery should be offered 6 weeks after the first clinical presentation (WSES, 2020).

Note: Compared with delayed cholecystectomy, early laparoscopic cholecystectomy is associated with a significant reduction in wound infection, length of hospital stay, operation duration, and improvement in quality of life. There was no difference in mortality rate, bile duct injury, bile leakage, overall complications, or conversion to open surgery (Song et al, 2016).

Choledocholithiasis (common bile duct stones)

GUIDELINES

British Society of Gastroenterology Guideline. (2017). *Updated guideline on the management of common bile duct stones.* Available at https://www. pubmed.ncbi.nlm.nih.gov/28122906/.
National Institute for Health and Clinical Excellence. (2014). *Gallstone disease and management. NICE clinical guideline 188.* Available at https://www.nice.org.uk/guidance/cg188.

Diagnosis

- Gallstones in the common bile duct should be suspected in patients with painful jaundice, acute cholangitis, acute pancreatitis, deranged LFT results or a dilated biliary tree.
- Classically patients will describe pain (in the right upper quadrant or epigastirum), jaundice, dark urine and pale stools

Management

- Patients with suspected common bile duct stones require emergency referral to secondary care
- Clearance of bile duct stones and laparoscopic cholecystectomy should be offered to people with symptomatic or asymptomatic common bile duct stones (NICE, 2014).
- Bile duct stones can be managed with either an endoscopic retrograde cholangiopancreatography followed by a laparoscopic cholecystectomy at a later date or a laparoscopic cholecystectomy with bile duct exploration performed at the same time.

Gallbladder Polyps

GUIDELINE

Foley, K. G., Lahaye, M. J., Thoeni, R. F., et al. (2022). *Management and follow-up of gallbladder polyps: Updated joint guidelines between the ESGAR, EAES, EFISDS and ESGE.* Available at https://pubmed.ncbi.nlm.nih.gov/34918177.

- Polypoid lesions of the gallbladder are found in 4% to 7% of patients who undergo abdominal ultrasound examination (Chou et al, 2017).
- Most polypoid lesions are benign, but a small number are malignant or premalignant. The likelihood of a polypoid

lesion being malignant or premalignant increases with polyp size.

Management

- Refer to secondary care to discuss laparoscopic cholecystectomy or polyp surveillance.
- Investigation and surveillance of gallbladder polyps should be with abdominal ultrasound examination.
- Cholecystectomy should be offered to patients with:
  - A gallbladder polyp 10 mm or larger
  - A gallbladder polyp and symptoms attributable to the gallbladder
  - A gallbladder polyp that grows by 2 mm or more in a 2-year surveillance period
  - A gallbladder polyp 6 to 9 mm in size and the presence of a risk factors for gallbladder cancer
- Risk factors for gallbladder malignancy include:
  - Age 60 years or older
  - Asian ethnicity
  - History of primary sclerosing cholangitis
  - Presence of sessile polypoid lesion (including focal gallbladder wall thickening >4 mm)
- Surveillance involves abdominal ultrasound examination at 6 months, 1 year, and 2 years.
- Surveillance is offered to the following patients
  - Gallbladder polyp 6 to 9 mm with no risk factors for gallbladder cancer
  - Gallbladder polyp 5 mm or smaller with risk factors for gallbladder cancer
- The following patients can be discharged from surveillance:
  - No growth of polyps over the 2-year surveillance period
  - Polyps that disappear during surveillance
  - Gallbladder polyp 5 mm or smaller with no risk factors for gallbladder cancer

Porcelain Gallbladder

GUIDELINE

European Association for the Study of the Liver Clinical Practice Guideline. (2016). *EASL clinical practice guideline on the prevention, diagnosis and treatment of gallstones.* Available at https://pubmed.ncbi.nlm.nih.gov/27085810/.

- This describes a condition in which there is calcification in the wall of the gallbladder.
- There is an association between gallbladder cancer and porcelain gallbladder, although the risk is much lower than previously thought (Morimoto et al, 2021).
- Patients with porcelain gallbladder should be referred to secondary care for consideration of laparoscopic cholecystectomy (EASL, 2016).

Adenomyomatosis

- This is a benign thickening of the wall of the gallbladder.
- If asymptomatic, this requires no further management.
- If associated with symptoms or if there are concerns about gallbladder malignancy, then referral to secondary care is indicated.

Diverticular Disease

GUIDELINE

National Institute for Health and Clinical Excellence. (2019). *Diverticular disease: Diagnosis and management. NICE clinical guideline 147.* Available at https://www.nice.org.uk/guidance/ng147.

Diverticulosis

- This describes the presence of asymptomatic diverticula in the colon.
- Diverticulosis is rare before 40 years of age; however, 50% of the population aged older than 50 years are affected, and 70% aged older than 80 years of age are affected (ACPBGI, 2014).
- About 4% of people with diverticulosis will develop acute diverticulitis (Shahedi et al, 2013).

Management

- Advise patients to maintain a healthy, balanced, high-fibre diet with adequate fluid intake.
- Patients are no longer advised to avoid seeds, nuts, popcorn, or fruit skins.
- Consider prescribing a bulk-forming laxative if there is constipation.
- Advise patients about exercise, smoking cessation, and weight loss (NICE, 2019).

PATIENT INFORMATION

Association of UK Dieticians. *Food fact sheet: Fibre.* Available at https://www.bda.uk.com/resourceDetail/printPdf/?resource=fibre.

Diverticular Disease

- This describes patients who have colonic diverticular disease who are symptomatic.
- Symptoms include lower abdominal pain, a change in bowel habit, blood or mucous in the stool, and abdominal bloating.
- Approximately 15% of people have rectal bleeding from their diverticula (ACPBGI, 2014).

Management

- Advise patients to maintain a healthy, balanced, high-fibre diet with adequate fluid intake.
- Patients are no longer advised to avoid seeds, nuts, popcorn, or fruit skins.
- Consider prescribing a bulk-forming laxative if there is constipation.
- Advise patients to exercise, stop smoking, and lose weight if they are overweight or obese (NICE, 2019).
- Patients with red flag symptoms for colorectal cancer (CRC) such as unexplained weight loss, rectal bleeding, iron-deficiency anaemia, and presence of an abdominal mass should be referred under the NICE 'suspected cancer: recognition and referral' pathway (see https://www.nice.org.uk/guidance/ng12/chapter/Recommendations-organised-by-site-of-cancer#lower-gastrointestinal-tract-cancers).

Further Management

- Some patients require elective bowel resection for diverticular disease. Indications for surgical resection include:
  - Frequent or severe recurrent episodes of acute diverticulitis
  - Symptoms affecting quality of life
  - Colonic stricture
  - Colonic fistula
  - Recurrent diverticular bleeding

PATIENT INFORMATION

Association of Coloproctology of Great Britain and Ireland. *Diverticular disease.* Available at https://www.acpgbi.org.uk/_userfiles/pages/files/conditions/diverticulardisease.pdf
Guts Charity. *Diverticular disease.* Available at https://gutscharity.org.uk/advice-and-information/conditions/diverticular-disease.

Diverticulitis

- Diverticulitis describes diverticula that become inflamed or infected.
- Classical symptoms include left iliac fossa pain, fever, and change in bowel habit.
- Complicated diverticulitis is most likely in patients having their first attack of diverticulitis.
- Acute complications of diverticulitis include abscess formation and colonic perforation.

Management

- Referral to hospital is not mandatory for all patients with acute uncomplicated diverticulitis.
- Emergency surgical admission should be arranged for patients with the following symptoms:
  - Uncontrolled abdominal pain

- Unable to tolerate oral fluids
- Unable to tolerate oral antibiotics
- Patients older than 65 years of age
- Patients who are frail, with significant comorbidities, and who are immunocompromised (NICE, 2019)
- Selected patients without significant comorbidities can be managed in primary care. Management includes:
  - A diet of clear liquids only. Reintroduce solid food as symptoms improve over 2 to 3 days.
  - Regular paracetamol for pain. Avoid nonsteroidal antiinflammatory drugs and opioid analgesics.
  - Offer broad-spectrum oral antibiotics to patients who are systemically unwell for 5 days (e.g., co-amoxiclav or cefalexin plus metronidazole or trimethoprim plus metronidazole) (NICE, 2019).
  - Reassess the patient within 48 hours or sooner.

Further Management

- Endoscopic investigation of the colon is usually recommended after an episode of acute diverticulitis, particularly if an endoscopy has not been performed in the past 3 years. Endoscopy is normally undertaken 6 weeks after the attack of diverticulitis.

Note: Endoscopic follow-up after diverticulitis is controversial. The rate of CRC in patients with complicated diverticulitis is between 7.9% and 10.8%; however, the rate of CRC in patients with computed tomography (CT)–confirmed uncomplicated diverticulitis is much lower at 0.5% to 1.2% (Schultz et al, 2020). European Society of Coloproctology guidelines state that endoscopy may not be required in this latter group (Schultz et al, 2020).

Rectal Bleeding

GUIDELINES

Royal College of Surgeons and Association of Coloproctology of Great Britain and Ireland. (2017). *Commissioning guide: Rectal bleeding.* Available at https://www.acpgbi.org.uk/about/news/295/commissioning_guide_rectal_bleeding_royal_college_of_surgeons_rcs_and_acpgbi_2017/.
National Institute for Health and Clinical Excellence. (2021). *Suspected cancer: Recognition and referral. NICE clinical guideline BG12.* Available at https://www.nice.org.uk/guidance/ng12/chapter/Recommendations-organised-by-site-of-cancer#lower-gastrointestinal-tract-cancers.

- Rectal bleeding is a common problem. In the United Kingdom, the 1-year prevalence in adults is about 10% (ACPGBI, 2017).
- Most rectal bleeding is caused by benign conditions such as haemorrhoids, anal fissure, or diverticular disease.

- Rectal bleeding can be a manifestation of more sinister problems such as inflammatory bowel disease (IBD) or CRC. Clinicians should take care not to miss proximal colorectal disease in the presence of benign anorectal pathology (ACPGBI, 2017).

  Note: Rectal bleeding has a positive predictive value for colorectal malignancy of 8% in patients aged older than 50 years (Astin et al, 2011).

Assessment

- Ask about perianal symptoms (pain, lump, prolapse, itch, leakage, incomplete evacuation, and discharge).
- Enquire about bleeding including, the colour of the blood (bright red, dark red) and where blood was observed (on the paper, coating the stool, or in the pan).
- Enquire about any family history of CRC and IBD.
- Ask about red flag symptoms including weight loss, symptoms suggestive of anaemia, and change in bowel habit.
- Perform an abdominal examination to exclude an abdominal mass.
- Examine the external anus. Spread the buttocks and look for fissures, prolapsed mucosa, and haemorrhoids.
- Perform a digital rectal examination (DRE). The cervix can commonly be palpated anteriorly in females. Haemorrhoids are vascular structures and cannot usually be palpated on DRE.
- If experience and logistics permit, undertake proctoscopy.

Investigation

- Blood tests are not routinely indicated in patients with rectal bleeding.
- Consider FBC if there are signs and symptoms of anaemia.
- Other bloods tests may be indicated if bleeding is associated with problems such as weight loss or a change in bowel habit.
- Offer quantitative faecal immunochemical testing (FIT) to the following patients:
  - >50 years with rectal bleeding and unexplained abdominal pain and or/ weight loss
  - 50 years and over with any of the following unexplained rectal bleeding
  - A FIT should be offered even if the person has previously had a negative FIT result through the NHS bowel cancer screening programme (NICE, 2023).
- If IBD is suspected in a young low-risk patient, consider a test for faecal calprotectin. A positive faecal calprotectin result has a high positive predictive value for finding IBD at colonoscopy.
- Tumour markers and faecal occult blood testing are not indicated in patients with rectal bleeding (ACPGBI, 2017)

Management

- Most bleeding resolves spontaneously. It is reasonable to manage low-risk patients with rectal bleeding with a 'watch and wait' policy (ACPGBI, 2017).

- Emergency surgical referral should be arranged in the presence of haemodynamic instability, significant blood loss, and the potential requirement for blood transfusion. (ACPGBI, 2017).
- Clinicians should consider an emergency referral in patients who are older, on anticoagulation medication, and unable to monitor bleeding.

Indications for Referral

- Patients with the following symptoms should be referred for an appointment within 2 weeks under the NICE 'suspected cancer: recognition and referral' pathway:
  - A FIT result of at least 10 micrograms of haemoglobin per gram of faeces
  - A rectal mass (NICE, 2023)
- A negative FIT should not exclude patients from referral for:
  - A strong family history of colorectal malignancy
  - Anxiety about colorectal malignancy
  - Persistent rectal bleeding despite treatment for haemorrhoids
  - Rectal bleeding in patients with a past history of pelvic radiotherapy
  - For assessment of suspected IBD (ACPGBI, 2017)

Perianal Disorders

Haemorrhoids

> **GUIDELINES**
>
> American Society of Colon and Rectal Surgeons Clinical Practice Guidelines. (2018). *Haemorrhoids*. Available at https://fascrs.org/healthcare-providers/education/clinical-practice-guidelines.
> National Institute for Health and Clinical Excellence. (2021). *NICE clinical knowledge summaries: Haemorrhoids*. Available at https://cks.nice.org.uk/topics/haemorrhoids.

- Haemorrhoids arise when the circular venous plexuses in the anus become persistently dilated.
- Haemorrhoids that originate above the dentate line are internal haemorrhoids. Haemorrhoids that originate below the dentate line are external haemorrhoids.
- Factors that contribute to the development of haemorrhoids include constipation, straining, ageing, heavy lifting, chronic cough, pregnancy, and childbirth (NICE, 2021).

Assessment

- It is important for the clinician to establish that haemorrhoids are the cause of a patient's symptoms and exclude the presence of more proximal and sinister colorectal disease.
- See the earlier 'Assessment of Rectal Bleeding' section.
- Bleeding classically presents as bright red blood on the toilet paper. Blood can also be seen in the toilet bowl or coating the faeces.

- Other possible symptoms include itching or irritation, a feeling of rectal fullness, discomfort, incomplete evacuation, and soiling.
- Ask about prolapse. Internal haemorrhoids can be classified according to their degree of prolapse
  - Grade I: project into the anal canal only
  - Grade II: prolapse on straining but reduce spontaneously
  - Grade III: prolapse on straining but require manual reduction
  - Grade IV: persistently prolapsed and cannot be reduced

Investigation

- See 'Investigation of Rectal Bleeding'.

Management

- Diet and lifestyle modification are the first-line treatments for all patients with symptomatic haemorrhoids (ASCRS, 2024).
- Recommend a diet with enough fluid and fibre intake so stools are soft and easy to pass.
- Advise that patients minimise time spent sitting on the toilet and straining.
- The anal region should be kept clean and dry.
- Consider prescribing a bulk-forming laxative if there is constipation.
- Consider prescribing a topical haemorrhoidal preparation (NICE, 2021).

Topical Haemorrhoidal Preparations

- A variety of topical treatments are available to manage the symptoms of haemorrhoids. These may contain one or a combination of mild astringents, lubricants, local anaesthetics, or corticosteroids.
- There is no evidence to suggest that one topical preparation is more effective than another, although lidocaine is the preferred topical anaesthetic agent.
- Generally, haemorrhoidal preparations should be used in the morning and night and after a bowel movement.
- Prolonged use of any agent is not recommended; anaesthetic-containing preparations may cause sensitisation of the anal skin. Corticosteroid-containing preparations should be used for no longer than 7 days because prolonged use may lead to skin atrophy, contact dermatitis, and skin sensitisation (NICE, 2021).

Indications for Referral

- Refer all patients for an urgent 2-week appointment if anal carcinoma or CRC is suspected.
- Indications for routine referral to secondary care include:
  - Patients who do not respond to conservative treatment
  - Third- or fourth-degree haemorrhoids that are too large for nonoperative measures (haemorrhoidectomy may be needed)
  - Combined internal and external haemorrhoids with severe symptoms (surgery may be required)
  - The presence of chronic irritation or leakage

- Large skin tags (surgical excision may be required) (NICE, 2021)
- In secondary care, most patients with grade I or II and selected patients with grade III internal haemorrhoids can be effectively treated with office-based procedures. Haemorrhoidal banding is typically the most effective option (ASCRS, 2018).
- Surgical options include haemorrhoidal artery ligation operation combined with rectal anorectopexy, formal haemorrhoidectomy, and stapled haemorrhoidectomy.

Thrombosed External Haemorrhoid

> **GUIDELINES**
>
> American Society of Colon and Rectal Surgeons Clinical Practice Guidelines. (2024). *Haemorrhoids*. Available at https://fascrs.org/ascrs/media/files/2024-Hemorrhoids-CPG.pdf.
> WSES-AAST. (2021). *Anorectal emergencies: WSES-AAST guidelines*. Available at https://www.ncbi.nlm.nih.gov/pmc/articles/PMC8447593.

- Symptoms include acute, severe anal pain. Patients may also report a perianal lump.

Assessment

- Spread the buttocks and inspect the anus.
- DRE is often intensely painful in patients with thrombosed haemorrhoids. A diagnosis can often be made without DRE.
- Examination may reveal an exquisitely tender lump that is blue or purplish in colour.

Management

- Patients are usually advised to manage their symptoms with oral analgesia, topical analgesia, and laxatives.
- Symptoms will take days to weeks to resolve.
- Incision and drainage of thrombus from an acutely thrombosed haemorrhoid is an option, but this can be complicated by bleeding.
  Note: There is scant evidence directing the management of this condition. Whereas ASCRS guidelines advise that patients may benefit from early surgical excision, WSES-AAST guidelines advise against the use incision and drainage of a thrombus.
- Patients may benefit from 0.3% nifedipine ointment.
  Note: A small randomised trial showed faster resolution of symptoms in patients managed with 0.3% nifedipine and 1.5% lidocaine ointment compared with topical lidocaine alone (Perrotti et al, 2001).

Anal Fissure

> **GUIDELINE**
>
> National Institute for Health and Clinical Excellence. (2021). *Anal fissure*. Available at https://cks.nice.org.uk/topics/anal-fissure.

- An anal fissure is a longitudinal tear in the skin of the anal canal.
- Symptoms include severe anal pain (usually when opening bowels) and bright red rectal bleeding.
- Anal fissures can be acute (<6-week history) or chronic (>6-week history).
- Anal fissures can be primary (thought to arise because of spasm of the internal anal sphincter causing localised ischaemia) or secondary (caused by conditions such as Crohn's disease, cancers, and sexually transmitted infection).

Assessment

- Spread the buttocks and inspect the anus.
- Ninety percent of anal fissures occur posteriorly in the midline.
- Patients with a chronic fissure may have a sentinel skin tag at the distal aspect of the fissure. In some patients, the internal anal sphincter muscle may be visible within the base of the fissure.
- If a there are multiple or lateral fissures or if the fissure has an irregular border, it should prompt investigation into an underlying cause.
- DRE is often intensely painful in patients with a fissure. A diagnosis can often be made without DRE.

Management

- Management consists of simple analgesia and lifestyle change that avoids constipation.
  Note: Almost half of patients with an acute anal fissure will resolve their symptoms with simple lifestyle changes (Stewart et al, 2017).
- Advise patinets to increase the amount of fibre and fluid in their diet.
- Advise taking paracetamol and ibuprofen for analgesia. Avoid opiate analgesia.
- Advise sitting in a shallow, warm bath several times a day (particularly after a bowel movement). This may help relieve pain.
- Recommend the anal region is kept clean and dry.
- Consider prescribing a bulking agent.
- Consider prescribing a topical anaesthetic for a few days. Avoid prolonged use because it can sensitise the anal skin (NICE, 2021).
- In secondary care, patients may be offered topical glyceryl trinitrate, topical diltiazem, calcium channel blockers, injection of botulinum toxin, and lateral internal sphincterotomy.

Referral to Secondary Care

- Referral is indicated in the following scenarios:
  - If anal cancer or CRC is suspected
  - To exclude a secondary cause for a fissure such as Crohn's disease
  - Older adult patients with a fissure
  - Patients who have continue to have an anal fissure despite adhering to lifestyle change

- Patients in whom the diagnosis is unclear or if spasm and pain make diagnosis impossible

Abdominal Wall and Groin Hernias

Inguinal Hernia

> **GUIDELINE**
>
> The HerniaSurge Group. (2018). *International guidelines for groin hernia management*. Available at https://www.britishherniasociety.org/groin-hernia-management.

- Groin hernias are very common. They are found in 27% to 43% of males and 3% to 6% of females (Kingsnorth & LeBlanc, 2003).
- Patients with symptomatic hernias should be offered surgery.
- Males with asymptomatic hernias can be offered watchful waiting, although it is worth noting that most hernias tend to become symptomatic over time.
  Note: One trial showed that 79% of males who were randomised to watchful waiting of their hernia eventually required hernia surgery over a 10-year follow-up period (Fitzgibbons et al, 2013).
- The risk of an inguinal hernia becoming incarcerated or strangulated is low, around 2% (Fitzgibbons et al, 2013).

Assessment

- The diagnosis of a groin hernia can be made by clinical examination in the majority of cases (HerniaSurge Group, 2018).
- Patients with suspected groin hernias should be examined with the patient standing up. A hernia is more likely to be evident in this position.
- Ensure both groins are examined as well as the scrotum to exclude other common groin lumps such as lymph nodes and testicular problems.
- It is not important to elicit if a hernia is direct or indirect; the management is the same.

Investigation

- The diagnosis of a groin hernia can be made by clinical examination in the majority of cases (HerniaSurge Group, 2018).
- Ultrasound scan is recommended as the first-line investigation for patients with groin pain or swelling of an unclear origin (HerniaSurge Group, 2018).

Management

- All male patients with inguinal hernias should be offered routine referral to secondary care.
- Surgery involves open or keyhole repair with a mesh. This is usually performed under general anaesthesia, but open repair can be performed under regional and local anaesthesia. Surgery is normally performed as a day case.

- Patients with irreducible and partially reducible inguinal hernias should be referred to secondary care on an urgent basis.
- All groin hernias in females should be 'urgent outpatient referrals' because of the increased rate of strangulation.

Femoral Hernia

- Femoral hernias are more common in females.
- Femoral hernias are more likely to become incarcerated or strangulated than inguinal hernias.

Assessment

- Patients with suspected groin hernias should be examined with the patient standing up. A hernia is more likely to be evident in this position.
- Femoral hernias are classically described as being below and lateral to the pubic tubercle.
- In practice, it can be difficult to differentiate between inguinal hernia and femoral hernias in females.

Investigation

- Ultrasound scan is recommended as the first-line investigation or patients with groin pain or swelling of an unclear origin (HerniaSurge Group, 2018).

Management

- Urgent outpatient referral is recommended in females with groin hernias

Umbilical and Epigastric Hernias

- Umbilical hernias are found in the midline in the umbilicus.
- Epigastric hernias are in the midline between the umbilicus and xiphoid process.

Assessment

- Most hernias can be diagnosed from clinical examination alone (European Hernia Society and Americas Hernia Society, 2020).
- Patients with suspected abdominal wall hernias should be examined with the patient initially standing up. A hernia is more likely to be evident in this position.
- Patients with epigastric or umbilical hernias should have their body mass index (BMI) measured.

Investigation

- Ultrasound or CT scan can be used to identify a hernia when the diagnosis is unclear (European Hernia Society and Americas Hernia Society. 2020)

Management

- Referral to secondary care is advised to discuss elective surgical repair.
- Watchful waiting appears to be safe.
- Patients are advised to stop smoking 4 to 6 weeks before surgery and lose weight (aim to get BMI <35 kg/m^2) before elective surgery (European Hernia Society and Americas Hernia Society, 2020).

Vascular Problems

Venous Disease

- Venous disease occurs when valves within the veins become incompetent, allowing blood to reflux.
- Venous insufficiency can occur in the superficial or deep veins of the legs.

Assessment

- Entirely expose the patient's lower limbs. Have them remove all footwear.
- Examine the patient standing up and then supine. Varicosities will be more evident when they are upright.
- Signs of venous disease include varicosities, limb oedema, lipodermatosclerosis (chronic hardening and discolouration of the skin, typically at the ankles and distal leg), venous eczema, and ulceration (commonly in the gaiter area).
- Examine the arterial system to exclude a problem related to peripheral arterial disease (PAD).

- It is not necessary to perform specialist bedside test such as the tourniquet test. In secondary care, venous disease is evaluated using duplex ultrasound examination.

Management

- Give lifestyle advice, including:
  - Weight loss
  - Light or moderate exercise
  - Avoiding prolonged periods of sitting and standing
  - Elevating the legs whilst resting
- Advise patients on meticulous skin care and foot awareness. Patients with venous insufficiency have impaired wound healing, and minor skin issues can quickly develop into infection and ulceration.
- Advise application of an emollient twice per day.
- Consider prescribing compression stockings after PAD has been excluded (avoid in patients with an ankle brachial pressure index [ABPI] ≤0.8).
- Explain that class 2 stockings may be more effective than class 1 but are less well tolerated (see Chapter 20 for more details).
- For management of skin changes or ulcers in the context of varicose veins see Chapter 20.

Indications for Referral

- Patients with venous skin disease
- Patients with poor symptom control
- Patients who require compression stockings with an ABPI of 1.5 or greater
- Many areas have specific referral criteria for varicose veins, but NICE recommends that referral be considered for:
  - Symptomatic veins
  - Thrombophlebitis
  - Skin changes, including active or healed ulceration
- Treatment options for superficial venous insufficiency in secondary care include radiofrequency ablation, endovenous laser treatment, and surgery (tie of the saphenofemoral or saphenopopliteal junction and stripping of the long or short saphenous vein [or both veins]).
- Treatment option for varicosities includes surgical avulsion of varicosities and ultrasound-guided foam sclerotherapy.
- The mainstay of deep venous insufficiency is compression hosiery.

Peripheral Arterial Disease

GUIDELINE

National Institute for Health and Clinical Excellence. (2022). *NICE clinical knowledge summaries: Peripheral arterial disease.* Available at https://cks.nice.org.uk/topics/peripheral-arterial-disease.

- PAD results from the narrowing or occlusion of peripheral arteries because of atherosclerotic disease.

- It is associated with the same risk factors as other cardiovascular disease, including increasing age, smoking, obesity, hypertension, diabetes mellitus, and hypercholesterolaemia.
- Limb ischaemia may be acute or chronic.

Assessment

- Entirely expose the patient's lower limbs. Have them remove all footwear.
- Signs of chronic arterial insufficiency include gangrene and ulcerations (classically seen in toes). Some patients may have a 'sunset foot' (dusky red discolouration of the forefoot that blanches with elevating the legs).
- Examine all pulses (from the aorta to the feet).
- Measure the ABPI.
  - An ABPI less than 0.9 suggests PAD.
  - An ABPI less than 0.5 suggests the patient is at risk of critical limb ischaemia. Refer urgently.
  - A value between 0.9 and 1.3 makes PAD less likely.
  - A value greater than 1.3 suggests arterial stiffening, particularly in patients with diabetes mellitus or renal failure.

  Note: NICE advises not to exclude PAD in patients with diabetes mellitus based on a normal or increased ABPI alone.

Diagnosis

- In primary care, the diagnosis is made from a combination of symptoms and clinical examination. A number of terms are used to describe PAD, including:
  - *Intermittent claudication*, which is pain in a group of muscles (classically the calves, thighs, or buttocks) precipitated by activity. The pain usually resolves within minutes with rest. This is a form of chronic limb ischaemia.
  - *Rest pain*. This is constant pain usually in the forefoot. Symptoms are usually helped by gravity. Patients commonly describe having to hang their legs over the edge of bed or having to sleep in a chair.
  - *Chronic limb-threatening ischaemia*. This term has superseded *critical limb ischaemia*. This describes the end stage of PAD. The patient has rest pain, gangrene, and lower limb ulceration of more than 2 weeks' duration.
  - *Acute limb ischaemia*. This is usually caused by acute blockage of a blood vessel(s). This can be caused by an embolus (caused by atrial fibrillation or a proximal aneurysm) or local thrombosis. This may occur in an individual with no history of PAD. Signs and symptoms include an acute onset of severe pain in a limb; the limb is pale, pulseless, and cold. In latter stages, there is paraesthesia, paralysis, and pain on squeezing the limb muscles.
  - *Chronic limb ischaemia*. This term encompasses a number of scenarios of PAD from intermittent claudication up to critical limb-threatening ischaemia.

Management

- Offer treatment for secondary prevention of cardiovascular disease, including:
  - Smoking cessation
  - Advice on diet and exercise

- Lipid modification with a statin
- Management of hypertension
- Management of diabetes
- Antiplatelet therapy (NICE recommend clopidogrel 75 mg OD as first-line treatment.)
- Advise patients on meticulous foot care and foot awareness. In patients with vascular disease, minor foot trauma can quickly escalate into life- and limb-threatening issues.
- Encourage patients to exercise as much as possible (ideally for 30 minutes three to five times each week). Urge patients to walk up to their claudication distance and if possible to try to incrementally extend this.
- If available, offer a supervised exercise programme (2 hours of supervised exercise per week for 3 months).
- See Chapter 20 for management of arterial ulcers.

Indications for Referral

- Referral to a vascular surgeon is indicated for patients who are:
  - Symptomatic despite risk factor modification and lifestyle change
  - Requiring ongoing opiate pain killers
  - In whom there is doubt about the diagnosis
- *Urgent* referral is indicated for patients with:
  - Rest pain and evidence of ulceration or gangrene
  - ABPI below 0.5
- Management in secondary care may involve endovascular treatment with angioplasty or stenting and/or arterial bypass surgery.
- Some patients may be offered naftidrofuryl oxalate if the above are declined or are not appropriate.

PATIENT INFORMATION

Circulation Foundation. *Peripheral arterial disease.* Available at https://www.circulationfoundation.org.uk/help-advice/peripheral-arterial-disease.

Vascular Society for Great Britain and Ireland. *Peripheral arterial disease.* Available at https://www.vascularsociety.org.uk/patients/conditions/7/peripheral_arterial_disease.

References

Astin, M., Griffin, T., Neal, R. D., Rose, P., & Hamilton, W. (2011). The diagnostic value of symptoms for colorectal cancer in primary care: A systematic review. *The British Journal of General Practice: The Journal of the Royal College of General Practitioners, 61*(586), e231–e243. https://doi.org/10.3399/bjgp11X572427.

Association of Coloproctology of Great Britain and Ireland. (2014). *Commissioning guide for colonic diverticular disease.* Retrieved from https://www.acpgbi.org.uk/resources/62/commissioning_guide_for_colonic_diverticular_disease.

B., Gallo, G., Rossi, G., Abu-Zidan, F., Agnoletti, V., de'Angelis, G., de'Angelis, N., Ansaloni, L., Baiocchi, G. L., Carcoforo, P., Ceresoli, M., Chichom-Mefire, A., ... Catena, F. (2021). Anorectal

emergencies: WSES-AAST guidelines. *World Journal of Emergency Surgery: WJES, 16*(1), 48. https://doi.org/10.1186/s13017-021-00384-x

Commissioning guide for colonic diverticular disease. Royal College of Surgeons (RCS) and Association of Coloproctology of Great Britain and Ireland (ACPGBI) (2014). https://www.acpgbi.org.uk/resources/62/commissioning_guide_for_colonic_diverticular_disease

Commissioning guide for rectal bleeding. Royal College of Surgeons (RCS) and Association of Coloproctology of Great Britain and Ireland (ACPGBI) (2017). https://www.acpgbi.org.uk/_userfiles/import/2014/03/Commissioning-Guide-for-Rectal-Bleeding-Dec-2017.pdf

Chou, S. C., Chen, S. C., Shyr, Y. M., & Wang, S. E. (2017). Polypoid lesions of the gallbladder: Analysis of 1204 patients with long-term follow-up. *Surgical Endoscopy, 31*(7), 2776–2782. https://doi.org/10.1007/s00464-016-5286-y.

Diverticular disease: Diagnosis and management. NICE guidelines [NG147]. (2019). https://www.nice.org.uk/guidance/ng147

EASL Clinical Practice Guidelines on the prevention, diagnosis and treatment of gallstones. (2016). *Journal of Hepatology, 65*(1), 146–181. https://doi.org/10.1016/j.jhep.2016.03.005

Fitzgibbons, R. J., Ramanan, B., Arya, S., Turner, S. A., Li, X., Gibbs, J. O., Reda, D. J., & Investigators of the Original Trial. (2013). Long-term results of a randomized controlled trial of a nonoperative strategy (watchful waiting) for men with minimally symptomatic inguinal hernias. *Annals of Surgery, 258*(3), 508–515. https://doi.org/10.1097/SLA.0b013e3182a19725

Gurusamy, K. S., & Davidson, B. R. (2014). Gallstones. *BMJ (Clinical research ed.), 348*, g2669. https://doi.org/10.1136/bmj.g2669.

Henriksen, N. A., Montgomery, A., Kaufmann, R., Berrevoet, F., East, B., Fischer, J., Hope, W., Klassen, D., Lorenz, R., Renard, Y., Garcia Urena, M. A., & Simons, M. P. (2020). Guidelines for treatment of umbilical and epigastric hernias from the European Hernia Society and Americas Hernia Society. *British Journal of Surgery, 107*(3), 171–190. https://doi.org/10.1002/bjs.11489

Kingsnorth, A., & LeBlanc, K. (2003). Hernias: Inguinal and incisional. The *Lancet, 362*(9395), 1561–1571. https://doi.org/10.1016/S0140-6736(03)14746-0

Morimoto, M., Matsuo, T., & Mori, N. (2021). Management of Porcelain Gallbladder, Its Risk Factors, and Complications: A Review. *Diagnostics (Basel, Switzerland), 11*(6), 1073. https://doi.org/10.3390/diagnostics11061073

National Institute for Health and Care Excellence. (2021). NICE Clinical Knowledge Summaries: Haemorrhoids. https://cks.nice.org.uk/topics/haemorrhoids/

National Institute for Health and Care Excellence. (2022). NICE Clinical Knowledge Summaries: peripheral arterial disease. https://cks.nice.org.uk/topics/peripheral-arterial-disease/

NICE. (2014). Gallstone disease: Diagnosis and management. Clinical guideline [CG188]. https://www.nice.org.uk/guidance/cg188

Perrotti, P., Antropoli, C., Molino, D., De Stefano, G., & Antropoli, M. (2001). Conservative treatment of acute thrombosed external hemorrhoids with topical nifedipine. *Diseases of the Colon & Rectum, 44*(3), 405–409. https://doi.org/10.1007/BF02234741.

Pisano, M., Allievi, N., Gurusamy, K., Borzellino, G., Cimbanassi, S., Boerna, D., Coccolini, F., Tufo, A., Di Martino, M., Leung, J., Sartelli, M., Ceresoli, M., Maier, R. V., Poiasina, E., De Angelis, N., Magnone, S., Fugazzola, P., Paolillo, C., Coimbra, R., ... Ansaloni, L. (2020). 2020 World Society of Emergency Surgery updated guidelines for the diagnosis and treatment of acute calculus cholecystitis. *World Journal of Emergency Surgery: WJES, 15*(1), 61. https://doi.org/10.1186/s13017-020-00336-x

Schultz, J. K., Azhar, N., Binda, G. A., Barbara, G., Biondo, S., Boermeester, M. A., Chabok, A., Consten, E. C. J., van Dijk, S. T., Johanssen, A., Kruis, W., Lambrichts, D., Post, S., Ris, F., Rockall, T. A., Samuelsson, A., Di Saverio, S., Tartaglia, D., Thorisson, A., Winter, D. C., ... Angenete, E. (2020). European Society of Coloproctology: Guidelines for the management of diverticular disease of the colon. *Colorectal Disease*, *22*(Suppl. 2), 5–28. https://doi.org/10.1111/codi.15140.

Shahedi, K., Fuller, G., Bolus, R., Cohen, E., Vu, M., Shah, R., Agarwal, N., Kaneshiro, M., Atia, M., Sheen, V., Kurzbard, N., van Oijen, M. G. H., Yen, L., Hodgkins, P., Erder, M. H., & Spiegel, B. (2013). Long-term risk of acute diverticulitis among patients with incidental diverticulosis found during colonoscopy. *Clinical Gastroenterology and Hepatology: The Official Clinical Practice Journal of the American Gastroenterological Association*, *11*(12), 1609–1613. https://doi.org/10.1016/j.cgh.2013.06.020.

Song, G.-M., Bian, W., Zeng, X.-T., Zhou, J.-G., Luo, Y.-Q., & Tian, X. (2016). Laparoscopic cholecystectomy for acute cholecystitis: Early or delayed?: Evidence from a systematic review of discordant meta-analyses. *Medicine, 95*(23), e3835. https://doi.org/10.1097/MD.0000000000003835

Stewart, D. B., Gaertner, W., Glasgow, S., Migaly, J., Feingold, D., & Steele, S. R. (2017). Clinical practice guideline for the management of anal fissures. *Diseases of the Colon and Rectum*, *60*(1), 7–14. https://doi.org/10.1097/DCR.0000000000000735.

Williams, E., Beckingham, I., El Sayed, G., Gurusamy, K., Sturgess, R., Webster, G., & Young, T. (2017). Updated guideline on the management of common bile duct stones (CBDS). *Gut, 66*(5), 765–782. https://doi.org/10.1136/gutjnl-2016-312317

10

Musculoskeletal Problems

John MacLean

CHAPTER CONTENTS

Osteoarthritis

GUIDELINE

National Institute for Health and Care Excellence. (2022). *Osteoarthritis in over 16s: Diagnosis and management. NICE clinical guideline 226.* Available at http://www.nice.org.uk/guidance/ng226.

- The aims of management are to:
  - Enable patients to actively participate in their care and access further information.
  - Control symptoms (mainly pain and stiffness).
  - Prevent progression of joint damage.
  - Reduce disability and improve function.

Management Strategy

- Make a holistic assessment of the impact of osteoarthritis on the patient in terms of:
  - Function, occupation, and leisure activities
  - Quality of life
  - Mood and sleep
  - Relationships
  - Comorbidities
- Elicit the patient's understanding of the illness and concerns.
- Discuss the risks and benefits of treatment options.

- Formulate a management plan with the patient based on the above and taking account of the patient's values and preferences.
- Screen for mental health issues, including depression, which is more common in patients with long-term disability.
  Management can be divided into three domains (Table 10.1).

Education and Self-Management

- Address concerns and counter any misconceptions (e.g., that the disease inevitably progresses to joint replacement). Patient-centred consultations result in better outcomes and better use of resources (e.g., fewer unhelpful investigations).
- Explain the disease in appropriate language and back it up with an offer of written information.

PATIENT INFORMATION

Versus Arthritis. Available at https://www.versusarthritis.org/about-arthritis/conditions/osteoarthritis/.

- Encourage exercise but explain that they may experience an initial increase in pain:
  - Local muscle strengthening
  - General aerobic exercise

TABLE 10.1 Management of Osteoarthritis

Core treatment	These should be considered for all patients.	Education Exercise Weight loss for the overweight
Relatively safe pharmaceutic options	These should be considered before adjunctive treatments.	Paracetamol Topical NSAIDs
Adjunctive treatments	This refers to treatments which have less proof of efficacy or involve more risk to the patient.	Pharmaceutical • NSAIDs • Opioids • Intraarticular steroids • Capsaicin self-management • Local heat and cold • Assistive devices Other nonpharmacologic • Supports and braces • Shock-absorbing shoes and insoles • TENS • Manual therapy • Surgery

NSAID, Nonsteroidal antiinflammatory drug; *TENS,* transcutaneous electrical nerve stimulation.

- Refer to physiotherapy for exercise according to local policies, including group classes to maintain motivation.
- Encourage weight loss in overweight patients. This improves general quality of life and physical function and reduces pain.

Relatively Safe Pharmaceutical Options

- Recommend paracetamol. Regular doses, namely 1 g four times daily, might be better than taking a dose *as required.*
- For some joints, such as the knee, recommend topical nonsteroidal antiinflammatory drugs (NSAIDs) before progressing to adjunctive drugs with their associated risks.

Adjunctive Nonpharmacologic and Nonsurgical Management

- Consider the following for pain relief:
  - Local application of heat or cold
  - Referral for manipulation or stretching for knee osteoarthritis together with therapeutic exercise
  - Transcutaneous electrical nerve stimulation (TENS) may have a place with less evidence for acupuncture and no evidence for electrotherapy
- Refer to the most appropriate agency according to local policies (e.g., physiotherapy or occupational therapy) for:
  - Assessment for bracing, joint supports, or insoles in those with biomechanical joint pain or instability
  - Assistive devices such as walking sticks

- Advise on footwear. Shock-absorbing shoes (trainers) and insoles (which can be purchased from pharmacies) may help weightbearing joints when there is evidence of abnormal biomechanical loading.
- Advise the patient to keep active and to pace oneself, take planned rest periods, and avoid bursts of overactivity.
- Monitor mental health, particularly depression. If present, treating it not only improves mood but also results in less pain and improved function at 12 months.

Adjunctive Pharmacologic Management

- Use along with nonpharmacologic treatments and therapeutic exercise.
- Prescribe either a weak opioid or an oral NSAID (see the NSAID section) depending on patient preferences and comorbidities. Do not use strong opioids.
- Consider a topical NSAID for knee osteoarthritis with or without other joints.
- Educate the patient in the self-management of analgesics so they can step up or down the scale of treatment:
  - Recommend that NSAIDs be used for the shortest period possible.
  - Explain that paracetamol or co-codamol can be used with ibuprofen but that co-codamol should *never* be taken with paracetamol because it contains the same drug.
  - Ensure the patient is not taking more than one NSAID, including over-the-counter (OTC) preparations (e.g., aspirin).

- Consider intraarticular steroid injections but not hyaluronic acid in those with severe pain.
- Consider topical capsaicin.
- Do not prescribe glucosamine or chondroitin.
  Newer pain treatments include nerve growth factor antibodies such as tanezumab with variable results.

Disability

- Consider the patient's need for aids (e.g., bath aids) and refer as appropriate.
- Consider eligibility for benefits (e.g., attendance allowance, a disabled driver's badge) and refer to the appropriate agency for advice.
- Consider the need for support and rehabilitation. Refer, according to local circumstances, to social services, a rehabilitation team, or hospital-based multidisciplinary team.

Radiographs

- Plain radiographs are not routinely indicated in the diagnosis or management of osteoarthritis. Imaging has a role in confirming the severity of disease when considering or planning surgery. Radiography appearances correlate poorly with the symptoms. Radiography may be considered also when soft tissue calcification is suspected and when it will determine treatment (e.g., steroid injection or when there is diagnostic doubt).

Referrals to a Specialist

- Joint replacement surgery is a clinically beneficial and cost-effective treatment for patients with severely affected functional disease. Consider referral for joint replacement surgery when a patient experiences joint symptoms, whether pain, stiffness, or reduced function, that substantially impact their quality of life and have not responded to core and adjunctive treatments. Referral is best made before prolonged functional limitation and severe pain become established.
- Follow local referral thresholds, which vary, but age, gender, smoking, obesity, and comorbidities should not be barriers to referral. Do not refer for arthroscopic washout or debridement because there is no evidence that these reduce pain and improve function.

Postoperative Care

Patients occasionally ask their general practitioners (GPs) about their return to normal activities.

- Advise the patient who has had a hip replacement not to cross the legs or drive for 6 weeks. The danger of dislocation is greatest in the first 6 weeks and occurs when the hip is flexed, especially if it is internally rotated and adducted.
- Advise patients that they may resume activities, including walking, swimming, bicycling, and tennis, *after 6 weeks*, provided they take care not to fall. Contact sports and use of ladders are not advised.

Recurrence of Pain

- Arrange for radiography, erythrocyte sedimentation rate (ESR), and white blood cell count in any patient with a hip prosthesis who develops pain. This may show loosening, infection, stress fracture, or dislocation. Refer any of these to the surgeon urgently. Refer anyway if the pain does not settle with rest. Any of these may be present despite a normal radiograph.

GUIDELINE

Hunter, D. J., & Bierma-Zeinstra, S. (2019). Osteoarthritis. *Lancet, 393,* 1745–1759.

Low Back Pain

GUIDELINE

National Institute for Health and Care Excellence. (2016). *Low back pain and sciatica in over 16s: Assessment and management.* NICE clinical guideline 59. Available at http://www.nice.org.uk/guidance/NG59.

- Low back pain (LBP) can be defined as:
  - Acute LBP: duration of 6 weeks or less
  - Subacute LBP: duration of 6 to 12 weeks
  - Chronic LBP: duration of 3 months or more
- LBP is extremely common. At any one time, 15% of adults have it, and 60% will have it some time in their lives (Mason, 1994). Back pain is the most common cause of long-term sickness: 52 million working days are lost each year from back pain.
- Mechanical LBP is self-limiting: 80% to 90% of patients recover spontaneously within 3 months.
- Consider using a risk stratification tool such as the STarT Back risk assessment tool (https://www.keele.ac.uk/startmsk).
- At presentation, triage patients into one of the three following groups based on history and examination:
  - Mechanical back pain, which has a good outcome
  - Nerve root compression, which may require more complex or intense input
  - Possible serious spinal pathology—look for *red flags* (see upcoming discussion) and act accordingly

- Note any psychological or social influences that might retard recovery (so-called *yellow flags*).

Aims of Management

- Reduce pain and the length of sickness in mechanical back pain.
- Identify early the small minority with serious pathology needing immediate or urgent attention.
- Prevent acute back pain becoming chronic.

Managing Acute Mechanical Low Back Pain

- Features of mechanical back pain include:
  - Presentation at age 20 to 55 years
  - Pain felt over lumbosacral area, buttocks, or thighs
  - Pain that alters with posture and activity
  - The patient is well
- Take time to listen and examine, explain, and reassure. These have beneficial effect on pain and anxiety.
- Encourage continued activity, including work if appropriate. Bedrest worsens outcome and should only be taken if pain is severe and then for no longer than necessary.
- Do not routinely offer imaging.

Pharmacologic Management

- Prescribe analgesics or NSAIDs at the lowest dose for the shortest time. Combine this with an exercise programme.
- Avoid prescribing muscle relaxants (e.g., diazepam). They control pain, but the abuse potential and the availability of other analgesic options mean that it should not be common practice to prescribe them.
- Avoid prescribing gabapentin and opioids.
- Ensure the patient has a medium-firm mattress (5 on the European Committee for Standardisation scale). This has been shown to be more effective than a firm one.
- Demonstrate stretching exercises or give written instructions.
- Consider group exercise programmes, which increase motivation and adherence.
- There is no evidence to support the use of corsets, foot orthotics, electrotherapy, or acupuncture.
- Mobilisation exercises or massage may be beneficial as part of an overall exercise programme. See the Chartered Society of Physiotherapy's video exercises for back pain (https://www.csp.org.uk/conditions/back-pain/video-exercises-back-pain).
- Offer a follow-up consultation after 2 to 6 weeks.
  - If activity and function are improving, encourage return to normal activities even if pain is still present. Stress that activity will not damage the back.

- If not improving, advise graded return to normal activity and set a return date to work.
- If not improving, also consider referral to another health professional with expertise in LBP, usually a physiotherapist or possibly a manipulative therapist.
- Reassess for *red flags* (to come).
- Reassess for *yellow flags* (to come). If present, be positive, schedule regular reviews, encourage a programme of activity, and consider early referral.
- If there has been a failure to progress at 6 weeks, then continue and intensify current management and consider referral to specialist services.

Psychosocial Blocks to Recovery (Yellow Flags)

- Yellow flags include:
  - A belief that back pain is harmful or potentially disabling
  - Fear-avoidance behaviour (avoiding a movement or activity because of misplaced anticipation of pain) and reduced activity levels
  - A tendency to low mood and withdrawal from social interaction
  - An expectation that passive treatments rather than active participation will help
  - Awaiting compensation
  - A history of absence from work for back pain or other problems
  - Poor job satisfaction, long hours, or heavy work
  - An overprotective family or a lack of support at home
- Note that these yellow flags should not be used pejoratively. They are a guide to patients in whom early intervention and early return to work are especially important. Consider a combined physical and psychological approach, including cognitive-behavioural therapy.

Management of Chronic Low Back Pain

- The prevalence of LBP is not increasing, but the level of disability and claims for long-term sickness benefits are. The management of chronic LBP therefore encompasses several approaches:
  a. Appropriate referral for physical treatments (see upcoming discussion)
  b. Principles of chronic pain management
  c. Attention to psychosocial issues
- Recommend regular physical exercise. This should start as soon as possible in the course of the illness. A light mobilisation programme for patients who have had back pain for 8 to 12 weeks has been shown to improve outcomes initially and at 3 years (Hagen, Eriksen, & Ursin, 2000).
- Treat underlying anxiety or depression if present.

- Consider prescribing a tricyclic antidepressant (TCA) at low doses even if depression is not present (Staiger et al, 2003).
- Explore work-related issues. If return to former employment is unlikely, advise the patient to see the disability employment adviser at the job centre.
- Consider referral to a multidisciplinary team; this can be effective in resistant cases (Guzmán et al, 2001).

Nerve Root Compression

- Mechanical back pain can be referred down the leg, so not all sciatica arises from a prolapsed disc; nerve root compression is more likely if pain extends down to the foot. Conversely, not all prolapsed discs cause sciatica because they can be demonstrated in 50% of asymptomatic adults.
- Sciatica arising from a prolapsed disc that causes significant disability has a lifetime prevalence of 5%.
- Recognising nerve root compression is important because surgery leads to quicker recovery than natural resolution, although there may be no difference in long-term outcomes (Peul et al, 2007).
- At presentation, test for limitation of straight leg raising. If straight leg raising is not impaired and pain does not radiate below the knee, then nerve root compression is very unlikely (Vroomen, de Krom, & Knotterus, 1999).
- Look for neurologic deficit from L5 to S1 compression, which includes loss of sensation over the lateral border of the lower leg and foot, weakness of dorsiflexion and plantarflexion of foot, and impairment of the ankle reflex. In L3 to L4 compression, the knee reflex may be impaired.
- Manage sciatica as you would acute LBP.
- Refer patients whose pain is not settling (the timescale will depend on local circumstances) or when there is increasing neurologic deficit.

Referrals

Whom to refer to will depend on local availability and agreed care pathways: physiotherapist, pain clinic, multidisciplinary team, orthopaedic physicians, or orthopaedic surgeons.

Failure to Progress in Acute Low Back Pain

- All guidelines are consistent in recommending early referral (≤2 weeks) for physiotherapy or manipulation to prevent acute LBP becoming chronic. Conversely, it is now clear that even in sciatica, epidural corticosteroid injection offers no long-term benefit, although there may be transient benefit at 3 weeks (Arden et al, 2005).
- Be prepared to discuss manipulation; many patients take themselves to osteopaths or chiropractors, and many physiotherapists practise a related treatment, mobilisation. The evidence for manipulation is of low quality,

but it may lead to quicker recovery in the first few weeks without making any difference to long-term outcomes (Koes et al, 1996).
- There is insufficient evidence for physical agents and passive modalities (e.g., ice, heat, short-wave diathermy, massage, ultrasound, TENS, acupuncture), but they remain popular.

Failure to Progress With Neurologic Symptoms or Signs and Other Serious Situations

- Do not exclude patients with a high body mass index (BMI) or significant psychological issues from a surgical opinion.
- Evidence of benefit from discectomy, which may be long term, is accumulating for patients with disc herniation, spinal stenosis, and spondylolisthesis (Gibson, 2007).
  - *Sciatica.* The ideal timing of referral to an orthopaedic surgeon of patients with sciatica which is not improving is not clear.
  - *Cauda equina syndrome* (see upcoming discussion). Refer immediately to an orthopaedic surgeon.
  - *Other red flags.* Refer urgently when appropriate and, if a malignancy is suspected, refer urgently according to suspected cancer guidelines.

Radiographs

- Explain to patients with mechanical LBP why radiographs are unhelpful: degenerative changes are common; most disorders are of soft tissue, which cannot be shown on radiograph; and the dose of radiation is high (60 times that of a chest radiograph) (Royal College of Radiologists, 2003).
- Consider radiographs in the presence of red flags, alongside urgent referral.

Possible Serious Spinal Pathology

- Red flags include:
  - Cauda equina syndrome (features include urinary retention, bilateral neurologic symptoms and signs, saddle anaesthesia—urgent referral is indicated)
  - Significant trauma (risk of fracture)
  - Weight loss (suggestive of cancer)
  - History of cancer (suggestive of metastases)
  - Fever (suggestive of infection)
  - Intravenous drug use (suggestive of infection)
  - Steroid use (risk of osteoporotic collapse)
  - Patient aged over 50 years (cancer is unlikely before this age)
  - Severe, unremitting nighttime pain (suggestive of cancer)
  - Pain that gets worse when the patient is lying down (suggestive of cancer)

Older Adults With Acute Back Pain

These patients are a special case because osteoporotic collapse and malignancy are more likely, and they need early radiograph. Half have a definite abnormality, and 10% have a malignancy (Frank, 1993).

Advice and Exercises for Low Back Pain

The following exercises are helpful for problems and pain affecting the back and are taken from Versus Arthritis - https://www.versusarthritis.org/about-arthritis/exercising-with-arthritis/exercises-for-healthy-joints/exercises-for-the-back/

- Pay attention to sitting, lifting, and bending to avoid aggravating pain and to prevent recurrence.
  - *Sitting.* Avoid prolonged sitting. A rolled towel in the small of the back may ease pain.
  - *Lifting.* Always lift with a straight back and bent knees.
  - *Bending.* Avoid spending too long at a task that requires bending (e.g., ironing).
- Exercise regularly.
  - Do stretching exercises to maintain flexibility daily. You may start these early on in an attack and should keep them up long term.
  - Do muscle-strengthening exercises daily. You should start these as your pain improves and keep them up long term.
  - Take up aerobic exercise for general fitness (e.g., swimming).
- Suitable exercises (there are many others):
  - Starting position: on all fours with hands shoulder width apart, arms and thighs vertical:
    1. Arch the back and look down. Then lower the stomach towards the floor, hollowing the back.
    2. Slowly walk the hands around to one side, back to the starting position, and then around to the other side.
    3. Raise one hand off the floor and reach underneath your body as far as you can. On the return, swing the arm out to the side as far as you can; then return to the starting position. Follow the moving hand with the eyes. Repeat with the other arm.
    4. Draw alternate knees to the opposite elbow.
    5. Stretch one arm forward in front, at the same time stretching the opposite leg out behind. Repeat on the other side.
    6. Swing the seat from side to side.

All exercises should be repeated 10 times. Exercises that hurt should be set aside and returned to with fewer repetitions on another occasion.

PATIENT INFORMATION

The National Back Pain Association. BackCare. *Welcome to BackCare* https://backcare.org.uk.
 NHS. *Back pain.* Available at https://www.nhs.uk/conditions/back-pain.

Neck Pain

- Although most episodes of neck pain resolve with or without treatment, 50% of individuals will experience ongoing or recurrent episodes; most likely are those with poor coping skills, poor work satisfaction, a sedentary lifestyle, concomitant back pain, or a history of previous neck injury.
- The principles of management of LBP also apply to neck pain.
- Triage neck pain into mechanical, nerve root compression (often termed *radiculopathy*), and potential serious pathology (*red flags*).
- In mechanical neck pain, keeping active is more effective than immobilisation.
- Similar medications may be prescribed.
- Psychosocial factors are important (see earlier).
- Imaging is not routinely indicated (see *red flags*).
- Manipulation or mobilisation may be effective in the short term (Gross et al, 2004).
- Acupuncture is not effective (Trinh et al, 2006).

Mechanical Pain

- Recognise by:
  - Aged 18 to 55 years
  - Absence of signs of radiculopathy or red flags
  - Made worse by posture or activity
- Advise the patient to stay active.
- Collars have little to no evidence of reduction of symptoms.
- Give regular analgesia. Either paracetamol or NSAIDs is required as an additional or alternate analgesic. Some evidence for benefit from short-term muscle relaxants in acute episodes.
- There is no to limited evidence for manipulation, acupuncture, traction, or electrotherapy.
- There is some evidence for massage therapy.
- There is good evidence for exercise programmes but no evidence or superiority of individual programmes.
- Treat hyperextension injuries (including whiplash injuries) in the same way but avoid a collar because this prolongs symptoms.

Daily Stretching and Strengthening Exercises

Advise the patient to hold the neck for 10 seconds in each of the six positions (right and left lateral flexion and rotation, flexion and extension) within the pain-free range. Repeat 10 times. (Based on the ARC information leaflet 'Pain in the Neck.')

Radiculopathy

- Distinguish radiculopathy from neck pain that is referred to the shoulder and arm.

- Look for the following signs, though their sensitivity and specificity have not been adequately assessed:
  - Diminished reflexes (triceps, biceps, supinator)
  - Diminished power
  - Diminished sensation along dermatomes
  - Axial compression test. Extend the neck and rotate the head to the side of the pain; then apply pressure to the head. Reproducing pain or paraesthesiae in the arm signifies likely radiculopathy.
- Treat as for mechanical neck pain but refer if there is no improvement after 4 weeks. Refer earlier if there is loss of power and refer immediately if deterioration is rapid. However, warn the patient that surgery is no better than conservative treatment except in severe cases (Kadanka et al, 2002).

Red Flags

- Red flags for malignancy, infection, and inflammation are as for LBP.
- A red flag specific for neck pain is evidence of cervical myelopathy (the equivalent of the cauda equina syndrome). Neck pain may be absent, but the syndrome should be suspected when any of the following features are present:
  - Sensory disturbances in the upper and lower limbs
  - Weakness in the upper and lower limbs
  - Clumsiness and gait disturbance
  - Spasticity of the lower limbs (the upper limbs may be normal, spastic, or flaccid)
  - Increased tendon reflexes
  - Lhermitte sign: paraesthesiae in the limbs on neck flexion indicate neck instability and warrant *immediate* admission.
- Refer patients with one or more red flags urgently for a specialist opinion.

PATIENT INFORMATION

Cohen, S. P. (2015). Epidemiology, diagnosis, and treatment of neck pain. *Mayo Clinic Proceedings, 90*(2):284–299.
   NHS. *Neck pain.* Available at https://www.nhs.uk/conditions/neck-pain-and-stiff-neck/.
   Versus Arthritis. *Neck pain: Causes, exercises, treatments.* https://www.versusarthritis.org/about-arthritis/conditions/neck-pain/.

Problems With Upper Limbs

Acute Shoulder Pain

Acute Onset With Injury

REVIEW

Mitchell, C., Adebajo, A., Hay, E., & Carr, A. (2005). Shoulder pain: Diagnosis and management in primary care. *British Medical Journal, 331,* 1124–1128.

- For patients with clinical fracture or dislocation suspected from history and initial clinical examination: send to the emergency department (ED).
- If the radiograph is normal at ED: control pain for 3 weeks with analgesia and a sling.
  - If pain and movement are both improved, refer for physiotherapy.
  - If pain is improved but not movement, refer urgently to an upper limb specialist (fracture clinic) as suspected rotator cuff tear. Repair, if needed, should be performed within 6 to 8 weeks of the injury.

Acute Onset Without Injury

- If there is a sudden onset of severe pain, then refer to the ED. This may indicate acute decalcification of an area of calcification in the rotator cuff, which needs urgent decompression.
- If the situation is less desperate, then obtain radiographs.
  - If normal, consider giving local anaesthetic and steroid injection and advise on cuff-strengthening exercises (or refer to physiotherapy for this advice). If this fails, refer to a shoulder specialist clinic. If it helps substantially but is followed by relapse, give further injections with a maximum of three per year.
  - If abnormal, refer according to diagnosis (see upcoming discussion).

Arthritis of Acromioclavicular Joint or Glenohumeral Joint

- If symptoms are mild, then give analgesia with or without an NSAID, heat, or shoulder exercises or refer to physiotherapy.
- If symptoms are more severe, then support as above and refer to Outpatient Department (OPD).

Calcification in the Rotator Cuff

- Refer to OPD. These patients are more likely to need surgery at some stage. They may benefit from a subacromial injection of local anaesthetic and steroid meanwhile.

Red Flags for Systemic Disease

- Investigate further if the patient is systemically unwell (e.g., with fever or weight loss), has a history of cancer, has arthritis elsewhere, or has a mass or neurologic symptoms or signs in that arm.

Chronic Shoulder Pain

Is It Acromioclavicular Joint Pain?

- Characteristics include:
  - Pain is localised to the acromioclavicular joint (ACJ).
  - The joint may be swollen and tender with crepitus.
  - Abduction is painful in the final 20 degrees.
  - There is a positive 'scarf' test result.
- Inject local anaesthetic and steroid and give analgesia. If not better in 2 weeks, refer to physiotherapy. If still not better, check the diagnosis and refer.

Is It a Rotator Cuff Lesion?

- Characteristics include:
  - Pain is usually felt at the deltoid insertion.
  - Any or all movements are painful.
  - Active movements are more painful than passive movements.
  - Pain is felt on resisted active elevation (this is the impingement sign).
- If pain is mild, then give analgesia and advice on cuff-strengthening exercises. If there is no improvement after 3 weeks, refer to physiotherapy (Green, Buchbinder, & Hetrick, 2003). If physiotherapy is unhelpful, give a sub-acromial injection of corticosteroid and local anaesthetic.
- If pain is moderate or severe, refer to physiotherapy. If physiotherapy is unhelpful, give a subacromial injection of corticosteroid and local anaesthetic:
  - If pain is improved but there is weakness, refer urgently as a suspected rotator cuff tear.
  - If pain is not improved, refer.
  - If pain and power improve substantially but return, give further injections up to a maximum of three per year.

Is It Chronic Capsulitis (Frozen Shoulder)?

- Characteristics include:
  - There is tenderness anteriorly between the coracoid process and the head of the humerus.
  - All movements are painful and restricted, whether active or passive, but there is less pain on resisted active movement (when the joint does not move).
  - Characteristically, the loss of external rotation is the most marked, there is no crepitus, and there is no arthritis elsewhere.
- Explain the nature of the condition and the fact that spontaneous resolution can be expected, with a mean duration of 30 months but longer in those with diabetes. However, explain that some long-term restriction of movement is usual (Dias, Cutts, & Massoud, 2005).
- Order mobilisation physiotherapy, designed to keep the shoulder mobile within the limits of pain (Green et al, 2003).
- At the same time, give a single steroid plus Local Anaesthetic (LA) injection into the glenohumeral joint (GHJ). The earlier the injection is given, the more effective it is (Dias et al, 2005).
- Refer refractory cases that have not resolved after 30 months for consideration of manipulation under anaesthesia or arthroscopic release.

Is It Glenohumeral Joint Arthrosis?

- The characteristics are the same as in chronic capsulitis, but crepitus may be felt, and there may be arthritis elsewhere.
- Confirm with a radiograph. Management depends on both the degree of pain and functional loss.
  - If mild, give analgesia and advice on exercises.
  - If moderate or severe, refer with a view to replacement surgery.

Is the Glenohumeral Joint Unstable?

- Characteristics include:
  - There may be a history of subluxation or dislocation.
  - There are two tests for this:
    1. Fix the shoulder girdle with one hand; with the other hand, try to rock the head of the humerus backward and forward in the glenoid fossa.
    2. Hold the arm abducted to 90 degrees with the upper arm pointing forward. Does external rotation cause apprehension and pain?
- Refer for consideration of specialist physiotherapy or surgery.
- Note: Nerve root compression in the neck frequently presents as shoulder pain, coexists with it, and can cause it!
- Note: Young sports people with shoulder pain frequently have occult instability; refer them readily.

Simplified Guide to Cover Most Cases of Shoulder Pain

- If the patient is unwell or has other disorders that could cause shoulder pain, investigate further.
- If the pain is acute and the patient cannot raise the arm actively but you can raise it passively, refer urgently as a suspected rotator cuff tear.
- If there is a history of partial or complete dislocation, refer for assessment of instability.
- Otherwise, decide between:
  - ACJ pain (tender over the ACJ with restriction of moving the arm across the front of the chest — 'scarf' test)
  - GHJ pain (active and passive movements of the shoulder painful and restricted)
- In both these conditions, recommend:
  - Analgesia and rest until the acute pain eases
  - Exercises within the limits of pain to keep the joint mobile

Exercises for the Shoulder

Flexibility

- Demonstrate pendular exercises.
  1. Stand up and lean forward with arm of affected side hanging perpendicularly.
  2. Sweep the arm around in a circle within the pain-free range. Do this 20 to 30 times.
  3. As time goes on, increase the range of the movement and length of time.

Strengthening the Rotator Cuff

1. Hold your arm outstretched at shoulder height and out to the side.
2. Bring your arm forward and then up; push to the back and then down to the starting position.
3. Repeat 10 times. As time goes on, build up to doing three sets of 10 repetitions.

PATIENT INFORMATION

Hermans, J., Luime, J. J., Meuffels, D. E., Reijman, M., Simel, D. L., & Bierma-Zeinstra, S. M. (2013). Does this patient with shoulder pain have rotator cuff disease? The Rational Clinical Examination systematic review. *Journal of the American Medical Association, 28,* 310(8):837–847.

NHS. *Shoulder pain.* Available at https://www.nhs.uk/conditions/shoulder-pain/.

Versus Arthritis. *Shoulder pain.* Available at https://www.versusarthritis.org/about-arthritis/conditions/shoulder-pain.

Tennis Elbow (Lateral Epicondylitis)

PATIENT INFORMATION

NHS. *Tennis elbow: Symptoms.* Available at https://www.nhs.uk/conditions/tennis-elbow/.

Versus Arthritis. *Elbow pain: Causes, exercise, treatments.* https://www.versusarthritis.org/about-arthritis/conditions/elbow-pain/

- This is a painful condition caused by overuse with resultant microtears of the tendons of the forearm muscles (particularly Extensor Carpi Radialis Brevis (ERCB)) as they attach to the lateral epicondyle.
- There is limited evidence of a local inflammatory reaction.
- Symptoms include local pain and tenderness and weakened grip strength.

Treatment

- Nonsurgical: up to 95% success within 1 year.
  - Initial rest with reduction in precipitating activities. Check sports technique and equipment (e.g., tennis racquet grip size).
  - Analgesia with or without NSAIDs (as an adjunct analgesic).
  - Physiotherapy. See the Chartered Society of Physiotherapy's 'Exercise advice for tennis elbow' (https://www.csp.org.uk/public-patient/rehabilitation-exercises/tennis-elbow).
  - Consider an epicondylar clasp or brace.
  - Corticosteroid injections may offer initial relief of symptoms, but evidence suggests they are no better than physiotherapy after 6 weeks.
  - Platelet-rich plasma (PRP) has no proven benefit.
- Surgical: Refer after a failed trial on nonsurgical treatment and only after 6 to 12 months.

Carpal Tunnel Syndrome

PATIENT EDUCATION

NHS. *Carpal tunnel syndrome.* Available at https://www.nhs.uk/conditions/carpal-tunnel-syndrome/.

Versus Arthritis. *Carpal tunnel syndrome: Causes, symptoms, treatment.* Available at https://www.versusarthritis.org/about-arthritis/conditions/carpal-tunnel-syndrome/.

- Carpal tunnel syndrome is compression neuropathy of the median nerve at the wrist.
- It is more common when there is repetitive hand or wrist use and in pregnancy and those with diabetes and rheumatoid arthritis (RA).
- Symptoms include numbness, pain, tingling, and weakness in the hand.
- The diagnosis is largely clinical with or without nerve conduction studies.

Treatment

- Advise the patient to rest the joint if possible and avoid provoking activities.
- Advise the patient to try a night splint to reduce the flexion of the joint.
- Consider corticosteroid injection.
- Refer for surgical treatment if any of the following are present:
  - There is thenar wasting or constant sensory impairment.
  - Symptoms are severe.
  - There has been no improvement after 3 months.
- Consider oral steroids while waiting for the appointment. There is evidence of benefit after 2 weeks.

De Quervain Tenosynovitis

- Consider injection of steroid into the tendon sheath, though accurate placing of the needle is difficult.

Ganglion

- Explain to the patient that the lesion is harmless, that 40% resolve spontaneously, and that surgery has its problems.
  - Excision does not always relieve pain.
  - Recurrence after surgery is common.
  - The scar may be unsightly.
- Consider aspiration with a wide-bore needle under local anaesthesia with or without steroid instillation.
- Refer for surgery if they are painful.

Problems With the Lower Limbs

Acute Knee Injury

- The Ottawa Knee Rules significantly reduce the need for radiography after acute knee injury, and it is reliable in children as in adults (Bulloch et al, 2003). Patients with major trauma are not suitable candidates for the use of the decision rule.
- The economic impact of adopting this approach could be a cost saving to the NHS as well as a reduction in waiting times and an improvement in efficiency (Davies et al, 2020).
- The rules state that a knee radiography series is only required for knee injury patients with any of these findings:
  - Age 55 years or older
  - Isolated tenderness of the patella (i.e., no bone tenderness of the knee other than the patella)
  - Tenderness at the head of the fibula
  - Inability to flex to 90 degrees

- Inability to bear weight both immediately and when examined (they should be able to take four steps [i.e., take their weight on each leg twice even if they limp])

If There Is No Fracture

- Mobilise as soon as pain permits.
- Encourage quadriceps exercises (see upcoming discussion).
- Provide suitable analgesia.

Anterior Knee Pain

Where There Is a Past History of Injury

- Refer to the next fracture clinic if pain and effusion have persisted for more than 2 weeks.
- If there are no grounds for immediate referral, arrange for radiography. Request anteroposterior, lateral, and skyline views.
- If the radiography results are abnormal, refer to the next fracture clinic. This applies whether the fracture is of the patella or a flake of bone from an osteochondral fracture.
- If the radiography results are normal, refer to orthopaedic outpatients if there is a good history of patella dislocation or the patella is unstable on examination.
- If neither of these applies, give advice (see upcoming discussion) and review after 8 weeks. Most young patients with anterior knee pain have improved spontaneously in that time (Heintjes et al, 2003b).

Where There Is No History of Injury

- Examine for gross abnormalities that might warrant immediate attention.
- Reassure the patient if it is Osgood–Schlatter disease (see upcoming discussion). Otherwise advise as below.

Patients Still in Pain After 8 Weeks (With or Without History of Injury)

- Arrange for radiography if not already done.
  - If the radiography results are abnormal, refer to OPD for assessment.
  - If the radiography results are normal, refer for physiotherapy. If there is still no progress, refer to OPD for assessment. Advise the patient that it may mean specialist physiotherapy or a brace rather than surgery.

General Advice for Patellofemoral Pain

1. Avoid provoking activities (e.g., stairs, walking up- and downhill, the breaststroke kick, skiing, cycling, exercise bikes, and high-impact aerobics).
2. Recommend quads exercises (see upcoming discussion) and hamstring stretching exercises. There is some evidence that exercise may reduce anterior knee pain (Heintjes et al, 2003a).
3. Recommend simple analgesics. NSAIDs may reduce pain in the short term but not after 3 months.

Knee Exercises

- Stretching the hamstrings:
  1. Stand up with the affected leg slightly in front.
  2. Place both palms over the kneecap and push toward the ground. Keep this position for 30 seconds.
  3. Repeat four times. As time goes on, try to increase the stretch by pointing your toes upward.
- Strengthening the quadriceps:
  1. Lying down on your back, lift the leg with the knee straight to a position about 45 degrees off the horizontal.
  2. Hold this position for a count of 10 seconds.
  3. Lower the leg; then rest.
  4. Repeat 10 times. As time goes on, build up to doing three sets of 10 repetitions.

Steroid Injections at the Knee

- Consider injections for:
  - Iliotibial band or anserine bursitis
  - The knee joint when a clinical diagnosis has been made (e.g., patients with symptomatic knee osteoarthritis unsuitable or waiting for knee replacement)

Acute Ankle Injury

- The Ottawa Ankle Rule reduces the need for radiographs after ankle injury by 30% to 40% (Table 10.2) (Bachmann et al, 2003). Note that the rule is very good at identifying patients who do not need radiography (high sensitivity). It is poor at identifying those who have a fracture (low specificity).
- An *ankle radiograph* is required if there is any pain in the malleolar zone and any of the following apply:
  - There is bone tenderness at the posterior edge or tip of the lateral malleolus.
  - There is bone tenderness at the posterior edge of the medial malleolus.
  - The patient is unable to weight bear both at injury and when seen.

TABLE 10.2	Reliability of the Ottawa Ankle Rules for Identifying Ankle and Foot Fractures or Avulsion Fractures		
Patient Group	Sensitivity (95% CI), %	Specificity (Interquartile Range), %	Likelihood Ratio[a]
All patients	96 (94–99)	26 (19–34)	0.10
Ankle injuries	98 (96–99)	40 (30–48)	0.08
Midfoot injuries	99 (97–100)	38 (25–70)	0.08

[a]Likelihood ratio for a negative result.

CI, Confidence interval.

- A *foot radiograph* is required if there is pain in the mid-foot zone and any of the following apply:
  - There is bone tenderness at the navicular.
  - There is bone tenderness at the base of the fifth metatarsal.
  - The patient is unable to weight bear both at injury and when seen.
- The immediate treatment of an ankle sprain (as for any injured joint or limb) is rest, ice, compression, and elevation (RICE). Of these, compression appears to be the most important and, with elevation, must be maintained for at least 48 hours (Smith, 2003). Ice should be applied no more than 20 minutes at a time three times a day, and the skin should be separated from the ice by a wet towel (Institute for Clinical Systems Improvement, 2003). It is an approach based on experience rather than evidence.
- Analgesia, support with mobilisation, immobilisation, and surgical repair are all used in inversion injuries of the ankle. There is no robust evidence to guide the clinician in their use although the use of support and early mobilisation seems to result in faster recovery and better long-term outcomes (Kerkhoffs et al, 2002).

Rehabilitation After Ankle Injuries

- Recommend active mobilisation to restore proprioception. This can be achieved by regular exercises.
  - Imagine writing the alphabet with the foot, first capitals and then small letters.
  - Balance on the injured leg while moving the free leg forward and backward and side to side, initially with the eyes open and then with the eyes shut.
  - Use a wobble board.

Heel Pain

Plantar Fasciitis

- Characteristics include:
  - Isolated plantar heel pain on initiation of weight bearing either in the morning on rising or after a period of sitting
  - Pain that tends to decrease after a while but increases as time on the feet increases
- Examine to confirm heel tenderness and to check the range of movements. There may be associated tightness of the Achilles tendon.
- Do not radiograph. The presence of a calcaneal spur does not alter treatment.
- Advise the patient about weight reduction, if appropriate, and the use of an orthotic insole.
- Give analgesics. There is no evidence that NSAIDs are more effective than simple analgesics.
- Advise the patient about stretching exercises (plantar fascia and Achilles tendon).
- Refer to a podiatrist if there is no improvement after 6 weeks.
- The benefit of steroid injection is limited and likely to be temporary if the underlying cause is not identified.

There is evidence of benefit from shockwave application if it is available (Rompe et al, 2003).
- Symptomatic relief and stretching can be achieved by rolling a bottle of frozen water along the length of the sole.

Plantar Stretching for Plantar Fasciitis

1. Sit with the affected foot crossed over the other knee.
2. Grasp the toes and pull toward the shin until the plantar fascia is stretched.
3. Hold each stretch for a count of 10 and repeat 10 times three times a day for 8 weeks.

Achilles Tendinopathy

> **REVIEW**
>
> Maffulli, N., Longo, U. G., Kadakia, A., & Spiezia, F. (2020). Achilles tendinopathy. *Foot and Ankle Surgery, 26*(3), 240–249.

- Now considered as a failure of the natural healing process to repetitive 'micro' injury rather than an inflammatory aetiology
- Characteristics include:
  - An insidious onset leading to chronic posterior heel pain and swelling
  - Worsened pain with activity and pressure from shoes
  - Swelling medially and laterally to the insertion of the Achilles tendon
- There is insufficient evidence to determine which treatment is most appropriate. However, the following are commonly tried:
  - Eccentric exercises.
  - Simple analgesia. The condition is not one of inflammation, and there is no reason to prefer an NSAID (Khan et al, 2002).
  - Shockwave therapy.
  - There is little evidence for the use of PRP (Kearney 2021).

Achilles Tendon Rupture

- There may be a history of a sharp snap felt in the tendon on exertion or on injury (e.g., slipping off a ladder). Up to 20% of ruptures are missed (Maffulli, 1999).
- Consider the possibility of rupture in those with an acute history (as discussed earlier) and all those who have a longer standing Achilles swelling or ankle injury that is slow to resolve.
- Diagnose rupture by lying the patient face down with the feet over the end of the couch. Squeeze the calf firmly. If the tendon is intact, this will cause plantar flexion of the foot. If the tendon is ruptured, there will be, at most, a small flicker of the foot (Thompson test).
- Refer any patient with a suspected rupture to be seen within 24 hours.

Problems With the Feet

Bunions

- Although a percentage of bunions are inherited by an autosomal dominant gene, this is of variable penetrance and hence not a reason for early referral or assessment.
- Examine to exclude heel valgus deformity and flatfoot and refer to a podiatrist if either is found. Orthoses may help reduce pain (Ferrari, 2003). While awaiting the appointment, teach the patient calf and foot exercises.
- Refer only those whose lives are severely affected by the bunion. They should be aware that:
  - After the operation, they will not be able to wear a shoe for 8 weeks.
  - Recovery of function will take at least 6 months.

Hallux Rigidus

- Advise the patient to wear a shoe with a rigid sole or to insert a rigid insole into the shoe.
- Refer if pain is interfering with work or sleep. Advise the patient that surgery is similar to bunion surgery, as is the recovery time.

Metatarsalgia

- Examine for a high arch and the presence of corns or calluses beneath the metatarsal heads.
- Refer to a podiatrist.
- Advise the patient to wear a metatarsal pad on the foot (just behind the site of the pain) or an adhesive pad inserted into the shoe to relieve the pressure on the metatarsal heads.
- Refer patients not responding and patients with severe lancinating pain radiating down the cleft between two toes (Morton neuroma).

Steroid Injections in Soft Tissue Lesions

- The poor quality of many studies means that evidence of long-term benefit of steroid injections is lacking. However, they are used because clinical experience demonstrates at least short-term relief for which there is evidence (Speed, 2001).
- The following potential harms are found in injections of the shoulder (Speed & Hazelman, 2001) and similar figures apply to injections in other sites:
  - Infection in 1 in 14,000 to 50,000 injections
  - Tendon rupture in fewer than 1%
  - Local scarring in fewer than 1%
- Discuss with the patient the benefits and harms.
- Familiarise yourself with the common techniques.

Indications

- Intensive use of other approaches for at least 2 months has failed.
- Rehabilitation is inhibited by symptoms.

Good Practice

- Obtain the patient's consent.
- Check that you can define the local anatomy.
- Select the finest needle that will reach the lesion.
- Clean your hands and the patient's skin.
- Use a no-touch technique.
- Use short-acting or medium-acting corticosteroid preparations in most cases, with local anaesthetic.
- Injection should be peritendinous; avoid injection into tendon substance.
- The minimum interval between injections should be 6 weeks.
- Use a maximum of three injections at one site.
- Soluble preparations may be useful in patients who have had hypersensitivity or a local reaction to a previous injection.
- Record the details of the injection.
- Do not repeat if two injections do not provide at least 4 weeks of relief.

Postinjection Advice

- Warn the patient of early postinjection local anaesthesia and to avoid initial overuse.
- Advise resting for at least 2 weeks after injection and avoid heavy loading for 6 weeks.
- The patient should inform the doctor if there is any suggestion of infection or other serious adverse event.

Contraindications to Corticosteroid Injection in Soft Tissue Lesions

- If pain relief and antiinflammatory effects can be achieved by other methods
- Local or systemic infection
- Coagulopathy
- Tendon tear
- Young patients

Oral Nonsteroidal Antiinflammatory Drugs

> **REVIEW**
>
> Machado, G. C., Abdel-Shaheed, C., Underwood, M., & Day R. O. (2012). Non-steroidal anti-inflammatory drugs (NSAIDs) for musculoskeletal pain. *British Medical Journal, 29, 372,* n104

- NSAIDs have good analgesic action, but many patients with acute or chronic pain can be managed with paracetamol. There is little additional benefit from the use of opioids such as codeine and the risk of common side effects such as nausea and constipation or more serious such as dependence. NSAIDS have an antiinflammatory action which is beneficial in controlling swelling and stiffness, as well as pain, in inflammatory diseases

such as RA and spondyloarthropathies and in some cases advanced osteoarthritis.
- NSAIDs have significant adverse effects, including gastrointestinal (GI), renal, and cardiovascular (increased risk of myocardial infarction, hypertension, and worsening of heart failure), particularly in older adults.

Which Oral Nonsteroidal Antiinflammatory Drug?

- The clinical effects of NSAIDs vary from patient to patient. There are important differences between NSAIDs in their relative cardiovascular and GI toxicity.
- Older nonselective NSAIDs such as ibuprofen, diclofenac, and naproxen inhibit both cyclooxygenase (COX)-1 and COX-2 enzymes.
- Newer selective COX-2 (coxibs) inhibit COX-2 enzymes, which are part of the prostaglandin-mediated pain response, and have a lower risk of serious GI effects than traditional NSAIDs. However, this advantage may be lost if prophylactic low-dose aspirin is also prescribed.
- Of the traditional NSAIDs, low-dose ibuprofen (1.2 g/day) has the lowest GI toxicity.
- Coxibs increase the risk of thrombotic events and are therefore contraindicated in patients with established cardiovascular disease. Diclofenac has the same thrombotic risk as coxibs.
- Low-dose ibuprofen and naproxen 1000 mg/day have the lowest risk of thrombotic events.
- The choice of NSAID, therefore, should take account of the individual's risk profile.

Topical Nonsteroidal Antiinflammatory Drugs

- There is some evidence of benefit in osteoarthritis, especially of the knee (Derry et al, 2016).
- There is no benefit of combining oral and topical NSAIDs (Simon et al, 2009).
- There is no increase in GI or cardiovascular effects compared with placebo (Honvo et al, 2019).
- There was good pain relief in acute soft tissue injuries in a Cochrane review (Derry et al, 2016).

Adverse Drug Reactions

- Upper GI disease: peptic ulceration, bleeding, nonulcer dyspepsia
- Fluid retention, leading to aggravation of heart failure
- Renal failure, precipitated in preexisting renal impairment
- Hypersensitivity
- Worsening of hypertension control

Contraindications and Cautions

- Absolute contraindications to all NSAIDs include:
  - Active peptic ulceration

- Hypersensitivity (rhinoconjunctivitis, bronchospasm, urticaria, angioedema, and laryngeal oedema) to aspirin or another NSAID; avoidance is essential to prevent life-threatening reactions
- Pregnancy (third trimester)
- Severe heart failure
- Absolute contraindications to coxibs include:
  - Ischaemic heart disease
  - Cerebrovascular disease
  - Peripheral arterial disease
  - Moderate heart failure
- Cautions for all NSAIDs include:
  - Breastfeeding—largely because of manufacturer warnings. The British National Formulary (BNF) states the amounts in breast milk for most NSAIDs are insignificant. See individual NSAIDs in Appendix 3 of the BNF.
  - Renal, cardiac, or liver failure—renal failure may worsen; monitor urea and electrolytes (U&Es).
  - Asthma—worsening of asthma may be caused by prescribed or OTC NSAIDs.
  - Coagulation defects, including anticoagulation therapy.
  - Older adults.
  - Previous peptic ulceration.
  - Concomitant use of medications that increase GI risk (e.g., steroid therapy or anticoagulants).
- Cautions for the use of coxibs include:
  - Left ventricular dysfunction
  - Hypertension
  - Oedema for any other reason
  - Patients with risk factors for heart disease

Prescribing Practice

- Before prescribing an oral NSAID, consider using a topical NSAID.
- Weigh the risks and benefits (Table 10.3) for the individual and involve the patient in the decision.
- Prescribe the lowest effective dose for the shortest period to control symptoms.
- If the patient has not responded after 3 weeks, consider changing to an NSAID from another class.
- Advise patients to take their tablets with meals and to report dyspepsia immediately.
- For patients at high risk of developing GI complications, whether prescribing a traditional NSAID or a coxib, coprescribe a gastroprotective drug. Use a proton pump inhibitor (PPI), though side effects (colic and diarrhoea) may limit its use. Misoprostol is an alternative. Old age is one such high-risk factor. Indeed, National Institute for Health and Care Excellence (NICE) (2014) guidance on osteoarthritis recommends the routine prescription of a PPI for all patients taking oral NSAIDs or coxibs.
- Review the patient's continued need for NSAIDs regularly.
- Check the patient's existing medication, especially for anticoagulants.

TABLE 10.3 Comparative Risks of Traditional Nonsteroidal Antiinflammatory Drugs and Coxibs (National Prescribing Centre, 2007)

	Traditional NSAID	Coxibs
Thrombotic risk	RRs compared with placebo are diclofenac, 1.63[a] (equivalent to a coxib); low-dose ibuprofen, 1.51 (not statistically significant); and naproxen, 0.92 (not statistically significant)	RR 1.42 NNH compared with placebo = 300 per annum The risk remains constant for the period of use
GI risk	RRs compared with placebo (from RCTs) are diclofenac, 1.7; ibuprofen, 1.2; and naproxen, 1.8; risk is highest during the first week	RR compared with traditional NSAIDs: 0.39; however, coxibs still carry some GI risk, probably equivalent to that of low-dose ibuprofen

[a]Meaning that diclofenac increases the risk of a thrombotic event by 63%. The absolute increase in risk depends on the baseline risk.
GI, Gastrointestinal; NNH, number needed to harm (the number who need to take the drug for one of them to have an excess adverse effect); NSAID, nonsteroidal antiinflammatory drug; RCT, randomised controlled trial; RR, relative risk.

Classes of Nonsteroidal Antiinflammatory Drugs

- Salicylates: aspirin, diflunisal
- Acetic acids: diclofenac, etodolac, indomethacin, sulindac, tolmetin
- Propionic acids: fenbufen, fenoprofen, flurbiprofen, ketoprofen, ibuprofen, naproxen, tiaprofenic acid
- Fenamic acids: flufenamic, mefenamic
- Enolic acids: piroxicam, tenoxicam
- Nonacidic acids: nabumetone
- Selective COX-2 inhibitors: celecoxib, etoricoxib

Monitoring Patients Taking Disease-Modifying Antirheumatic Drugs

See (Table 10.4) and Appendix 12.

Biologic Therapy Monitoring

- Patients receiving biologicals are monitored in secondary care. Disease-modifying antirheumatic drugs (DMARDs) may be coprescribed; if so, monitoring should be in line with the recommendation for the DMARDs.
- Patients receiving biologicals are at increased risk of serious infections. They also have an increased risk of malignancies and possibly autoimmune diseases, including demyelinating and lupuslike syndromes.
- Therefore, for GPs, it is more important to be alert for the appearance of symptoms suggestive of these complications than to rely on routine monitoring.
- Warn patients of the risk of infection and advise them to report symptoms other than minor illnesses.
- Pay particular attention to the risk of tuberculosis. If the patient develops a productive cough or haemoptysis, weight loss, and fever, stop treatment and send a sputum sample to be tested for acid-fast bacilli.
- Warn patients who are not immune to varicella of the need to avoid contact with chickenpox and shingles and of the need to report any inadvertent contact.

- Ensure that the patient has had a single immunisation against pneumococcus and annual influenza vaccine.
- If the patient develops a lupuslike rash, take blood for antinuclear antibodies (ANAs) and double-stranded DNA (dsDNA) binding and inform the rheumatologist.

Gout

GUIDELINE

National Institute for Health and Care Excellence. (2019). *Gout: diagnosis and management.* NICE guideline [NG219] Published: 09 June 2022 Available at https://www.nice.org.uk/guidance/ng219.

PATIENT INFORMATION

Versus Arthritis. *Gout: Causes, symptoms, treatments.*

Aims of Management

- To terminate an attack
- To prevent recurrent attacks
- To prevent complications

Treatment of the Acute Attack

- Consider the possibility of septic arthritis and refer urgently if this is suspected.
- Acute attacks can be very painful, so aim to provide rapid relief of inflammation and pain.
- Nonpharmacologic:
  - Advise resting of the affected joint(s).
  - Advise the application of a cold pack.
- Pharmacological
  - Prescribe a fast-acting NSAID at the maximum dose provided there are no contraindications.
  - Advise that the NSAID should be continued until symptoms subside and for 1 to 2 weeks thereafter.
  - Prescribe additional analgesia in the form of opiates if needed for severe pain.

TABLE 10.4	Disease-Modifying Antirheumatic Drugs, Usual Doses, and Selected Toxicity[a]	
Drug	**Usual Maintenance Dose**	**Toxicity**
Methotrexate	7.5–15 mg/week	GI symptoms, stomatitis, rash, alopecia, infrequent myelosuppression, hepatotoxicity, rare but serious (even life-threatening) pulmonary toxicity
Sulfasalazine	1000 mg twice or three times daily	Rash, myelosuppression (infrequent), GI intolerance
Leflunomide	Maintenance, 10–20 mg once daily	Hepatotoxicity, myelosuppression, GI symptoms, rashes (including Stevens–Johnson syndrome, toxic epidermal necrolysis)
Cytokine modulators, anti-TNF drugs (etanercept, adalimumab, infliximab)	Etanercept, weekly or fortnightly SC injection Infliximab IV infusion every 8 week Adalimumab fortnightly SC injection	Infections, sometimes severe, including tuberculosis, septicaemia, and hepatitis B reactivation; hypersensitivity reactions, including lupus erythematosus–like syndrome, pruritus, injection-site reactions, and blood disorders, myelosuppression; worsening heart failure
Hydroxychloroquine	200 mg twice daily	Rash (infrequent), diarrhoea, retinal toxicity (rare)
Injectable gold salts	25–50 mg IM every 2–4 week	Rash, stomatitis, myelosuppression, thrombocytopenia, proteinuria
Oral gold	3 mg/day or twice daily	Same as injectable gold but less frequent, plus frequent diarrhoea
Azathioprine	50–150 mg/day	Myelosuppression, hepatotoxicity (infrequent), early flulike illness with fever, GI symptoms, elevated LFT results
Penicillamine	250–750 mg/day	Rash, stomatitis, loss of taste, proteinuria, myelosuppression, infrequent but serious autoimmune disease

[a]See the British National Formulary for full list of adverse effects.
GI, Gastrointestinal; *IM,* intramuscular; *IV,* intravenous; *LFT,* liver function test; *SC,* subcutaneous; *TNF,* tumour necrosis factor.

- Patients with comorbidity
  - For patients at increased risk of GI complications, follow advice under the NSAID section about the use of a PPI or consider an alternative.
  - For patients on a diuretic for hypertension, consider changing to another hypertensive.
  - For patients with heart failure, do not stop the diuretic.
  - For patients with heart failure or renal failure, limit the use of NSAID or consider an alternative.
- Alternatives to nonsteroidal antiinflammatory drugs
  - Prescribe colchicine at a dose of 500 μg two to four times per day. Do not use higher doses because of the risk of adverse effects (vomiting, diarrhoea, and abdominal cramps). The drug should be stopped when the attack abates or if side effects outweigh the benefit. Caution is urged in breastfeeding; older adults; and in patients with hepatic or renal impairment, GI disease, and cardiac disease.
  - Prescribe prednisolone 35 mg/day until the attack is settling; then reduce to zero so that the total course is 7 to 10 days.
- Patients Not responding to the above
  - Consider an intraarticular injection of methylprednisolone (40 or 10 mg for a small joint) as a single dose.

Management After an Attack

- Review the patient at 4 to 6 weeks.
- Educate the patient regarding self-management. Advise the patient to start treatment *as soon as possible* after the onset of any future attacks and to have a standby supply of NSAID or alternative.
- Assess all patients for conditions associated with hyperuricaemia:
  - Obesity
  - Alcohol consumption
  - Blood pressure
  - Hyperlipidaemia
  - Diabetes
  - Renal failure
- Investigations
  a. Uric acid. Check this after the attack has settled because it may be lowered during an attack. An increased level does not prove the diagnosis nor does a low level exclude it. The main value is in determining and monitoring prevention.
  b. Blood tests. Check renal function, serum glucose, and cholesterol.
  c. Consider joint aspiration when the diagnosis is in doubt (e.g., knee monoarthritis when the differential diagnosis may be gout or pseudogout [urate crystals

and calcium pyrophosphate dihydrate crystals seen, respectively, on microscopy]). Send the aspirate immediately in a plain glass bottle for polarising microscopy (by prior arrangement).

d. Radiographs are rarely helpful but can sometimes confirm pseudogout (chondrocalcinosis seen on plain films) or demonstrate joint damage from chronic gout, which is more likely to happen as an insidious process in the elderly.

Prevention of Recurrence and Complications

- Explain the nature of the condition, which is that gout is a long-term condition with progression to joint damage. Discuss the causes, signs, and symptoms of gout.
- Promote self-management to reduce ongoing joint destruction.
- Advise patients that:
  - The NICE guidelines state that 'the current evidence base to support specific dietary advice is limited'.
  - They should lose weight if they are obese.
  - They should restrict alcohol to recommended limits.
  - They should maintain a fluid intake over 2 L/day.
  - Consider stopping drugs that reduce uric acid excretion or reduce them to the lowest effective dose. They are aspirin (though not low-dose aspirin used in cardiovascular protection), thiazides, and loop diuretics.
- Consider drug prophylaxis according to the following indications:
  - Multiple or troublesome flares
  - Those with stage 3 to 5chronic kidney disease
  - Polyarticular gout
  - The presence of tophi
  - Clinical or radiologic signs of chronic gouty arthritis
  - Recurrent uric acid renal stones
- Asymptomatic hyperuricaemia is not considered an indication for drug prophylaxis.
- Wait until the acute attack has subsided for at least 2 to 4 weeks before starting prophylaxis; otherwise the attack may be prolonged.

Use of Urate-Lowering Therapy

- Start with a low dose and use monthly serum urate levels to titrate dose increases as tolerated.
- Aim for urate below 360 μmol/L or below 300 μmol/L when there are tophi or chronic gouty arthritis.
- Choose either:
  - Allopurinol—fewer side effects. Start at 100 to 200 mg and then increase over weeks until target serum uric acid levels are achieved. The usual dose around 300 mg but can increase to maximum of 900 mg; then give it in three divided doses.
  - Febuxostat—more effective. Start at 80 mg and increase to 120 mg once daily after 4 weeks.

- Prevention of gout flares when starting prophylactic treatment
  - Use colchicine while dose titration is taking place.
  - If contraindicated, use NSAIDs (with PPI cover) or oral prednisolone.

Indications for Referral

- Septic arthritis is suspected: referral is urgent.
- The diagnosis is uncertain.
- There is a suspicion of an underlying systemic illness (e.g., RA or connective tissue disorder).
- Gout occurs during pregnancy or in a young person (younger than 25 years of age).
- They have chronic kidney disease stage 3b to 5.
- Treatment is contraindicated, not tolerated, or ineffective.

PATIENT EDUCATION

Versus Arthritis. *Gout: Causes, symptoms, treatments*. https://www.versusarthritis.org/about-arthritis/conditions/gout/

Rheumatoid Arthritis

GUIDELINES

Aletaha, D., & Smolen, J. S. (2018). Diagnosis and management of rheumatoid arthritis: A review. *Journal of the American Medical Association, 320*(13), 1360–1372.
    Allen, A., Carville, S., McKenna, F., & Guideline Development Group. (2018). Diagnosis and management of rheumatoid arthritis in adults: Summary of updated NICE guidance. *British Medical Journal (Clinical research ed.), 362*, k3015. National Institute for Health and Care Excellence. (2018, Updated 2020). *Rheumatoid arthritis in adults: Management. NICE clinical guideline 100.* Available at https://www.nice.org.uk/guidance/ng100.

Background

RA
- A chronic, disabling autoimmune disease
- Affects 1% of the UK population
- Female:male ratio is 3:1
- Early age of onset (younger than 40–60 years)
- Presents to primary care with joint pain and swelling, particularly of the hands and feet

Aims of Management

- Fast specialist referral is essential to confirm the diagnosis, undertake appropriate investigations, and start early drug treatment.
- Target treatment to achieve remission or as low disease activity as possible.
- Suppress or minimise disease progression.
- Control symptoms (pain and stiffness).
- Preserve function.
- Minimise drug side effects.

- Provide patient education and promote independence and quality of life through a multidisciplinary team approach.

The General Practitioner

- The GP has a continuing role in managing patients in the long term within protocols shared with secondary care. The GP also has a role in managing the illnesses that accompany RA.
- Patients with RA have an increased risk of cardiovascular disease and mortality.
- Patients with RA have an increased risk of osteoporosis.

Referral to Secondary Care

- Refer when there is suspected persistent synovitis in which the small joints of the hands or more than one joint are affected.

Initial Investigations

GPs should not delay referral waiting on the following results or if these initial investigations are negative but refer on clinical suspicion alone. While these results should be interpreted by a specialist, if ordered by the GP, the results will be available at the specialist consultation

- Inflammatory markers (ESR, C-reactive protein [CRP]).
- Rheumatoid factor.
- Radiographs of the hands and feet as a baseline for disease progression. This may not help in diagnosis because erosions are not present in early disease.
- Anti-CCP (cyclic citrullinated peptide) antibodies (NICE, 2018). This is highly specific (>95%) for RA at all stages of the disease. This means that a positive finding makes the diagnosis almost certain. However, the sensitivity is not sufficiently high in early disease (45%–60%) to rule out disease.
- Full blood count (FBC) should be done because the anaemia of chronic disease is common and to get a baseline because some DMARDs and biologicals affect the blood count.
- Liver function tests (LFTs) should be done because some DMARDs and biologicals affect the liver.
- U&Es and dip testing of urine should be done because some DMARDs and biologicals affect renal function.

Pharmacologic Treatment

Drug treatment is now based on a 'treat-to-target strategy' (NICE 2018).

Disease activity can be measured by tools (e.g., Disease Activity Score 28 (DAS-28)) which use a combination of clinical assessment (number of swollen, tender joints and overall pain) together with inflammatory markers (ESR, CRP). These measurements can be used to monitor disease activity.

Treatment target is remission or as low disease activity as possible, especially if baseline assessment indicated positive anti-CCP antibodies or erosions on radiograph.

Symptom and Pain Control

- NICE 2018 found very limited evidence for the use of paracetamol, opioids, and TCAs, so these drugs have been removed from the guidelines.
- Use either traditional or COX-2 NSAIDs if not contra-indicated (GI, liver, and cardiorenal toxicity).
- Use the lowest effective dose with PPI cover and review regularly for adverse effects.

Disease-Modifying Antirheumatic Drugs

- These should be by choice and management by specialists and ideally started within 3 months of persistent symptoms.
- These include 'conventional' DMARDs as well as targeted and biologic DMARDs.
- First-line conventional drugs include methotrexate, leflunomide, and sulfasalazine.
- Consider hydroxychloroquine for milder disease.
- Consider a combination of the above agents when remission has not been achieved.
- Move to second- or third-line treatments with biologics as per treatment algorithm (Aletaha & Smolen, 2018).
- Consider short-term use of glucocorticoids (oral, intramuscular, or intraarticular) when starting treatment to improve symptoms.
- Specialists may consider stepping down treatment in patients maintained in remission for at least 1 year but be prepared to escalate if symptoms relapse.

Nondrug Management

- Education, physiotherapy, and related interventions remain at the centre of care.
- Constantly review patients not under the care of the multidisciplinary hospital team for the need for referral to any of the following:
  - Physiotherapists—for education, exercise programmes, and splints
  - Occupational therapists—for mobility and daily living aids
  - Nurse specialists
  - Orthotic and prosthetic departments
  - Podiatrists
  - Orthopaedic surgeons

Education

- Education improves knowledge, symptom control, adherence, and self-management.
- Consider every consultation an opportunity to educate the patient.
- Provide information leaflets.

Spondyloarthropathies

GUIDELINE

National Institute for Health and Care Excellence. (2017). *Spondyloarthritis in over 16s: diagnosis and management. NICE guideline [NG65] Published: 28 February 2017 Last updated: 02 June 2017.* https://www.nice.org.uk/guidance/ng10065.

- The spondyloarthropathies are a group of inflammatory conditions with shared features which are generally classified as axial or peripheral disease. While associated with the human leukocyte antigen (HLA) B27 tissue type, there is no single diagnostic test, resulting in a delayed or incorrect diagnosis. The category includes:
  - Axial disease: ankylosing spondylitis (AS)
  - Peripheral disease: reactive arthritis (usually after a bowel or genitourinary infection), psoriatic arthritis, enteropathic arthritis (associated with inflammatory bowel disease [IBD])

Aims of Management

- Make the diagnosis early; the average delay in diagnosis is 8.5 years (NICE, 2018).
- Control symptoms (pain, stiffness, and disability).
- Prevent deformity and disability.
- Manage nonskeletal complications: fatigue, anterior uveitis, pulmonary and thoracic restriction (AS), aortic incompetence (AS), and IBD.

Diagnosis and Referral

- No single test has been shown to diagnose or exclude disease.
- Symptoms can be diverse with both musculoskeletal and extraarticular features.
- Early diagnosis is important to establish an exercise programme and to start effective pharmacotherapy to prevent deformity.
- Typical features include:
  a. Axial: LBP for more than 3 months in those aged younger than 45 years if they have four of the following (NICE, 2018):
     - LBP for less than 35 years
     - Waking in the later part of the night
     - Buttock pain
     - Improvement with exercise or NSAIDs
     - First-degree relative with AS
     - Current or past arthritis
  b. Peripheral
     - Those with enthesitis, especially if at multiple sites
     - Those with uveitis, IBD, psoriasis, or GI or genitourinary infection
- Investigations
  a. Inflammatory markers (CRP and ESR) are frequently increased but may be normal.

  b. HLA-B27 does not confirm the diagnosis because the background incidence is 6% to 8% in the general population. However, a negative result makes the diagnosis unlikely because 95% of patients with AS have positive results.
  c. Radiographs of the sacroiliac joints give a high dose of radiation with little benefit because diagnostic changes take years to develop. Magnetic resonance imaging is more accurate than radiographs.

Management

- Axial
  - NSAIDs at the lowest effective dose. If there no benefit, consider switching to an alternate NSAID. Consider DMARDs as second-line treatment.
  - Referral to a specialist physiotherapist for a structured exercise programme. Consider hydrotherapy. Refer to other therapists such as occupational therapy or podiatry.
- Peripheral
  - Treat the associated disease (e.g., psoriasis, colitis). Consider DMARDs and corticosteroid injection in monoarthritis.
  - Refer to specialist therapists as discussed earlier.
- Consider regular (every 2 years) assessment of bone mineral density (hip better than spinal because of the presence of spinal calcification).
- Educate patients about 'flare episodes' and develop an individual management plan which should include self-care (e.g., exercise) and quick access to specialist care, including doctors and nurses regarding medications and therapists.

PATIENT INFORMATION

National Ankylosing Spondylitis Society. About AS. Available at https://nass.co.uk/National Axial Spondyloarthritis Society (nass.co.uk).
    Versus Arthritis. *Ankylosing spondylitis: Symptoms, causes, treatments.* https://www.versusarthritis.org/about-arthritis/conditions/ankylosing-spondylitis/.

Connective Tissue Diseases

- The connective tissue diseases (CTDs) are:
  - Systemic lupus erythematosus (SLE)
  - Scleroderma or systemic sclerosis
  - Polymyositis
  - Dermatomyositis
  - Sjögren syndrome
  - Raynaud disease
- The term *connective tissue diseases* covers a group of autoimmune, inflammatory diseases of unknown cause but with a genetic background affecting multiple systems that have a variable presentation and course and whose features overlap. They are strongly associated with several autoantibodies.

In addition to genetic factors, certain environmental factors have been implicated, including exposure to ultraviolet light and viral infections. A drug-induced lupuslike disease has been recognised as a reaction to medications such as chlorpromazine, hydralazine, and isoniazid.

- The term *mixed CTD* is used to describe the clinical picture in which there are features of various CTDs.
- CTDs are more common in females younger than 50 years.
- Complications can be serious and fatal and include:
  - Pulmonary hypertension
  - Pulmonary fibrosis
  - Renal failure
  - Anaemia

Diagnosis

- Many features, especially early in the disease, are nonspecific, including:
  - Arthralgia usually without synovitis
  - Raynaud disease with cold or numb fingers and toes, especially in cold weather
  - Skin rash: malar rash in SLE or on the face or hands in dermatomyositis
  - Generally feeling unwell, fatigue, muscle weakness, and a mild fever
- A group practice with 8000 patients may have 50 to 80 patients with Sjögren syndrome, 4 patients with SLE, and 4 to 8 with other CTDs. They are uncommon, but GPs have a special role in both diagnosis and treatment because of their multisystem and chronic nature.
- Evidence-based guidelines are not available for CTDs in general; however, many of the management issues overlap with those of other inflammatory rheumatic conditions already mentioned.

Investigations

a. FBC: leucopenia, lymphopenia, thrombocytopenia, or haemolysis suggests a CTD.
b. Urine dipstick and U&Es to screen for renal disease.
c. Creatine kinase.
d. ESR and CRP are usually raised in patients with CTDs (but note that the CRP is often normal in SLE in the absence of infection).
e. Serum ANAs are is positive in more than 90% of CTDs; however, they should *not* be relied on as a diagnostic test in the absence of clinical features because are positive in 5% of the general population and more than 30% of people with RA.

Management

- There is no cure for CTDs. Treatment aims to manage symptoms and prevent further tissue damage (e.g., pulmonary fibrosis, renal failure).
- Refer suspected cases early to a rheumatologist for diagnosis and a management plan.

- Screen for and manage other cardiovascular risk factors (e.g., hypertension), especially when renal disease is present or high-dose steroid therapy is used.
- Drug treatment includes the use of oral corticosteroids, tumour necrosis factor blockers, and other biologics and other immunosuppressants such as methotrexate and azathioprine as well as the older established antimalarial drugs such as hydroxychloroquine.

Osteoporosis

GUIDELINES

Compston, J., McClung, M., & Leslie, W. (2019). Osteoporosis. *Lancet, 393*, 364–376.
   SIGN. (2021). Osteoporosis: assessing the risk of fragility fracture Guidance NICE. Available at https://www.nice.org.uk/guidance/cg146.

- Osteoporosis is the most common disease of bone and twice as common in females as males. It is defined as ' a systemic skeletal disease characterised by low bone mass and microarchitectural deterioration in bone tissue, with a consequent increase in bone fragility and susceptibility to fracture' (Anonymous, 1993).
- Although hip and vertebral fractures are most common, osteoporosis is a systemic disease with fracture risk increased at all skeletal sites.
- Most fractures occur in patients with lesser degrees of demineralisation (osteopenia) through interaction with other risk factors.
- A fragility fracture occurs on minimal trauma (e.g., falling when standing on the ground) after the age of 40 years in a typical site, including the vertebral bodies, distal radius, proximal femur, or proximal humerus.
- It has been estimated that half of all hip fractures could have been prevented if osteoporosis could be avoided.

Definitions of Osteopenia and Osteoporosis

GUIDELINE

World Health Organization. (1994). Assessment of fracture risk and its application to screening for postmenopausal osteoporosis. Report of a WHO Study Group. *World Health Organization technical report series, 843*, 1–129.

- These conditions are defined by the result of dual-energy radiograph absorptiometry (DXA) measurements of bone mineral density (BMD):
  - T score below −2.5 = *osteoporosis.* The BMD is greater than 2.5 standard deviations below the young adult mean.
  - T score between −1 and −2.5 = *osteopenia.* The BMD is between 1 and 2.5 standard deviations below the young adult mean.
  - T score above −1 = *normal.*
- It is important to remember that BMD is only one of a number of risk factors for fracture.
- When more than one site is scanned, the lowest score is used.

General Principles

- Fracture liaison services 'pick-up' those at higher risk after a fragility fracture and provide a cost-effective, tested model for the assessment and further management of these individuals.
- Diagnosis is based on case finding—namely, identifying those likely to be at risk because of either a previous fragility fracture or the presence of significant clinical risk factors in postmenopausal females or males older than the age of 50 years.
- The risk of future fracture is used as a *guide* to further management. Clinical judgement still has a place. Calculators do not take account of a tendency to falls, the greater prognostic risk attached to vertebral relative to other fractures, or the greater risk after more than one fragility fracture.
- There is geographic variation in how services are organised and which specialty leads them. The GP's role, referral routes, and prereferral workup vary accordingly, and local protocols need to be observed.
- Assessment in general practice includes the search for a possible cause of secondary osteoporosis and a differential diagnosis, according to the individual's age, sex, and clinical features.
- Take a history, perform an examination, and order investigations appropriate to the individual's clinical picture.
- Refer younger males with osteoporosis for further investigation because there is a greater chance of secondary osteoporosis in this group.

Procedures Proposed in the Investigation of Osteoporosis

- Perform the following investigations:
  - Blood cell count, ESR or CRP, serum calcium, albumin, creatinine, phosphate, alkaline phosphatase, and liver transaminases
  - Serum 25-hydroxy vitamin D
  - Thyroid function tests (TFTs)
  - Bone densitometry (DXA), which is the key investigation

- Consider the following investigations if indicated by history and examination:
  - Lateral radiographs of the lumbar and thoracic spine or DXA-based vertebral imaging
  - Protein immunoelectrophoresis and urinary Bence Jones proteins
  - Serum testosterone, sex hormone–binding globulin, follicle-stimulating hormone), luteinizing hormone (in males)
  - Serum prolactin
  - Screening tests for coeliac disease
  - New measures to enhance fracture risk assessment include trabecular bone score, lateral spine DXA, and computed tomography to detect previously undiagnosed vertebral fractures. Measurements of muscle mass and function can assist in predicting falls risk.

Approach to Prognosis and Intervention

- Be alert to patients at risk with a previous fragility fracture or significant clinical risk factors (see upcoming discussion).
- Use the Fracture Risk Assessment Tool (FRAX) tool to assess the patient's 10-year probability of a major osteoporotic fracture (https://frax.shef.ac.uk/FRAX/). The tool places the patient in one of three bands: low, intermediate, or high risk.
- The UK National Osteoporosis Guidelines Group suggests using FRAX without BMD assessment to estimate fracture risk. (The US National Osteoporosis Foundation advises BMD measurement in all females older than 65 years of age and males older than 70 years of age).
- *Intermediate risk.* Arrange for a DXA scan because the results may alter management. Recalculate the risk using the FRAX tool and the result of the DXA. The tool will now place the patient in one of two bands: low or high risk.
- *Low risk.* Give general advice (see upcoming discussion).
- *High risk.* Offer pharmacologic intervention (see upcoming discussion).

Clinical Risk Factors for Osteoporosis

- Age
- Sex
- Low BMI ($\leq$19 kg/m^2)
- Previous fragility fracture, particularly of the hip, wrist, and spine, including morphometric vertebral fracture
- Parental history of hip fracture
- Current glucocorticoid treatment (any dose by mouth for $\geq$3 months)
- Current smoking
- Alcohol—dose dependent; risks start at daily intake of 3 or more units
- Causes of secondary osteoporosis, including:
  - RA
  - Untreated hypogonadism in males and females
  - Prolonged immobility
  - Organ transplantation
  - Type I diabetes

- Hyperthyroidism
- GI disease
- Chronic liver disease
- Chronic obstructive pulmonary disease
- Falls (not used in the FRAX calculation)

General Management

- For those with irreversible risk factors, management is lifelong. Despite advances in the assessment and treatment options available, treatment rates are low (and possibly falling) in those with a high fracture risk. The key to the treatment of osteoporosis is to reduce the incidence of fragility fractures by increasing the 'strength' of the bony skeleton or decreasing the frequency of falls.
- Assess the risk of falls and refer to local falls prevention services as appropriate.
- Lifestyle intervention
  - Encourage regular weight-bearing impact physical activities such as dancing plus resistance exercises (lifting weights).
  - The results of studies evaluating the effects of calcium and vitamin D are inconsistent. However, current advice is a diet that provides a daily intake of 1000 mg calcium and 800 IU of vitamin D_3. The recommended calcium intake can be achieved with 1 pint of semi-skimmed milk plus one of 3 oz of hard cheese, three slices of white bread (or six of wholemeal bread), one small pot of yoghourt, or 3 oz of canned sardines. The National Osteoporosis Society has a list of calcium and vitamin D contents, which can be useful for vegans and religious observances.
  - Give the same dietary advice to those receiving pharmacologic intervention.
  - Prescribe calcium and ergocalciferol 1 tablet twice daily to housebound older adults.
- Pharmacologic intervention:
  - Pharmacologic treatment is appropriate for high-risk patients when secondary causes have been excluded or treated and when the benefit outweighs the risk and contraindications.
  - Placebo-controlled trials suggest a reduction in fracture risk of 30% to 70% for vertebral fractures and up to 50% for hip fractures.
  - Fracture risk reduction is related to the individual patient's risk rather than the choice of a particular medication.

Bisphosphonates

- Prescribe alendronate as a first-line agent because of a good evidence base for the prevention of fractures at several sites and its cost-effectiveness. Risedronate and zoledronic acid are alternatives. Alendronate is suitable in both males and females for the:
  - Treatment of postmenopausal osteoporosis: 10 mg/day or 70 mg once weekly

- Treatment of osteoporosis in males: 10 mg/day
- Prevention of postmenopausal osteoporosis: 5 mg/day
- Prevention and treatment of corticosteroid-induced osteoporosis: 5 mg/day but 10 mg/day for postmenopausal females not receiving hormone replacement therapy

The Practicalities of Prescribing Bisphosphonates

- Advise the patient to swallow the tablets whole with plenty of water half an hour before breakfast and to remain upright for half an hour afterwards.
- Correct disturbances of calcium and mineral metabolism (e.g., vitamin D deficiency, hypocalcaemia) before starting. Monitor serum calcium concentration during treatment.
- Advise the patient on good dental hygiene during and after treatment to avoid the rare complication of osteonecrosis of the jaw. If remedial dental treatment is needed, advise the patient to consider having it done before starting alendronate.
- If alendronate is not tolerated or contraindicated, consider an alternative bisphosphonate such as risedronate. If this is not tolerated, consider intravenous bisphosphonate or the monoclonal antibody RANK (receptor activator of nuclear factor-κB) ligand inhibitor denosumab. Other treatment options include raloxifene (an alternative for postmenopausal osteoporosis; advise the patient it does not reduce menopausal vasomotor symptoms), teriparatide, and abaloparatide. There is little study evidence for combining treatments, but using different medicines sequentially has shown some benefit.
- Bisphosphonates have similar contraindications and side effects. If GI side effects are prominent, a weekly formulation (alendronate 70 mg or risedronate 35 mg) may be tried.
- Contraindications to bisphosphonates are:
  - Abnormalities of the oesophagus that delay emptying (alendronate, risedronate)
  - Inability to stand or sit upright for at least 30 minutes
  - Hypocalcaemia
  - Pregnancy
  - Breastfeeding
- Bisphosphonates should be used with caution if there is:
  - Another upper GI problem
  - Significant renal failure (creatinine clearance <30 mL/ min). Treatment should be reviewed after 3 years with intravenous zoledronate and after 5 years of oral bisphosphonate. Continuing treatment beyond this period is generally recommended for those with a history of hip or vertebral fracture, those who have had a fracture on treatment, those taking corticosteroids, and people older than age 75 years.

Corticosteroid-Induced Osteoporosis

- Keep doses of oral corticosteroids as low as possible and courses as short as possible.
- Consider the risk of osteoporosis in patients with cumulative doses from intermittent courses. Long-term use of

high-dose inhaled corticosteroids may also carry a risk, especially in those at high risk of developing osteoporosis independent of the concomitant steroid use.

PATIENT INFORMATION

Royal Osteoporosis Society. *Osteoporosis Charity UK*. Available at http://theros.org.uk.
   Versus Arthritis. *Osteoporosis: Causes, symptoms, treatment*. https://www.versusarthritis.org/about-arthritis/conditions/osteoporosis/

Polymyalgia Rheumatica

SYSTEMATIC REVIEWS

Buttgereit, F., Dejaco, C., Matteson, E. L., & Dasgupta, B. (2016). Polymyalgia rheumatica and giant cell arteritis: A systematic review. *Journal of the American Medical Association, 315*(22), 2442–2258.
   González-Gay, M. A., Matteson, E. L., & Castañeda, S. (2017). Polymyalgia rheumatica. *Lancet, 390*(10103), 1700–1712.

GUIDELINE

Weyand, C. M., & Goronzy J. J. (2014). Clinical practice. Giant-cell arteritis and polymyalgia rheumatica. *New England Journal of Medicine, 371*(1), 50–57.

Management Objectives

- To control symptoms of stiffness and pain (plus associated constitutional symptoms such as fatigue and weight loss)
- To reduce the risk of the complication of temporal arteritis (TA)
- To minimise the risks of steroid therapy

Diagnosis

AMERICAN COLLEGE OF RHEUMATOLOGY AND EUROPEAN LEAGUE AGAINST RHEUMATISM CLASSIFICATION CRITERIA FOR POLYMYALGIA RHEUMATICA, 2012

Patients aged 50 years or older with bilateral shoulder aching and abnormal C-reactive protein concentrations or erythrocyte sedimentation rate plus at least 4 points (without ultrasonography) or 4 points or more (with ultrasonography) from the following criteria:
- Morning stiffness for >45 minutes (2 points)
- Hip pain or restricted range of motion (1 point)
- Absence of rheumatoid factor or anticitrullinated protein antibodies (2 points)
- Absence of other joint involvement (1 point)
- If ultrasonography is available, at least one shoulder with subdeltoid bursitis, biceps tenosynovitis, or glenohumeral synovitis (either posterior or axillary) and at least one hip with synovitis or trochanteric bursitis (1 point)
- If ultrasonography is available, both shoulders with subdeltoid bursitis, biceps tenosynovitis, or glenohumeral synovitis (1 point)

FEATURES OF POLYMYALGIA RHEUMATICA

- Bilateral diffuse, morning shoulder with or without upper arm or neck pain or stiffness for more than 45 to 60 minutes
- Worse after rest or prolonged inactivity
- General fatigue and malaise
- Onset of illness less than 2 weeks in duration
- Initial ESR above 40 mm/h
- Age older than 50 years
- Female:male ratio is 2:1
- Depression or weight loss
- More prevalent in Northern European populations

Investigations

- Check ESR (>40 mm/h) or CRP (>6 mg/dl). Note that the ESR may be normal in 20% of cases (especially in younger patients). Both are strongly associated with disease activity.
- Consider tests to rule out alternative diagnoses as appropriate:
  - TFTs for hypothyroidism
  - Creatinine kinase for polymyositis and statin-induced myositis
  - CXR, as malignancy, especially lung cancer, can cause polymyalgia
  - Protein electrophoresis to exclude multiple myeloma

Initial Management

- Check FBC; a normocytic normochromic anaemia is common.
- Measure weight and blood pressure) and check serum glucose before starting steroids.
- Oral prednisolone is the mainstay of treatment.
- The dose range is from 10-15 mg daily until remission of disease, reducing slowly to maintenance dose prescribed for patients weighing more than 80 kg in the absence of risk factors for side effects such as osteoporosis and diabetes and lower doses for patients weighing less than 60 kg.
- The patient's symptoms improve significantly within 1 week and often within 72 hours with an improvement in pain, a reduction in the length of morning stiffness, and a fall in the elevated ESR or CRP.
- If there is no response to steroids, review alternative diagnoses as above plus:
  - Cervical spondylosis (the most common differential diagnosis)
  - RA
- Consider increasing the dose of prednisolone if you have confidently excluded other diagnoses.
- Conventional immunosuppressive agents such as methotrexate can be used when there are significant steroid side effects or where steroids are ineffective or the symptoms relapse after tapering or stopping.

Maintenance Steroid Therapy

- Although randomised trial evidence is limited, both the American College of Rheumatology (ARC) and European League Against Rheumatism (EULAR) suggest maintaining the prednisolone dosage for 3 to 4 weeks and then progressively tapering the dose.
- For prednisolone doses of 15 mg, reduce to 12.5 mg after 2 to 4 weeks, then to 10 mg for 4 to 6 weeks, and then by 1 mg every month thereafter. This will depend on the absence of a return of symptoms and can be guided by ESR or CRP measurement.
- Relapse is common (20%–55% in the first year) during the average duration of the disease of 2 to 3 years and seen more commonly with rapid reductions in dosage or when the dose of prednisolone is reduced to less than 5 mg. ARC and EULAR suggest returning to the pre-relapse dose and a slower reduction over 4 to 8 weeks to the dose at which the relapse occurred.

Referral

- Refer patients when:
  - Symptom control requires a high maintenance dose of steroids or the patient develops significant adverse steroid effects on lower doses (immunosuppressive drugs such as methotrexate may be considered).
  - There is doubt about the diagnosis, particularly when there is synovitis and anaemia suggestive of RA.

Patient Education

Versus Arthritis. *Polymyalgia rheumatica (PMR):Causes, symptoms, treatments.* Available at https://www.versusarthritis.org/about-arthritis/conditions/polymyalgia-rheumatica-pmr/.
- Advise patients to seek urgent attention if they develop symptoms suggestive of giant cell arteritis (GCA):
  - Unilateral headache
  - Tenderness in the scalp
  - Jaw claudication (facial pain on chewing)
- Advise patients about the risks of steroids (see upcoming discussion) and precautions to take.

Temporal Arteritis

- TA is the most common form of GCA, but other arteries may be involved. After headache or pain in the temple, the next most common syndrome is jaw claudication.
- It is almost exclusively a disease of White people.
- A normal ESR or CRP or a negative temporal artery biopsy does not rule out the disease. The chance of obtaining a positive biopsy after 1 week of steroid therapy falls to 10% (Pountain & Hazleman, 1995).
- Steroid therapy should not be delayed pending the results of investigations because untreated GCA carries a risk of visual loss in 40% of patients.

DIAGNOSTIC CRITERIA FOR TEMPORAL ARTERITIS
American College of Rheumatology

At least three criteria must be met:
1. Age at disease onset of 50 years or older
2. New headache, either of new onset or new type of localised pain in the head
3. Abnormal temporal artery, with tenderness to palpation or decreased pulsation
4. Elevated erythrocyte sedimentation rate (>50 mm/h)
5. Biopsy evidence of vasculitis with predominance of mononuclear cell infiltration or granulomatous inflammation, usually with multinucleated giant cells

---

Initial Management

- *Likely clinical diagnosis according to albumin–creatinine ratio (ACR) criteria with visual loss:* If vision is impaired, give prednisolone up to 60 mg immediately and make an urgent referral to an ophthalmologist. If there is likely to be a delay, continue the dose daily.
- *Likely clinical diagnosis according to ACR criteria without visual loss:*
  - Take blood for an ESR, CRP, and FBC.
  - Start prednisolone 40 mg/day.
  - See the patient after 48 hours.
- If there is no response, review the diagnosis.
- *Suspected diagnosis:* Check ESR or CRP, start steroids at 40 mg/day, and arrange for the patient to be seen within 48 hours by a rheumatologist or ophthalmologist.
- Opinion varies on the use of routine temporal artery biopsy. Follow local guidance regarding referral.

Maintenance Treatment

SYSTEMATIC REVIEW

Buttgereit, F., Dejaco, C., Matteson, E. L., & Dasgupta, B. (2016). Polymyalgia rheumatica and giant cell arteritis: A systematic review. *Journal of the American Medical Association, 315*(22), 2442–2458.

- Reduce gradually to maintenance dose of 7.5-10 mg daily. Many patients require treatment for at least 2 years and in some patients it may be necessary to continue long-term low dose corticosteroids.
- Consider methotrexate if there are frequent relapses.

Steroids

Adverse effects develop in up to 50% of patients. The risk is positively associated with the dose.
- Educate the patient about the risks:
  - Weight gain
  - Hypertension

- Osteoporosis
- Development of diabetes or worsening of diabetic control
- Infection risk
- Risk of GI perforation in combination with NSAIDs
- Adrenal suppression
- Ensure the patient has an up-to-date steroid card.
- Follow guidance on steroid-induced osteoporosis.
- Advise the patient not to stop steroids suddenly.
- Advise the patient that it may be necessary to increase the dose of steroids during intercurrent illness and to seek medical advice.
- Warn the patient to avoid contagious contacts with chickenpox and shingles (there is a risk of fatal disseminated chickenpox if not immune). Advise them to seek urgent medical advice if they are exposed. Obtain specialist advice if such exposure occurs.
- Consider testing immune status for chickenpox when commencing steroid therapy.
- Check weight, blood pressure, and urine (or blood) for glucose every 3 months.
- Patients who take long-term corticosteroids are at an additional risk of osteoporosis. An overall risk assessment should include increasing age, low body mass index and low bone mineral density in addition to the traditional clinical risk factors such as a personal/family history of fractures, alcohol consumption and cigarette smoking.
- Recommend pneumococcal and flu vaccinations.

Fibromyalgia

GUIDELINE

Bair, M. J., & Krebs, E. E. (2020). Fibromyalgia. *Ann Intern Med, 172*(5), ITC33–ITC48.

- Fibromyalgia is a distinct syndrome of widespread, chronic pain associated with fatigue, sleep disturbance, and often cognitive symptoms such as memory and concentration. It may coexist with other chronic illnesses such as chronic back pain and irritable bowel syndrome.
- The mechanism for the pain is thought to be a disorder of pain regulation and central sensitisation.
- The prevalence is a female:male ratio of 2:1 and is less common in those who are regularly active, not overweight, and whose sleep and mood disturbance have been treated.
- Criteria for diagnosis (ARC Wolfe et al, 1990; revised 2010):
  1. A history of widespread pain: pain must be present in four of five body regions (the four quadrants of the body and in the spine)
  2. Presence of somatic symptoms such as headache, abdominal pain, bloating, dizziness, and paraesthesia
  3. Scores of greater than 7 on the Widespread Pain Index and greater than 5 on Symptom Severity Score
  4. Symptoms that have been present for over 3 months

Management

- Exclude rheumatologic, neurologic, and endocrine disorders on clinical examination.
- No specific laboratory tests are diagnostic and are used to rule out other conditions as above.
- Management should aim to maintain or improve function, manage symptoms, and improve overall quality of life.
- Explain the nature of the condition (do not dismiss the underlying pathology), which is that there is no serious pathology and that pain arises from abnormal processing of pain signals.
- Emphasise the benefits of self-management strategies, especially around activity, sleep hygiene, stress management, weight reduction, and a generally healthy active lifestyle.
- Coexistent mood disorders should be identified and treated independently.
- Formal supervised (and thus social) graduated exercise programmes and formal cognitive-behavioural therapy have been shown to be beneficial.
- Pharmacologic options include TCAs (particularly amitriptyline), duloxetine, and gabapentin/pregabalin. Simple analgesics have not been shown to be clinically effective, and stronger opioids should be avoided.
- A Cochrane review found some benefit with acupuncture but no benefit from massage-like therapies or any specific diets.

PATIENT INFORMATION

Versus Arthritis. *Fibromyalgia: Causes, symptoms, treatment.* https://www.versusarthritis.org/about-arthritis/conditions/fibromyalgia/

Further Reading

Aker, P. D., Gross, A. R., Goldsmith, C. H., & Peloso, P. (1996). Conservative management of mechanical neck pain: Systematic overview and meta-analysis. *British Medical Journal (Clinical Research Ed.), 313*, 1291–1296.

Alamo, M., Moral, R., & de Torres, L. (2002). Evaluation of a patient-centred approach in generalised musculoskeletal chronic pain/fibromyalgia patients in primary care. *Patient Education and Counseling, 48*, 23–31.

Bachmann, L. M., Kolb, E., Koller, M. T., Steurer, J., & ter Riet, G. (2003). Accuracy of Ottawa ankle rules to exclude fractures of the ankle and mid-foot: Systematic review. *British Medical Journal (Clinical Research Ed.), 326*, 417–419.

Bahlas, A., Ramos-Remos, C., & Davis, P. (1998). Clinical outcome of 149 patients with polymyalgia rheumatica and giant cell arteritis. *Journal of Rheumatology, 25*, 99–104.

Bird, H. A., Esselinckx, W., Dixon, A. S., Mowat, A. G., & Wood, P. H. (1979). An evaluation of criteria for polymyalgia rheumatica. *Annals of Rheumatic Diseases, 38*, 434–439.

Bisset, L., Beller, E., Jull, G., Brooks, P., Darnell, R., & Vicenzino, B. (2006). Mobilisation with movement and exercise, corticosteroid injection, or wait and see for tennis elbow: Randomised trial. *British Medical Journal (Clinical Research Ed.), 333*, 939–941.

Busch, A. J., Barber, K. A., Overend, T. J., Peloso, P., & Schachter, C. L. (2007). Exercise for treating fibromyalgia syndrome. *The Cochrane Database of Systematic Reviews*, (4), CD003786.

Casimiro, L., Barnsley, L., Brosseau, L., Milne, S., Robinson, V. A., Tugwell, P., & Wells, G. (2005). Acupuncture and electroacupuncture for the treatment of rheumatoid arthritis. *The Cochrane Database of Systatic Reviews*, (4), CD003788, doi:10.1002/14651858. CD003788.pub2.

Clinical Knowledge Summaries. (2009). *How do I treat someone with polymyalgia rheumatica?* National Library for Health. Retrieved from www.cks.library.uk/polymyalgia.

Digiovanni, B. F., Nawoczenski, D. A., Lintal, M. E., Moore, E. A., Murray, J. C., Wilding, G. E., & Baumhauer, J. F. (2003). Tissue-specific plantar fascia-stretching exercise enhances outcomes in patients with chronic heel pain. A prospective, randomized study. *The Journal of Bone and Joint Surgery*, 85, 1270–1277.

Elyan, M., & Khan, M. (2008). Does physical therapy still have a place in the treatment of ankylosing spondylitis? *Current Opinion in Rheumatology*, 20, 282–286.

Fairbank, J. (2008). Prolapsed intervertebral disc. *British Medical Journal (Clinical Research Ed.)*, 336, 1317–1318.

Hazard, R. G., Haugh, L. D., Reid, S., McFarlane, G., & MacDonald, L. (1997). Early physician notification of patient disability risk and clinical guidelines after low back injury: A randomized, controlled trial. *Spine (Phila Pa 1976)*, 22, 2951–2958.

Holdcraft, L. C., Assefi, N., & Buchwald, D. (2003). Complementary and alternative medicine in fibromyalgia and related syndromes. *Best Practice & Research: Clinical Rheumatology*, 17, 667–683.

Janssens, H. J., Janssen, M., van de Lisdonk, E. H., van Riel, P. L., & van Weel, C. (2008). Use of oral prednisolone or naproxen for the treatment of gout arthritis: A double-blind, randomised equivalence trial. *Lancet*, 371, 1854–1860.

Karjalainen, K., Malmivaara, A., Van Tulder, M., Roine, R., Jauhiainen, M., Hurri, H., & Koes, B. (2000). Multidisciplinary rehabilitation for fibromyalgia and musculoskeletal pain in working age adults. *The Cochrane Database of Systematic Reviews*, (2), CD001984.

Kay, T. M., Gross, A., Goldsmith, C., Santaguida, P. L., Hoving, J., Bronfort, G., & Cervical Overview Group. (2005). Exercises for mechanical neck disorders. *The Cochrane Database of Systematic Reviews*, (3), CD004250.

Koes, B. (2009). Corticosteroid injection for rotator cuff disease. *British Medical Journal (Clinical Research Ed.)*, 338, 245–246.

Koh, W. H., Pande, I., Samuels, A., Jones, S. D., & Calin, A. (1997). Low dose amitriptyline in ankylosing spondylitis: A short term, double blind, placebo controlled study. *Journal of Rheumatology*, 24, 2158–2161.

Kovacs, F. M., Abraira, V., Pena, A., Martín-Rodríguez, J. G., Sánchez-Vera, M., Ferrer, E., Ruano, D., Guillén, P., Gestoso, M., Muriel, A., Zamora, J., Gil del Real, M. T., & Mufraggi, N. (2003). Effect of firmness of mattress on chronic non-specific low-back pain: Randomised, double-blind, controlled, multicentre trial. *Lancet*, 362, 1599–1604.

Kyle, V., & Hazleman, B. (1989a). Treatment of polymyalgia rheumatica and giant cell arteritis. I. Steroid regimens in the first two months. *Annals of the Rheumatic Diseases*, 48, 658–661.

Kyle, V., & Hazleman, B. (1989b). Treatment of polymyalgia rheumatica and giant cell arteritis. II. Relation between steroid dose and steroid-associated side effects. *Annals of the Rheumatic Diseases*, 48, 662–666.

Kyle, V., & Hazleman, B. (1993). Clinical and laboratory course of polymyalgia rheumatica/giant cell arteritis after the first two months of treatment. *Annals of the Rheumatic Diseases*, 52, 847–850.

Lin, E. H., Katon, W., Von Korff, M., Tang, L., Williams, J. W., Jr, Kroenke, K., Hunkeler, E., Harpole, L., Hegel, M., Arean, P., Hoffing, M., Della Penna, R., Langston, C., Unützer, J., & IMPACT Investigators. (2003). Effect of improving depression care on pain and functional outcomes among older adults with arthritis: A randomized controlled trial. *JAMA: The Journal of the American Medical Association*, 290, 2428–2429.

Maddison, P., & Huey, P. (2006). *Rheumatic diseases: Serological aids to early diagnosis: Arthritis Research Campaign: Reports on the rheumatic diseases series 5: Topical reviews*. Retrieved from www.arc.org.uk.

Mayo Clinic. (2008). *Rheumatoid arthritis*. Retrieved from www.mayoclinic.com/health/rheumatoid-arthritis/DS00020/DSECTION511.

Nachemson, A., & Jonsson, E. (Eds.). (2000). *Neck and back pain*. Philadelphia, PA: Lippincott Williams & Wilkins.

National Institute for Health and Care Excellence. (2004). *Dyspepsia: Managing dyspepsia in adults in primary care*. Retrieved from https://www.nice.org.uk/guidance/cg184.

National Institute for Health and Care Excellence. (2008b). *Adalimumab, etanercept and infliximab for ankylosing spondylitis (no. 143)*. London: Technology Appraisal Guidance.

National Library for Health. (2008). *Clinical knowledge summaries: Gout management*. Retrieved from https://cks.nice.org.uk/topics/gout/.

New Zealand Guideline Group. (2004). *Management of dyspepsia and heartburn*. Retrieved from www.nzgg.org.nz.

Nichol, G., Stiell, I. G., Wells, G. A., Juergensen, L. S., & Laupacis, A. (1999). An economic analysis of the Ottawa knee rule. *Annals of Emergency Medicine*, 34, 438–447.

O'Malley, P. G., Balden, E., Tomkins, G., Santoro, J., Kroenke, K., & Jackson, J. L. (2000). Treatment of fibromyalgia with antidepressants: A meta-analysis. *Journal of General Internal Medicine*, 15, 659–666.

Sieper, J., & Rudwaleit, M. (2005). Early referral recommendations for ankylosing spondylitis (including pre-radiographic and radiographic forms) in primary care. *Annals of the Rheumatic Diseases*, 64, 659–663.

Silver, T. (1999). *Joint and soft tissue injection, injecting with confidence* (2nd ed.). London: Radcliffe Medical Press.

Towheed, T. E., Maxwell, L., Anastassiades, T. P., Shea, B., Houpt, J., Robinson, V., Hochberg, M. C., & Wells, G. (2005). Glucosamine therapy for treating osteoarthritis. *The Cochrane Database of Systematic Reviews*, (2), CD002946, doi:10.1002/14651858. CD002946.pub2

Tulder, M., Malmivaara, A., Esmail, R., et al. (2000). Exercise therapy for low back pain (Cochrane Review). In *The Cochrane Library*. Oxford: Update Software. Issue 2. https://pubmed.ncbi.nlm.nih.gov/11064524/

Uçay, I. (2008). Antibiotic prophylaxis before invasive dental procedures in patients with arthroplasties of the hip and knee. *Journal of Bone and Joint Surgery*, 90, 833–838.

UK BEAM Trial Team. (2004). United Kingdom back pain exercise and manipulation (UK BEAM) randomised trial: Effectiveness of physical treatments for back pain in primary care. *British Medical Journal (Clinical Research Ed.)*, 329, 1377–1381.

Verdugo, R. J., Salinas, R. S., Castillo, J., & Cea, J. G. (2003). Surgical versus non-surgical treatment for carpal tunnel syndrome. *The Cochrane Database of Systematic Reviews*, (3), CD001552. Retrieved from www.thecochranelibrary.com.

Verhaar, J., Walenkamp, G., Kester, A., van Mameren, H., & van der Linden, T. (1993). Lateral extensor release for tennis elbow. A prospective long-term follow-up study. *Journal of Bone and Joint Surgery*, 75, 1034–1043.

Waddell, G., Feder, G., & Lewis, M. (1997). Systematic reviews of bed rest and advice to stay active for acute low back pain. *British Journal of General Practitioners*, 47, 647–652.

References

Anonymous. (1993) Consensus development conference: Diagnosis, prophylaxis, and treatment of osteoporosis. *American Journal of Medicine, 94*, 646–650.

Arden, N. K., Price, C., Reading, I., Stubbing, J., Hazelgrove, J., Dunne, C., Michel, M., Rogers, P., Cooper, C., & WEST Study Group (2005). A multicentre randomized controlled trial of epidural corticosteroid injections for sciatica: The WEST study. *Rheumatology, 44*, 1399–1406.

Aletaha, D., & Smolen, J. S. (2018). Diagnosis and management of rheumatoid arthritis: A review. *Journal of the American Medical Association, 320*(13), 1360–1372.

Bulloch, B., Neto, G., Plint, A., Lim, R., Lidman, P., Reed, M., Nijssen-Jordan, C., Tenenbein, M., Klassen, T. P., Bhargava, R., & Pediatric Emergency Researchers of Canada (2003). Validation of the Ottawa knee rule in children: A multicenter study. *Annals of Emergency Medicine, 42*, 48–55.

Derry, S., Conaghan, P., Da Silva, J. A., Wiffen, P. J., & Moore, R. A. (2016). Topical NSAIDs for chronic musculoskeletal pain in adults. *The Cochrane Database of Systematic Reviews 4*, CD007400. doi:10.1002/14651858.CD007400.pub3.

Dias, R., Cutts, S., & Massoud, S. (2005). Frozen shoulder. *British Medical Journal (Clinical Research Ed.), 331*, 1453–1456.

Ferrari, J. (2003). *Bunions*. Clinical Evidence. Retrieved from www.clinicalevidence.com.

Frank, A. (1993). Low back pain. *British Medical Journal (Clinical Research Ed.), 306*, 90.

Gibson, J. (2007). Surgery for disc disease. *British Medical Journal (Clinical Research Ed.), 335*, 949.

Green, S., Buchbinder, R., & Hetrick, S. (2003). Physiotherapy interventions for shoulder pain. *Cochrane Database of Systematic Reviews*, (2), CD004258, Retrieved from www.thecochranelibrary.com.

Gross, A. R., Hoving, J. L., Haines, T. A., Goldsmith, C. H., Kay, T., Aker, P., Bronfort, G., & Cervical overview group (2004). Manipulation and mobilisation for mechanical neck disorders. *The Cochrane Database of Systematic Reviews*, (1), CD004249.

Guzmán, J., Esmail, R., Karjalainen, K., Malmivaara, A., Irvin, E., & Bombardier, C. (2001). Multidisciplinary rehabilitation for chronic low back pain: Systematic review. *British Medical Journal (Clinical Research Ed.), 322*, 1511–1516.

Hagen, E., Eriksen, H., & Ursin, H. (2000). Does early intervention with a light mobilization program reduce long-term sick leave for low back pain? *Spine (Phila Pa 1976), 28*, 2309–2316.

Heintjes, E., Berger, M. Y., Bierma-Zeinstra, S. M., Bernsen, R. M., Verhaar, J. A., & Koes, B. W. (2003a). Exercise therapy for patellofemoral pain syndrome. *The Cochrane Database of Systematic Reviews*, (4), CD003472. Retrieved from www.thecochranelibrary.com.

Heintjes, E., Berger, M. Y., Bierma-Zeinstra, S. M., Bernsen, R. M., Verhaar, J. A., & Koes, B. W. (2003b). Pharmacotherapy for patellofemoral pain syndrome. *The Cochrane Database of Systematic Reviews*, (3), CD003470. Retrieved from www.thecochranelibrary.com.

Honvo, G., Leclercq, V., Geerinck, A., Thomas, T., Veronese, N., Charles, A., Rabenda, V., Beaudart, C., Cooper, C., Reginster, J. Y., & Bruyère, O. (2019). Safety of topical non-steroidal anti-inflammatory drugs in osteoarthritis: Outcomes of a systematic review and meta-analysis. *Drugs Aging, 36*(Suppl. 1), 45–64. doi:10.1007/s40266-019-00661-0.

Institute for Clinical Systems Improvement. (2003). *Ankle sprain*. Bloomington, MN. Retrieved from www.ngc.gov/anklesprain.

Kerkhoffs, G. M., Rowe, B. H., Assendelft, W. J., Kelly, K., Struijs, P. A., & van Dijk, C. N. (2002). Immobilisation and functional treatment for acute lateral ankle ligament injuries in adults. *The Cochrane Database of Systematic Reviews*, (3), CD003762.

Khan, K. M., Cook, J. L., Kannus, P., Maffulli, N., & Bonar, S. F. (2002). Time to abandon the 'tendinitis' myth. *British Medical Journal (Clinical Research Ed.), 324*, 626–627.

Koes, B. W., Assendelft, W. J., van der Heijden, G. J., & Bouter, L. M. (1996). Spinal manipulation for low back pain: An updated systematic review of randomized clinical trials. *Spine (Phila Pa 1976), 21*, 2860–2871.

Maffulli, N. (1999). Rupture of the Achilles tendon. *The Journal of Bone and Joint Surgery, 7*, 1019–1036.

Mason, V. (1994). *The prevalence of back pain in Great Britain*. London: OPCS HMSO.

National Prescribing Centre. (2007). *Cardiovascular and gastrointestinal safety of NSAIDs*. MeReC extra issue No 30. Retrieved from www.npc.co.uk/MeReC_Extra/2008/no30_2007.html.

Peul, W. C., van Houwelingen, H. C., van den Hout, W. B., Brand, R., Eekhof, J. A., Tans, J. T., Thomeer, R. T., Koes, B. W., & Leiden-The Hague Spine Intervention Prognostic Study Group (2007). Surgery versus prolonged conservative treatment for sciatica. *The New England Journal of Medicine, 356*, 2245–2256.

Pountain, G., & Hazleman, B. (1995). Polymyalgia rheumatica and giant cell arteritis. *British Medical Journal (Clinical Research Ed.), 310*, 1057–1059.

Rompe, J. D., Decking, J., Schoellner, C., & Nafe, B. (2003). Shock wave application for chronic plantar fasciitis in running athletes. A prospective, randomized, placebo-controlled trial. *American Journal of Sports Medicine, 31*, 268–275.

Royal College of Radiologists. (2003). *Making the best use of a department of clinical radiology* (5th ed.). London: RCR.

Simon, L. S., Grierson, L. M., Naseer, Z., Bookman, A. A. M., & Shainhouse, Z. J. (2009). Efficacy and safety of topical diclofenac containing dimethyl sulfoxide (DMSO) compared with those of topical placebo, DMSO vehicle and oral diclofenac for knee osteoarthritis. *Pain, 143*, 238–245. doi:10.1016/j.pain.2009.03.008.

Smith, G. (2003). Sprains and soft tissues injuries: Do you know the latest priorities? *The New Generalist, 1*(4), 21–22.

Speed, C. (2001). Corticosteroid injections in tendon lesions. *British Medical Journal (Clinical Research Ed.), 323*, 382–386.

Speed, C., & Hazelman, B. (2001). *Shoulder pain. Clinical evidence.* London: BMJ Publishing Group.

Staiger, T. O., Gaster, B., Sullivan, M. D., & Deyo, R. A. (2003). Systematic review of antidepressants in the treatment of chronic low back pain. *Spine (Phila Pa 1976), 28*, 2540–2545.

Vroomen, P., de Krom, M., & Knotterus, J. (1999). Diagnostic value of history and physical examination in patients suspected of sciatica due to disc herniation: A systematic review. *Journal of Neurology, 246*, 899–906.

Wolfe, F., Smythe, H. A., Yunus, M. B., Bennett, R. M., Bombardier, C., Goldenberg, D. L., Tugwell, P., Campbell, S. M., Abeles, M., & Clark, P. (1990). The American College of Rheumatology 1990 criteria for the classification of fibromyalgia: Report of the multicenter criteria committee. *Arthritis and Rheumatology, 33*, 160–172.

11

Neurologic Problems

Kate Robinson

CHAPTER CONTENTS

Headache

Headaches account for 4.4% of consultations in primary care and 30% of neurology outpatient appointments. Headaches are a cause of pain and disability, a substantial societal burden, and an important cause of absence from work and school.

For details of assessment of headaches, refer to the guidelines box or National Institute for Health and Care Excellence (NICE) Pathways. The British Association for the Study of Headache (BASH) has produced an updated 'headache management system' aimed at both clinicians and patients, containing guidance which is both of class A quality and appears in at least two guidelines at the international level.

GUIDELINES

British Association for the Study of Headache. (2019). *National headache management system for adults 2019*. Retrieved from https://headache.org.uk/wp-content/uploads/2023/02/bash-guideline-2019.pdf.

National Institute for Health and Care Excellence. (2012; updated 2015). *Headaches in over 12s: Diagnosis and management. NICE clinical guideline 150*. Retrieved from https://www.nice.org.uk/guidance/CG150.

Scottish Intercollegiate Guidelines Network. (2023). *Pharmacological management of Migraine. Guidelines no. 155*. Retrieved from https://www.sign.ac.uk/media/2077/sign-155-migraine-2023-update-v3.pdf.

- Most of the time, a thorough history will suffice to confidently diagnose a primary headache condition. A normal neurologic examination is helpful in excluding a secondary headache condition when the history is suggestive of migraine or tension headache but not other headache types. When a positive diagnosis of primary headache has been made:
  a. A patient-centred approach to the management of primary headache should be sought, including explanation of diagnosis, reassurance that serious underlying pathology has been excluded, discussion about options for management, and the offering of written information (including support groups).
  b. Headache diaries are useful in both diagnosis of headache and monitoring the effectiveness of headache interventions, as well as recognition of impact.
  c. Early discussion on the risks of medication overuse should be prioritised.
  d. Recognition of the impact of the condition on daily life is essential to validate the patient's lived experience.
- Do not refer people diagnosed with tension-type, migraine, or cluster headaches for neuroimaging solely for reassurance.

Migraine (With or Without Aura)

- The most disabling of the primary headache conditions, migraine occurs in 15% of the UK adult population and results in more than 100,000 absences every working day.
- Chronic migraine, in which a person has 15 days or more with symptoms per month for 3 consecutive months or more, affects 2% of the population.

After the Diagnosis Has Been Made

- Explain that the majority of patients can be successfully treated, but finding the best treatment can take time.
- Discuss lifestyle changes that might make a difference (see later).
- Discuss the possibility of nondrug therapies (see later).
- Make a follow-up appointment at a time calculated to give the patient a chance to have had three or four further attacks.

Initial, Complementary, and Lifestyle Management

- Patient expectations should be addressed, with emphasis on control of symptoms via a trial-and-error approach rather than cure.
- A discussion to identify potential triggers can be helpful. Food triggers should only be accepted if migraine symptoms occur within 6 hours of ingestion, the association can be repeated, and avoidance reduces frequency of attacks.
- Encourage physical fitness, provided exercise does not trigger attacks.
- Stop combined oral contraceptives (COCs) in any female whose migraine starts or worsens when taking them, especially if focal symptoms develop; there is an increased risk of cerebral thrombosis.
- Patient self-report questionnaires such as Headache Impact test (HIT-6) can be used to assess quality of life.
- Cognitive-behavioural therapy should be considered when there is significant associated disability.
- Evidence exists for benefit from acupuncture in patients with chronic migraine, and NICE suggests considering this if first-line drug prophylaxis is unsuitable or ineffective.
- Riboflavin 400 mg/day may be effective in reducing migraine frequency and intensity for some people.
- Limited evidence exists for benefit from manual therapy such as chiropractic treatment; NICE highlights the risk of cervical artery dissection or stroke with neck manipulation.

Acute Treatment

- A stratified approach (in which treatment is aligned to symptom severity) is now favoured over the traditional stepwise approach because of better health outcomes and improved cost-effectiveness.
- Use of drugs in the acute attack is only useful for headache and nausea symptoms, not aura. Their effectiveness should be judged by improvement or resolution of symptoms within 2 hours.
- Opioids should be avoided because of a risk of medication overuse, and ergots should be avoided because of comparably poor efficacy and worse side effect profile.
- Antiemetics should be considered even in the absence of nausea and vomiting because absorption of oral analgesics is enhanced.

- Reconsider the diagnosis in a patient who uses rescue medication more than once per week.
  NICE guidelines suggest:
- A first-line choice of combination therapy (triptan plus nonsteroidal antiinflammatory drug [NSAID] or triptan plus paracetamol), taking into account the patient's preference, comorbidities, and risk of adverse events. Monotherapy, if preferred, can be used. Options include a triptan, NSAID (e.g., ibuprofen 400–600 mg qds (four times daily)), aspirin (900 mg stat (single dose)) or paracetamol (1 g stat).
- For people aged 12 to 17 years, consider a nasal triptan in preference to an oral triptan.
- Aspirin should not be offered to patients younger than 16 years of age because of the association with Reye syndrome.
- Rimegepant, an oral calcitonin gene-related peptide (CGRP) antagonist, has recently been approved by NICE for the acute treatment of migraine when there is intolerance to or treatment failure of NSAIDs and paracetamol combination and at least two triptans.
- In patients who respond and then relapse, repeat the medication that worked earlier provided that doing so does not exceed the dosage limits. All triptans are associated with a return of symptoms within 48 hours in 20% to 50% of those who initially responded. In those who can be predicted to relapse, give naproxen 500 mg or tolfenamic acid 200 mg, along with sumatriptan 100 mg.
- For people in whom oral preparations (or nasal preparations in those aged 12–17 years) for the acute treatment of migraine are ineffective or not tolerated:
  a. Offer a nonoral preparation of metoclopramide or prochlorperazine.
  b. Consider adding a nonoral NSAID or triptan if these have not been tried.

Antiemetics

Scottish Intercollegiate Guidelines Network (SIGN) and BASH suggest use of:
- Prochlorperazine 3- to 6-mg buccal tablets, domperidone 10 mg orally, or 30 mg rectally for nausea and vomiting
- Metoclopramide 10 mg or domperidone 20 mg as prokinetics to promote gastric emptying

Use of Triptans

- Triptans vary in individual response and tolerability. NICE recommends starting with sumatriptan 50-100 mg and try one or more alternative if ineffective. When vomiting prevents oral administration, intranasal or subcutaneous versions should be tried over 'melt' preparations. BASH advises that an alternative triptan be tried after two treatment failures.
- Triptans should be taken at the start of the headache phase, ideally when the pain is less severe. Triptans appear to be ineffective if administered during the aura.

- Triptans are contraindicated in patients with cardiovascular and cerebrovascular disorders and severe hepatic impairment.
- Triptans are not indicated for hemiplegic, basilar, or ophthalmoplegic migraine; it is unlicensed for use in those older than 65 years of age.
- Warn patients regarding side effects (tingling, heat, heaviness, pressure, or tightness in any part of the body, including the chest and throat); discontinue if side effects are intense or flushing, dizziness, or vomiting occurs.

Prophylaxis

- Consider prophylaxis in patients whose life is sufficiently disturbed by attacks. Whereas BASH recommends offering it to patients with four or more migraine episodes per month, NICE recommends considering prophylaxis when episodes are prolonged or severe, or there is more than one episode a week.
- Discuss the benefits and risks of prophylactic treatment, taking into account the person's preferences, comorbidities, and risk of adverse events, as well as the impact of the headaches on quality of life.
- NICE recommends use of propranolol, topiramate, or amitriptyline as first-line agents.
  - Propranolol: Initially 80 mg/day (either 40 mg bd (twice daily) or 80 mg MR od (once daily)). The dosage may be increased to 160 mg/day and subsequently to 240 mg/day if necessary (either in divided doses or once daily if MR (modified release)). BASH, however, recommend the use of atenolol 25 to 100 mg bd or metoprolol 50 to 100 mg bd over propranolol.
  - Topiramate: Initially 25 mg at night for 1 week; then increase in steps of 25 mg at weekly intervals. The usual dosage is 50 to 100 mg/day in two divided doses, and the maximum dosage is 200 mg/day. Not licensed for patients younger than 18 years of age.
    - Advise female patients with childbearing potential that topiramate is associated with fetal malformations and can impair the effectiveness of hormonal contraception. Ensure female patients are on appropriate contraception.
    - The drug should not be stopped rapidly. If the patient has any visual problems, reduce and stop the drug as rapidly as possible while seeking urgent advice from an ophthalmologist; acute myopia and secondary angle-closure glaucoma can occur.
  - Amitriptyline: 10 to 150 mg at night. This is likely to be especially helpful in patients with a combination of migraine and tension headaches.
- In addition, BASH also recommends candesartan 2 to 16 mg (unlicensed).
- Titrate each drug up to the effective or maximum recommended dose.

- Try each for 6 to 8 weeks at full dose before abandoning it, using a headache diary to assess impact.
- Continue an effective medication for 6 months before considering if remission has been achieved and a two- to three-month tapering withdrawal could be tried.
- If both topiramate and propranolol are unsuitable or ineffective, NICE suggest considering a course of up to 10 sessions of acupuncture over 5 to 8 weeks.
- Use only one prophylactic drug at a time except as an extreme measure, although the combination of a beta-blocker and amitriptyline may be useful in patients who also have tension-type headaches.
- Alternative options:
  a. *Rimegepant* has been recently approved by NICE. It can be used when three or more traditional preventatives have been ineffective and the patient has 4 to 15 episodes per month.
  b. *Antidepressants.* Venlafaxine 75 to 150 mg/day is an unlicensed alternative. To avoid misunderstanding, explain that you are not giving them for their antidepressant effect.
  c. *Sodium valproate* is helpful both in migraine and tension-type headache. Initially 200 mg bd, increased if necessary to 1.5 g in divided doses. It is licensed.
  d. *Calcium channel blockers.* Nifedipine, verapamil, and diltiazem are thought to be effective in conventional doses, but there is a lack of evidence, and they are unlicensed.
- Do not use ergots or gabapentin.
- When the above are unsuitable or ineffective, referral can be made for consideration of an CGRP monoclonal antibody (e.g., galcanezumab, erenumab, fremanezumab injections; eptinezumab infusion), methysergide, or Botox treatment.
- There is some evidence to support greater occipital nerve block in chronic migraine, though research is ongoing.

Botulinum Toxin Type A

NICE has recommended the use of Botox as an option for prophylaxis of headache in adults with chronic migraine (defined as headaches on at least 15 days per month of which at least 8 days are with migraine) with both of the following:
- That have not responded to at least three prior pharmacological prophylaxis therapies
- Whose condition is appropriately managed for medication overuse (NICE, 2012)

Migraine in Females of Reproductive Age

Menstrual Migraine

- Suspect menstrual migraine if migraine occurs predominantly between 2 days before and 3 days after the start of menstruation in at least two of three menstrual cycles. Use a headache diary to diagnose.
- If standard acute treatment fails to give an adequate response, consider intermittent prophylaxis.
- *Frovatriptan* (2.5 mg twice a day) or *zolmitriptan* (2.5 mg twice or three times a day) on the days migraine is expected is recommended by NICE (off-label use). Warn the patient that they may experience rebound headache after stopping the triptan.
- *An NSAID*, traditionally mefenamic acid 500 mg tds (three times daily) or naproxen, starting 2 days before the migraine is expected and ending after the risk has passed, usually 2 to 3 days after the onset of menses. Although widely used, there is limited evidence for this.
- *Oestrogen supplementation.* Targeted oestrogen supplementation can be considered but is not recommended by NICE, SIGN, or BASH, and there is risk of rebound attacks.
- *Females already on COCs.* Consider the tricycle regimen to reduce the frequency of menstruation to once every 10 weeks (i.e., take the pill continuously for 9 weeks rather than 3 followed by the usual 7-day pill-free interval). If migraine with aura occurs while the patient is on COCs, it must be stopped.

Migraine and Oral Oestrogens

- *Migraine with aura.* NICE advise not to use combined hormonal contraceptives for contraception in females with migraine with aura. This supports the UKMEC (UK Medical Eligibility Criteria for Contraceptive Use) advice that this would present an unacceptable risk to the individual because of increased risk of ischaemic stroke.
- *Migraine without aura.* Use the COC up to the age of 35 years, provided there are no other risk factors for vascular disease and the patient is not using ergotamine.
- *Menopause.* Use hormone replacement therapy (HRT) if indicated. There is no evidence that its use increases stroke risk, although the migraine itself may be exacerbated. If so, consider changing HRT, and SIGN suggests if taking oral HRT to consider transdermal as an alternative.

Migraine in Pregnancy and Lactation

- Most females find that their migraines improve in pregnancy. In those still troubled by attacks, the treatment options are limited.
- Offer paracetamol as first-line treatment for acute treatment. Consider use of sumatriptan or ibuprofen as second-line treatment. Do not prescribe aspirin or opiates. For nausea, metoclopramide and domperidone are unlikely to cause harm throughout pregnancy and lactation.
- Be wary of making a new diagnosis of migraine in a pregnant female patient. Cerebral venous thrombosis may mimic migraine.

- In lactating females, use paracetamol, ibuprofen, diclofenac, and/or domperidone. Sumatriptan is probably safe.
- Seek specialist advice if prophylactic treatment is needed during pregnancy. This is not commonly required.

Cluster Headaches (Migrainous Neuralgia)

Despite similarities in presentation, cluster headaches are much rarer than migraine and more likely to be found in middle-aged male smokers. Key features include restlessness rather than motion sensitivity, strictly unilateral headache, and ipsilateral autonomic features (e.g., lacrimation, nasal congestion or rhinorrhoea, eyelid drooping).

Acute Treatment

- Discuss the need for neuroimaging for people with a first bout of cluster headache with a specialist.
- *Parenteral triptans* (e.g., sumatriptan subcutaneously or zolmitriptan 5 mg intranasally (IN) off-label use) relieve pain in 73% to 96% of people within 15 minutes.
- *100% oxygen* at a flow rate of at least 12 L/min through a nonrebreathing mask and reservoir bag for 10 to 20 minutes aborts an attack in some people. If found to be useful in accident and emergency (A&E), arrange provision of home and ambulatory oxygen.
- Do not offer paracetamol, NSAIDs, opioids, ergots, or oral triptans.

Prevention

- Attacks are so devastating that prevention is needed in most cases.
- Consider *verapamil 80 mg* tds, increasing as high as 320 mg tds for prophylaxis during a bout of cluster headache. Seek specialist advice regarding dosage regimes. BASH recommends an electrocardiogram at baseline, after any dose increase, or at 6-month intervals if stable (risk of atrioventricular block). It will stop two-thirds of episodes after attacks begin.
- Seek specialist advice for cluster headache that does not respond to verapamil. Greater occipital nerve block is considered an effective alternative.

PATIENT ORGANISATION

Organisation for the Understanding of Cluster Headache (OUCH). Pyramid House, 956 High Road, London, N12 9RX. Tel: 01646 651979. Available at http://www.ouchuk.org.

Nonmigrainous Headache

- A history and simple examination (blood pressure, fundi, and a search for focal neurologic signs) permit a clinical diagnosis in most patients. The erythrocyte sedimentation rate may be needed in patients older than 50 years of age to exclude giant cell arteritis. Cervical spondylosis, sinusitis, intracranial haemorrhage, and other conditions of which headache is a symptom need treatment in their own right.
- *Analgesic headache* may complicate management and is most likely to occur in patients taking analgesics combined with benzodiazepines or opioids.

Tension-Type Headache

- Exclude conditions which can be associated with tension-type headache, including cervical spondylosis, poor neck posture, temporomandibular joint dysfunction, sinus pain, and eye muscle disorders.
- Explore the tensions in the patient's life; screen for depression.
- Explain that the condition is real and benign and that treatment aims at reducing the frequency and severity of symptoms rather than cure. Reassurance is very important.
- Advise exercise (tension-type headache is more commonly seen in sedentary people) and consider physiotherapy, cognitive-behavioural therapy, or relaxations techniques. Acupuncture may be useful.
- Consider sparing use of aspirin, paracetamol, or an NSAID as acute treatment but do not offer opioids.
- Consider prophylaxis in those whose attacks are severe or occur on 2 or more days per week:
  - NICE suggests offering a trial of amitriptyline (off-label use) to those with frequent episodic or chronic tension headaches, in whom conservative measures are insufficient. A significant effect can be expected in 25% to 50% of patients.
- Aim to tail off prophylactic treatment after 4 to 6 months if remission has occurred.

Medication-Overuse Headache

- Establish the diagnosis. Headache may be daily or at least 15 days per month in people overusing acute relief medication for an underlying headache disorder. This does not occur in people using analgesia for other painful conditions such as arthritis. Consider it in patients who have taken simple analgesics on 15 days per month or more for at least 3 months or who have taken a triptan, ergotamine, opioids, or combination analgesics for 10 days per month or more for at least 3 months.
- Explain the diagnosis to the patient. Patients are often hard to convince, especially the minority whose headaches take up to 2 months without analgesics to resolve.
- Explain that it is treated by withdrawing overused medications. Advise people to stop taking all overused acute headache medications for at least 1 month and to stop abruptly rather than gradually.
- Advise that headache symptoms are likely to get worse in the short term (2–10 days) before they gradually improve (12 weeks) and that there may be associated withdrawal symptoms. Offer close follow-up and support.

- Consider specialist referral or advice if using strong opioids, the patient has relevant comorbidities, or in patients in whom repeated attempts at withdrawal have been unsuccessful. Relapse is common with 40% estimated to relapse within 1 year (Anonymous, 2010).
- Consider prophylactic treatment for the underlying primary headache disorder in addition to stopping overused medication.
- Review the diagnosis of medication-overuse headache and further management at 4 to 8 weeks after the start of withdrawal of overused medications.
- Withdrawal headaches can be managed with naproxen 250 mg tds or 500 mg bd. Some specialists recommend a prolonged period of this treatment for 3 to 4 weeks and not repeated, but there are no studies to support this. When nausea and vomiting are present, antiemetics can be used.

Chronic Daily Headache

This is said to exist when headache lasts for at least 4 hours and occurs at least 15 days a month. Most patients have one or more of the following: migraine, tension-type headache, or analgesic-overuse headache. Management is of the underlying cause. If analgesic-overuse headache is present, tackle that first.

Chronic Paroxysmal Hemicrania

- These are repeated attacks of unilateral headache lasting less than 45 minutes.
- Indomethacin 25 to 75 mg tds, reducing to 25 mg/day, should prevent attacks. Indeed, if it does not, reconsider the diagnosis.

Exertional and Coital Headache

- Give an NSAID or propranolol before attacks after a pattern is established. This should be a diagnosis of exclusion, having ruled out subarachnoid bleeding, for example.

Severe Headache of Sudden Onset

- Refer urgently if the first attack is sufficiently severe to present acutely. It may be a subarachnoid haemorrhage, presaging a more severe bleed.

Increased Intracranial Pressure

- This is rarely the cause of headache in a patient without vomiting, papilledema, or neurologic signs. However, exceptions occur.
- Refer patients with a short history of headache (<4 months), especially if it is localised, worse on waking, worse on coughing or straining, and especially in older patients.

Epilepsy

GUIDELINES

National Institute for Health and Clinical Excellence. (2022). *Epilepsies in children, young people and adults. NICE clinical guideline 217.* Retrieved from https://www.nice.org.uk/guidance/ng217/resources/epilepsies-in-children-young-people-and-adults-pdf-66143780239813.
Scottish Intercollegiate Guidelines Network. (2015; revised 2018). *Diagnosis and management of epilepsy in adults. SIGN guideline no. 143.* Retrieved from https://www.sign.ac.uk/media/1079/sign143_2018.pdf.

Management of a Major Seizure

1. Protect the patient from injury: cushion the head, remove glasses, and move away from nearby hazards when possible.
2. Prevent onlookers from restraining the seizing patient or putting anything in their mouth.
3. Do not give drugs initially; the seizure is likely to have stopped before they can act. Give drugs if the seizure continues without signs of abating after 5 minutes or if three seizures occur within 1 hour.
4. When seizure stops, check their airway and put the person in the recovery position.
5. Check the patient's cardiovascular and neurologic status.
6. Admit any patient with a seizure if:
   - There is suspicion that the seizure is secondary to other illness.
   - This is their first seizure.
   - The patient fails to recover completely after the seizure (other than feeling sleepy).
   - There is status epilepticus.

Emergency Management of Prolonged or Repeated Seizures, Including Status Epilepticus, in the Community

- Initiate treatment if a seizure lasts longer than 5 minutes or there are more than three in 1 hour:
  1. Check ABCs (airways, breathing, and circulation).
  2. Provide high-flow oxygen if available.
  3. Check the blood glucose with a test strip.
  4. NICE recommends administering buccal midazolam as first-line treatment for children, young people, and adults in the community. Use rectal diazepam if preferred or if buccal midazolam is not available.
- *Adults*:
  - Administer buccal midazolam 10 mg first line.
  - Rectal diazepam as an alternative: 10 to 20 mg rectally, repeating 15 minutes later if necessary.
- *Children.* Give buccal midazolam: 0.5 mg/kg, to a maximum of 10 mg. The British National Formulary (BNF) for Children suggests:
  - 0 to 3 months: 0.3 mg (300 μg)/kg up to a maximum of 2.5 mg
  - 3 months to 1 year: 2.5 mg
  - 1 to 5 years: 5 mg

- 5 to 10 years: 7.5 mg
- 10 to 18 years: 10 mg
- All doses can be repeated once after 10 minutes if necessary.
- At the time of writing, midazolam oromucosal solution is not licensed for use in children younger than 3 months of age, and some preparations of rectal diazepam are not licensed for children younger than 1 year of age.

5. Call an ambulance (this will depend on response to treatment, the individual's situation, and any personalised care plan), particularly if:
   - Seizure is continuing 5 minutes after the emergency medication has been given.
   - The patient has a history of frequent episodes of serial seizures or status epilepticus.
   - This is the patient's first seizure.
   - There are difficulties monitoring the person's ABCs.

- *Convulsive status epilepticus* exists when a convulsive seizure continues for a prolonged period (>5 minutes) or when convulsive seizures occur one after the other with no recovery in between. This is a medical emergency.

Subsequent Management

- A single seizure is not necessarily epilepsy. The risk of a second seizure occurring within 2 years is about 50%. After a second seizure, the risk of a third is about 70% (Rugg-Gunn & Sander, 2012). Initial screening generally takes place in A&E with onward referral for specialist assessment. Some patients may present to their general practitioners (GPs) after these events.
- Urgently refer for neurologic assessment to be seen, if possible within 2 weeks, because of the need to exclude an underlying cause and because of the implications for work and driving. Refer more urgently if there are multiple seizures or focal neurologic signs. The only patient who need not be referred is a child aged 18 months to 5 years who has recovered promptly from a febrile convulsion.
- The NICE guideline recommends that referral without drug treatment should be the norm. Initiation of antiepileptic treatment should only be considered in exceptional circumstances after discussion with specialist services.
- After the diagnosis of epilepsy has been made and a decision taken about drug treatment, the role of the GP depends on who else is on the team. An epilepsy nurse specialist may be best suited to act as key worker, but the GP is best placed to see the epilepsy in the context of the patient's other medical needs and is the only professional in the community available out of hours.
- Whoever undertakes it, follow-up must be structured, with a review at least annually and defaulters sought out. Depression and anxiety should be screened for.
- Repeat prescriptions of drugs and a policy of waiting until a patient complains of problems are inadequate. The NICE guideline recommends that the care plan be in writing; that it should be agreed by professionals, patient, and carers; and that it should include details of

how to access care, about drug treatment (including benefits and possible adverse effects), and about lifestyle issues (e.g., employment, driving, and swimming).
- Re-referral is needed when:
   a. Control is poor or the drugs are causing side effects.
   b. Seizures have continued for 5 years.
   c. There are pointers to a previously unsuspected cause for the seizures.
   d. Concurrent illness complicates management.
   e. There is concern over epilepsy or its treatment causing cognitive impairment.
   f. The patient needs preconceptual advice.
   g. The patient needs withdrawal of antiepileptic drugs (AEDs).

Initial Management

- Find out how much the patient and their family or carers understand about epilepsy and answer their questions. Issues to include in discussions are:
   a. *Support.* Offer verbal and written information about epilepsy and signpost to support groups (see box).
   b. *Risk management.* Discuss first aid and safety at home, school, and work.
   c. Prognosis. In 80% of patients with epilepsy, seizures can be controlled with drug treatment (Rugg-Gunn & Sander, 2012).
- Acknowledge the distress and anger the patient and family feel at the disruption this diagnosis has brought to their lives.
- *Driving.* Advise the patient of the need to notify the Driver and Vehicle Licensing Agency (DVLA; in the United Kingdom) and the insurance company of any seizure, however minor. Document this advice. A licence is likely to be withdrawn until one of the following applies:
   a. The patient is free from seizures for 1 year.
   b. The patient's seizures in the past year have been while asleep *and* the patient has had seizures while asleep for more than 3 years with no seizures while awake in that time. Seizures at the time of waking or falling asleep count as 'daytime' seizures.
- *Employment.* Advise the patient not to work at heights or near dangerous machinery. An HGV (Heavy Goods Vehicle) or PSV (Public Service Vehicle) licence will be lost until the patient is seizure free for 10 years.
- *Lifestyle.* Stress the positive side of how few changes there need to be. Swimming is possible provided someone else is present who could save the person's life if necessary, provided the patient is not in one of the higher risk categories (see later). Avoid bathing a baby alone. Cycling in traffic is probably unwise. Counsel the patient about disclosing the diagnosis to their friends and employers.

Epilepsy Society. Chesham Lane, Chalfont St Peter, Bucks SL9 ORJ. Helpline: 01494 601400 for details of local groups and as an excellent source of information. Available at http://www.epilepsysociety.org.uk.

The Joint Epilepsy Council's website has links to all the UK and Irish patient organisations: Available at http://www.jointepilepsycouncil.org.uk.

The Danger of Swimming

- The danger of swimming for a patient with epilepsy varies according to clinical situation, as follows, compared with the general population:
  - All types of epilepsy: ×15
  - Prevalent epilepsy: ×18
  - Epilepsy and learning disability: ×26
  - Temporal lobe excision performed: ×41
  - Epilepsy and in institutional care: ×97

Drug Treatment

- Epilepsy is not a single condition but rather an umbrella term for a number of conditions. First-line treatment and adjuvant therapy are outlined by NICE based on the type of epilepsy diagnosed. This will be a specialist decision following discussion with the patient and their family or carers to include risks and side effects.
- Treatment with an AED is generally started after the second epileptic seizure and diagnosis is confirmed with a specialist. Exceptions to this do occur.
- Consistent use of the same manufacturer's preparations is recommended.
- NICE recommend monotherapy whenever possible. If this fails, monotherapy with a different drug is advised. Only when control is not achieved with any first-line drug should an add-on drug be given as well.
- Antiepileptic treatment is associated with a small increased risk of suicidal thoughts and behaviour. Patients and caregivers should be alert to signs of this throughout treatment (Medicines and Healthcare Products Regulatory Agency, 2008).
- Be alert to the use of sodium valproate in females of childbearing age because of the risk of congenital malformation and neurodevelopmental effects. All females of potential childbearing age *must* be on the Pregnancy Prevention Programme (PPP; see later).

NICE Recommendations for Treatment in Epilepsy

- *Tonic–clonic or generalised seizures*
  - First-line treatment in all but females of reproductive age: sodium valproate; initially 300 mg bd, increased gradually (in steps of 150–300 mg) every 3 days. Usual maintenance is 1 to 2 g. Maximum is 2.5 g with specialist advice.
  - First-line treatment in females of reproductive age and second-line treatment in all others: lamotrigine (initially 25 mg od as monotherapy, increased fortnightly to 100–200 mg/day) or levetiracetam.
  - Adjunctive treatment options include clobazam, lamotrigine, levetiracetam, perampanel, sodium valproate (except females of reproductive age), or topiramate.
- *Focal seizures*
  - First-line treatment: lamotrigine or levetiracetam
  - Second-line treatment: carbamazepine (initially 100–200 mg once or twice daily, increased slowly (100–200 mg every 2 weeks); usual dose is 0.8 to 1.2 g/day in divided doses), oxcarbazepine, or zonisamide
  - Adjunctive treatment options include carbamazepine, lacosamide, lamotrigine, levetiracetam, oxcarbazepine, topiramate, and zonisamide.
- *Petit mal or absence seizures*
  - First-line treatment is ethosuximide, second-line or add-on treatment is sodium valproate, and third-line or add-on treatment is lamotrigine or levetiracetam.
- *Myoclonic seizures*
  - Sodium valproate or levetiracetam in females of reproductive potential.

Practical Points

- *Adverse effects.* Before starting a new drug, note the adverse effects listed, for instance, in the BNF, and discuss them with the patient.
- *Compliance.* Explain the importance of not missing doses and especially of not stopping treatment abruptly. Poor compliance may be a sign that the patient does not fully accept the diagnosis.
- *Alcohol.* Explain that moderate drinking of 1 to 3.5 units per day twice a week has no effect on seizure control; 1 to 2 units a day is probably safe. Heavier drinking may induce a seizure and interact with AEDs.
- *Drugs bought over the counter*
  a. *Aspirin.* Warn patients taking sodium valproate against taking intermittent aspirin. It displaces valproate from protein-binding sites and so potentiates it. If regular aspirin is needed, the dose of valproate may need to be reduced to allow for this.
  b. *St John's wort.* It reduces plasma concentrations of carbamazepine and phenytoin.

Special Considerations for Epilepsy in Females

- Careful counselling, with their partners if appropriate, about contraception, conception, pregnancy, and breast-feeding should be required.
- *Sodium valproate and the PPP*
  - Valproate must no longer be used in any female able to have children unless they have a PPP in place.
  - There must be an annual review with a specialist, including a risk acknowledgement form signed by the patient.
  - This is because of the high risk of birth defects (1 in 10: spina bifida and malformations of the face, skull, limbs, heart, kidneys, urinary tract, and sexual organs)

and developmental disorders (4 in 10). The is also evidence of a link to increased risk of autistic spectrum disorders and attention-deficit hyperactivity disorder.

- *Planning pregnancy and pregnancy*
  - Early specialist referral is indicated, ideally before conception, for advice regarding the risks and benefits of medication adjustment. The risks associated with inadequate seizure control are considered more detrimental to foetuses than use of AEDs. For unplanned pregnancies, patients should be advised not to stop any AEDs and be referred urgently.
  - Offer all females taking AEDs 5 mg of folic acid daily. This should be continued throughout first trimester.
  - The risk of seizure during labour is low but sufficient to recommend delivery in an obstetric led unit.
  - Vitamin K is indicated for the baby on delivery (1 mg intramuscularly) because of the risk of neonatal haemorrhage associated with AEDs.
  - Most females on monotherapy should be encouraged to breastfeed. If the patient is on combination therapy or has other risk factors, such as premature birth, seek specialist advice.
- *Contraception and AED therapy*
  - Enzyme-inducing AEDs may reduce the effect of COCP, POP, and progesterone implants.
  - Enzyme inducers have no effect on intrauterine devices (IUD; copper coil or Mirena) or depot medroxyprogesterone injection. There is a possible impact to the effectiveness of norethisterone enanthate (Noristerat) injection.
  - If using COC, increased doses of oestrogen are required.
  - Emergency contraception: IUD is the preferred option. Otherwise use of levonorgestrel at double dose (3 g as a single dose) as soon as possible within the first 72 hours.
  - Refer to Faculty of Sexual and Reproductive Healthcare (FSRH) Drug interactions with hormonal contraception, May 2022. for further details https://www.fsrh.org/documents/ceu-clinical-guidance-drug-interactions-with-hormonal/.

Follow-up

- NICE recommends that a structured routine review in general practice should take place once a year with specialist review depending on individual circumstances. This should include:
  a. *Seizure control and adverse effects of treatment.* Encourage the use of a seizure diary to record seizure frequency and severity, seizure type for those who have more than one type of seizure, and any changes in pattern since the last review.
  b. *Social or psychological issues* related to epilepsy. These may include driving, work, family planning, attitude to diagnosis, and depression.
  c. *Review drug compliance* by checking the frequency of repeat prescriptions. Ensure person understands risks of poor control of seizures and sudden unexpected death in epilepsy (SUDEP) (see later).

d. *Person's information needs.* This may involve signposting to websites (see earlier) or information sources such as https://www.Patient.co.uk where a range of information leaflets are available.
e. *Carer skills.* Review knowledge of first aid for people having a seizure and any agreed treatment protocols for the treatment of prolonged or recurrent seizures.
f. *Other considerations.* SIGN does not recommend routine blood tests as part of review.
g. *Adverse effects of anticonvulsant drugs.* See Box 11.1.

Avoiding Sudden Unexpected Death in Epilepsy

- The deaths of 500 people a year in the United Kingdom are attributed to SUDEP.
- In adults, 33% of these deaths are thought to be avoidable and the result of inadequate treatment.
- Failure to collect prescriptions for AEDs has been identified as a warning sign (Neligan, Bell, & Sander, 2011).
- To reduce this risk, observe the following rules:
  - Titrate a drug up to the maximum tolerated dose or until seizures are controlled.
  - When discontinuing a drug, titrate a new drug up to an effective dose first and then tail off the old drug slowly. The only exception to this is a patient having a life-threatening reaction to a drug, in which case abrupt cessation (with immediate introduction of a new drug) is justified.

Stopping Treatment

- Specialist advice is wise before withdrawing drugs in a patient who has been free from seizures for a number of years. Ultimately, it is the patient who must make the decision, weighing the problems of drug taking against

---

• BOX 11.1 **Adverse Effects of Anticonvulsant Drugs**

Acute: Rash (usually seen shortly after starting the drug). Tail off the drug. If combined with fever and lymphadenopathy, the rash may represent a severe hypersensitivity syndrome. Usually starts between 1 and 8 weeks of exposure. Multiple organ failure can occur. If the patient is systemically ill, admit.

Chronic: Weight gain and sedation are the adverse effects most commonly complained of. Check that the patient is taking the lowest effective dose of as few drugs as possible. There is some evidence that the quality of life is better on the newer drugs, but the NICE review did not consider the evidence to be strong. It is clear that each drug has a different side effect profile, and individuals respond to a drug in different ways. A small increased risk of suicidal thoughts and behaviour has been reported.

Some AEDs are known to reduce bone mineral density and increase fracture risk with long-term use. SIGN recommend dietary and lifestyle advice be given at review to minimise the risk of osteoporosis. Consider supplementation for those at increased risk.

AED, Antiepileptic drug; *SIGN,* Scottish Intercollegiate Guidelines Network.

the upset of a further seizure with its implications for driving, employment, and family distress.

- SIGN recommends this be discussed with patients who have been seizure free for at least 2 years. A risk table is found within the SIGN guideline to aid discussions.
- In adults with epilepsy who have been seizure free for 2 years, about 60% will have no further seizures when medication is withdrawn (Anonymous, 2003).
- There is an increased likelihood of recurrence if the patient:
  - Has had epilepsy since childhood
  - Requires more than one medication to control epilepsy
  - Had seizures while on medication
  - Has myoclonic or tonic-clonic seizures
  - Has had an abnormal electroencephalogram in the past year (Anonymous, 2003)
- Reduction should be gradual, and SIGN recommends that for those taking carbamazepine, lamotrigine, phenytoin, sodium valproate, or vigabatrin, the dose should be reduced by 10% every 2 to 4 weeks.
- *Driving when stopping medication.* The DVLA recommends that patients should be advised not to drive during withdrawal and for 6 months after cessation of treatment. Patients must be counselled regarding the need to satisfy driving regulations before resuming driving if a seizure does occur.

Parkinson Disease

GUIDELINES

National Institute for Health and Clinical Excellence. (2017). *Parkinson's disease in adults. NICE clinical guideline 71.* Retrieved from https://www.nice.org.uk/guidance/ng71.
   National Institute for Health and Clinical Excellence. (2023). *Parkinson's disease. Clinical knowledge summaries.* Retrieved from https://cks.nice.org.uk/topics/parkinsons-disease/.
   Scottish Intercollegiate Guidelines Network. (2010). *Diagnosis and pharmacological management of Parkinson's disease. SIGN guideline 113.* Retrieved from https://www.parkinsons.org.uk/sites/default/files/2018-10/SIGN%20guideline%20Diagnosis%20and%20pharmacological%20management%20of%20Parkinson%27s.pdf.

- Parkinson disease (PD) is a progressive neurodegenerative condition resulting from the loss of dopamine-containing cells in the substantia nigra. The disease should be confirmed by a specialist in all cases and patients referred untreated.
- Parkinsonism is a clinical syndrome involving bradykinesia plus one or more of the following: tremor (4-6 Hz when at rest), rigidity, and postural instability. PD is the most common form of parkinsonism. The diagnosis of PD also involves the absence of atypical features, a slow clinical progression, and response to drug treatment.
- Other causes of 'parkinsonism' include drug-induced, cerebrovascular disease, other forms of dementia, multisystem atrophy, and supranuclear palsy.

- Clinical diagnosis has poor specificity in the early stages of PD. Regular specialist review is needed to review the patient's diagnosis and response to treatment.
- Routine use of functional imaging is not recommended by SIGN but may be considered by specialists in certain situations. Single-photon emission computed tomography can be considered as an aid to clinical diagnosis in patients in whom there is uncertainty between PD and nondegenerative parkinsonism or tremor.
- Acute dopamine challenge testing is not recommended in the diagnosis of PD.

Management

- The diagnosis of PD has huge medical, psychological, and social implications for the patient and family. The medical aspects of care should be shared between the specialist and GP. The role of primary care in management of confirmed PD has been outlined by NICE Clinical Knowledge Summaries (CKS).
- GPs should enable appropriate access to:
  a. A PD specialist physician, generally a neurologist or a geriatrician
  b. A PD specialist nurse if available
  c. Speech and language therapy, physiotherapy, occupational therapy, social services, community nursing, continence and urology specialists, palliative care specialists, and psychology and mental health services
  d. The Parkinson's Disease Society local branch and regional support (see box)
- Liaise with specialist services, particularly in relation to changes in medication. Only start or alter antiparkinsonian medication on the advice of a specialist. Ensure that changes to repeat medications are made promptly. Titrate therapy between specialist reviews according to the recommendations of secondary care.
- Do not suddenly stop any antiparkinsonian medication because doing so can precipitate acute akinesia or neuroleptic malignant syndrome.
- Identify worsening motor symptoms and motor complications (which may be caused by the disease itself or by antiparkinsonian medication) and manage them appropriately. This usually requires specialist advice or an interim referral.
- Identify and appropriately manage nonmotor symptoms and complications, which may be caused by the disease itself or by antiparkinsonian medication.
- Manage comorbidities. Avoid or use with caution any drugs that could exacerbate parkinsonism or interact with antiparkinsonian medications. For example, avoid use of metoclopramide, prochlorperazine, and antipsychotics.
- Advise care staff in nursing or residential homes of the need for correct timing of antiparkinsonian medication.
- Offer a regular medication review, including adherence and adverse effects.
- Other considerations:
  - *Financial benefits.* Many patients are eligible for benefits for the disabled.

- *Carers.* Assess, and reassess, the ability of the carer to cope.
- *Driving.* Advise drivers to notify the DVLA (in the United Kingdom) and their insurance company at the point of diagnosis.

SELF-HELP GROUPS

Parkinson's Care and Support UK has information on exercise, physiotherapy, social groups, counselling, finances and COVID. Available at https://parkinsonscare.org.uk.

The Parkinson's Disease Society. 215 Vauxhall Bridge Road, London SW1V 1EJ. Tel: 020 7931 8080. This has information for patients and carers and organises local groups. Helpline: 0808 800 0303; Available at http://www.parkinsons.org.uk.

Nondrug Treatment

- Ensure that the patient's individual needs are met holistically, referring on to all applicable multidisciplinary team members as required.
- Signpost any informal carer(s) to appropriate support, including information on respite care.
- Encourage physical activity when possible, especially that which may aid balance and gait (e.g., the Alexander technique).
- Support the patient to create a PD passport if they are considering travelling (digital and printable versions available from Parkinsons' Europe at https://www.parkinsonseurope.org).

Drug Treatment

- Choice of medication is a specialist decision and should be made by taking into account patient preferences.
- Drug therapy does not prevent disease progression but improves most patients' quality of life.
- When initiating treatment, patients should be advised about its limitations and possible side effects. About 5% to 10% of patients with PD respond poorly to treatment.
- Claims that certain drugs are neuroprotective and should be started before the development of disabling symptoms are not supported by clinical evidence.
- The old practice of 'drug holidays' is contraindicated because sudden cessation may give rise to acute akinesia or to neuroleptic malignant syndrome.
- It is not possible to identify a universal first-choice therapy for early PD or as adjuvant therapy for later PD according to guidelines.
- Early disease can be considered the point at which a diagnosis of idiopathic PD has been made and a clinical decision has been made to start treatment (based on a functional disability requiring symptomatic treatment). Possible first-choice therapies are levodopa, non–ergot-derived dopamine agonists, or monoamine oxidase B inhibitors. Most people eventually require levodopa.
- Later disease refers to people with PD taking levodopa who have developed motor complications. Possible first

choice therapies are dopamine agonists, monoamine oxidase B inhibitors, and catechol-O-methyltransferase (COMT) inhibitors.

Treatment Options for Early Parkinson Disease

- *Levodopa*
  - Given with a dopa decarboxylase inhibitor to reduce peripheral availability of levodopa and reduce side effects such as nausea, vomiting, and cardiovascular effects. Examples are co-beneldopa and co-careldopa. Slow-release preparations may also reduce side effects.
  - Use the lowest effective dose to maintain good function to reduce the development of motor complications. This may include individual realistic goal setting with specialist team (e.g., being able to walk to the shop).
  - Warn patients about the immediate side effects (e.g., nausea, postural hypotension, sleepiness). Give the tablets after food to avoid nausea. Be aware, however, that a protein meal can compete with levodopa for absorption. If an antiemetic is needed, use domperidone. Check the standing blood pressure before and after starting the drug.
  - Over time, the response to treatment may decrease, and motor complications may occur in approximately 40% of patients after 4 to 6 years, including motor fluctuations, such as unpredictable switching between 'on' and 'off' states, wearing off between doses, and dose failures, or dyskinesia, such as athetosis (slow, writhing motions of fingers and hands) and dystonia (involuntary spasms of muscle contraction that cause abnormal movements and postures) occur.
  - There is some debate about use of levodopa as first-line treatment, and some specialists use alternative first-line treatments to delay starting levodopa and thereby reduce the onset of disabling dyskinesia.
- *Dopamine agonists*
  - These are used as monotherapy as either oral or transdermal preparations. Transdermal (e.g., rotigotine) are useful if swallowing is difficult or there is a high pill burden. These are found to be slightly less effective than levodopa in terms of treating motor impairment and disability, but they may delay motor complications.
  - Two groups exist:
    1. Non–ergot-derived dopamine receptor agonists (e.g., pramipexole, ropinirole, and rotigotine). These can be used as first-line treatment.
    2. Ergot-derived dopamine receptor agonists (e.g., bromocriptine, cabergoline, and pergolide). Both NICE and SIGN advise these are not used as first-line treatment because of the risk of fibrotic reactions (pulmonary, retroperitoneal, and pericardial). Specific baseline investigations and follow-up is recommended if used, and these are outlined in the BNF and SIGN guidance. Be alert for symptoms such as persistent cough, chest pain, cardiac failure, and abdominal pain.

- Patients should be warned that treatment with dopamine agonists and levodopa is associated with:
    1. Impulse control disorders (including pathological gambling, binge eating, and hypersexuality)
    2. Excessive daytime somnolence (inform patients of the implications for driving and operating machinery)
- Other side effects include hallucinations, especially in older people, and postural hypotension, often worse at the start of treatment.
- Dopamine agonists are very likely to cause initial nausea or vomiting and domperidone may be needed.
- *Monoamine oxidase B inhibitors*
    - Examples are rasagiline and selegiline.
    - NICE and SIGN state may be considered as a first-choice therapy. When used as a monotherapy:
        1. They have been found to improve motor symptoms, improve activities of daily living, and delay the need for levodopa. It is less clear whether they delay the onset of motor complications.
        2. Dopaminergic side effects such as dyskinesia, hallucinations, or vivid dreaming may occur or worsen.
        3. A levodopa-sparing effect has been demonstrated (i.e., a lower dose is required).
- *Other drugs available*
    a. *Anticholinergics.* Occasionally used when tremor predominates. They are not recommended as first-choice treatment because of limited efficacy and the propensity to neuropsychiatric side effects.
    b. *Amantadine.* SIGN found there to be insufficient evidence to support its use in early PD. Relatively weak efficacy and mechanism of action have not been established.

Treatment Options in Later Parkinson Disease

- Most people with PD will develop, with time, motor complications and will eventually require levodopa. Adjuvant drugs to take alongside levodopa have been developed with the aim of reducing motor complications and improving quality of life.
- There are three main strategies when managing motor complications:
    - Manipulation of oral or topical drug therapy
    - More invasive drug treatments (e.g., apomorphine infusions or intraduodenal levodopa)
    - Neurosugery, most commonly deep brain stimulation
- Patients with complex and disabling motor complications should be reviewed regularly by their specialist team. In the later stages of disease, as nonmotor complications begin to dominate quality of life, the withdrawal of some drugs is often appropriate. These decisions should be made by specialist in consultation with carers and patients.
- The following options may be considered in people with advanced PD:
    a. *Oral COMT inhibitors* (e.g., entacapone). These may aid reduction of 'off' time in patients who have motor fluctuations but have an increased risk of daytime somnolence and impulse control disorders.
    b. *Monoamine oxidase (MAO)-B inhibitors* (selegiline or rasagiline).
    c. *Oral amantadine.* This may be used for dyskinesias but has several side effects, including confusion, hallucinations, insomnia, nightmares, and dry mouth. SIGN does not recommend this in early disease.
    d. *Subcutaneous apomorphine* (a potent dopamine agonist) may be offered in severe motor complications under specialist supervision, either as intermittent bolus or continuous infusion. Side effects include nausea, vomiting, and orthostatic hypotension. Sublingual apomorphine rescue therapy has recently been approved in the United States but has not yet made it to the United Kingdom.

Nonmotor Complications of Parkinson Disease

- It is important to be alert to nonmotor symptoms at patient reviews and manage them appropriately. An extensive list of these is available in NICE CKS, which includes postural hypotension, falls, and pain.
- *Depression* is of particular importance.
    - Depression may be part of the disease rather than a reaction to the disease. Mood disorders, including depression, are thought to affect up to 50% of patients. There is significant overlap in symptoms of depression, cognitive impairment, and PD, which makes diagnosis difficult. Screening using self-rating or clinician rating scales may be of benefit. Information from relatives and carers should also supplement any assessment.
    - In general terms, treatment of depression is the same as those without PD. There is limited evidence from trials, but selective serotonin reuptake inhibitors (SSRIs) are most frequently used. Prescribers should be aware that SSRIs can worsen motor symptoms such as restless legs, periodic limb movements, and rapid eye movement (REM) sleep disorder.
    - Tricyclic antidepressants (TCAs) may be more effective than SSRIs, but use is limited because of adverse effects of the medication. Both classes should be avoided if a patient is takin MAO-B inhibitors and with caution if using a COMT inhibitors. Seek specialist advice if necessary.
- *Dementia* is more common in people with PD.
    - Treatable causes should be investigated and treated (e.g., acute infection and depression).
    - Consider safely reducing or discontinuing (on specialist advice if necessary) any drugs which may be causing or worsening symptoms. This includes antimuscarinics such as tricyclic antidepressants, tolterodine or oxybutynin, H2 antagonists such as ranitidine, benzodiazepines, amantadine, and dopamine agonists.
    - Refer for specialist assessment and management.

PATIENT INFORMATION

Parkinson's UK. (2013). *Parkinson's dementia information sheet.* Retrieved from https://www.parkinsons.org.uk/sites/default/files/2018-10/FS58%20Parkinson%27s%20dementia%20WEB.pdf .

- *Psychosis* is a key neuropsychiatric feature of PD and is associated with a high degree of disability. This includes hallucinations, delusions, and paranoid beliefs.
  - Management should include treating any reversible causes and reviewing medication.
  - Liaise with specialist services early.
  - Mild symptoms that are well tolerated may not need treatment. More severe symptoms may require gradual withdrawal of precipitating antiparkinsonian medications or the use of an atypical antipsychotic.
  - Evidence supports the use of clozapine but this requires weekly blood monitoring, which may be difficult in some patients. There is some evidence of benefit from quetiapine, but it is not licensed for treatment of psychosis in patients with PD.
- *Excessive daytime somnolence* is found in up to 54% of patients with PD. The aetiology is believed to be multifactorial, and it increases with age.
  - Management should centre around finding a reversible cause such as depression, poor sleep hygiene, and drugs associated with altered sleep pattern.
  - Other conditions associated with PD that may affect sleep include restless legs syndrome, periodic leg movement of sleep, nocturnal akinesia, and nocturia.

Palliative Care of Terminal Patients

- End-stage PD can be considered when there is severe, progressive worsening of motor symptoms and its complications (e.g., on-off phenomenon, falls) or nonmotor complications (e.g., dementia, hallucinations, weight loss, aspiration pneumonia).
  - Treat symptoms of the dying process as per any other terminal illness.
  - Be aware that communication difficulties (including reduced facial expressions) may affect your ability to detect they are in pain.

Main Drugs to Avoid in Parkinson Disease

- *Antipsychotics* (e.g., chlorpromazine, haloperidol, flupentixol). Atypical antipsychotics may be less likely to cause problems. Use clozapine cautiously.
- *Antiemetics* (e.g., metoclopramide, prochlorperazine). Use domperidone.
- *Baclofen* may cause agitation and confusion. Use with caution.

Stroke

GUIDELINES

National Clinical Guideline for Stroke for the United Kingdom and Ireland. (2023). Available at https://www.strokeguideline.org/contents/?_gl=1*1eeteg7*_up*MQ..*_ga*MTU1ODgyNDE2MC4xNzE5MDU4MTA1*_ga_EE3BZMVLRT*MTcxOTA1ODEwNC4xLjAuMTcxOTA1ODEwNC4wLjAuMA.

National Institute for Health and Care Excellence. (2019; updated 2022). *Stroke and transient ischaemic attack in over 16s: Diagnosis and initial management. NICE clinical guideline 128.* Retrieved from http://www.nice.org.uk.

- Stroke is a preventable and treatable disease. Stroke is the third largest cause of death in the United Kingdom, and it is estimated that 10% of the world's population dies from a stroke.

Acute Stroke

- NICE recommends that all people with suspected stroke be admitted directly to a specialist stroke unit after initial assessment, either from the community or from A&E. In certain circumstances, this may be inappropriate (e.g., the patient is already in the terminal stage of another illness).
- Admit by dialling 999 (in the United Kingdom), without seeing the patient if necessary. This will trigger the local protocol for the management of acute stroke.
- Assessment of the patient by paramedics using a validated tool such as FAST (see later) to diagnose stroke or transient ischaemic attack (TIA) is supported by NICE stroke quality standards. People with persistent neurologic symptoms who screen positive using a validated tool in whom hypoglycaemia has been excluded and who have a possible diagnosis of stroke should be transferred to specialist stroke unit within 1 hour. When available, give supplemental oxygen to those whose oxygen saturations are less than 95% unless there are contraindications.
- Patients with acute stroke should receive brain imaging within 1 hour of arrival in hospital if they meet the indications for immediate imaging. These include:
  - Those who are candidates for thrombolysis (i.e., they are within 3 hours of the start of symptoms, although SIGN highlights evidence for up to 4.5 hours) or early anticoagulation
  - Patients taking anticoagulants or with a bleeding tendency
  - Those with a depressed level of consciousness (Glasgow Coma Scale score <13)
  - Those with progressive or fluctuating symptoms
  - Those with signs of alternative pathology: neck stiffness, papilloedema, or fever
  - Those whose stroke begins with severe headache of sudden onset

FAST (Face, Arm, Speech, Time)

This was initially developed to aid paramedics to recognise people with stroke but has become a widely publicised part of the Act F.A.S.T. campaign which was launched in the United Kingdom in 2009 to aid public awareness:

- Face: Ask the patient to smile. Is there a new droop of the mouth or eye on one side?
- Arm: a new inability to hold one arm out for 5 seconds compared with the other arm
- Speech: new slurred speech or new inability to understand or say words
- Time: time to dial 999 immediately if you see any of these signs

Longer-Term Management

- Follow-up arrangements should be based on individual need and response to treatment. It is recommended to have a primary care review within 6 weeks of discharge, again at 6 months, and then annually.
- Management should include:
  - Assess the need for further specialist review, advice, information, support, and rehabilitation.
  - Assess social care needs over time, including carer needs.
  - Assess healthcare needs.
  - Check and optimise lifestyle measures and drug treatments for secondary prevention.
- Ensure involvement of the community rehabilitation team if they are not already involved. This team will manage the rehabilitation process but may need support from the GP.
- Check that a multidisciplinary assessment has been performed, including assessment of consciousness level, swallowing, speech, pressure sore risk, nutritional status, cognitive impairment, movement, and handling needs.
- *Depression.* Monitor for depression with a screening questionnaire. Mood disturbance is common after stroke and includes depression, anxiety, and emotional lability. Consider a therapeutic trial of an SSRI if depression is present and continue it for at least 6 months if a benefit is achieved.
- *Fatigue.* Fatigue caused by stroke disease is typically not relieved with rest. Exclude other causes before making the diagnosis. Management centres around planned coping mechanisms.
- *Cognitive impairment* should be screened for.
- *Mouth care.* Patients who are unable to care for their own oral hygiene should have their teeth and gums brushed three times daily followed by the application of lip balm.
- *Central poststroke pain.* Pharmacologic options include a trial of amitriptyline, gabapentin, or pregabalin.
- *Bowel and bladder problems.* Disturbance of control of excretion is common in the acute phase of a stroke and remains a problem for a significant minority of patients. Support and continence aids should have been put in place before discharge, including carer training, but this requires ongoing support in the community.
- *Sexual dysfunction.* Phosphodiesterase inhibitors can be used after 3 months after a stroke, provided that blood pressure is controlled.
- For further information on specific issues, refer to NICE CKS Stroke: Long-term care and support.

Secondary Prevention

- *Lifestyle changes.* Patients should be encouraged to be physically active, including balance specific exercises at least twice per week. Diet should include five or more portions of fruit and vegetables daily, with two portions of oily fish a week and reduced salt intake if the patient has hypertension. Alcohol intake should be moderated to include no more than 14 units of alcohol per week spread over at least 3 days.
- Smoking should be stopped immediately.
- *Antiplatelet therapy.* After 2 weeks on high-dose aspirin 300 mg once daily, those with ischaemic stroke should be started on 75 mg clopidogrel as first-line treatment or 75 mg of aspirin and 200 mg of dipyridamole bd as second-line treatment, lifelong.
- *Blood pressure.* After the initial phase of the stroke is over (usually about 2 weeks), control any hypertension to achieve a target blood pressure of <130/80 mm Hg (<125 mm Hg systolic at home). Treatment of hypertension in the immediate poststroke period is thought to potentially cause extension of stroke.
- *Atrial fibrillation (AF).* Those who are found to be in AF (whether paroxysmal or permanent) should be anticoagulated after 2 weeks of antiplatelet therapy unless there are contraindications or informed dissent.
- *Cholesterol.* Statin therapy is recommended for all people after an ischaemic stroke, to be initiated 48 hours after onset of symptoms. NICE recommend any high-strength statin, aiming for a low-density lipoprotein level of less than 1.8 mmol/L.
- *Carotid artery surgery.* All patients with ischaemic disease should be assessed for carotid disease, and those with greater than 50% stenosis should be referred within 7 days for endarterectomy or angioplasty.
- *Contraception and HRT.* Contraception must not be oestrogen-containing. HRT can be given as usual, although transdermal delivery may be preferred if hypertensive.
- *Obstructive sleep apnoea.* All patients should be screened because of the strain of untreated disease on the cardiovascular system.

Other Routine Matters

- Explain the prognosis if requested. About 65% of patients are likely to achieve independence, but the GP can modify this figure according to the individual patient's clinical state. Patients with a better prognosis are those who are continent, who have regained power on the affected side within 1 month, and who are progressing towards walking within 6 weeks. Improvement is likely to continue for some months.
- *Driving.* Explain that the patient should not drive for at least 1 month after a stroke or TIA or 3 months for recurrent TIA. The DVLA does not need to be informed unless there is residual neurologic deficit after 1 month (including visual and cognitive sequelae).
- *Influenza.* Arrange for annual immunisation, as well as pneumococcal immunisation in those aged 65 years and older.
- Check that the patient knows about the relevant statutory and voluntary organisations.
- Arrange relief admissions and other support for the carers (e.g., attendance allowance) in consultation with the stroke team.

Transient Ischaemic Attack

- A TIA is a sudden focal neurologic disturbance lasting less than 24 hours. Early recurrent stroke is common. It is estimated that 10% to 15% have a second TIA or cerebrovascular accident in the first week, with a high proportion being in the first 48 hours (Markus, 2007).
- Check that the symptoms are caused by a TIA. Up to 50% of presentations are TIA mimics. Differentiate TIA from:
  a. Transient cerebral symptoms caused by hypoperfusion from cardiac disease.
  b. Cerebral tumour. Patients with sensory TIAs, jerking TIAs, loss of consciousness, or speech arrest should be assumed to have a tumour until proved otherwise.
  c. Epilepsy. A careful history of the attacks from an observer is important.
  d. Migraine.
  e. Traumatic brain injury.
  f. Subdural haematoma.
  g. Subarachnoid haemorrhage.
- Note that a patient with a TIA that seems to be in the vertebrobasilar distribution, as manifested, for instance, by vertigo, bilateral visual loss, or diplopia, should be managed in the same way as one with a TIA in the carotid distribution.
- Do not use the clinical prediction tool ABCD2 to assess for risk of stroke or urgency of referral in those with suspected TIA.
- ABCD2 and the newer ABCD3 have been shown to discriminate poorly between low and high risk of stroke after TIA, putting high-risk patients at risk of harm.
- All cases of TIA should now be considered potentially high risk for subsequent stroke.
- Admission also required when uncontrolled AF is present or if a TIA has occurred in a patient taking warfarin because urgent computed tomography is required to rule out a bleed.

Other Measures

- *Aspirin.* Give 300 mg/day to be started immediately unless contraindicated and continue while awaiting specialist assessment. Consider use of a proton pump inhibitor if there is a history of dyspepsia associated with aspirin. If there is a contraindication or history of intolerance to aspirin, then advice should be sought urgently from the local stroke team. Patients who are already taking low-dose aspirin should continue on this dose rather than increase to 300 mg.
- *Long-term antiplatelet therapy.* Initiated in secondary care after diagnosis. Generally, clopidogrel 75 mg (unlicensed use) is used. NICE recommends use of a combination of aspirin 75 mg/day and dipyridamole MR 200 mg bd if clopidogrel is not tolerated. Aspirin 75 mg alone can be used if clopidogrel and dipyridamole are both not tolerated or contraindicated.
- *Secondary prevention.* Manage as for stroke.
- *Driving.* Advise as for stroke.

Recurrent Transient Ischaemic Attacks

- If the TIA occurred in a patient already taking aspirin 75 mg/day, options include changing to clopidogrel.
- Check that a treatable cardiac or carotid cause has been excluded.
- Tighten control of other risk factors for stroke (e.g., blood pressure, cholesterol, glucose).
- Admit if the TIAs assume a crescendo pattern.
- Refer if recurrent attacks continue despite these measures.

PATIENT ORGANISATIONS

The Stroke Association. Stroke House, 240 City Road, London EC1V 2PR. Helpline: 0845 30 33 100 www.stroke.org.uk.
  Local Stroke Clubs can be accessed through the community rehabilitation team.

Motor Neurone Disease

GUIDELINE

Motor Neurone Disease Association. *Evidence-based clinical guidelines in MND.* Available at https://www.mndassociation.org/professionals/management-of-mnd/best-practice-guidelines-pathways (choose 'For professionals' and then 'For GPs').

- Refer every patient for confirmation of the diagnosis.
- Explain what little is known about the disease. Offer referral to the Motor Neurone Disease (MND) Association's regional care development adviser.
- Support the patient and family as you would in any terminal illness. The median survival time is only 3 to 4 years, with older patients having the worst prognosis. Always make a further appointment rather than waiting for the patient or family to contact you with a problem.
- *Ventilation.* Discuss at an early stage with the patient and the family the fact that ventilation may become necessary. Noninvasive ventilation (i.e., via facemask) at night only in those with good bulbar function prolongs life by a median of 7 months with improvement in the quality of life (McDermott & Shaw, 2008). If bulbar function fails, tracheostomy or ventilation may become necessary. Discuss this well before it becomes necessary; there is often no time to discuss it with them during a crisis.
- *Nutrition.* In the early stages of dysphagia, refer to a speech therapist and a dietician. Offer referral for consideration of insertion of a gastrostomy tube or a nasogastric tube *before* the patient becomes weak through malnutrition. Standard criteria for tube feeding are when more than 10% of premorbid weight has been lost or when the patient finds eating an ordeal because of choking or because it takes too long (McDermott & Shaw, 2008).
- Refer for physiotherapy, occupational therapy, speech therapy for help with speech as well as eating, district

nursing, and social work assistance as appropriate. In each case, do this proactively, not when a serious problem has developed.

- *Driving.* Patients are required to inform the DVLA at the point of diagnosis. They may continue until weakness or cognitive decline becomes impairing.
- *Hospice care.* Introduce this idea well before it is needed. Short-term admission as respite care will establish a link with the hospice and help the patient to make a decision about what they want to happen in the terminal stages.
- *Drug treatment.* Riluzole is recommended by NICE for patients with the amyotrophic lateral sclerosis form of MND (NICE, 2001). Treatment should be initiated by a specialist, but it can then be supervised under a shared-care arrangement with GPs. Riluzole reduces the rate of decline rather than increasing strength and prolongs life by an average of 3 to 4 months.

End-of-Life Care in Motor Neurone Disease

- Treat palliative issues such as pain and dribbling as per usual palliative principles.
- *Dry mouth.* Try pineapple chunks or apple or lemon juice to stimulate saliva.
- Consider referral for tracheostomy for sputum retention or stridor or for recurrent aspiration of food or drink.
- *Choking spasms.* Give sublingual lorazepam (0.5–2.5 mg) and leave a supply with the patient for future occasions. They relieve the laryngeal spasm associated with inhalation of food, drink, or saliva.
- *Respiratory failure.* Consider referral for ventilatory support if the quality of life is otherwise sufficiently good. Be prepared to ease the distress of more prolonged dyspnoea with oral morphine (start with 2.5 mg four to six times per day and titrate up) while the patient is able to swallow and subcutaneous morphine in the terminal stage. More than 90% of patients die in their sleep as a result of increasing hypercapnia. Choking to death is not seen in clinical practice (McDermott & Shaw, 2008).

PATIENT ORGANISATION

Motor Neurone Disease Association. PO Box 246, Northampton NN1 2PR. Tel: 08457 626262. Available at http://www.mndassociation.org.

Multiple Sclerosis

GUIDELINE

National Institute for Health and Clinical Excellence. (2014). *Multiple sclerosis in adults: Management. NICE clinical guideline no. 186.* Retrieved from https://www.nice.org.uk/guidance/cg186.

Increasing evidence shows that Epstein–Barr virus is a major risk factor for the development of multiple sclerosis (MS) (Bjornevik et al, 2022).

- The NICE guidance sets out the following principles:
    a. The diagnosis should be made rapidly by a specialist neurologist, and every patient, after being diagnosed, should have access to neurologic and specialist neurologic rehabilitation services as the need arises.
    b. The patient should be actively involved in all decisions. To do this, the patient needs clear verbal and written information.
    c. The patient and any family or other carers need emotional as well as practical support from the medical services.
    d. Whenever the patient is assessed, attention should be paid to all 'hidden' factors (e.g., emotional state, fatigue, bladder, and bowel problems) as well as to the presenting symptom. The NICE guidance includes a useful checklist of issues to consider.
    e. The GP should be proactive in the prevention of avoidable morbidity (e.g., contractures, inhalation, pressure sores, renal infections).
- The MS Society's booklet for GPs stresses the role of the GP as the patient's advocate. GPs may not know how to manage every problem raised by this complex illness, but they should know someone who does and should make the referral.
- Even if the patient is already authorised to self-refer directly, the GP may be needed to expedite the appointment if the first offer of an appointment is not sufficiently prompt.

Prognosis

- MS follows an unpredictable course but a better prognosis is associated with:
    - Young age at onset
    - Female gender
    - A relapsing and remitting course
    - Initial symptoms: sensory or optic neuritis
    - First manifestations affecting only one central nervous system region
    - High degree of recovery from initial bout
    - Longer interval between first relapses
    - Low number of relapses in the first 2 years
    - Less disability at 5 years after onset
- Explain what is known about the disease and how good the prognosis is; the average life expectancy is 25 years after onset of the disease. Five years after diagnosis, approximately 70% of people are still employed, and 50% need some help with walking. Approximately 25% of patients have a nondisabling form of MS, but up to 15% of patients are severely disabled within a short period (Confavreux, Vukusic, & Moreau, 2000). Point out the positive prognostic features (see earlier box) if they apply.

Management of Acute Relapses

- About 70% of relapses are monofocal.
- Diagnose a relapse if new symptoms develop or existing symptoms worsen and last for longer than 24 hours and occur after a stable period of longer than 1 month.
- Before treatment, possible precipitants, particularly infections, should be sought. Urine dipstick should be done on all patients.
- Liaise with the specialist team; frequency of relapse may influence decisions regarding disease-modifying treatment.
- At the start of an acute disabling relapse, give methylprednisolone 500 mg orally daily for 5 days after discussion with the patient of the risks and benefits. Intravenous treatment may be necessary if the relapse is severe enough to warrant admission or the patient cannot tolerate oral steroids.
- Give gastric protection with a protein pump inhibitor.
- Also consider what help the patient needs in the way of care and equipment because of the relapse and whether referral to the specialist neurologic rehabilitation service is needed.
- Giving the same dose intravenously is not feasible in primary care because the high-dose intravenous preparation should be given over 30 minutes.
- Steroids can hasten recovery, but there is no evidence that the long-term course is altered.
- No more than three courses should be given in 1 year.
- Do not give patients a prescription for steroids to keep on standby.

Disease-Modifying Treatment

- The aim is to reduce the frequency and severity of relapses; there is increasing emphasis on reducing the 'invisible' lesions on magnetic resonance imaging.
- All patients with relapsing–remitting disease with active disease (defined as two or more clinical relapses in the previous 2 years) should be considered for treatment.
- For those patients with inflammatory primary progressive MS, Ocrevus has now been approved.
- For those patients with secondary progressive MS, Mayzent has now been approved.

First-Line Treatments

- There are currently five first-line drugs, the beta-interferons (Avonex, Betaferon, Extavia, and Rebif) and glatiramer acetate (Copaxone). These should be started and supervised by a consultant neurologist, preferably one with a specialist interest in MS.
- All drugs must be given by injection.
- Flulike symptoms are common with both beta-interferon and glatiramer acetate after treatment. These lessen over time. Injection site reactions are also common.
- Any female receiving disease-modifying therapy (e.g., interferon) must stop treatment for at least 12 months before trying to conceive.

Second-Line Therapies

- NICE recommends natalizumab is an option only for the treatment of patients with rapidly evolving severe relapsing–remitting MS (NICE, 2007). Fingolimod is the first oral therapy for patients with MS and has also been approved by NICE as an option in the treatment of highly active relapsing–remitting MS (NICE, 2012). In expert centres, other treatments may be considered.
- *Other treatment.* Sativex oromucosal spray, a cannabis extract, is licensed for use in the United Kingdom on a named patient basis, via specialists, for moderate to severe spasticity. Percutaneous venoplasty is no longer supported by NICE because of risk of serious complications and lack of efficacy.

Regular Review

- Check that there is a key worker to whom the patient has immediate access and who is coordinating all members of the multidisciplinary team. If there is no such person then, by default, the role falls to the GP.
- *Fatigue*, which is common and not the same as sleepiness. The fatigue may be physical or mental, so the patient can concentrate for only a short period of time. Check for an underlying cause (e.g., depression, chronic pain, disturbed sleep). The most useful manoeuvre is to explain that the fatigue is real and that it is a part of the syndrome. Amantadine, modafinil, and an SSRI are all options for drug treatment (unlicensed).
- *Spasticity.* Treat any precipitating cause, such as infection or pain. Otherwise management should be supervised by the specialist rehabilitation service. The components of a treatment programme are:
  a. Stretching exercises by a physiotherapist, patient, or family
  b. A skeletal muscle relaxant. Baclofen or gabapentin is often used as first-line treatment; if they fail, tizanidine, diazepam, or dantrolene is an option. Start low and increase the dose slowly. Up to 100 mg/day of baclofen may be required. If stopping, reduce the dose over several weeks. Abrupt withdrawal of baclofen may result in hallucinations or seizures.
  c. Consider an evening dose of diazepam if spasms or clonus interfere with sleep.
  d. Gabapentin can be considered but is unlicensed.
  e. Refer if spasticity is still uncontrolled for consideration of other treatments. This may include use of Sativex (cannabis extract) spray or botulinum toxin as an intramuscular injection.
- *Weakness.* Refer to the specialist rehabilitation service for training in exercises and techniques to maximise strength.
- *Contractures.* These may develop around any joint whose muscles are weak or spastic. Contractures lead to further reductions in mobility and difficulties in handling. Prevent them by instructing the patient or carer in passive stretching of the joint. Refer to the specialist team if a contracture does develop.

- *Pressure sores.* Check that all wheelchair users have been assessed for pressure sore risk and that appropriate preventive measures are in place.
- *Depression and anxiety.* A major depressive episode occurs in more than 50% of patients with MS at some stage. Search for it and treat it as actively as in a patient without MS.
- *Emotionalism.* Consider a trial of an antidepressant (a TCA or SSRI).
- *Dysphagia.* If the patient has bulbar signs (dysarthria, ataxia, or abnormal eye movements) or if has had a chest infection, assess swallowing formally.
- *Dysarthria.* If communication is affected, refer to a speech and language therapist.
- *Pain* may be neuropathic or musculoskeletal. The former needs a trial of carbamazepine, gabapentin, or amitriptyline; the latter needs physiotherapy and analgesics.
- *Visual problems* that are not corrected with glasses need assessment by an ophthalmologist. Optic neuritis is the commonest cause of visual loss.
- *Cognitive impairment*, if suspected, should be formally assessed and the results used to inform the management of every aspect of the patient's care.
- *Bladder problems.* See later.
- *Constipation.* Can usually be managed with adequate fluid, bulk laxatives, and stool softeners. More severe constipation may require osmotic agents, bowel stimulants, anal stimulation, suppositories, or enemas.
- *Sexual problems.* The precise nature of the sexual dysfunction will determine the treatment. Physical difficulty from spasticity may be alleviated by premedication with baclofen, and a fast-acting anticholinergic such as oxybutynin may calm urinary urgency. Sexual dysfunction should not be automatically attributed to MS. It may be necessary to investigate hormonal levels and to obtain urologic or gynaecologic consultation. Manual lubrication with gel is a ready solution to vaginal dryness. Erectile dysfunction may be treated by sildenafil at NHS expense in the United Kingdom. If it fails, older treatments may succeed (vacuum devices, intracavernous injections, or a penile implant).
- *The health and state of mind of all carers* should also be explored.

The Bladder

- *Urgency.* See whether access to the toilet can be made easier and give an anticholinergic (e.g., oxybutynin or tolterodine).
- *Minor incontinence.* Consider desmopressin for nighttime incontinence. It works by reducing the volume of urine produced. The same dose once in any 24-hour period may be useful to tide a patient over a time when there is no toilet within reach (e.g., on a journey). Padding may help a patient of either sex.
- *More severe incontinence*, occurring more than once a week: refer to a continence service. The patient needs ultrasound assessment for a residual urine and consideration of intermittent or even long-term catheterisation. Meanwhile, supply pads for females and penile drainage devices for males.
- *Urinary infection.* After treated, order an ultrasound scan for residual urine, if not already performed. Residuals in excess of 15 mL are abnormal. If the residual is above 50 mL or if there have been more than three confirmed infections in a year, refer to a continence service. If catheterisation is needed, intermittent self-catheterisation is better than an indwelling catheter if the patient can manage it.

Other Issues

- *Pregnancy* does not appear to influence the course of the disease overall. There may be fewer relapses during the pregnancy with a slight increase in the risk of relapse after delivery.
- *Vitamin D.* Deficiency is a risk factor for development of MS; if low, it should be treated.
- *Immunisations.* Patients should have all routine immunisations as well as an annual influenza vaccination. Advise that flu itself is more likely to trigger a relapse than getting the vaccine. There is no evidence that they precipitate relapse. Avoid live vaccines if the patient is taking steroids or disease-modifying antirheumatic drugs.
- *Employment.* Check that the patient knows about the assistance that is available from disability employment advisors and the Access to Work scheme in the United Kingdom.

End-of-Life Care

Although MS is not often fatal in itself, life is shortened by an average of 6 to 11 years, and it may complicate a death from another condition. See the section on MND for a discussion of end-of-life care.

PATIENT ORGANISATION

The Multiple Sclerosis (MS) Society. 372 Edgware Road, London NW2 6ND. National helpline: 0808 800 8000. Available at http://www.mssociety.org.uk.

Huntington Disease

- The diagnosis of Huntington disease (HD) should always be made by a specialist.
- Genetic testing may be requested by people who are at risk because of their family history. The arguments in favour and against testing are complex, and the discussion is best handled by experienced staff at a genetics centre.
- Management should be in the hands of a specialist team, but the GP may be the first person to detect a new problem and needs to understand the principles of management.
- No NICE guidelines yet exist.

Management

- Involuntary movements may be helped by three groups of drugs: neuroleptics, benzodiazepines, and dopamine depleting agents. They have the problems, respectively, of parkinsonism and tardive dyskinesia, drowsiness and ataxia, and depression and sedation. Some patients can be managed by ensuring an environment free from stress, with padding of chair and bed and weights on the wrists and ankles to reduce movements.
- The impairment of voluntary movements does not respond to medication, but useful improvement can be achieved by behavioural methods. Dysphagia can improve with a change of food type, usually to a slightly more liquid food, and by developing a habit of eating slowly. A speech therapist can help with speech and dysphagia. An occupational therapist can make the home safer for a patient at risk of falling.
- The problems posed by cognitive impairment can be reduced by training the family to communicate with the patient in a simple way. Explain that a patient who seems to be unaware of their disability may have a neurologic basis for the unawareness and is not 'just being difficult'.
- The specific psychiatric disorders that are associated with HD, namely depression, mania, and obsessive-compulsive disorder, may respond to the same treatment as would be appropriate for a patient without HD.

Coping With the Cognitive Impairment

- Explain to the family and the patient, if the impairment is not too advanced, the principles of coping with cognitive impairment.
- Explain that HD has certain specific problems and suggest solutions to them:
  a. *Difficulty with initiating and organising tasks.* Use lists and prompt the patient to do things.
  b. *Perseveration of thoughts or actions.* Gently ease the patient on to something else.
  c. *Impulsivity and irritability.* Reduce stress with a regular schedule; respond with calmness and try to find out what has prompted it.
  d. *Difficulty with attention.* Do one thing at a time.
  e. *Lack of insight.* This is a feature of the disease, not a sign that the patient is being difficult.
- Advise the patient of the need to notify the DVLA in the United Kingdom and insurance company of the condition after it has been diagnosed (though not when a genetic diagnosis has been made in an asymptomatic patient).
- Raise the question of an advance directive. It can be a great help if the patient decides certain key issues and records the decisions when still competent to do so. Some key issues are preferred place of terminal care when the need arises, whether to be given a gastrostomy tube when no longer able to swallow, and whether to be resuscitated when in a terminal state.

- Check what the family has been told about who else is at risk of developing the disease and what decision has been made about genetic testing. Record this in the patient's records.

Paraplegia

Every patient with paraplegia will be under the care of a consultant. The GP, however, is likely to be the doctor to whom certain problems present. A proactive approach can make a difference to the patient's quality of life.

Spasticity

- Four types of oral drugs are licensed for the treatment of spasticity in the United Kingdom. These are benzodiazepines, baclofen, dantrolene, and tizanidine. In 2000, *Drugs and Therapeutics Bulletin* reported that tizanidine was slightly better tolerated than other oral drugs (baclofen and diazepam) and caused less muscle weakness (Anonymous, 2000).
- Attempts to control troublesome spasticity should include referral for consideration of intrathecal injection of baclofen, botulinum toxin, or nerve blocks.

Urinary Tract Infection

- Always confirm suspected urinary tract infections (UTIs) with a midstream urine specimen.
- Do not give antibiotics if the patient is catheterised unless there are systemic symptoms.

Autonomic Dysreflexia

- This is reflex sympathetic overactivity, giving rise to vasoconstriction, resulting in hypertension, severe headache, visual disturbance, anxiety, and pallor. The parasympathetic system slows the heart and causes flushing and sweating above the lesion. It only occurs in patients with lesions above T6. This should be considered a medical emergency.
- If this occurs, do the following:
  a. Sit up the patient.
  b. Remove the cause (e.g., distended bladder, UTI, loaded colon, or anal fissure). If catheterising or

disimpacting, allow the lidocaine jelly at least 2 minutes to act. Both activities can exacerbate autonomic dysreflexia. If flushing a catheter through, use fluid at body temperature.

c. It is essential that prompt action is taken to reduce blood pressure to avoid serious or life-threatening complications. Do not ignore headaches. Give nifedipine 10 mg sublingual. Get the patient to bite the capsule. Alternatively, use glyceryl trinitrate, one to two sprays sublingually. Note that patients with spinal injuries may normally have low blood pressure (e.g., 90/60 mm Hg), and an increase to a 'normal' level of 120/80 mm Hg may represent a significant elevation.

d. Monitor the blood pressure at least every 5 minutes. It may fluctuate rapidly. If hypotension occurs, lie down the patient and raise the legs.

e. Admit urgently to hospital if not settling.

f. If it does settle, warn the patient that it may recur as the medication wears off and that they should call for help at the first sign of recurrence (NHS Scotland, 1999).

Pressure Ulcers

- Avoid prolonged immobilisation in the same position (i.e., for >2 hours).
- Identify pressure areas and protect them.
- Ensure that someone inspects at risk areas daily (the ischii, sacrum, trochanters, and heels).
- Refer for an exercise programme to retain posture and muscle strength.
- Refer to a dietician to ensure adequate nutrition.
- Treat sores or ulcers intensively and admit early if not resolving (e.g., within 2–4 weeks).

Psychological Aspects

- Be aware of the fact that the patient may have:
  a. A severe grief response to the loss of function and independence
  b. A feeling of fear and vulnerability
  c. Difficulties with their changing relationships with those around them
- Be prepared to raise the issue of sexuality. Avoid the temptation to think of the individual as asexual. Sexual function and fertility are possible with appropriate support. Recommend publications from the Spinal Injuries Association (see box).

ADVICE FOR PATIENTS AND PROFESSIONALS

Spinal Injuries Association. SIA House, 2 Trueman Place, Oldbrook, Milton Keynes MK6 2HH. Helpline: 0800 980 0501. Available at http://www.spinal.co.uk.

Essential Tremor

SYSTEMATIC REVIEW

Deuchl, G., Raethjen, J., Hellriegel, H., & Elble, R. (2011). Treatment of patients with essential tremor. *Lancet Neurology*, *10*(2), 148–161.

- Ask what effect the tremor is having. A quarter of those who consult about tremor retire early or change jobs because of it.
- Check regular medications and, thyroid function and screen for alcohol misuse or dependence.
- *Mild cases.* Patients may choose not to take any medication. Check that they are not exacerbating the tremor with, for instance, caffeine. They may have noticed the improvement given by alcohol that is seen in 50% to 70% of patients.
- *Cases in which the patient is more bothered.* Propranolol and primidone have established efficacy and produce a mean tremor reduction of about 50%.
  - Use propranolol 40 mg 2-3 times daily, increased to 80-160 mg daily for maintenance.
  - Primidone 50 mg/day initially, increased gradually over 2 to 3 weeks if necessary. Side effects are common and frequently dose limiting (e.g., drowsiness, dizziness, or disequilibrium).
- *Patients not responding to propranolol or primidone or in whom they are contraindicated.* Consider one of the following: atenolol, sotalol, alprazolam, topiramate, or gabapentin, although the evidence of efficacy is less convincing.
- *Severe cases uncontrolled by medication.* Consider referral for neurosurgery. Deep brain stimulation has shown significant reductions in tremor, but further studies are required. Botulinum toxin injection has been used in some studies, but limited evidence exists to support its use.

References

Anonymous. (2000). The management of spasticity. *Drugs and Therapeutics Bulletin, 38,* 44–46.

Anonymous. (2003). When and how to stop antiepileptic drugs in adults. *Drugs and Therapeutics Bulletin, 41,* 41–43.

Anonymous. (2010). Management of medication overuse headache. *Drug and Therapeutics Bulletin, 48,* 2–6.

Bjornevik K, Cortese M, Healy B, Kuhle J, Mina M, Leng Y, Elledge S, Niebuhr D, Scher A, Munger K and Ascherio A (2022). Longitudinal analysis reveals high prevalence of Ebstein-Barr virus associated with multiple sclerosis. *Science,* 375 (6578), 296–301.

Confavreux, C., Vukusic, M. D., Moreau, M. D., & Adeleine, P. (2000). Relapses and progression of disability in multiple sclerosis. *New England Journal of Medicine, 343,* 1430–1438.

Markus, H. (2007). Improving the outcome of stroke. *BMJ (Clinical research ed.), 335,* 359–360.

McDermott, C. J., & Shaw, P. J. (2008). Diagnosis and management of motor neurone disease. *BMJ (Clinical research ed.), 336,* 658–662.

Medicines and Healthcare Products Regulatory Agency. (2008). *Antiepileptics: Risk of suicidal thoughts and behaviour.* MRHA. Retrieved from https://www.gov.uk/drug-safety-update/antiepileptics-risk-of-suicidal-thoughts-and-behaviour.

Neligan, A., Bell, G. S., & Sander, J. W. (2011). Sudden death in epilepsy. BMJ (Clinical research ed.), *343,* d7303.

NHS Scotland. (1999). *The Queen Elizabeth National Spinal Injuries Unit. Management of autonomic dysreflexia.* Retrieved from www.spinalunit.scot.nhs.uk.

NICE technology appraisal guidance 20. Guidance on the use of Riluzole for the treatment of motor neurone disease. (2001). (TA20). Retrieved from www.nice.org.uk.

NICE technology appraisal guidance 254. Fingolimod for the treatment of highly active relapsing-remitting multiple sclerosis. (2012). (TA254). Retrieved from www.nice.org.uk.

NICE Technology Appraisal Guidance 260. Botulinum toxin type A for the prevention of headaches in adults with chronic migraine. (2012). Retrieved from www.nice.org.uk.

Rugg-Gunn, F. J., & Sander, J. W. (2012). Management of chronic epilepsy. *BMJ (Clinical research ed.), 345,* e4576.

Scolding N, Barnes D, Chataway J, Chaudhuri A, Coles A, Giovannoni G, Miller D, Rashid W, Schmierer K, Silber E and Zajicek J. (2015). Association of British Neurologists revised guidelines for prescribing in multiple sclerosis. Retrieved from www.theabn.org.uk.

12

Women's Health

Kate Robinson

CHAPTER CONTENTS

Dysmenorrhoea

GUIDELINE

Royal College of Obstetricians and Gynaecologists. (2012). *The initial management of chronic Pelvic pain. 'Green Top' guideline 41*. Retrieved from https://www.rcog.org.uk/media/muab2gj2/gtg_41.pdf.

Primary Dysmenorrhoea

- Dysmenorrhoea is common. In about 20% of women, it is severe enough to interfere with daily activities.
- Dysmenorrhoea is more common in women with an early age of menarche and a longer duration of menstruation and in those who smoke.
- Reassure the patient that this is not a sign of disease. An examination of the abdomen is worthwhile as part of that reassurance as well as to exclude gross pelvic pathology. The need for a vaginal examination depends on the individual circumstances. It should be performed if the patient is sexually active.
- Give a nonsteroidal antiinflammatory drug (NSAID), alone or in addition to an analgesic. These work by inhibiting the synthesis of prostaglandins, and if the cycle is regular, it should be started the day before the onset of menstruation until pain subsides. They are effective in up to 70% of cases. Examples are ibuprofen 1200 mg/day, mefenamic acid 750 to 1250 mg/day, or naproxen, although adverse effects may be more common with the latter (Marjoribanks, Proctor, & Farquhar 2006).
- Simple analgesics such as paracetamol can be helpful, especially in patients in whom NSAIDs are contraindicated.
- Consider a trial of the combined oral contraceptive (COC). It is commonly used despite the lack of evidence either way about its benefit.
- Complementary and alternative therapy options:
  a. *Thiamine* 100 mg/day. In one study, it was more effective than placebo (Gokhale, 1996).
  b. *Toki-shakuyaka-san*, an herbal remedy, which may reduce pain after 6 months.
  c. Acupressure, which may be as effective as ibuprofen and high-frequency transcutaneous electrical nerve stimulation.
- Lifestyle and self-help techniques which could be helpful include smoking cessation, warmth to the abdomen, lying supine, tea, and warm baths.
- *Women who are still in pain.* Consider referrals for all those not responding.

Secondary Dysmenorrhoea

- Examine vaginally. Take a high vaginal swab (HVS) and swabs for *Chlamydia* spp.
- Refer for laparoscopy women in whom there is suspicion of pelvic pathology.
- *Chronic pelvic pain.* This affects about one in six women. It is a symptom with a number of contributory factors, including gynaecologic factors and nongynaecologic factors (e.g., irritable bowel syndrome, nerve entrapment) as well as psychological and social factors.
  - Allow enough time for the female patient to tell her story.
  - Recommend a pain diary and review.
  - Refer women who also have dyspareunia and low-grade pain throughout the cycle; they may have subclinical endometriosis, adenomyosis, or low-grade pelvic inflammatory disease (PID) despite a normal pelvic examination.
- Otherwise, treat symptomatically as for primary dysmenorrhoea, although symptom control is less likely to be successful.
- A levonorgestrel-releasing intrauterine device (LNG-IUD) may be beneficial, especially as up to 50% of women will be amenorrhoeic after 12 months. This option depends on the suitability for the patient (Vercellini et al, 1999).
- *Intrauterine device (UD).* Consider removing an intrauterine contraceptive device, if present.
- Refer all women, if the pain persists, to a gynaecologist.

Endometriosis

GUIDELINES

The European Society of Human Reproduction and Embryology. (2022). *Guideline on the management of women with endometriosis*. Retrieved from http://www.eshre.eu/Guidelines-and-Legal/Guidelines/Endometriosis-guideline.aspx.
   National Institute for Health and Care Excellence. (2023). *CKS endometriosis*. Available at http://cks.nice.org.uk/endometriosis.

- It is common for women to experience a significant delay in diagnosis, with almost 50% having symptoms for more than 10 years before receiving confirmation (Ballard et al, 2006). The explanation for this is multifactorial, including nondisclosure of symptoms because of embarrassment and not wanting to appear acopic at a physiological process, and the normalisation of pain by healthcare professionals.
- In addition to dysmenorrhoea, consider the diagnosis particularly in those with deep dyspareunia, chronic pelvic pain, ovulation pain, subfertility, or cyclical bowel or urinary symptoms with or without bleeding.
- A detailed history is key. Include not only exploration of presenting symptoms listed earlier but also the identification of any risk factors and potential complications (e.g., subfertility, depression).
- Risk factors for endometriosis (Coleman & Overton, 2015) are as follows:
  - Early menarche
  - Late menopause
  - Delayed childbearing

- Nulliparity
- Family history
- Vaginal outflow obstruction
- White ethnicity
- Low body mass index (BMI)
- Autoimmune disease
- Late first sexual encounter
- Smoking
- Laparoscopy remains the gold standard for diagnosis. Refer patients in whom you suspect the diagnosis because the examination is likely to be normal. Transvaginal ultrasound examination is sometimes helpful; pelvic magnetic resonance imaging and measurement of CA-125 are not routinely recommended in primary care.
- *When endometriosis has been diagnosed*, treatment should be guided by a number of factors, including the wishes of the female patient, the severity and duration of symptoms, requirements for fertility, previous treatment, and any abnormalities identified on pelvic ultrasound or clinical examination.
- Patients not wishing to become pregnant should consider:
  a. *COC*. First-line treatment is usually a monophasic COC containing 30 to 35 μg of ethinyloestradiol and either norethisterone or levonorgestrel. A 3-month trial of this treatment is recommended. Studies support the use of continuous oral contraceptives as a more effective treatment than cyclic prescribing, of dysmenorrhoea, chronic pelvic pain, and dyspareunia, as well as a reduction in endometriomas (Muzii et al, 2016).
  b. *Progestogens*. All forms of progesterone-only contraception appear to be effective in the treatment of patients with endometriosis-associated pain. The mode of administration can be guided by the patient. Evidence suggests that the LNG-IUS reduces pain and that it is maintained for at least 3 years. Efficacy is similar to that of gonadorelin analogues (Brown et al, 2010).
  c. *Gonadorelin analogues* are considered second-line treatment, should only be prescribed under the supervision of a gynaecologist, and are available in a number of different preparations (e.g., Goserelin subcutaneous injection every 28 days; Buserelin intranasal every day). Oral contraceptives should be stopped before starting treatment, and a nonhormonal form of contraception should be recommended because ovulation may occur if the treatment is interrupted at any point. Usual treatment is a single course of up to 6 months' duration, though there is some evidence for repeated and shorter duration courses. It is important to warn patients about the possibility of menopause-type symptoms with this treatment, which may necessitate addback treatment in the form of tibolone (licensed) or hormone replacement therapy (HRT) (continuous combined, off licence).
  d. *Danazol* is an androgen and is no longer recommended except as a last resort because of severe side effects of acne, weight gain, muscle cramps, oedema, and irreversible voice changes (Anonymous, 1999;

Pattie et al, 1998). Nonhormonal contraception is essential if the patient is sexually active.
  e. *Aromatase inhibitors*. These can be used off-label in combination with any other medical or surgical treatment, when pain is refractory.
- Patients wishing to become pregnant:
  a. Consider using NSAIDs, as in primary dysmenorrhoea.
  b. Refer for consideration of surgical ablation or excision of endometriosis. This is an effective alternative to medical management (Sutton et al, 1994).

PATIENT ADVICE

Endometriosis UK. 10-18 Union Street, London SE1 1SZ; helpline: 0808 808 2227; Retrieved from https://www.endometriosis-uk.org.
    Royal College of Obstetricians and Gynaecologists. (2016). *Endometriosis: Information for you*. Retrieved from https://www.alliance-scotland.org.uk/wp-content/uploads/2024/03/Endometriosis-Information-sheet-FINAL-2.pdf.

Menorrhagia

GUIDELINES

National Institute for Health and Clinical Excellence. (2021). *Heavy menstrual bleeding. NICE clinical guideline* 88. Retrieved from https://www.nice.org.uk/guidance/ng88/resources/heavy-menstrual-bleeding-assessment-and-management-pdf-1837701412549.
    National Institute for Health and Care Excellence. (2023). *CKS menorrhagia*. Retrieved from https://cks.nice.org.uk/topics/menorrhagia-heavy-menstrual-bleeding/management/management/.

- Menorrhagia is regular, excessive menses occurring over consecutive cycles in an otherwise normal menstrual cycle which interferes with the female patient's quality of life. Objectively, this has been quantified as a loss of more than 80 mL of blood per month (Duckitt & Collins, 2008).
- Two-thirds of women who have a blood loss of more than 80 mL per month have to limit their normal activities and have anaemia.
- Menorrhagia is suggested by a history of bleeding that cannot be controlled with tampons alone and by having to get up during the night to change.

The presence of other menstrual symptoms may influence a female patient's assessment of the severity of her blood loss. Fifty percent of patients referred for menorrhagia have depression or anxiety as their primary problem (Anonymous, 1994a). One in 20 women aged 30 to 55 years consults her general practitioner (GP) each year with menorrhagia (Royal College of Obstetricians and Gynaecologists (RCOG), 1999) with one-third of women quantifying their periods as heavy.

- In 40% to 60% of women, no underlying cause is found.

Clinical Assessment

- Check that there is no intermenstrual or postcoital bleeding.
- Check that there are no other menstrual symptoms, such as pain or pelvic pressure, which might suggest an underlying pathology.
- Check that the patient has had a recent smear as offered by the current recall system.
- Ascertain the impact the bleeding is having on the patient's life.
- Do not perform a pelvic and abdominal examination unless the history suggests an underlying pathology, initial treatment has proved ineffective, or an IUD is being considered. Perform swabs if infection is suspected.
- Check haemoglobin; two-thirds of patients will be anaemic. Do not routinely check ferritin.
- Do not routinely measure female hormones.
- Exclude hypothyroidism only if there are signs or symptoms.
- Consider haematologic abnormalities (e.g., von Willebrand disease or thrombocytopenia), especially in women who have a family history of easy bleeding or who have bled heavily since the menarche.
- Consider referral for pelvic ultrasonography if there is a palpable uterus (routine) or pelvic mass (urgent). Consider referral for transvaginal ultrasonography if there is coexisting dysmennorhoea to suggest adenomyosis.
- Refer to a gynaecologist for assessment if any of the following are present:
  a. The patient is older than 45 years of age.
  b. There is suspicion of an organic cause (fibroids, pelvic pain, dyspareunia).
  c). There is any postcoital, intermenstrual, or irregular bleeding, or any sudden change in blood loss.
  d. Medical treatment is unsuccessful.

Treatment

- *LNG-IUD(Mirena).* This appears to be the most effective nonsurgical treatment (National Institute for Health and Clinical Excellence (NICE), 2007), is licensed for the treatment of menorrhagia. and is now suggested as the preferred first-choice treatment in all but those with fibroids larger than 3 cm or causing distorted uterine cavities or adenomyosis. The patient should be warned that irregular bleeding may occur in the first 6 months and that progestogen-type adverse effects are possible, including breast tenderness, acne, and headaches. A pelvic examination is needed before insertion.
- *Tranexamic acid.* Start on the first day of each cycle and continue until heavy bleeding has ceased. Tranexamic acid 1g 4 times daily (QDS) decreases bleeding by up to 70% (NICE, 2007).
- *NSAIDs.* Give mefenamic acid 500 mg tds (3 times daily) or naproxen 500 mg bd (twice daily). Taken shortly before or at the start of menstruation and continued during heavy loss, they can decrease bleeding by 20% to 50%. They are especially useful if there is dysmenorrhoea.

- *The COC* is commonly used, but there is insufficient evidence at present to adequately assess its effectiveness (NICE, 2007). It is especially useful if there is also dysmenorrhoea and if contraception is required.
- *Progestogens.* Give oral norethisterone for 21 days of each cycle (days 5–26). Giving it for the second half of each cycle only is no better than placebo (Lethaby, Irvine, & Cameron 2001). This is not an effective form of contraception. Alternatively, any form of progesterone-only contraception may be used.
- *Cu-IUD.* If a copper IUD is in situ, either give an NSAID or an antifibrinolytic or change to an LNG-IUD.
- *Women not responding.* Consider referral for:
  a. Ultrasound examination and if inconclusive, hysteroscopy to exclude endometrial polyps and other pathology such as fibroids. Also consider endometrial sampling in patients older than 40 years of age.
  b. Endometrial ablation or hysterectomy. Endometrial ablation has a shorter hospital stay and less time off work, but a proportion of women will have further bleeding and will require further surgery (Gannon et al, 1991). It is not suitable for women who may wish to conceive in future.
  c. *Gonadotropin-releasing hormone (GnRH) analogues* are effective at treating menorrhagia but have significant side effects. They should not be initiated in primary care and are time limited in their use.

PATIENT ADVICE

Wirral University Teaching Hospital website. Retrieved from https://www.wuth.nhs.uk/media/18090/pl00829-heavy-periods.pdf.

Flooding

- Give norethisterone as one of the following:
  a. 15 mg bd for 2 days, then 10 mg bd for 2 days, then 15 mg once daily for 2 days, followed by 10 mg once daily for 14 days. The patient should expect a bleed 2 to 3 days after stopping the norethisterone
  b. 20 mg bd for 5 days

Delaying a Period

- Give norethisterone 5 mg bd or tds 3 days before the expected period. If this fails, double the dose on the next occasion. Continue it until it is convenient to have the period. The next period can be expected 2 to 3 days after stopping norethisterone.

Irregular Periods

Teenagers

- *Reassure* the patient that irregular periods are common after the menarche and that a regular cycle will probably establish itself without treatment.

- *If the patient is sufficiently bothered.* Give a progestogen cyclically, from day 10 to day 25 or day 1 to day 21, for 3 months. There is, however, no reason to think that this will speed up the establishment of normal periods.
- The *COC* can be considered, especially if contraception is required or the patient has dysmenorrhoea.
- *Very infrequent periods.* These girls need assessment (see later discussion).

Women in Their Reproductive Years

- Exclude pregnancy.
- Check whether irregular periods or amenorrhoea have always been a feature. They may have polycystic ovary syndrome (PCOS) (see later).
- Check whether the irregularity is caused by the progestogen-only pill (POP).
- Look for weight loss, excessive exercise, recent stress, hirsutism, galactorrhoea, and infertility.
- Take blood for thyroid function tests (TFTs), prolactin, free androgen index, luteinising hormone (LH), and follicle-stimulating hormone (FSH) on day 2 of the cycle.
- If results are normal and the patient wishes to become pregnant, consider referral for clomiphene.
- If the results are normal and pregnancy is not desired, COC or cyclical progestogens can be considered.
- If the results are abnormal, refer to an endocrinologist or gynaecologist as appropriate.

Older Women

- Distinguish the irregularity caused by ovarian failure from the pathological pattern of intermenstrual bleeding (IMB), which should be referred.
- Consider cyclical progestogens if the patient is sufficiently bothered.
- The COC regulates bleeding and provides contraception. The known risks of thrombosis and breast carcinoma should be discussed with the patient and documented.
- HRT can be considered if there are other symptoms of menopause and the bleeding is not pathological.

Postmenopausal Women

GUIDELINE

National Institute of Health and Care Excellence. (2021). *Suspected cancer: Recognition and referral. NICE clinical guideline 12.* Retrieved from https://www.nice.org.uk/guidance/ng12/resources/suspected-cancer-recognition-and-referral-pdf-1837268071621.

- Postmenopausal bleeding is generally accepted as an episode of bleeding 12 months or more after the last period.
- Refer (along a suspected cancer pathway) if:
  a. There has been any unexplained postmenopausal bleeding in a female aged older than 55 years (consider the same if aged younger than 55 years)

  b. Women on tamoxifen, especially if they have been on it for more than 5 years. There is a fourfold increase in incidence in endometrial cancer.
- For the management of bleeding in women taking HRT, see the section on HRT.

Intermenstrual Bleeding

- Examine the following:
  a. For anaemia
  b. The pelvis for abnormalities with a bimanual examination
  c. The cervix for abnormalities and take swabs
  d. The vulva and vagina
- Check the patient's smear history and past results.
- Take a pregnancy test if appropriate.
- Refer urgently (along a suspected cancer pathway) any female with abnormalities on examination suspicious for cancer.
- Consider urgent referral for any patient with persistent IMB despite normal examination findings.
- *Premenstrual spotting.* Reassure the patient if the loss is light and premenstrual. It is probably caused by failure of the corpus luteum and should settle within a few cycles. Give cyclical progestogens on days 12 to 26 (i.e., in the luteal phase) to women sufficiently troubled by the symptoms.
- *Women on the COC.* Check compliance. If the examination is normal and bleeding persists, consider changing the pill (see section on COC).
- *Women with an IUD*
  a. Take endocervical swabs and a HVS.
  b. If there is no infection, remove the IUD but remember to discuss alternative contraception.
  c. Reassess in 3 months.

Postcoital Bleeding

- Ascertain the patient's smear history, including any visits to colposcopy and the outcome and treatment (if known).
- Enquire about risk factors for cervical cancer, including family history and smoking status.
- Assess risk of sexually transmitted infections and arrange swabs when appropriate.
- Examine the abdomen and pelvis, including a bimanual and assessment for lymphadenopathy.
- Refer urgently (along a suspected cancer pathway) any female whose cervix appears consistent with cervical cancer, without awaiting an up-to-date smear.

Amenorrhoea

REVIEW

National Institute of Health and Care Excellence. (Updated 2022). *Clinical knowledge summaries: Amenorrhoea.* Retrieved from https://cks.nice.org.uk/topics/amenorrhoea/.

Primary Amenorrhoea

When to Refer

- Age 13 years and no secondary sexual characteristics
- Age 15 years with normal secondary sexual characteristics
- Puberty for 5 years or more without menarche
- At any age if:
  - Growth retardation, suspicion of androgen excess, hyperprolactinaemia, thyroid disease (to endocrinology)
  - Suspected genital tract malformation (to gynaecology)
  - Suspected eating disorder (to mental health services, paediatrics, or both)

Secondary Amenorrhoea

- Secondary amenorrhoea exists when a female has not menstruated for 6 months, having had a previously established cycle.
- In the history, note particularly:
  a. Any weight loss (if the patient's weight is <45 kg and she is of average height, she is unlikely to menstruate).
  b. Contraception. Amenorrhoea may occur with use of the LNG-IUD, with depot medroxyprogesterone, or after use of the COC.
  c. Excessive exercise (suggestive of relative energy deficiency in sport).
  d. Recent stress.
  e. The character of the cycles before the amenorrhoea.
- Exclude pregnancy.
- Take blood for LH and FSH, free testosterone, prolactin, oestradiol, and TFTs.
- Refer to a gynaecologist or endocrinologist as appropriate if any of the following are present:
  a. The FSH and LH are persistently high and the patient is younger than 40 years of age. This indicates premature ovarian failure.
  b. The free testosterone is raised. This suggests PCOS (see later); or
  c. The prolactin is over 1000 mIU/L or 500 to 1000 mIU/L on two occasions. This suggests a pituitary adenoma. This includes females who are taking drugs that can cause hyperprolactinaemia (e.g., selective serotonin reuptake inhibitors (SSRIs)).
  d. The oestradiol is low.
  e. There is a recent history of uterine or cervical surgery. This may indicate Asherman syndrome.
- Osteoporosis risk needs to be considered in patients with persistent amenorrhoea. Measurement of bone density may be required, and if symptoms have persisted over 12 months, then consideration should be given to treatment with cyclical combined HRT (off-label use). Advice on adequate dietary intake of calcium should be given.
- Contraception should be discussed because there remains a small theoretical risk of pregnancy if the patient is sexually active.

Polycystic Ovary Syndrome

> **GUIDELINES**
>
> National Institute of Health and Care Excellence. (2023). *Clinical knowledge summaries: Polycystic ovary syndrome.* Retrieved from https://cks.nice.org.uk/topics/polycystic-ovary-syndrome/.

- Polycystic ovaries are a common ultrasound finding, affecting up to 33% of females of reproductive age in the United Kingdom, only one-third of whom have clinical or biochemical features of PCOS.
- The characteristic features include:
  a. Truncal obesity
  b. Oligomenorrhoea, amenorrhoea, or dysfunctional uterine bleeding
  c. Hirsutism
  d. Acne
  e. Raised serum-free testosterone or free androgen index
  f. Male-pattern hair loss
- Patients with PCOS are twice as likely to develop diabetes (Wild et al, 2000). By the age of 40 years, up to 40% will have type 2 diabetes (Lord, Flight, & Norman, 2003). These patients have a higher prevalence of features associated with metabolic syndrome, including hypertension, dyslipidaemia, visceral obesity, insulin resistance, and hyperinsulinaemia.

Diagnosis

Consider the diagnosis if two of the following three criteria are met:

a. Polycystic ovaries on USS (Ultrasound scan) (either 12 or more follicles in at least one ovary or increased ovarian volume (>10 mL). The diagnosis can be made in the absence of polycystic ovaries on USS, and the appearance of polycystic ovaries on USS, without the other criteria, is not enough to make the diagnosis.
b. Oligo- or anovulation. This is suggested by menstrual cycles longer than 35 days or more than 10 periods a year.
c. Clinical or biochemical signs of hyperandrogenism. Clinical signs include acne, hirsutism, and androgenic alopecia. The biochemical confirmation required is a raised total or free testosterone. Sex hormone binding globulin (SHBG) may be low and is a proxy for hyperinsulinaemia. Free androgen index (total testosterone/SHBG × 100%) measures the amount of physiologically active testosterone and may be increased. Note: An increased LH-to-FSH ratio is no longer considered useful in the diagnosis because of its inconsistency, but measurement can be helpful in excluding premature ovarian failure; biochemical testing requires cessation of hormonal contraception for at least 3 months.

- Exclude adrenal hyperplasia, hyperprolactinaemia, androgen-secreting tumours, and Cushing syndrome. If the latter is suspected on clinical grounds, refer to an endocrinologist.

- Check TFTs, serum prolactin, and free testosterone. If there is clinical evidence of hyperandrogenism and the total testosterone is greater than 5 nmol/L, check the level of 17-hydroxyprogesterone.
- If one of the criteria b or c above is met but not the other, order a pelvic USS for ovarian cysts. Do not request this for adolescents.

Management

- Explain what little is known about the syndrome: that the pituitary produces excess LH, which stimulates the ovary to produce excess testosterone, which in turn causes acne and hirsutism. Associated with this is a tendency to insulin resistance, manifested by weight gain and the development of diabetes.
- *Cardiovascular disease risk.* Check the serum lipids, blood pressure, waist circumference, and BMI regularly in females older than 35 years of age. NICE recommends calculating the cardiovascular risk score, but it should be noted that cardiovascular risk calculators have not been validated in those with PCOS. Hypertension should be treated, but lipid-lowering agents should only be introduced by a specialist. Advise on weight loss, diet, and exercise as appropriate.
- *Diabetes.* Screen all females with PCOS every 1 to 3 years for impaired glucose tolerance and type 2 diabetes. Initially offer to all females an oral glucose tolerance test, fasting glucose or HbA1c. Consider repeating this annually for females at higher risk (impaired glucose tolerance, strong family history of diabetes, BMI >30 kg/m^2 or >25 kg/m^2 in Asian females and those with a history of gestational diabetes).
- *Nonalcoholic fatty liver disease (NAFLD).* The risk of NAFLD is increased because of the metabolic effects of PCOS and should be investigated if appropriate.
- *Snoring.* Ask about snoring and sleep apnoea. PCOS appears to be a risk factor independently of BMI in sleep apnoea.
- *Weight.* Advise about weight loss through diet (especially with a low–glycemic index diet) and exercise. Loss of weight has been reported to result in resumption of ovulation, improvement in fertility, increased SHBG, and reduced risk of diabetes and cardiovascular disease.
- *Psychological impact.* Do not neglect this aspect. Screen for depression and anxiety and be alert to risk of psychosexual problems and eating disorders caused by a negative body image.

Management of Symptoms

- *Acne.* See section on acne. COCs should be considered alongside topical retinoids and antibiotics. Co-cyprindiol (e.g., Dianette) should not be considered first-line treatment because of the risk of adverse events.
- *Hirsutism.* Physical methods of hair removal (e.g., waxing, IPL (Intense pulsed light)) and topical treatment with eflornithine may be helpful but do not treat the underlying cause. Eflornithine has been reported

as resulting in marked improvement in 32% of females. Females who are overweight should be advised to lose weight. First-line drug treatment is with a combined hormonal contraception containing ethinylestradiol, though a desogestrel-containing COC may be as effective. Dianette (cyproterone acetate and ethinylestradiol) is the only licensed COC for moderate to severe hirsutism, but it should be avoided in females with increased risk of venous thromboembolism (VTE). Second-line treatments include spironolactone, finasteride, GnRH analogues, and metformin; these should be started by secondary care (NICE 2020). Contraception is required while patients are taking spironolactone because there is a theoretical risk of feminising male foetuses (Farquhar et al, 2000). Warn that benefit is unlikely before about 6 months of any of these treatments.
- *Lack of regular periods.* This may predispose to endometrial hyperplasia and later carcinoma. The United Kingdom's Royal College of Gynaecologists (RCOG) recommends that a withdrawal bleed should be induced every 3 to 4 months with progestogens (for at least 12 days) or the COC. Females who have less frequent bleeding should be referred for a transvaginal USS to assess for endometrial thickness and referred for assessment if it is thicker than 10 mm. Females who do not have withdrawal bleeds should be referred to a gynaecologist.
- *Lack of ovulation.* Refer to a gynaecologist. Metformin 500 mg tds, though unlicensed for this use, can induce ovulation and reduce fasting insulin concentrations, blood pressure, and low-density lipoprotein cholesterol. However, the RCOG states that 'long term use of insulin sensitising agents cannot as yet be recommended'. Patients are increasingly aware and ask for metformin treatment, but this is ahead of the evidence and outside the product licence (Harborne et al, 2003).
- *Infertility.* Refer. A combination of metformin and clomiphene is more effective than either alone. Both laparoscopic electrocautery and ovarian drilling have been shown to have long-term benefits in ovulation and normalisation of serum androgens.

SELF-HELP GROUP

Verity. *The polycystic self-help group.* Retrieved from http://www.verity-pcos.org.uk.

Vaginal Discharge

GUIDELINE

National Institute of Health and Care Excellence. (2019). *Clinical knowledge summaries: Vaginal discharge.* Retrieved from https://cks.nice.org.uk/topics/vaginal-discharge/.

- Ask about the type of discharge, the timing, whether it smells, whether it itches, and whether there is pelvic pain.

- Ask if the female uses any vaginal products, such as washes or douches.
- Many females self-diagnose thrush or bacterial vaginosis and purchase over-the-counter treatments. Ask what has been tried and the effect (if any).
- Ask the female what she thinks it is and, when asking whether it seems related to sexual activity, ask tactfully about the number of sexual partners.
- Examine the vulva and test the vaginal pH using narrow-range pH paper. There are no grounds for a *routine* bi-manual or speculum examination nor for a swab. However, bimanual examination is needed if the history raises the possibility of pelvic infection; swabs are needed in those at risk of sexually transmitted infections (STIs) and in those in whom the clinical picture does not suggest bacterial vaginosis or candida.
- In those who are low risk of STIs and who decline examination, treatment can be given based on clinical history.
- *Interpretation of findings*
  - Smelly white discharge with pH greater than 4.5: bacterial vaginosis
  - White curdy discharge, usually with vulval soreness and itch, erythema, possibly fissuring, satellite lesions, and pH less than 4.5: candidiasis
  - Smelly yellow or green frothy discharge with pH greater than 4.5, perhaps with dysuria: *Trichomonas* infection
- When the clinical picture is not typical of bacterial vaginosis nor of candidiasis or the patient is younger than 25 years of age or has had a new sexual partner in the previous year, take swabs:
  - HVS for *Trichomonas* spp., the clue cells of bacterial vaginosis, and *Candida* spp.
  - Endocervical swab for chlamydia and gonorrhoea testing with nucleic acid amplification test
- Patients with STIs are best managed in the GUM (Genito-urinary medicine) clinic.

Management of *Candida*

GUIDELINE

British Association for Sexual Health and HIV. (2020). National guideline for the management of vulvovaginal candidiasis. *International Journal of STD & AIDS, 3*(12), 1124–1144. Retrieved from http://www.bashh.org (choose 'Guidelines').

- Give general advice to avoid local irritants and avoid tight-fitting synthetic clothing (Bingham, 1999).
- Treat only if the patient is symptomatic.
- Prescribe a topical imidazole. Cure rates are 80% to 95%. Give it either as a single dose or as a short course at night, usually for 3 nights. Oral imidazoles are no more effective (Watson et al, 2002), but they have more side effects. In addition, they are contraindicated in pregnancy.
- *Male partners.* There is no evidence to support the treatment of asymptomatic male sexual partners (Bisschop et al, 1986). Sexual intercourse does not need to be avoided unless it is uncomfortable for the female.

- COC. Do not stop the COC. Its use is not associated with candidiasis.
- *Pregnancy.* Asymptomatic colonisation is more common in pregnancy (30%–40%). Treat symptomatic patients with topical azoles, but a longer course may be necessary. Clotrimazole 500 mg pessary at night for up to 7 nights is the recommended first-line treatment.

Recurrent Candidiasis

- Recurrent candidiasis is when there are four or more symptomatic episodes per year.
- Check the urine for glucose approximately 2 hours after a meal or glucose load. Note that this would be inadequate as a screening test for diabetes in any other situation.
- Exclude other risk factors, including iron-deficiency anaemia, thyroid disease, frequent antibiotic use, corticosteroid use, and immunodeficiency.
- Screen for other vaginal infections.
- Treatment choice should be guided by whether it is suspected that there is recurrence with a good or complete response to prior treatment or recurrence because of poor or partial response to treatment.
  a. Good or complete response
    - Fluconazole susceptible. Suppressive therapy with induction (150 mg three times per week); then weekly 150 mg fluconazole for 6 months
    - Fluconazole resistance. 100,000 IU Nystatin pessaries for 14 nights
  b. Poor or partial response
    - Fluconazole or azole resistance. 100,000 IU Nystatin pessaries for 14 nights
    - Nystatin resistance. 600 mg boric acid pessaries for 14 nights
    - Failure of the above. Consider alternative diagnoses.
- Consider giving cetirizine 10 mg/day for 6 months or montelukast 10mg od for 6 months. Allergy may be an important component, especially in females with atopy.
- Candida *of the gut.* There is no evidence to suggest that eradication of *Candida* from the gut is helpful.
- *Probiotics or* Lactobacillus. Evidence does not support the use of oral or topical *Lactobacillus* in prevention of vulvovaginal candidiasis.
- *Alteration of vaginal pH.* Suggest a trial of a pH lowering agent (e.g., AciGel).
- *Yoghurt, honey, and tea tree essential oil.* Insufficient evidence.

Management of Bacterial Vaginosis

GUIDELINE

British Association for Sexual Health and HIV. (2012). *UK national guideline for the management of bacterial vaginosis.* Retrieved from http://www.bashh.org.uk. (choose 'Guidelines').

- Bacterial vaginosis is characterised by a reduction in lactobacilli and an overgrowth of predominantly anaerobic organisms (*Gardnerella vaginalis, Mycoplasma hominis, Prevotella* spp., *Mobiluncus* spp.).
- Approximately 50% of females with the condition are asymptomatic.
- It is not regarded as sexually transmitted. It can arise and remit spontaneously in females regardless of sexual activity. However, it is more common in females liable to STIs.
- *Partners.* No evidence has been found supporting the treatment of partners of females affected by bacterial vaginosis (Potter, 1999).
- Treatment is indicated for:
  a. Symptomatic females.
  b. Pregnant females with a history of recurrent miscarriage.
  c. Females undergoing termination of pregnancy. They are at greater risk of PID if the bacterial vaginosis is untreated.
- Give metronidazole 400 to 500 mg bd for 5 to 7 days, intravaginal metronidazole gel (0.75%) once daily for 5 days, metronidazole 2 g as a single oral dose, or intravaginal clindamycin cream (2%) once daily for 7 days. The cure rate is 70% to 80%.
- *Pregnancy and lactation.* Symptomatic females in pregnancy should be treated with metronidazole. Lactating females should be treated with intravaginal metronidazole.

Pelvic Inflammatory Disease

> **GUIDELINE**
>
> British Association for Sexual Health and HIV. (2019). *UK national guideline for the management of pelvic inflammatory disease.* Retrieved from https://www.bashh.org/resources/6/pid_2019/.

- PID is usually the result of ascending infection, with *Neisseria gonorrhoeae* and *Chlamydia trachomatis* being identified as causative agents in 25% of cases. *Mycoplasma genitalium*, anaerobes, and other organisms commonly found in the vagina may also be implicated. Having an IUD fitted conveys an increased risk for the first 4 to 6 weeks after insertion.
- PID has a high morbidity rate: about 20% of affected females become infertile, 20% develop chronic pelvic pain, and 10% of those who conceive have an ectopic pregnancy (Metters et al, 1998).
- Repeated episodes of PID are associated with a four- to sixfold increased risk of permanent tubal damage (Hillis et al, 1997).
- PID may be asymptomatic.
- About 10% to 20% of females with PID will develop right upper quadrant pain and perihepatitis (Fitz-Hugh–Curtis syndrome).
- A delay of only a few days in receiving treatment markedly increases the risk of long-term sequelae (Hillis et al, 1993). Because of this and the lack of definitive diagnostic criteria,

a low threshold for the empirical treatment of patients with PID is recommended.

Diagnosis

- Symptoms can include fever, lower abdominal pain, deep dyspareunia, abnormal bleeding, abnormal vaginal, or cervical discharge. On examination, there may be cervical excitation and adnexal tenderness.
- Clinical diagnosis is correct in only 65% to 90% of cases compared with laparoscopy. Even laparoscopy can miss mild cases, but it remains the most reliable investigation. In the United Kingdom, it is not recommended in all cases but should be performed when there is diagnostic doubt.
- If not referring, perform the following:
  a. Endocervical swabs for gonococcus and *Chlamydia*. Negative microbiological test results do not exclude a diagnosis of PID; in at least 50% of cases, no specific organism is identified. Screen for the same diseases in all sexual partners.
  b. Urinalysis, pregnancy test, and MSU (Mid-stream urine) specimen to look for other causes of lower abdominal pain.
  c. Blood for erythrocyte sedimentation rate or C-reactive protein.
- Recommend rest and provide adequate analgesia.
- Recommend that unprotected intercourse be avoided until the female and her partner(s) have completed treatment and follow-up. If it is not possible to screen for gonorrhoea and chlamydia in the sexual partner(s) give empirical treatment for both gonorrhoea and chlamydia (Haddon et al, 1998; Groom et al, 2001).
- If an IUD is in situ and is the preferred method of contraception, leave it in place. Remove it only if the condition fails to respond to treatment and other causes of pain have been excluded (Teisala, 1989; Larsson & Wennergren, 1981; Soderberg & Lingren, 1981).
- Drug treatment is one of the following:
  a. Ofloxacin 400 mg bd plus metronidazole 400 mg bd for 14 days
  b. In females at high risk of gonococcal infection: ceftriaxone 1000 mg intramuscularly as a single dose; then 14 days of oral doxycycline 100 mg bd and metronidazole 400 mg bd
  c. Moxifloxacin 400 mg once daily (OD) for 14 days (most effective against *M. genitalium*)
- Review daily in case admission becomes necessary.

Admission

- Admit patients if:
  a. The illness is severe, including pyrexia greater than 38°C.
  b. The patient is not responding after 3 days of oral therapy.
  c. The patient is unable to tolerate oral drugs.
  d. A pelvic mass is present, suggestive of tubo-ovarian abscess.

e. The patient is pregnant.

f. There is diagnostic uncertainty.

g. The patient has an immunodeficiency.

h. The patient is above the usual age for PID. An alternative diagnosis (e.g., ovarian carcinoma) is more likely.

Follow-up for All Patients

- Review within 72 hours. Refer if there is little improvement.
- Review again in 4 weeks to:
  a. Ensure there is adequate clinical response.
  b. Ensure there was compliance with the antibiotics.
  c. Trace, investigate, and treat the female's partner(s) if an STI is diagnosed. A study found that 60% of contacts had relevant infections and that in most of them, it was asymptomatic (Kamwendo et al, 1993). Consider referral to a GUM clinic for contact tracing.
  d. Stress the significance of the disease and the sequelae.
- Discuss with the patient her need for safer sex.
- Advise the patient to ask for antibiotic cover (e.g., doxycycline 200 mg stat or metronidazole 2 g stat) if she ever needs a termination of pregnancy or a dilatation and curettage.
- Advise the patient to seek advice promptly if the symptoms return.

PATIENT INFORMATION

Royal College of Obstetricians and Gynaecologists. *Acute pelvic inflammatory disease.* Retrieved from http://www.rcog.org.uk (search on 'Acute pelvic inflammatory disease').

Premenstrual Syndrome

GUIDELINES

National Institute for Health and Care Excellence. (2019). *Clinical knowledge summaries: premenstrual syndrome.* Available at http://cks.nice.org.uk/premenstrual-syndrome.
    Royal College of Obstetricians and Gynaecologists. *Premenstrual syndrome, management. Green-Top guideline no. 48.* Retrieved from http://www.rcog.org.uk/guidance.

- Ninety-five percent of females have symptoms related to their menstrual cycles; in 5%, they are disabling. More than 150 symptoms have been reported.
- The diagnosis depends not on the type of symptom but on the timing of the symptoms and their cyclicity, as well as the degree of impairment. Symptoms are present 1 to 14 days before menstruation and disappear at the onset or by the day of the heaviest flow. A symptom-free week should follow. If behavioural symptoms persist throughout the cycle, then consider a psychological or psychiatric disorder. If daily activities (e.g., work, interpersonal

relationships) are unaffected, it is likely to represent physiological menstrual symptoms.

- Ask the patient to keep a prospective menstrual and symptom diary for at least 2 months. She can score symptoms according to their severity.
- Listen sympathetically. It is a real entity. This alone can be therapeutic.
- Give simple advice.
  a. *Dietary advice.* Explain that some females seem more sensitive to blood sugar changes at this time of the cycle, and this may be the cause of food cravings, panic reactions, irritability, and aggression. Advise patients to reduce their refined sugar intake as well as their caffeine intake. Small, frequent carbohydrate snacks seem effective in about 30% of females. Moderate any alcohol.
  b. *Stress management.* Explain that although it is not the cause of the syndrome, stress is harder to cope with during the premenstrual period. Relaxation methods, yoga, meditation, and exercise can be of benefit.
  c. *Regular exercise.* A recent systematic review has shown that regular exercise programmes may confer benefit in females with premenstrual syndrome (PMS) in terms of global, psychological, and behavioural symptoms (Pearce et al, 2020). Forty-five minutes of low- to moderate-aerobic exercise (50%–70% of maximum) three times a week has been shown to reduce symptoms.
  d. *Dietary supplements.* Many are used, but good evidence is lacking. Those with proven benefit include calcium and vitamin D, *Vitex agnus castus* L, and saffron, and some benefit has been shown with *Ginko biloba*, evening primrose oil, lemon balm, curcumin, and wheatgerm. More research is required for all. Vitamin B_6 has mixed results and should be limited to 10 mg/day because of potential neurotoxicity at higher doses.

Therapeutic Options

- *SSRIs.* Consider using an SSRI either continuously or in the luteal phase alone. There is good evidence of their efficacy (Wyatt et al, 2002). Side effects may limit their acceptability, and their use is off-label. Females should be advised of the potential risks of SSRIs in pregnancy and the likelihood of PMS symptom abatement and should discontinue them if planning to conceive or become pregnant.
- *Breast tenderness, bloating, and irritability* may be improved by taking spironolactone 100 mg/day from day 12 until the onset of menstruation. Consider bromocriptine 1.25 mg bd for breast tenderness; however, adverse effects are common.
- *Cognitive-behavioural therapy.* Consider for all who are severely affected.
- *NSAIDs* given for 7 days before menses and 4 days after the onset have been shown to improve a number of symptoms but not breast tenderness.

- *Oestrogens* may improve or in some cases worsen the situation. The COC can prove helpful, especially in those females requiring contraception. The best evidence is for drospirenone-containing COC, and continuous rather than cyclical use is recommended. A lower dose of oestrogen, as HRT, may help some females, but cyclical progestogens must also be used in females with an intact uterus, and the need for contraception should be considered.
- *Danazol* 200 mg bd has been shown to be effective. Adverse effects are common (masculinisation and weight gain) with continuous use but may not occur with luteal phase use alone. Contraception is essential because of its virilising effects on female foetuses.

Note: Progestogens have been found unhelpful in the treatment of patients with PMS.

Patients Not Responding

- Refer to a gynaecologist for the consideration of suppression of ovarian function. Treatment options include high-dose danazol, high-dose oestrogen, GnRH analogues with add back HRT, or hysterectomy and bilateral oophorectomy.

PATIENT SUPPORT

National Association for Premenstrual Syndrome. Retrieved from http://www.pms.org.uk.

Ovarian Cancer Screening

- Many women request screening for ovarian cancer on the basis of their family history. Some useful figures can be used to reassure many women (Table 12.1).
- There is currently no national screening programme for ovarian cancer. Despite early promising results, the UK Collaborative Trial of Ovarian Cancer Screening has so far failed to show clear-cut evidence of benefit from a universal screening programme.
- Results of the UK Familial Ovarian Cancer Screening Study indicate that females at 'higher risk' who choose to delay or decline prophylactic bilateral salpingo-oophorectomy may be suitable for 4-month screening.

TABLE 12.1 Ovarian Cancer Risk

First-Degree Relatives With Ovarian Cancer (n)	Lifetime Risk of Developing Ovarian Cancer (%)
0	1
1	5
2	15
>2	50?

using the Risk of Ovarian Cancer Algorithm (Rosenthal et al, 2017). More than 4000 high-risk females were screened for 3 years; 90% of ovarian cancers were successfully detected. Research is ongoing. Females at 'higher risk' are those with any of the following:

a. Two or more first-degree relatives with ovarian cancer
b. One first-degree relative with ovarian cancer and one first-degree relative with breast cancer diagnosed before 50 years of age
c. One ovarian cancer and two breast cancers diagnosed before 60 years of age in first-degree relatives
d. Known *BRCA-1* or *BRCA-2* mutations in the family
e. Three colorectal cancers, at least one diagnosed before 50 years of age, and one ovarian cancer, all first-degree relatives of each other
f. Affected relatives with any of the above combinations who are related by second-degree through an unaffected male and there is an affected sister (i.e., paternal transmission is occurring)

Note: A first-degree relative is a parent, sibling, or child. A second-degree relative is a grandparent, aunt or uncle, or cousin.

- *Weak family history.* Females with one close relative with epithelial ovarian cancer diagnosed before the age of 50 years may also wish to be referred for advice but may not be offered regular screening.

PATIENT INFORMATION

Cancer Research UK. *Ovarian cancer screening*. Retrieved from https://www.cancerresearchuk.org/about-cancer/ovarian-cancer/getting-diagnosed/screening.

Gestational Trophoblastic Hydatidiform Mole and Choriocarcinoma

GUIDELINE

Royal College of Obstetricians and Gynaecologists. (2022). *The management of gestational trophoblastic disease. Green-Top clinical guideline no. 38.* Retrieved from https://obgyn.onlinelibrary.wiley.com/doi/full/10.1111/1471-0528.16266.

- Gestational trophoblastic disease is uncommon in the United Kingdom, with a calculated incidence of 1 per 714 live births. The incidence is highest in females from Asia (incidence, 1 per 387 live births) compared with non-Asian females (incidence, 1 per 752 live births).
- In the United Kingdom, there is an effective registration and treatment programme with high cure rates.
- After the diagnosis of hydatidiform mole has been made, follow-up is needed for between 6 months and 2 years. The aim is to detect the occurrence of choriocarcinoma.
- After treatment, serum estimations of levels of human chorionic gonadotrophin (hCG) levels should be performed according to protocols from the regional expert units (London, Sheffield, and Dundee).

- The COC pill and hormone replacement are safe to use when hCG levels have reverted to normal.
- Females should be advised not to conceive until the hCG level has been normal for 6 months or follow-up has been completed (whichever is the sooner). The risk of further recurrence is 1 in 55. After any further pregnancy, urine and blood samples should be taken to exclude disease recurrence.
- Females who undergo chemotherapy should not attempt to conceive until 1 year after completion of treatment. More than 80% of females receiving chemotherapy achieve successful subsequent pregnancy, although the chance of return to fertility is substantially reduced if high-dose chemotherapy is used.
- Refer all females with persistent bleeding:
  a. After the evacuation of retained products of conception
  b. After normal pregnancy
  c. After miscarriage
- Send for histology any products of conception passed at home.
- If no products of conception are available, check hCG 4 weeks after the loss of the pregnancy.

PATIENT INFORMATION

The Hydatidiform Mole and Choriocarcinoma UK information service. (n.d.) Retrieved from http://www.hmole-chorio.org.uk. Royal College of Obstetricians and Gynaecologists. (n.d.) *Molar pregnancy and gestational trophoblastic disease, RCOG patient information.* Retrieved from http://https://www.rcog.org.uk/for-the-public/browse-our-patient-information.

SCREENING CENTRES

Trophoblastic Tumour Screening and Treatment Centre. Charing Cross Hospital, Department of Oncology, Fulham Palace Road, London, England W6 8RF. Tel. 020 8846 1409
　Trophoblastic Tumour Screening and Treatment Centre. Weston Park Hospital, Whitham Road, Sheffield, England S10 2SJ. Tel. 0114 226 5202.
　Hydatidiform Mole Follow-up (Scotland). Ninewells Hospital, Department of Obstetrics and Gynaecology, Dundee, Scotland DD1 9SY. Tel. 01382 632748.

Menopause

Establishing the Diagnosis

- No investigations are routinely indicated. FSH levels fluctuate markedly during perimenopause and so are of limited value in symptomatic females in whom a clinical history can form the basis of diagnosis. They are not reliable in those taking combined hormonal contraception or high-dose progestogen. There is little place for LH, oestradiol, and progesterone estimation in clinical practice (Hope et al, 1999).

- Consider taking serial FSH measurements in the following circumstances:
  a. Females with symptoms before the age of 40 years because of the implications of premature ovarian failure.
  b. Females with symptoms who have had a hysterectomy with ovarian conservation. They are at risk of an early menopause.
- Take FSH levels:
  a. Four to 8 weeks apart when the female is not taking HRT or hormonal contraception. FSH levels of greater than 30 IU/L are generally considered to be in the postmenopausal range.
  b. On day 2 or 3 of menses in females with menstrual bleeding. A FSH level of 10 to 12 IU/L is considered to be increased (American Association of Clinical Endocrinologists, 1999).
- *Abnormal bleeding.* Refer females, without starting HRT, if they give a history of abnormal bleeding (e.g., sudden change in menstrual pattern, IMB, postcoital bleeding, postmenopausal bleed; Hope et al, 1999; Korhonen et al, 1997).

Initial Management

- Counsel females about menopause. Ideally, all perimenopausal females should be given the opportunity to discuss menopause, with particular reference to the symptomatology, common misconceptions, and treatment options.
- Take the opportunity to discuss lifestyle issues (smoking cessation, diet, and exercise).
- *Osteoporosis.* Identify patients at high risk of osteoporosis and investigate and treat if appropriate. HRT is no longer indicated for the prevention of osteoporosis except in those with early menopause.
- *Vasomotor symptoms*
  a. *HRT* is extremely effective in controlling these symptoms (MacLennan et al, 2001). Because of the possible harms, use the lowest effective dose for the shortest time possible (see later).
  b. *SSRIs and related drugs.* A meta-analysis has found some evidence of benefit, with paroxetine performing best. However, even paroxetine reduced flushes by only one or two a day compared with placebo (Nelson et al, 2006).
  c. *Gabapentin.* A trial of 12 weeks of 900 mg/day reduced the hot flash composite score by 54% against 31% with placebo (Guttuso et al, 2003). The use of gabapentin for menopause is currently restricted to specialist centres.
  d. *Diet.* Discuss the limited evidence suggesting that phytoestrogens may be helpful in relieving vasomotor symptoms (Anonymous, 1998; Scambia et al, 2000). They are plant substances, found in soya beans, chickpeas, red clover, and cereals, that stimulate the oestrogen receptors.

e. *Consider clonidine* for those unable to take HRT or an SSRI.

f. *Black cohosh*, with or without other natural remedies, has been shown to be ineffective (Newton et al, 2006).

- *Vaginal dryness.* Treatment options include:
  a. HRT (see later)
  b. Local oestrogens. These can be given per vagina daily until symptoms have ceased and then twice weekly for as long as is needed to control symptoms. Systemic progestogens do not need to be given alongside local oestrogens because there is no evidence that they cause endometrial proliferation, and they can be given alongside systemic HRT if required. Females with contraindications to systemic HRT or whose symptoms are not controlled with standard dosing should be discussed with a specialist.
  c. Vaginal lubricants. These include KY Jelly and Replens (a nonhormonal aqueous moisturiser) and Senselle (a water-based lubricant), although the latter two are not available on the NHS in the United Kingdom.
- *Urinary symptoms*
  a. Symptoms related to urogenital atrophy respond to oestrogen by any route. Maximum benefit will not be seen for at least the first month and may take up to 1 year (Cardozo et al, 1998).
  b. Stress incontinence is unlikely to respond to oestrogen replacement therapy alone. Refer patients who are sufficiently troubled to a gynaecologist.
- *Psychological symptoms.* Psychological symptoms may relate to a female's hormonal status but, equally, menopause may become a 'scapegoat' for patients with underlying emotional problems (Hunter, 1996). Counselling may be helpful, but many patients improve when their physical symptoms improve (Gath & Iles, 1990). Depression may need treatment in its own right. Cognitive-behaviour therapy should be considered.

Hormone Replacement Therapy

GUIDELINES

Greater Manchester Medicines Management Group. (2023). *Hormone replacement therapy guidance for menopause management. Based on NHS Stockport CCG HRT guidance for menopause management.* Retrieved from https://gmmmg.nhs.uk/wp-content/uploads/2023/03/GM-HRT-Guidance-for-Menopause-Management-final-v1.0-approved-for-GMMMG-website.pdf.
National Institute for Health and Care Excellence. (2019). *Menopause: Diagnosis and management. NICE clinical guideline 23.* Retrieved from https://www.nice.org.uk/guidance/ng23/resources/menopause-diagnosis-and-management-pdf-1837330217413.

HRT may be indicated in the following:
- Females with an early menopause (before age 45 years), mainly for the prevention of osteoporosis. It may also give some protection in this young age group against cardiovascular disease. It is usually given until age 50 years.

- Females younger than the age of 65 years with severe vasomotor and other symptoms of menopause who understand the risks and are prepared to take HRT for a limited period. Analysis of Women's Health Initiative results has shown no increase in breast cancer, myocardial infarction, or stroke in females younger than 60 years of age who use HRT for 5 years or less (Rossouw et al, 2007).
- Record that the risks of HRT have been explained and an informed decision taken by the patient.
- Review the decision at least annually.

Benefits and Risks

Benefits

- *Symptom relief.* Improvement in vasomotor symptoms occurs in a few weeks and in vaginal symptoms in 3 months. Improvement in mental function is less certain. The mental health of females with vasomotor symptoms seems to improve on HRT, but those without vasomotor symptoms worsen, with poorer physical functioning and lower energy levels compared with those on placebo (Hlatky et al, 2002). Overall, HRT does not improve the quality of life (Hays et al, 2003).
- *Osteoporosis.* Combined HRT protects against hip fracture in unselected postmenopausal females and reduces the risk of all fractures. This represents five fewer hip fractures per 10,000 person years, a number needed to treat of 2000 for 1 year (Rossouw et al, 2002). In females at high risk of fracture, the absolute benefit is greater. The benefit is dose related (Table 12.2). However, the benefit on fracture risk is lost within 3 years of stopping HRT (Heiss et al, 2008).
- *Prevention of carcinoma of the colon.* HRT appears to reduce the risk of developing colonic carcinoma by 20% (relative risk (RR), 0.80; 95% confidence interval (CI), 0.74–0.86) (Nelson et al, 2002).

TABLE 12.2	Minimum Doses of Oestrogen Needed for Bone Conservation	
Drug	Dosage	Frequency
Oestradiol	1–2 mg	Daily[a]
Oral conjugated equine oestrogens	0.625 mg	Daily
Transdermal oestradiol patch	50 mg	Daily
Oestradiol gel	1.5 g (two measures)	Daily
Oestradiol implants	50 mg	Every 6 months

[a]Although 1 mg or 2 mg of oral oestradiol can be used for prevention of osteoporosis, the bone-protective effect is dose related. Some products are licensed for osteoporosis prevention at 2 mg only, but others are licensed at 1 mg and 2 mg.

Harms

- *Cardiovascular disease.* HRT does not increase risk of cardiovascular disease when given to females younger than the age of 60 years nor does it affect the risk of dying from cardiovascular disease. If cardiovascular risk factors are well managed, then they are not in themselves a contraindication to using HRT. Oral oestrogen appears to be associated with a small increased risk of stroke in the context of a very low baseline risk in females younger than the age of 60 years. There is no increased risk seen with the transdermal route.
- *Breast cancer.* The use of combined HRT in healthy postmenopausal females is associated with an increase in breast cancer risk (RR, 1.24; 95% CI, 1.01–1.54) (Rossouw et al, 2002), but this is not the case with oestrogen-only treatment. The increase in risk is related to the duration of treatment and decreases again after cessation.
- *Endometrial cancer.* Unopposed oestrogen is associated with an extra 5 cases per 1000 females over 5 years. The use of combined preparations reduces, but does not eliminate, this risk with an estimated risk of 2 extra cases per 1000 females over 10 years.
- *Ovarian cancer.* Long-term combined or oestrogen-only HRT is associated with a small increased risk of ovarian cancer. This excess risk disappears within a few years of stopping HRT.
- *VTE.* Oral HRT increases the risk of VTE, but transdermal HRT does not increase risk above the baseline population risk. Consider the transdermal route for females with additional risk factors for VTE, including BMI above 30 kg/m^2. Consider referring females who are at high risk of VTE (e.g., because of a family history of hereditary thrombophilia or VTE) to a haematologist for assessment.
- *Dementia.* The effect of HRT on dementia risk is unknown.

Other Issues to Discuss

- Explain that taking HRT means that cyclical bleeding will return if the female has an intact uterus and a cyclical preparation is used. Irregular bleeding is common with continuous preparations.
- Explain that evidence from randomised trials suggests that HRT does not cause extra weight gain in addition to that normally gained at the time of menopause (Norman et al, 2001).

Contraindications

- Oestrogen replacement therapy is absolutely contraindicated in very few patients. Even in females in whom treatment appears contraindicated, oestrogen therapy may be prescribed under supervision of a specialist menopause clinic if the female's symptoms are particularly severe (Rees & Purdie, 1999).
- Absolute contraindications include:
  a. Acute-phase myocardial infarction, pulmonary embolism, or deep vein thrombosis
  b. Active endometrial or breast cancer
  c. Pregnancy
  d. Undiagnosed breast mass
  e. Uninvestigated abnormal vaginal bleeding
  f. Severe active liver disease

Note: Many contraindications given in prescribing data sheets are derived from high-dose COCs and are, in the view of most experts, not applicable to HRT (Rees & Purdie, 1999).

- HRT use in females with comorbidity (relative contraindications):
  a. *History of thromboembolic disease.* Females with a personal or family history of thromboembolism should be offered screening for thrombophilia before starting. Those with a personal history of VTE should not take HRT unless the female decides that, for her, the benefits outweigh the risks (RCOG, 2004). She may choose prophylactic anticoagulation, though that has its own risks. Transdermal oestrogen with LNG-IUD is considered a good choice if HRT is desired. A specialist opinion is wise in those with thrombophilia.
  b. *Past history of endometrial cancer.* Refer females who want to consider HRT to the appropriate specialist. Although conventional advice is that oestrogens are contraindicated, small studies of endometrial cancer survivors have not shown an adverse effect on survival.
  c. *Diabetes and gallbladder disease.* Use a transdermal preparation.
  d. *Liver disease.* Refer to a specialist clinic.
  e. *Endometriosis.* Refer to a specialist clinic.
  f. *Fibroids.* HRT may enlarge fibroids, causing heavy or painful withdrawal bleeds. Warn patients to report pain or pressure effects on the bladder or bowel.
  g. *Migraine* is not a contraindication to HRT. There is no evidence that the risk of stroke is increased by the use of HRT in females with migraine (Bousser et al, 2000). Transdermal oestrogen is recommended, and if required, progesterone should be given continuously.
  h. *Hypertension.* There is no evidence that HRT raises blood pressure (Rees & Purdie, 1999), but transdermal delivery is recommended.
  i. *Perimenopausal depression.* History of postnatal depression and PMS are risk factors. Avoid androgenic progestogens (e.g., norethisterone, medroxyprogesterone) and instead consider micronised progesterone and dydrogesterone.
  j. *Hyperlipidaemia.* Those with raised triglycerides should be offered transdermal rather than oral oestrogen, and if required, micronised progesterone. Those with normal triglycerides who are otherwise low risk and younger than 60 years should be offered oral oestrogen-containing HRT because of its beneficial effects on total cholesterol, low-density lipoprotein, and high-density lipoprotein levels.

Initial Assessment

- Take a history and assess the female patient's menopausal status.

- Check for contraindications to HRT therapy, especially a history of breast cancer or VTE.
- Check blood pressure, BMI, and serum lipids.
- Advise female patients about breast awareness. Check that mammography screening is in place if older than 50 years. Mammography is not needed before commencing HRT unless a female is at high risk of breast cancer (Hope et al, 1999).
- Check that regular cervical screening is taking place.
- Give lifestyle advice, as discussed earlier.

Treatment

Oestrogens

- Start at the lowest possible dose of oestrogen (especially in older females, who tend to get more oestrogenic side -effects) and increase at 3-month intervals if necessary to achieve optimum symptom control.
- Give oestrogens continuously, and only give them without progestogens if the female has had a hysterectomy.

Progestogens

- These must be added for endometrial protection in females with a uterus. Most products contain either C-19 derivatives (norethisterone, levonorgestrel), which are more androgenic, or C-21 derivatives (medroxyprogesterone acetate, dydrogesterone) which are less androgenic.
- Change to a less androgenic preparation if the patient is troubled by progestogenic side effects.

Perimenopausal Females With an Intact Uterus

- Use a cyclical regimen (monthly or every 3 months). The majority of females will have a bleed towards the end of the progestogen phase.

Postmenopausal Females With an Intact Uterus

- Use one of the following:
  a. A cyclical regimen
  b. A continuous combined regimen. Continuous regimens induce an atrophic endometrium and so do not produce a withdrawal bleed, although irregular bleeding can occur in the first 4 to 6 months. Bleeding should be investigated if it persists for longer than 6 months, becomes heavier rather than less, or occurs after amenorrhoea.
  c. Tibolone. This combines oestrogenic and progestogenic activities and weak androgenic activity. It is indicated for the treatment of patients with vasomotor symptoms and osteoporosis prophylaxis. It must only be started at least 1 year after menopause. There is evidence that it improves libido (Kokcu et al, 2000). However, it also confers higher risk of stroke compared with standard HRT.

Alternative Modes of Delivery

- *Oestrogen implants.* Repeat every 4 to 8 months. Occasionally, vasomotor symptoms can return despite supraphysiological plasma concentrations of oestradiol (tachyphylaxis).

Check plasma oestradiol levels have returned to normal (<1000 pmol/L) before inserting a new implant.
- *Transdermal patches and gels.* These avoid the first-pass metabolism in the liver and deliver a more constant level of hormone. Patches come as either reservoir or matrix patches. Skin reactions are less common with the matrix patches.
- *LNG-IUD.* The LNG-IUD is now licensed for 4 years' usage for the delivery of progestogen to protect the endometrium. A 5-year follow-up concludes that the LNG-IUD effectively protects against endometrial hyperplasia (Varila, Wahlstrom, & Rauramo, 2001). It provides contraception, and it is the only way a nonbleed regimen may be achieved in the perimenopause.

Managing the Side Effects of Hormone Replacement Therapy

Bleeding

Patients on HRT should only be referred urgently if the bleeding continues after the HRT has been stopped for 4 weeks.

Bleeding on Cyclical Combined Therapy

- Check when the bleeding occurs. These regimens should produce regular predictable bleeds starting towards or soon after the end of the progestogenic phase.
- Consider poor compliance, drug interactions, or gastrointestinal upset.
- Try stopping HRT to see if it is the cause of the bleeding.
- If bleeding problems are caused by HRT, alter the progestogen:
  a. *Heavy or prolonged bleeding.* Increase the dose or duration of progestogen or change the type of progestogen to a more androgenic type (see earlier discussion).
  b. *Bleeding early in the progestogenic phase.* Increase the dose or change the type of progestogen.
  c. *Painful bleeding.* Change the type of progestogen.
  d. *Irregular bleeding.* Change the regimen or increase the dose of progestogen.
- *No bleeding* whilst taking a cyclical regime reflects an atrophic endometrium and occurs in 5% of females, but pregnancy needs to be excluded in perimenopausal females.
- Refer if there is:
  a. A change in the pattern of withdrawal bleeds and breakthrough bleeding that persists for more than 3 months
  b. Unexpected or prolonged bleeding that persists for more than 4 weeks after stopping HRT: refer urgently

Bleeding on Continuous Combined Therapy or Tibolone

- Explain to patients that the risk of bleeding is 40% in the first 4 to 6 months.
- Make sure the patient was at least 1 year postmenopausal before she started the regimen.
- Bleeding beyond 6 months requires further investigation.
- Bleeding that occurs after a period of amenorrhoea requires further investigation.

Oestrogen-Related Side Effects

- Oestrogenic side effects include fluid retention, bloating, breast tenderness and enlargement, nausea, headache, leg cramps, and dyspepsia.
- Encourage the patient to persist with therapy for 12 weeks because most side effects resolve with time.
- For persistent side effects, consider one of the following:
  a. Reducing the dose
  b. Changing the oestrogen type (swap between the two main forms of oestrogen: oestradiol and conjugated equine oestrogens)
  c. Changing the route of delivery
- *Nausea and gastric upset.* Change the timing of the oestrogen dose (e.g., try taking it with food or at bedtime).

Progestogen-Related Side Effects

- Progestogen-related side effects tend to occur in a cyclical pattern during the progestogenic phase of cyclical HRT. Continuous combined products contain lower doses of progestogens, and side effects are less likely. Side effects include fluid retention, breast tenderness, headaches, mood swings, depression, acne, lower abdominal pain, and backache.
- Encourage the patient to persist with therapy for about 12 weeks because some side effects will resolve.
- Various changes in the progestogens may be helpful, but remember not to reduce the dose or duration below that which protects the endometrium. Options include:
  a. Reduce the duration but not below 10 days per cycle.
  b. Reduce the dose of progestogen.
  c. Change the progestogen type (either C-19 or C-21 derivatives; see earlier).
  d. Change the route of progestogen (oral, transdermal, vaginal, or intrauterine).
  e. Reduce the frequency of how often the progestogen is taken by switching to a long-cycling regimen, in which progestogens are administered for 14 days every 3 months. This is only suitable for females with scant periods or who are postmenopausal.
  f. Change to a continuous combined therapy which often reduces progestogenic side effects with established use, but it is only suitable for postmenopausal females.

Follow-up of Females on Hormone Replacement Therapy

- See after 3 months and then every 6 months thereafter.
- Check for compliance, bleeding patterns, and side effects.
- Check that the patient is up to date with her cervical smears and mammograms.

  Note: There is no need to check the blood pressure except as good practice in any well-person screening.

How Long to Continue

- *Symptomatic relief.* Guidelines recommend that HRT be given 'for the shortest possible time', but there is no way of predicting how long this is. Most authorities recommend that HRT given for symptom relief be stopped within 5 years. In the World Health Organization trial,

HRT was stopped after 5.7 years. Half the females with vasomotor symptoms at the start of the trial reported moderate or severe symptoms after stopping (Ockene et al, 2005). If troublesome symptoms recur on withdrawal, HRT can be restarted for 6 to 12 months at a time.

- *Osteoporosis prevention when no more appropriate alternatives exist.* Five years of treatment is the minimum period for which benefit has been shown, yet after this, the risks, especially of breast cancer, increase. The fact that the benefit rapidly drops off after stopping HRT must be set against the risks associated with longer term use.

Stopping Treatment

- HRT may be stopped abruptly or gradually. There is no evidence that either approach is better in terms of preventing the return of symptoms.
- For gradual reduction, reduce the strength of oestrogen every 1 to 2 months, then take it on alternate days for 1 to 2 months, and then stop. At this stage:
  - If using a calendar pack, take alternate tablets from the pack so that the regimen includes progestogen for the second half of the cycle.
  - If using a patch, cut the patch in half once the lowest dose has been reached. If using the half patch cyclically, use the progestogen-containing half patch for the second half of the cycle.
- Review after a few months. If troublesome symptoms have recurred, consider restarting therapy at the lowest possible dose and titrating up as necessary. If only local symptoms persist, use a vaginal preparation.
- *Stopping HRT before surgery.* The RCOG does not consider that this is necessary but recommends prophylactic measures instead, including antithromboembolic stockings and low-molecular-weight heparin (RCOG, 2004).

Hormone Replacement Therapy and Contraception

- Perimenopausal females cannot be assumed to be infertile.
- Routine HRT preparations do not suppress ovulation and are not contraceptive.
- Contraception should be continued for 1 year after the last menstrual period (LMP) for females older than 50 years or for 2 years after the LMP for females younger than the age of 50 years.
- Perimenopausal females may use:
  a. Barrier methods, Cu-IUD or LND-IUD, as well as HRT
  b. Low-dose COC instead of HRT
  c. The POP, possibly combined with HRT, although there are theoretical concerns that the oestrogen component of HRT may interfere with the action of the POP on the cervical mucus (Pitkin, 2000).

When Has Menopause Occurred When Masked by Hormone Replacement Therapy or Combined Oral Contraceptives?

- It is important to know this so that a realistic idea of how long the female needs to remain on contraception can be calculated (see earlier discussion); 80% of females are post-menopausal by the age of 54 years (Anonymous, 1994b).

- Discontinue HRT or COC for 6 to 8 weeks; then check FSH and repeat after a further 4 to 8 weeks (Gebbie, 1998). If both FSH levels are above 30 IU/L, stop contraception after 1 further year. If a spontaneous period occurs or FSH is less than 30 IU/L, continue contraception and repeat the test in 1 year.
- *Females on the POP.* Check the FSH without stopping the POP.

The Role of Testosterone

RECOMMENDATIONS

British Menopause Society. (n.d.) *Tool for clinicians: Testosterone replacement in menopause. Information for GPs and other health professionals.* Retrieved from https://thebms.org.uk/wp-content/uploads/2022/12/08-BMS-TfC-Testosterone-replacement-in-menopause-DEC2022-A.pdf.
British Menopause Society. (2023). *BMS statement on testosterone.* Retrieved from https://thebms.org.uk/2023/03/bms-statement-on-testosterone/#:~:text=healthcare%20professionals%20alike.-,British%20Menopause%20Society%20guidance%20follows%20NICE%20NG23%20which%20recommends%20that,plateaued%20out%20and%20are%20stable.

- Testosterone is indicated when low libido is not ameliorated with HRT alone.
- Before commencement
  - Exclude other causes (e.g., relationship issues, depression, medication side effects).
  - Test serum total testosterone (to ensure testosterone is not raised) and SHBG (a high level reduces therapeutic response to testosterone replacement, and low levels increase the chance of adverse effects).
  - Switch the patient from oral to transdermal oestrogen if applicable (minimal effect on SHBG).
  - Consider whether tibolone is a suitable alternative (age younger than 60 years, >12 months postmenopausal).
  - Advise the patient that any adjunctive treatment with testosterone is unlicensed.
  - Discuss possible side effects, including acne, generalised hirsutism, and increased hairiness at application site, but especially those which are irreversible (vocal deepening, clitoral hypertrophy, and male-pattern baldness).
- Suggested regimens
  - Testogel 2.5-g sachets: ⅛ of a sachet/day (5 mg/day, i.e., each sachet should last 8 days)
  - Tostran 2% in 60 g: one metered pump of 0.5 g = 10 mg on alternate days (each canister should last 240 days)
  - Testim 1% in 5 mL: 0.5 mL (5 mg) per day (each tube should last for 10 days)
  - Andro Feme 1% cream in 50 mL: 0.5 mL/day = 5mg/day (each tube should last 100 days). (This is available by private prescriptions only in the United Kingdom.)
- Application
  - Apply to the clean, dry skin of the lower abdomen or upper thigh. Allow it to dry before dressing or skin

contact with others. Avoid washing the application site for 2 to 3 hours.

Premature Ovarian Insufficiency

- Consider in females younger than the age of 40 years with irregular or absent periods in whom other pathology and pregnancy have been excluded.
- Confirm the diagnosis by testing FSH on two separate occasions 4 to 6 weeks apart. Do not test other parameters (e.g., antimullerian hormone). Refer if there is diagnostic uncertainty.
- Discuss the need for hormonal therapy for both cardiovascular and bone protection. Either HRT or combined hormonal contraception may be used.
- Discuss the need for ongoing contraception. About 5% to 10% of females may still ovulate until the usual age of menopause.

PATIENT ORGANISATION

British Menopause Society. 4-6 Eton Place, Marlow, Bucks SL7 2QA. Tel. 01628 890199; Retrieved from http://www.thebms.org.

Cervical Screening

GUIDELINES

GOV.UK. (n.d.) *A summary of updated national guidelines within the cervical screening programme.* Available at http://www.cancerscreening.nhs.uk (choose 'Cervical').
National Institute for Health and Care Excellence. (2022). *Clinical knowledge summaries: Cervical screening.* Retrieved from cks.nice.org.uk/cervical-screening.

- The incidence of cervical cancer is highest in females aged 30 to 34 years.
- The NHS screening programme requires that all females between the age of 25 and 64 years are offered a smear:
  - Aged 24.5 years: first invitation
  - 25 to 49 years: every 3 years
  - 50 to 64 years: every 5 years
  - 65 years and older. Only screen those who have not been screened since the age of 50 years and request one or who have had a recent abnormal test result.
- The advisory committee on cervical screening reviewed the policy on screening (June 2009) and concluded that there should be no change in policy on the age of starting screening and that the harms of screening before this age outweigh the benefits.
- Evidence for the programme
  a. In 2000, there were 2424 new registrations for invasive cervical cancer in England (National Statistics, 2000).
  b. Cervical cancer incidence fell by 42% between 1988 and 1997 (England and Wales). This decrease was directly related to the cervical screening programme (National Statistics, 2000).
  c. In 1995, there were 10.4 per 100,000 population of newly diagnosed cases. By 1999, this had fallen to

9.3 per 100,000 population (National Statistics, 1999).

d. Cervical cancer screening saves approximately 4500 lives in England and prevents 3900 cases per year in the United Kingdom (Peto et al, 2004; Sasieni et al, 1996).

- The major risk groups are:
  a. Females with many sexual partners or whose partners have had many partners
  b. Smoking, which doubles a female patient's risk
- Screening involves up to three stages:
  1. Samples are screened for high-risk human papillomavirus. Negative samples are kept on routine recall. Positive samples go to step 2.
  2. Liquid-based cytology is performed to check for early cellular abnormalities. If present, females are referred to step 3. If absent, recall is set to 12 months.
  3. Colposcopy is undertaken to diagnose cervical intraepithelial neoplasia (CIN) and differentiate high-grade lesions from low-grade abnormalities.
- Liquid-based cytology (LBC) has reduced the number of inadequate samples from more than 9% to 2.9% in 2008. Results are received faster, and there is less pressure on the workforce. The changeover to LBC was completed in October 2008 in the United Kingdom.
- Smears cannot be interpreted (inadequate) if the specimen is obscured by inflammatory cells or blood, does not contain the right type of cells, or is incorrectly labelled.
- See Table 12.3 for terminology used in cervical screening.
- Repeat an inadequate smear after between 6 weeks and 3 months. Repeating the smear within 6 weeks does not allow adequate tissue regrowth. Refer if there are two further inadequate smears, repeated at 3-month intervals (preferably midcycle).

Follow-up After Colposcopy and Treatment

- Follow-up at 6 months (by a gynaecologist).
- If the results are normal, then a smear should be performed yearly for up to 10 years (by a GP or gynaecologist).

<table>
<tr><td colspan="2">**TABLE 12.3** **Terminology Used During Cervical Screening**</td></tr>
<tr><td>**Cytological Terms**</td><td>**Histological Equivalent[a]**</td></tr>
<tr><td>Mild dyskaryosis</td><td>CIN 1 (mild dysplasia): outer third of the epithelium</td></tr>
<tr><td>Moderate dyskaryosis</td><td>CIN 2 (moderate dysplasia): one-third to two-thirds of the epithelium</td></tr>
<tr><td>Severe dyskaryosis</td><td>CIN 3 (severe dysplasia or carcinoma in situ): full-thickness of the epithelium with breakdown of the structure between the basement membrane and the epithelium</td></tr>
</table>

[a]The correlation between status on smear and on histology is not close.
CIN, Cervical intraepithelial neoplasia.

- If results are normal, then revert to smears every 3 years.
- Potential symptoms after treatment include:
  - *Periodlike pain.* Advise usual analgesia.
  - *Discharge.* Common; should settle quickly. Advise to seek help if offensive.
  - *Bleeding.* Common. Advise to seek help if heavy or persistent (>4 weeks).

Follow-up After Hysterectomy

- For patients with routine smears for 10 years before hysterectomy and negative for CIN at hysterectomy, vault cytology is not required.
- For patients with less than 10 years of routine smears before hysterectomy and negative for CIN at hysterectomy, a single-vault smear required; then no further follow-up is required.
- For patients with CIN present at hysterectomy but fully excised, vault smears at 6 and 18 months are needed; then no further follow-up is required if results are negative.
- For patients with CIN present at hysterectomy with incomplete or uncertain excision, follow-up as if the cervix were still in situ.

Further Reading

ALTS Group. (2003). A randomized trial on the management of low-grade squamous intraepithelial lesion cytology interpretations. *American Journal of Obstetrics and Gynecology, 188,* 1393–1400.

Austoker, J. (1994). Screening for cervical cancer. *BMJ, 309,* 241–248.

Beral, V., & Million Women Study Collaborators. (2003). Breast cancer and hormone-replacement therapy in the Million Women Study. *Lancet, 362,* 419–427.

Kinghorn, G. R., Duerden, B. I., & Hafiz, S. (1986). Clinical and microbiological investigation of women with acute salpingitis and their consorts. *British Journal of Obstetrics and Gynaecology, 93,* 869–880.

Luesley, D., & Leeson, S. (Eds.). (2004). Colposcopy and programme management: Guidelines for the NHS Cervical Screening Programme. NHS Cancer Screening Programmes (NHSCSP publication No. 20).

Miller, E. R., Pastor-Barriuso, R., Dalal, D., Riemersma, R. A., Appel, L. J., & Guallar, E. (2005). Meta-analysis: High-dosage vitamin E supplementation may increase all-cause mortality. *Annals of Internal Medicine, 142,* 37–47.

References

American Association of Clinical Endocrinologists. (1999). *AACE medical guidelines for clinical practice for management of menopause.* American Association of Clinical Endocrinologists. Retrieved from www.aace.com.

Anonymous. (1998). Alternatives for the menopause. *Bandolier,* 56–59.

Anonymous. (1994a). Surgical management of menorrhagia. *Drug and Therapeutics Bulletin, 32,* 70–72.

Anonymous. (1994b). Hormone replacement therapy. *Drug and Therapeutics Bulletin, 34,* 81–84.

Anonymous. (1999). Managing endometriosis. *Drug and Therapeutics Bulletin, 37*, 25–29.

Ballard, K., Lowton, K., & Wright, J. (2006). What's the delay? A qualitative study of women's experiences of reaching a diagnosis of endometriosis. *Fertility and Sterility, 86*, 1296–1301.

Bingham, J. S. (1999). What to do with patients with recurrent vulvovaginal candidiasis. *Sexually Transmitted Infections, 75*, 225–227.

Bisschop, M. P., Merkus, J. M., Scheygrond, H., & van Cutsem, J. (1986). Co-treatment of the male partner in vaginal candidosis: A double blind randomised controlled study. *British Journal of Obstetrics and Gynaecology, 93*, 79–81.

Brown, J., Pan, A., & Hart, R. J. (2010). Gonadotrophin-releasing hormone analogues for pain associated with endometriosis. *Cochrane Database of Systematic Reviews, 2010*, CD008475.

Bousser, M. G., Conard, J., Kittner, S., de Lignières, B., MacGregor, E. A., Massiou, H., Silberstein, S. D., & Tzourio, C. (2000). Recommendations on the risk of ischaemic stroke associated with use of combined oral contraceptives and hormone replacement therapy in women with migraine. The International Headache Society Task Force on Combined Oral Contraceptives & Hormone Replacement Therapy. *Cephalalgia, 20*, 155–156.

Cardozo, L., Bachmann, G., McClish, D., Fonda, D., & Birgerson, L. (1998). Meta-analysis of estrogen therapy in the management of urogenital atrophy in postmenopausal women: Second report of the Hormones and Urogenital Therapy Committee. *Obstetrics and Gynecology, 92*, 722–727.

Coleman, L., & Overton, C. (2015). GPs have key role in early diagnosis of endometriosis. *Practitioner, 259*(1780), 13–17, 2.

Farquhar, C., Lee, O., Toomath, R., & Jepson, R. (2000). Spironolactone versus placebo or in combination with steroids for hirsutism and/or acne. *Cochrane Database of Systematic Reviews*, (4), CD000194.

Gannon, M. J., Holt, E. M., Fairbank, J., Fitzgerald, M., Milne, M. A., Crystal, A. M., & Greenhalf, J. O. (1991). A randomised trial comparing endometrial resection and abdominal hysterectomy for the treatment of menorrhagia. *BMJ, 303*, 1362–1364.

Gath, D., & Iles, S. (1990). Depression and the menopause. *BMJ, 300*, 1287–1288.

Gebbie, A. E. (1998). Contraception for women over 40. In J. Studd (Ed.), *The management of the menopause, annual review* (pp. 67–80). London: Parthenon Publishing.

Gokhale, L. B. (1996). Curative treatment of primary (spasmodic) dysmenorrhoea. *Indian Journal of Medical Research, 103*, 227–231.

Groom, T. M., Stewart, P., Kruger, H., & Bell, G. (2001). The value of a screen and treat policy for *Chlamydia trachomatis* in women attending for termination of pregnancy. *Journal of Family Planning and Reproductive Health Care, 27*, 69–72.

Guttuso, T., Jr, Kurlan, R., McDermott, M. P., & Kieburtz, K. (2003). Gabapentin's effects on hot flashes in postmenopausal women: A randomized controlled trial. *Obstetrics and Gynecology, 101*, 337–345.

Haddon, L., Heason, J., Fay, T., McPherson, M., Carlin, E. M., & Jushuf, I. H. (1998). Managing STIs identified after testing outside genitourinary medicine departments: One model of care. *Sexually Transmitted Infections, 74*, 256–257.

Harborne, L., Fleming, R., Lyall, H., Norman, J., & Sattar, N. (2003). Descriptive review of the evidence for the use of metformin in polycystic ovary syndrome. *Lancet, 361*, 1894–1901.

Hays, J., Ockene, J. K., Brunner, R. L., Kotchen, J. M., Manson, J. E., Patterson, R. E., Aragaki, A. K., Shumaker, S. A., Brzyski, R. G.,

LaCroix, A. Z., Granek, I. A., Valanis, B. G., & Women's Health Initiative Investigators. (2003). Effects of estrogen plus progestin on health-related quality of life. *New England Journal of Medicine, 348*, 1839–1854.

Heiss, G., Wallace, R., Anderson, G. L., Aragaki, A., Beresford, S. A., Brzyski, R., Chlebowski, R. T., Gass, M., LaCroix, A., Manson, J. E., Prentice, R. L., Rossouw, J., Stefanick, M. L., & WHI Investigators. (2008). Health risks and benefits 3 years after stopping randomized treatment with estrogen and progestin. *JAMA, 299*, 1036–1045.

Hillis, S. D., Joesoef, R., Marchbanks, P. A., Wasserheit, J. N., Cates, W., Jr, & Westrom, L. (1993). Delayed care of pelvic inflammatory disease as a risk factor for impaired fertility. *American Journal of Obstetrics and Gynecology, 168*, 1503–1509.

Hillis, S. D., Owens, L. M., Marchbanks, P. A., Amsterdam, L. F., & Mac Kenzie, W. R. (1997). Recurrent chlamydial infections increase the risks of hospitalisation for ectopic pregnancy and pelvic inflammatory disease. *American Journal of Obstetrics and Gynecology, 176*, 103–107.

Hlatky, M. A., Boothroyd, D., Vittinghoff, E., Sharp, P., Whooley, M. A., & Heart and Estrogen/Progestin Replacement Study (HERS) Research Group. (2002). Quality-of-life and depressive symptoms in postmenopausal women after receiving hormone therapy: Results from the Heart and Estrogen/Progestin Replacement Study (HERS) trial. *JAMA, 287*, 591–597.

Hope, S., Rees, M., & Brockie, J. (1999). *Hormone replacement therapy – a guide for primary care*. Oxford: Oxford University Press.

Hunter, M. S. (1996). Depression and the menopause. *BMJ, 313*, 350–351.

Kamwendo, F., Johansson, E., Moi, H., Forslin, L., & Danielsson, D. (1993). Gonorrhea, genital chlamydial infection, and non-specific urethritis in male partners of hospitalized women treated for acute pelvic inflammatory disease. *Sexually Transmitted Diseases, 20*, 143–146.

Kokcu, A., Cetinkaya, M. B., Yanik, F., Alper, T., & Malatyalioğlu, E. (2000). The comparison of effects of tibolone and conjugated estrogenmedroxyprogesterone acetate therapy on sexual performance in postmenopausal women. *Maturitas, 36*, 75–80.

Korhonen, M. O., Symons, J. P., Hyde, B. M., Rowan, J. P., & Wilborn, W. H. (1997). Histologic classification and pathologic findings for endometrial biopsy specimens obtained from 2964 perimenopausal and postmenopausal women undergoing screening for continuous hormone replacement therapy. *American Journal of Obstetrics and Gynecology, 176*, 377–380.

Larsson, B., & Wennergren, M. (1981). Investigation of Cu-IUD for possible effect on frequency and healing of PID. *Contraception, 24*, 137–149.

Lethaby A, Irvine GA, Cameron IT. (2008). Cyclical progestogens for heavy menstrual bleeding. *Cochrane Database of Systematic Reviews*, Issue 1. Art. No.: CD001016. DOI: 10.1002/14651858. CD001016.pub2.

Lord, J. M., Flight, I. H. K., & Norman, R. J. (2003). Metformin in polycystic ovary syndrome: Systematic review and meta-analysis. *BMJ, 327*, 951–955.

MacLennan, A., Lester, S., & Moore, V. (2001). Oral oestrogen replacement therapy versus placebo for hot flushes. *Cochrane Database of Systematic Reviews*, (3). https://www.cochranelibrary.com/cdsr/doi/10.1002/14651858.CD002978/full.

Marjoribanks, J., Proctor, M. L., Farquhar, C. (2006). Nonsteroidal anti-inflammatory drugs for primary dysmenorrhoea. *Cochrane Database of Systematic Review*. Retrieved from www.library.nhs.uk (choose 'Cochrane library').

Metters, J. S., Catchpole, M., Smith, C., et al. (1998). *Chlamydia trachomatis: Summary and conclusions of CMO's Expert Advisory Group*. London: Department of Health.

Muzii, L., Di Tucci, C., Achilli, C., Di Donato, V., Musella, A., Palaia, I., & Panici, P. B. (2016). Continuous versus cyclic oral contraceptives after laparoscopic excision of ovarian endometriomas: A systematic review and metaanalysis. *American Journal of Obstetrics and Gynecology, 214,* 203–211.

National Institute for Health and Clinical Excellence. (2007). *Heavy menstrual bleeding. Clinical guideline 44.* Retrieved from www. nice.org.uk.

National Institute for Health and Clinical Excellence. (2020). *Hirsutism.* CKS. Retrieved from www.nice.org.uk.

National Statistics. (1999). MB1 No 28 Cancer statistics registrations 1995–1997; National Statistics MB1 No 30 Registrations of cancer diagnosed in 1999.

National Statistics. (2000). Health Quarterly Statistics 07, Autumn 2000.

Nelson, H. D., Humphrey, L. L., Nygren, P., Teutsch, S. M., & Allan, J. D. (2002). Postmenopausal hormone replacement therapy: Scientific review. *JAMA, 288,* 872–881.

Nelson, H. D., Vesco, K. K., Haney, E., Fu, R., Nedrow, A., Miller, J., Nicolaidis, C., Walker, M., & Humphrey, L. (2006). Nonhormonal therapies for menopausal hot flashes. *JAMA, 295,* 2057–2071.

Newton, K. M., Reed, S. D., LaCroix, A. Z., Grothaus, L. C., Ehrlich, K., & Guiltinan, J. (2006). Treatment of vasomotor symptoms of menopause with black cohosh, multibotanicals, soy, hormone therapy, or placebo: A randomized trial. *Annals of Internal Medicine, 145,* 869–879.

Norman, R. J., Flight, I. H. K., & Rees, M. C. P. (2001). Oestrogen and progestogen hormone replacement therapy for perimenopausal and post-menopausal women: Weight and body fat distribution. *Cochrane Database of Systematic Reviews,* (3). https://www.cochranelibrary.com/cdsr/doi/10.1002/14651858.CD001018/pdf/full

Ockene, J. K., Barad, D. H., Cochrane, B. B., Larson, J. C., Gass, M., Wassertheil-Smoller, S., Manson, J. E., Barnabei, V. M., Lane, D. S., Brzyski, R. G., Rosal, M. C., Wylie-Rosett, J., & Hays, J. (2005). Symptom experience after discontinuing use of estrogen plus progestin. *JAMA, 294,* 183–191.

Pattie, M. A., Murdoch, B. E., Theodoros, D., & Forbes, K. (1998). Voice changes in women treated for endometriosis and related conditions: The need for comprehensive vocal assessment. *Journal of Voice, 12,* 366–371.

Pearce, E., Jolly, K., Jones, L. L., Matthewman, G., Zanganeh, M., & Daley, A. (2020). Exercise for premenstrual syndrome: A systematic review and meta-analysis of randomised controlled trials. *BJGP Open, 4*(3), bjgpopen20X101032. doi:10.3399/bjgpopen20X101032.

Peto, J., Gilham, C., Fletcher, O., & Matthews, F. E. (2004). The cervical cancer epidemic that screening has prevented in the UK. *Lancet, 364,* 249–256.

Pitkin, J. (2000). Contraception and the menopause. *Maturitas, 1,* S29–S36.

Potter, J. (1999). Should sexual partners of women with bacterial vaginosis receive treatment? *British Journal of General Practice, 49,* 913–918.

Rees, M., & Purdie, D. W. (1999). *Management of the menopause.* BMS Publications. London: The Handbook of the BMS.

Rosenthal, A. N., Fraser, L. S. M., Philpott, S., Manchanda, R., Burnell, M., Badman, P., Hadwin, R., Rizzuto, I., Benjamin, E., Singh, N., Evans, D. G., Eccles, D. M., Ryan, A., Liston, R., Dawnay, A., Ford, J., Gunu, R., Mackay, J., Skates, S. J., Menon, U.,

... United Kingdom Familial Ovarian Cancer Screening Study collaborators. (2017). Evidence of stage shift in women diagnosed with ovarian cancer during phase II of the United Kingdom Familial Ovarian Cancer Screening Study. *Journal of Clinical Oncology, 35*(13), 1411–1420.

Rossouw, J. E., Anderson, G. L., Prentice, R. L., LaCroix, A. Z., Kooperberg, C., Stefanick, M. L., Jackson, R. D., Beresford, S. A., Howard, B. V., Johnson, K. C., Kotchen, J. M., Ockene, J., & Writing Group for the Women's Health Initiative Investigators. (2002). Risks and benefits of estrogen plus progestin in healthy postmenopausal women: Principal results from the Women's Health Initiative randomized controlled trial. *JAMA, 288,* 321–333.

Rossouw, J. E., Prentice, R. L., Manson, J. E., Wu, L., Barad, D., Barnabei, V. M., Ko, M., LaCroix, A. Z., Margolis, K. L., & Stefanick, M. L. (2007). Postmenopausal hormone therapy and risk of cardiovascular disease by age and years since menopause. *JAMA, 297,* 1465–1477.

Royal College of Obstetricians and Gynaecologists. (1999). *The initial management of menorrhagia. Evidence-based clinical guidelines, No. 1.* London: Royal College of Obstetricians and Gynaecologists.

Royal College of Obstetricians and Gynaecologists. (2004). Hormone replacement therapy and venous thromboembolism. Royal College of Obstetricians and Gynaecologists guideline no.19. Retrieved from www.rcog.org.uk.

Sasieni, P. D., Cuzick, J., & Lynch-Farmery, E. (1996). Estimating the efficacy of screening by auditing smear histories of women with and without cervical cancer. *British Journal of Cancer, 73,* 1001–1005.

Scambia, G., Mango, D., Signorile, P. G., Anselmi Angeli, R. A., Palena, C., Gallo, D., Bombardelli, E., Morazzoni, P., Riva, A., & Mancuso, S. (2000). Clinical effects of a standardised soy extract in postmenopausal women: A pilot study. *Menopause (New York, N.Y.), 7,* 105–111.

Soderberg, G., & Lingren, S. (1981). Influence of an IUD on the course of acute salpingitis. *Contraception, 24,* 137–143.

Sutton, C. J., Ewen, S. P., Whitelaw, N., & Haines, P. (1994). Prospective, randomized, double-blind, controlled trial of laser laparoscopy in the treatment of pelvic pain associated with minimal, mild, and moderate endometriosis. *Fertility and Sterility, 62,* 696–700.

Teisala, K. (1989). Removal of an IUD and the treatment of acute PID. *Annals of Medicine, 21,* 63–65.

Varila, E., Wahlstrom, T., & Rauramo, I. (2001). A 5-year study of the use of a levonorgestrel intra-uterine system in women receiving hormone replacement therapy. *Fertility and Sterility, 76,* 969–973.

Watson, M., Grimshaw, J., Bond, C., Mollison, J., & Ludbrook, A. (2002). Oral versus intra-vaginal imidazole and triazole anti-fungal treatment of uncomplicated vulvovaginal candidiasis (thrush). *Cochrane Database of Systematic Reviews,* (1). https://www.cochranelibrary.com/cdsr/doi/10.1002/14651858.CD002845/full.

Wild, S., Pierpoint, T., Mckeigue, P., & Jacobs, H. (2000). Cardiovascular disease in women with PCOS at long term follow up: A retrospective cohort study. *Clinical Endocrinology, 52,* 595–600.

Wyatt, K. M., Dimmock, P. W., O'Brien, P. M. S. (2002). Selective serotonin reuptake inhibitors for premenstrual syndrome. *Cochrane Database of Systematic Review. 2.* https://www.cochranelibrary.com/cdsr/doi/10.1002/14651858.CD001396/full.

13

Obstetric Problems

Kate Robinson & Adam Staten

CHAPTER CONTENTS

Prepregnancy Care

GUIDELINES

Medicines Health Regulatory Authority. (2023). *Valproate use by women and girls*. Retrieved from https://www.gov.uk/guidance/valproate-use-by-women-and-girls.
National Institute for Health and Clinical Excellence. (2022). *CKS miscarriage*. Retrieved from https://cks.nice.org.uk/topics/miscarriage/.

- Although prepregnancy counselling offers an opportunity to reinforce good health habits and identify potential problems for pregnancy early, there is no evidence from randomised controlled trials that women who attend such visits have better health or pregnancy outcomes. In one large cohort study, only a small proportion of women planning pregnancy followed the recommendations for nutrition and lifestyle (Inskip et al, 2009).

- General practitioners (GPs) may have the opportunity to identify risk factors before conception. This can be done either at a specific consultation or when the opportunity arises (e.g., as part of contraceptive care or when seeing patients with diabetes or hypertension).
- If a patient does present for a prepregnancy visit, this can be used as a time to encourage her to:
  a. Stop smoking.
  b. Start an appropriate dose of folic acid. (Explain that folic acid supplements have been shown to reduce the risk of neural tube defects (NTDs) by 50%–70%; Rush, 1994.)
  c. Avoid alcohol or at most take 2 units a week.
  d. Take a healthy diet, particularly avoiding soft cheeses and liver.
  e. Aim to achieve a healthy weight and body mass index (BMI).
- At the same time, the doctor can
  a. Consider the risk of inherited disorders.
  b. Assess existing medical conditions (e.g., hypertension, diabetes, epilepsy, hyperthyroidism).
  c. Assess whether the patient has an eating disorder or needs help with weight management.
  d. Check that the patient is immune to rubella.
  e. Check the patient has an up-to-date cervical smear.
  f. Warn the patient to avoid contact with chickenpox or exposed shingles. In the United States and Australia, varicella vaccination is offered to nonimmune women.

Genetic Disorders

- All couples should be referred for genetic counselling if they request it or there are risk factors that need further investigation. The list of identifiable conditions is increasing, and studies suggest that clinicians across specialties are poor at appreciating which conditions have identifiable genetic components (Harris et al, 1999).
- If there is any doubt, contact the nearest department of clinical genetics for advice. Children or adults with a major abnormality or disease, even if not at present thought to be genetic in origin, should have blood stored at a regional genetics laboratory for later analysis.
- Those at higher risk are:
  a. Couples with a personal or family history of an abnormality that is presumed to be genetic in origin. They should be referred for genetic counselling or have blood taken by the GP on the advice of the geneticist. Important examples are:
     - Cystic fibrosis
     - Huntington chorea
     - Duchenne and other muscular dystrophies
     - Polycystic kidneys

- Intellectual disability, which may be caused by fragile-X syndrome
  b. Couples belonging to a high-risk ethnic group (see later)
  c. *Older women.* The risk of having a baby with Down syndrome is 1 in 400 at age 35 years, increasing to 1 in 100 at age 40 years and 1 in 30 at age 45 years. Around the age of 37 years, the risk of chromosomal abnormality is greater than the risk of miscarriage after amniocentesis. Recommend the leaflet *Screening for Down's, Edwards' and Patau's syndromes* available from www.nhs.uk.
  d. *Consanguineous couples.* First-degree cousins have a slight but significant increase in congenital malformations. This is likely to be higher if there is a family history of congenital disease. White first-degree cousins should be offered screening for cystic fibrosis even when there is no family history.

Diseases in High-Risk Ethnic Groups

Sickle Cell and Thalassaemia

- Women from areas where malaria has been common are at increased risk of carrying the sickle cell or thalassaemia traits. These areas include Africa, the Caribbean, the Middle East, the Indian subcontinent, South America, South and Southeast Asia, and the Mediterranean.
- In the United Kingdom, all pregnant women are offered screening for thalassaemia using the mean corpuscular haemoglobin (MCH) measurement as part of the routine blood count.
- Female patients and potential fathers from an ethnic group at risk are also offered a test for sickle cell and related haemoglobin variants.
- At a prenatal consultation, a couple may choose to undergo screening because of the ethnic group to which they belong or because of a positive family history. When assessing ethnic origin, try to go back at least two generations. Discuss the appropriate test with the laboratory and send the completed Family Origin Questionnaire with the blood samples. This is available from the sickle cell and thalassaemia screening programme (http://sct.screening.nhs.uk; search for 'Family origin questionnaire').
- Refer to an obstetrician all couples who are both heterozygous for sickle cell or thalassaemia or when the mother is and the father's status is unknown.

PATIENT INFORMATION

Sickle Cell Society. 54 Station Road, London NW10 4UA. Tel: 020 8961 7795. Helpline: 0800 001 5660.@sicklecelluk on Instagram.
   UK Thalassaemia Society. 19 The Broadway, Southgate Circus, London N14 6PH. Tel: 020 8882 0011. Free advice line: 0800 731 109. Available at http://www.ukts.org.

Jewish Population: Tay–Sachs Disease

- Tay–Sachs disease is an incurable neurodegenerative disorder that begins around 6 months of age. Babies born with it live for only a few years. People of Ashkenazi (Eastern European) Jewish descent are at highest risk.
- Consider referral of both prospective parents to the regional genetics centre for testing for *Tay–Sachs* trait. One in 25 of Jewish descent is positive.

Previous Obstetric History

a. *Down syndrome.* Make certain that all patients who have had a previous pregnancy affected by Down syndrome have received genetic counselling regardless of the age at which they conceived.
b. *Previous miscarriages* (see later). Inform all patients, if asked, that the overall incidence of miscarriage is around 15%. However, patients whose last pregnancy was normal have a risk of miscarriage of only 5%, whereas patients whose last pregnancy ended in miscarriage have a 20% to 25% chance of a miscarriage (Regan et al, 1989). Patients with three consecutive miscarriages have a 40% chance of the next pregnancy ending in miscarriage.
c. *Recurrent miscarriages.* Refer to a gynaecologist for assessment all patients who have had three consecutive miscarriages before 10 weeks' gestation or one or more miscarriage if after 10 weeks' gestation. Reassure them, however, that they still have a 60% chance of a normal pregnancy and that it is common for no cause to be identified. Consider earlier referral if:
    - The patient requests it.
    - There is a family history of miscarriage or of congenital disease.
    - There is a relevant medical problem.
    - There is an urgency to achieve a live birth, as in older females.

Investigations to Consider Undertaking Before Referral for Recurrent Miscarriage

a. Pelvic ultrasonography
b. Luteinising hormone level on day 7
c. Blood group and antibodies
d. Anticardiolipin antibodies (immunoglobulin (Ig) M and IgG)
e. Lupus anticoagulant
f. Protein C, protein S, and factor V Leiden

Medical History

Hypertension

- This should be assessed before a patient gets pregnant, as it may be masked by the fall in blood pressure in the first half of pregnancy.

- Discuss the most appropriate drug with the relevant specialist before conception.
- See later discussion for more information.

Diabetes

- Explain that diabetes is associated with an increase in congenital abnormalities (about double) but that this can be decreased significantly by good control of the blood sugar before and during pregnancy (Steel et al, 1990; Nachum et al, 1999).
- See later discussion for more information.

Epilepsy

- Patients with epilepsy are more likely to have unplanned pregnancies because of contraceptive failure and twice as likely to have foetuses with foetal malformations.
- Not all malformations may be attributable to antiepileptic drugs (Fairgrieve et al, 2000).
    - Sodium valproate increases the risk of NTDs 50 times, to about 1.5%. Patients of childbearing potential should not be treated with valproate. When this is unavoidable, patients and prescribing clinicians must engage with the terms of the Pregnancy Prevention Programme.
    - With carbamazepine, the rate is 1%.
    - There are few data on the safety of newer drugs.
    - There is no convincing evidence that any one drug is safer than another.
- Discuss with the neurologist:
    - Whether to stop anticonvulsants in any patient who has been free of convulsions for 2 years; however, counsel the patient about the risks of untreated epilepsy in pregnancy. Convulsions may lead to stillbirth.
    - Whether to change anticonvulsants or reduce their dose in those in whom they cannot be stopped.
- Make it clear that even when taking anticonvulsants, there is a 90% chance of a normal outcome, prenatal diagnosis is effective in picking up NTDs (see later), and many defects can be corrected after birth.
- Ensure that all patients with epilepsy are offered:
    - *Folic acid.* Those continuing antiepileptic medication should take folic acid 5 mg/day from 3 months before conception until the end of the 12th week. Those stopping their drugs need only take 400 μg/day from 1 month before conception.
    - *An anomaly ultrasound examination* at 18 to 21 weeks.
    - *Vitamin K.* Give vitamin K 10 mg orally daily for the last 4 weeks of pregnancy to patients taking enzyme-inducing antiepileptic treatment.
- Educate the patient's partner about what to do if the patient has a seizure because epilepsy may be less predictable during pregnancy.

Asthma

- Asthma is one of the commonest chronic medical conditions, and around 5% of pregnant patients require asthma medication during pregnancy (Olesen et al, 1999).
- Asthma increases the risk of intrauterine growth restriction (IUGR) by 24% overall and by 47% in those with severe asthma (Bracken et al, 2003).
- Patients with asthma should continue their asthma medications, including preventers, because the risk of uncontrolled asthma poses a greater risk to the foetus than continuing preventive medication (Martel et al, 2005).

Other Medication

- A decision should be taken about the need to stop other drugs which are associated with foetal abnormalities (e.g., warfarin, lithium).
- The National Institute for Health and Clinical Excellence (NICE) guideline, *Antenatal and postnatal mental health: Clinical management and service guidance*, available on www.nice.org.uk, discusses the risks associated with psychotropic medication.

Psychiatric History

Mental illness is a common 'indirect' cause of maternal death. Seeking a history early in pregnancy and ensuring effective follow-up in late pregnancy and the early postnatal period are essential.

Infection

a. *Rubella.* All patients should have rubella antibodies tested before each pregnancy; immunity can be lost between one pregnancy and the next.
b. *Hepatitis B.* All patients should be offered screening for hepatitis B early in pregnancy because selective screening has been shown to miss cases of hepatitis B virus (HBV) because of the time pressures of routine clinical practice.
c. Listeria *spp.* Advise patients to avoid soft cheeses, chilled ready-to-eat foods (unless thoroughly reheated), and pâtés before and during pregnancy. They should avoid contact with sheep at lambing time and with silage. Advise patients to reheat food to steaming hot and thaw frozen foods in a microwave or refrigerator. Listeriosis is rare but can occur in outbreaks.
d. *Toxoplasmosis.* Patients contemplating pregnancy should be warned about the risks of handling soil, cat faeces, and raw meat and of eating undercooked meat and unwashed vegetables and fruit. About 80% of British patients are not immune at the time of pregnancy. Routine screening is not recommended.
e. *Human immunodeficiency virus (HIV).* All patients should be offered screening for HIV early in pregnancy by midwives or doctors trained in pre- and posttest counselling (Brocklehurst, 2000).
f. *Genital herpes and warts.* Management is only an issue in the last weeks of pregnancy.

Prenatal and Antenatal Advice

> **GUIDELINE**
>
> National Institute for Health and Clinical Excellence. (2023). *CKS pre-conception Advice and management*. Available at https://cks.nice.org.uk/topics/pre-conception-advice-management/.

Lifestyle

- *Alcohol.* Counsel patients to reduce their alcohol consumption to a minimum (at the most 1 or 2 units once or twice a week). Complete abstinence is now recommended by the Department of Health, the British Medical Association (BMA), the Royal College of Obstetrics and Gynaecology (RCOG), and the World Health Organization (WHO). However, the evidence relating to the possibility of foetal damage from very low levels of alcohol intake does not provide a clear answer about the risk. A more powerful argument in favour of total abstinence is that patients who drink a little in pregnancy may easily overstep the limits without realising it (Head to Head, 2007).
- *Smoking.* Rather than asking: *'Do you smoke?'* patients should be asked, *'What best describes your smoking—daily, every once in a while, or I don't currently smoke'?* All patients who smoke should be offered a smoking cessation intervention. Advise about the risks. Provide information. Assess willingness to quit. Assist to quit using a cognitive-behavioural intervention. Arrange for additional support if unsuccessful. Nicotine replacement therapy can be used if conservative measures are unsuccessful; however, other prescribed aids (e.g., bupropion, varenicline) are contraindicated. The prevalence of vaping in pregnancy is estimated to be between 1% and 7% (Calder et al, 2021), though research is scanty, and the effects are unknown.
- *Coffee.* Heavy coffee drinking ($\geq$8 cups a day) is associated with a tripling of the risk of stillbirth (odds ratio, 3.0; 95% confidence interval, 1.5–5.9) (Wisborg et al, 2003). A recent study found that caffeine intake as low as 200 mg (2 cups of coffee or 5 cups of tea or 5 cans of caffeinated fizzy drinks) was associated with a doubling of the rate of miscarriage and that lower intakes were not without risk (Weng, Odouli, & Li, 2008). However, a Danish randomised trial failed to show any effect on birth weight or length of gestation from reducing caffeine intake, suggesting

that the association of caffeine with poor outcomes may be attributable to one or more confounding factors (Bech et al, 2007).

- *Other drugs.* All patients should be asked about their use of prescription and nonprescription drugs. Patients using nonprescription drugs should be referred to the appropriate drug service for assistance in quitting.

Nutrition

- Recommend a balanced diet that is low in fat with adequate iron and fresh fruits and vegetables.
- Consumption of peanuts is now supported.
- Foods which should be avoided include:
  - Soft and blue cheeses, unpasteurised dairy, and pâté (see the earlier discussion of *Listeria*)
  - Liver (vitamin A toxicity)
  - Undercooked or cured meat or raw seafood (*Salmonella* risk)
  - High-mercury fish, including swordfish and tuna

Anaemia

- Check haemoglobin in all patients with a previous history or at high risk of anaemia, such as vegans, those with multiple pregnancies, and those with a short interval between pregnancies.
- Check the serum ferritin in patients who have a history of iron-deficiency anaemia even if the haemoglobin is normal.

Vitamin D

- All patients should be counselled about the importance of adequate vitamin D intake during pregnancy and whilst breastfeeding.
- All females should take 10 μg of vitamin D per day (e.g., Health Start Vitamins for female adults). Those particularly at risk of deficiency include:
  a. Females of South Asian, African, Caribbean, or Middle Eastern family origin
  b. Females who have limited exposure to sunlight, such as those who are predominantly housebound or usually remain covered when outdoors
  c. Females who eat a diet particularly low in vitamin D, such as those who consume no oily fish, eggs, meat, vitamin D-fortified margarine, or breakfast cereal
  d. Females with a prepregnancy BMI greater than 30 kg/m^2

Folic Acid

- Recommend that all females take 400 μg of folic acid a day from before conception until the end of the 12th week. This will prevent 95% of NTDs.
- Higher dose folic acid supplementation (5 mg/day) should be offered to patients who have one of the following:

- The patient or her partner is affected by spina bifida.
- The patient has had a previous pregnancy affected by NTDs.
- Patients taking epilepsy medication (see earlier).
- The patient has diabetes or coeliac disease.
- BMI greater than 30 kg/m^2.
- Patients with sickle cell disease or thalassaemia.

Vitamin A

- Advise all females to limit intake of vitamin A to 700 μg/day and not to eat liver or liver products (e.g., sausage or pâté) because of their high vitamin A content. High levels of vitamin A may be teratogenic, particularly for craniofacial, limb, eye, and central nervous system abnormalities.

Exercise

- Advise patients that beginning or continuing a moderate course of exercise during pregnancy is not associated with adverse outcomes.
- Inform patients about sports that have a danger, including contact sports, high-impact sports, and vigorous racquet sports that may involve the risk of abdominal trauma, falls, or excessive joint stress, and scuba diving, which may result in foetal birth defects and foetal decompression disease.

Sexual Intercourse in Pregnancy

- Advise patients that sexual intercourse in pregnancy is not known to be associated with any adverse outcomes.

Car Travel

- Advise about the correct use of seatbelts in pregnancy:
  a. Place the seatbelt above and below the bump, not over it.
  b. Use three-point seatbelts with the lap strap placed as low as possible beneath the 'bump', lying across the thighs with the diagonal shoulder strap above the bump lying between the breasts.
  c. Adjust the fit to be as snug as comfortably possible.

Travel Overseas

- Most airlines require a doctor's letter confirming the pregnancy is uncomplicated and the expected date of delivery after 27 weeks' gestation, and air travel is not allowed after 37 weeks' gestation (singleton) and 32 weeks' gestation (multiple).
- For advice about immunisation in pregnancy, see Appendix 18.

- *Malaria.* Pregnant patients are advised to avoid travel to malarious areas. However, advice is available for those whose travel is essential. See the Health Protection Agency's document *Malaria prevention guidelines for travellers from the UK* available at http://www.hpa.org.uk.

PATIENT INFORMATION AND SUPPORT

Bumps. (n.d.). *Best use of medicines in pregnancy.* Available at https://www.medicinesinpregnancy.org/Medicine—pregnancy.
Royal College of Obstetrics and Gynaecology. (2015). *Air travel and pregnancy.* Available at https://www.rcog.org.uk/for-the-public.

Routine Antenatal Care

GUIDELINES

Department of Health. (2017). *FGM safeguarding and risk assessment: Quick guide for health professionals.* Retrieved from https://assets.publishing.service.gov.uk/media/5a805c53e5274a2e8ab4fb48/FGM_safeguarding_and_risk_assessment.pdf.
National Institute for Health and Clinical Excellence. (2023). *CKS. Antenatal care—Uncomplicated pregnancy.* Retrieved from https://cks.nice.org.uk/topics/antenatal-care-uncomplicated-pregnancy/.

- The patient should be the focus of maternity care.
- Midwifery and GP-led models of maternity care are safe for low-risk patients.
- Patients with the following conditions may require specialist care:
  a. A current medical problem (e.g., diabetes, epilepsy, hypertension)
  b. A psychiatric disorder (taking medication)
  c. HIV or HBV infected
  d. An autoimmune disorder
  e. Obesity (BMI 30 kg/m^2 or more at first contact) or underweight (BMI <18.5 kg/m^2 at first contact)
  f. Patients with complex social factors, including lack of social support; substance misuse; recent migrant, asylum seeker, or refugee, illiteracy or non–English speaking; and victims of domestic abuse
  g. Multiple pregnancy
  h. Older than 40 years of age or younger than 20 years of age at booking
- Patients who have experienced any of the following in previous pregnancies also need specialist care:
  a. Recurrent miscarriage (three or more consecutive pregnancy losses) or a midtrimester loss
  b. Severe preeclampsia, HELLP (hemolysis, elevated liver enzymes, low platelet count) syndrome, or eclampsia
  c. Rhesus isoimmunisation or other significant blood group antibodies
  d. Uterine surgery, including caesarean section, myomectomy, or cone biopsy
  e. Antenatal or postpartum haemorrhage on two occasions
  f. Retained placenta on two occasions
  g. Puerperal psychosis
  h. Grand multiparity (more than six pregnancies)
  i. A stillbirth or neonatal death
  j. A small-for-gestational-age infant (<5th centile)
  k. A large-for-gestational-age infant (>95th centile)
  l. A baby weighing less than 2500 g or more than 4500 g
  m. A baby with a congenital anomaly (structural or chromosomal)
- Patients at risk of gestational diabetes should be offered an oral glucose tolerance test at 16 to 18 weeks' and 28 weeks' gestation. Those at high risk are patients with BMIs greater than 30 kg/m^2, previous gestational diabetes, a previous macrosomic baby, a family history of diabetes, and an ethnic origin with a high prevalence of diabetes. Those without any of these risk factors but who have glycosuria detected (2+ on one occasion, or 1+ on two or more occasions) should also be considered for testing.
- Patients at risk of preeclampsia should be referred for consultant-led care and commenced on aspirin. This includes patients with previous preeclampsia or hypertension in pregnancy; renal, autoimmune, or diabetic disease; nulliparity; multiple pregnancy or wide pregnancy interval (>10 years); age older than 40 years; and BMI greater than 35 kg/m^2.
- Risk factors for postnatal depression should be noted at this stage to facilitate earlier detection if it occurs. There is little evidence that it can be prevented by intervention in the antenatal period (NICE, 2014).
- Care providers should:
  a. Make sure that pregnancy care is patient centred and that they use effective communication skills to ensure that patients make informed choices about their care.
  b. Be aware that there is a huge amount of information presented to patients during pregnancy and they should provide written information and resources in plain language.
  c. Ensure patients are given an opportunity to discuss information at antenatal visits.
- Because of the increase in information to be processed by pregnant patients, early antenatal appointments should be scheduled to allow discussion time.

Booking: Before 12 Weeks' Gestation

a. Take a full medical, drug, social, psychological, family, and obstetric history.
b. Enquire about the patient's occupation and any concerns they may have.
c. Recommend the appropriate daily dose of folic acid until week 12 if the patient is not already taking it. Vitamin D supplementation is now recommended for all, and high-dose supplementation is recommended for those at high risk of deficiency. A Cochrane review has shown likely beneficial effects on risk of preeclampsia,

gestational diabetes, low birth weight, and severe postpartum haemorrhage (Palacios et al, 2019).

d. Assess risk and discuss the model of maternity care appropriate for the patient.

e. Estimate the estimated date of delivery. Offer early (10–13 weeks) ultrasound examination to determine gestation. Offer 18- to 20-week ultrasound examination for structural anomalies.

f. Provide information on diet and lifestyle. Routine iron supplementation is not recommended. Advise about reducing the risk of listeriosis, toxoplasmosis, and salmonellosis. Discuss the safe use of medicines.

g. Offer a smoking cessation programme if the patient is a smoker.

h. Check blood group and rhesus D status.

i. Offer screening for anaemia, red cell autoantibodies, HBV, HIV, rubella, asymptomatic bacteriuria, and syphilis. Tests for sickle cell trait and thalassaemia if at risk.

j. Offer screening for Down syndrome.

k. Measure BMI and blood pressure and test urine for proteinuria.

l. Assess for risk of preeclampsia, gestational diabetes, venous thromboembolism, and foetal growth restriction.

m. Sensitively enquire about the possibility of female genital mutilation when appropriate. A positive answer to either screening question should prompt formal risk assessment:
   1. Do you, your partner, or your parents come from a community where cutting or circumcision is practised?
   2. Have you been cut?

n. Assess psychosocial well-being. Ask about feelings and fears. Ask about relationships and supports. Consider asking about intimate partner violence. Ask the two screening questions for depression (see later), and if the answers are positive, ask if it is something the patient would like help with (NICE, 2007).

Follow-up Appointments

- Reducing the number of visits is not associated with worse outcomes except that patients may be less satisfied (Villar et al, 2001; Sikorski et al, 1996). Ten visits can provide essential care (booking and weeks 16, 18–20, 25, 28, 31, 34, 36, 38, and 40). Visits should be long enough to allow patients to have their concerns voiced and addressed. Some patients require more visits. Multiparous patients may need as few as six (booking and weeks 28, 34, 36, 38, and 41).

- Current evidence does *not* support the following *as routine*:
   a. Repeated maternal weighing
   b. Breast examination
   c. Pelvic examination
   d. Antenatal screening to predict postnatal depression using the Edinburgh Postnatal Depression Scale (EPDS)
   e. Iron supplementation

f. Screening for cytomegalovirus (CMV), hepatitis C virus, group B streptococcus, toxoplasmosis, bacterial vaginosis, and gestational diabetes mellitus

g. Formal foetal movement counting

h. Antenatal electronic cardiotocography

i. Ultrasound scanning after 24 weeks

j. Umbilical artery Doppler ultrasound scan (USS)

k. Uterine artery Doppler USS to predict preeclampsia

At Every Appointment Check

a. The patient's general health and psychosocial well-being

b. Blood pressure

c. Symphysis–fundal height, plotted in centimetres on a chart

d. Foetal movements or foetal heart sounds

e. Presentation (after 34 weeks' gestation)

Prenatal Diagnosis and Screening

Screening Tests

Pregnant patients should be offered screening for structural anomalies and chromosomal abnormalities by appropriately trained staff. If there is a family history of another genetic disorder, the patient should be referred to a specialist service for genetic counselling.

Structural Abnormalities

- *Ultrasonography* should be offered between 18 and 21 weeks' gestation. Routine ultrasonography can detect the more obvious forms of congenital abnormality (e.g., cranial and NTDs; severe skeletal dysplasia; abnormalities of the heart, chest, and abdominal organs). Hydrocephalus may be detected later. As technology and training improve, the range of anomalies detectable before birth continues to increase.

- *Fetoscopy.* Visualisation of the foetus is necessary for the assessment of some external malformations. It is also used for laser treatment of twin-to-twin transfusion syndrome.

Chromosomal Abnormalities

- In the United Kingdom, Down (trisomy 21), Edwards (trisomy 18), and Patau (trisomy 13) syndromes are routinely screened for.

- Patients need:
   a. To understand that screening is a risk assessment and not a diagnostic test.
   b. To be informed that diagnostic tests are invasive and have a risk of miscarriage.
   c. Information about the performance of a screening test based on *their* age because maternal age is a key component of all screening tests: younger patients (younger than 25 years of age) having screening tests will have a low screen positive rate (1%) and a 30% detection rate, but older patients (older than 40 years) will have a high screen positive rate (50%) and a 90%

detection rate (Three Centres Consensus Guidelines on Antenatal Care Project, 2001).

d. To be informed that most patients having a screen positive result do *not* have a Down syndrome–affected pregnancy.

Types of Screening Tests for Chromosomal Abnormalities

- A number of screening tests exist, yet availability varies between countries and centres. Check with your local maternity unit to confirm availability.
- Tests with detection rates greater than 75% and false-positive rates less than 3% are:
  - *Combined first trimester screening* (nuchal translucency at 11.5–14 weeks; human chorionic gonadotrophin (hCG) and pregnancy-associated plasma protein A (PAPP-A) at 8–12 weeks)
  - *Second trimester maternal serum screening* (*the quadruple test* (hCG, alpha fetoprotein (AFP), unconjugated oestriol (uE3), and inhibin A) performed between 14 and 20 weeks)
  - *The integrated test* (nuchal translucency, PAPP-A + hCG, AFP, uE3, and inhibin A).
  - *The serum integrated test* (PAPP-A + hCG, AFP, uE3, and inhibin A) can be performed between 11 and 20 weeks.
- The first, third, and fourth methods involve tests at different stages of pregnancy. A result is only reported when all tests have been performed.
- Cell-free foetal DNA testing can be used to detect chromosomal abnormalities. This is not offered on the NHS in the United Kingdom but is available commercially, and patients may choose to undertake this.

Diagnostic Tests for Chromosomal Abnormalities

- *Chorionic villus biopsy (CVB).* This is usually performed after 11 weeks' gestation and allows patients to consider termination of pregnancy in the first trimester, but it has a miscarriage rate of 1.2%. There is also a further 1% to 2% chance of needing an amniocentesis to establish the diagnosis. CVB performed before 10 weeks' gestation may rarely cause limb abnormalities (Lilford, 1991).
- *Amniocentesis.* This is usually performed at 15 to 16 weeks' gestation, which allows patients to consider termination by 20 weeks' gestation. It is associated with a miscarriage rate of 1%. Polymerase chain reaction technology allows results for Down and Edwards syndrome in 48 hours, usually backed by culture results for other chromosomal anomalies available 2 weeks later.

Problems in Pregnancy

Nausea and Vomiting

- Around 80% of pregnant patients experience nausea during the first trimester, and around 50% experience vomiting. These problems can vary from being minor to severe and disabling.
- Reassure the patient that most cases of nausea and vomiting settle by 20 weeks' gestation and that it does not harm the foetus.
- Consider over-the-counter or prescribed treatment if the vomiting has severe consequences on the quality of life (on day-to-day activities, including interfering with household activities, restricting interaction with children, greater use of healthcare resources and time lost off work). Ensure that patients remain adequately hydrated, avoid exhaustion, and consider the following (Jewell & Young, 2003):
  a. Acupressure at P6 (seabands) and ginger may be of benefit.
  b. Antihistamines (e.g., promethazine or cyclizine) or prochlorperazine reduce nausea and vomiting but can cause drowsiness. There is no evidence that they are teratogenic. NICE0 clinical knowledge summaries (CKS) advise metoclopramide or ondansetron as second-line options but advises that their use should not be continued beyond 5 days.
  c. Vitamin B_6 may be of benefit alone, but the evidence is not strong. There are concerns about the toxicity of B_6 at high dose. Limit the maximum daily dose to 10 mg.
- If associated with reflux, advise:
  a. Eating a biscuit before getting up
  b. Eating small frequent meals
  c. Taking a low-sodium, low-sugar antacid for heartburn
  d. Stopping iron if it is making symptoms worse
- Ranitidine was used in pregnancy for many years but is no longer available. Famotidine would be an alternative, but the manufacturer does not recommend its use in pregnancy.
- Proton pump inhibitors (PPIs) are now widely used in pregnancy. The manufacturer of omeprazole advises that it is safe in pregnancy, and this is the first-choice treatment. There is a lack of data for other PPIs.
- In late pregnancy, exclude UTI, preeclampsia, and surgical causes of vomiting.
- *Hyperemesis gravidarum.* Admit if the weight loss is more than 5% with ketosis; there is other evidence of dehydration; or if a patient has severe, intractable vomiting that you cannot control with oral antiemetics.

Heartburn

- Heartburn is common in pregnancy and becomes more common as the pregnancy progresses.
- Suggest lifestyle modifications (see later).
- Alginate antacids (e.g., Gaviscon). Liquid preparations are usually more effective than tablets.
- PPIs are now widely used in pregnancy. The manufacturer of omeprazole advises that it is safe in pregnancy, and this is the first-choice treatment. There is a lack of data for other PPIs. Ranitidine is no longer available, and the manufacture of famotidine advises against its use.

Pelvic Pain

- Symphysis pubis dysfunction is a collection of signs and symptoms of discomfort and pain in the pelvic area, including pelvic pain radiating to the upper thighs and perineum. It can be debilitating.
- There is no evidence that any treatment helps, but referral to a physiotherapist and pelvic support may be of value.

Vaginal Bleeding and Miscarriage

GUIDELINE

National Institute for Health and Clinical Excellence. (2023). *Ectopic pregnancy and miscarriage: Diagnosis and early management. NICE guideline 126.* Retrieved from https://www.nice.org.uk/guidance/ng126.

- *Rhesus status.* If a rhesus-negative patient bleeds, anti-D immunisation is recommended. The dose depends on the preparation used. Give it within 72 hours of the bleeding starting, but if a longer period has elapsed, it may still give some protection.

Ectopic Pregnancy

- Ectopic pregnancy is usually associated with mild vaginal bleeding as well as pain. A negative pregnancy test result (i.e., an hCG level <50 IU/L) virtually excludes it.
- Intrauterine pregnancies should be visible on transvaginal ultrasound examination when serum hCG exceeds 1000 IU/L.
- Admit any patient in whom the possibility of an ectopic is anything more than remote. It is the commonest cause of death in early pregnancy (MBBRACE-UK Maternal Report, 2022).

Suspected Miscarriage Up to 14 Weeks' Gestation

- If provided with appropriate counselling, most patients who miscarry in the first trimester choose expectant management. About 81% of them complete their miscarriage without intervention (Luise et al, 2002).
- Assess haemodynamic stability. Admit patients who are not haemodynamically stable.
- Perform a pregnancy test if pregnancy has not previously been confirmed.
- Perform an abdominal examination looking for tenderness; unilateral tenderness is suggestive of an ectopic pregnancy.
- If there is no abdominal pain or tenderness, perform a gentle pelvic examination for cervical motion tenderness or pelvic tenderness (suggestive of an ectopic pregnancy). Do not palpate for adnexal masses because doing so may risk rupturing an ectopic pregnancy.
- Consider a speculum exam to assess the cervical os and to exclude other causes of bleeding (e.g., ectropion).
- If they are over 6 weeks' gestation arrange admission to an early pregnancy assessment unit (EPAU); the urgency of admission depends upon the clinical situation.

- If they are less than 6 weeks' gestation:
  - Repeat a pregnancy test after 7 to 10 days to confirm miscarriage if bleeding stops before 6 weeks' gestation.
  - Arrange admission to the EPAU if bleeding continues beyond 6 weeks' gestation or if the patient develops signs suggestive of an ectopic pregnancy.
- If miscarriage is confirmed and has not completed, then management may be expectant, medical (with vaginal or oral misoprostol), or surgical (by manual vacuum aspiration under local anaesthetic or general anaesthetic).
- Patients who have been managed medically should take a pregnancy test 3 weeks later. If the result is still positive, they need to be reassessed for molar or ectopic pregnancy.
- Rhesus-negative patients who have undergone surgical management should be offered anti-D rhesus prophylaxis.

Follow-up After Miscarriage

- Arrange to meet all patients who have miscarried about 4 weeks afterwards. Be aware that these patients have experienced bereavement and may need counselling.
- Attend to all physical issues and the possible need for contraception. The traditional advice to have two normal periods before trying to conceive again may be more important to allow time for the grieving process than for any physical reason.
- Be aware that patients are distressed by the fact that no reason for the miscarriage can usually be given. Many feel unreasonable guilt and feel 'brushed off' by being reassured that miscarriage is common (Wong et al, 2003). Explain that early miscarriage is caused by either an abnormality of foetal development or a failure of implantation.
- Explain that one miscarriage is followed by a slight or even no increase in risk of subsequent miscarriages. Investigations are unlikely to be fruitful unless three or more pregnancies have miscarried. Having three consecutive miscarriages gives a patient a subsequent risk of 40%. Referral for investigation is then traditional, but earlier referral may be justified as discussed earlier.

PATIENT INFORMATION AND SUPPORT

The Miscarriage Association. 2 Otter Holt, Wakefield, West Yorkshire, WF4 3QE. Helpline: 01924 200799, administration 01924 200795 for leaflets about all aspects of miscarriage, ectopic pregnancy, and molar pregnancy. Available at http://www.miscarriageassociation.org.uk.
The Royal College of Obstetricians and Gynaecologists. (n.d.) *Patient information leaflet: Early miscarriage.* Retrieved from https://www.rcog.org.uk/for-the-public.

Suspected Miscarriage After 14 Weeks' Gestation

- The more advanced the pregnancy, the more advisable it is to admit the patient to hospital at the onset of bleeding, whether or not there has been pain.
- After 14 weeks' gestation, painless bleeding is caused by placenta praevia until proven otherwise.

- Bleeding with severe pain is likely to be caused by abruptio placentae.
- Do not do a vaginal examination in these patients.

> **PATIENT INFORMATION AND SUPPORT**
>
> Stillbirth and Neonatal Death Society. 10-18 Union Street, London SE1 1SZ. Helpline: 0808 164 3332. Retrieved from http://www.uk-sands.org.

Abdominal Pain

- Abdominal pain may be from a variety of causes, some of which are serious and which may present in an atypical way. Any cause which could occur outside pregnancy (e.g., renal calculus) must be considered.
- *In the first 20 weeks of pregnancy*, consider:
  a. Miscarriage
  b. Ectopic pregnancy
  c. Urinary infection
  d. Appendicitis
  e. Impaction of a retroverted uterus
  f. Red degeneration of a fibroid (the maximum incidence is at 12–18 weeks, but it may occur at any time)
  g. Torsion of an ovary or tube
  h. Haematoma of the round ligament
  i. Accident to an ovarian cyst
- *After 20 weeks of pregnancy*, consider, in addition:
  a. Labour
  b. Abruptio placentae
  c. Haematoma of the rectus abdominis
  d. Uterine rupture
  e. Dehiscence of the pubic symphysis

Infection or Contact With Infectious Disease

Rubella Contact

- Rubella is now very rare in many countries because of vaccination programmes. It should be confirmed by serology if suspected (see later).
- If a pregnant patient is infected with rubella, the risk to the foetus is greatest up to 11 weeks, but 30% of foetuses between 11 and 16 weeks are affected.
- Patients experiencing infection before 20 weeks' gestation should be referred to an obstetrician for risk assessment and counselling.
- If a pregnant patient is affected between 16 and 19 weeks' gestation, the risk of foetal damage is less than 2%. Deafness is the most likely problem. Risk after 20 weeks' gestation appears to be low.
- Accidental immunisation in pregnancy has not been associated with embryopathy.

Rubella Contact Before 16 Weeks' Gestation

If the pregnancy is less than 16 weeks' gestation, regardless of whether the patient has had rubella or the vaccination or antibodies were previously detected:

- Take blood for rubella antibodies.
  - If IgG is present and the blood was taken within 12 days of contact, inform the patient that she is immune and that there is little need to worry.
  - If IgG is present but the blood was taken more than 12 days after contact, request IgM levels. If IgM shows recent infection, discuss the risks of foetal abnormality and the question of termination of pregnancy.
  - If IgG is absent, repeat IgM 2 weeks later. If the patient has seroconverted, discuss the question of termination of pregnancy as earlier. The value of Ig in protecting the foetus is doubtful.
  - All IgG-negative patients should be immunised in the puerperium.

Note: If a patient contracts rubella and decides to continue the pregnancy, foetal blood sampling (from the umbilical vein) from 20 weeks' gestation onwards can indicate whether the baby has contracted it by assessing foetal IgM.

Note: IgM can persist for up to 1 year after rubella. Only act on an IgM result if it is consistent with the clinical picture or with a reliable history of exposure (Best et al, 2002).

Varicella (Chickenpox)

> **GUIDELINE**
>
> Royal College of Obstetricians and Gynaecologists. (2015). *Chickenpox in pregnancy. 'Green Top' clinical guideline 13.* Retrieved from https://www.rcog.org.uk/guidance/browse-all-guidance/green-top-guidelines/chickenpox-in-pregnancy-green-top-guideline-no-13/.

- A congenital varicella syndrome, including limb deformities and scarring, may occur in 1% to 2% of pregnancies in which the mother contracts chickenpox (though not shingles) up to, but not after, 20 weeks' gestation (RCOG, 2001).
- Exposure to chickenpox after 20 weeks' gestation and before 36 weeks' gestation does not appear to be associated with foetal abnormalities.
- In patients who *are* not known to be immune and who is in contact with chickenpox in the first trimester, check the varicella antibodies urgently and give varicella zoster immune globulin (VZIG) if the patient is not immune.
- Give acyclovir to a pregnant patient who develops chickenpox at a gestation of more than 20 weeks, starting within 24 hours of the appearance of the rash. Monitor all pregnant patients with chickenpox carefully; 10% develop pneumonia.
- Offer an ultrasound anomaly scan to patients contracting chickenpox before 20 weeks' gestation.
- If a mother contracts chickenpox in the 5 days before giving birth or within 2 days of giving birth, the baby should be given VZIG.

Cytomegalovirus

- CMV infection is now the commonest congenital infection worldwide. The birth incidence is between 0.2%

and 2.5%, and 10% of these infections will produce an affected neonate.
- Consequences of infection can include deafness and developmental disability; this is commoner with primary infection and occurs in up to 20% of cases.
- Two-thirds of congenital infections are thought to result from primary maternal infection and one-third from recurrent infection in the mother.
- Ganciclovir and valganciclovir are modestly effective in infected neonates but are associated with toxicity (Leung et al, 2022). They have not been proven to be of benefit if given to the mother during pregnancy.
- Advice to a patient who seroconverts to CMV during pregnancy is difficult, and such cases should be referred for tertiary centre advice.

Toxoplasmosis

- Toxoplasmosis causes foetal infection in about 15% of cases in the first trimester, increasing to 70% in the third. The risk of serious foetal damage if the foetus is infected is, however, greater in early pregnancy. Overall, up to 90% of infected babies escape long-term damage. Most maternal cases are asymptomatic. The incidence of children born with definite or probable toxoplasmosis is very low.
- Where there is concern, check serology as soon as possible after conception and monthly thereafter. IgM may stay positive for months; timing infection in relation to pregnancy stage requires IgG avidity testing at the National Reference Laboratory.
- In the case of infection, the patient may be offered USS and amniocentesis to detect foetal abnormality and foetal blood sampling between 20 and 24 weeks' gestation. Even if foetal blood sampling demonstrates foetal infection, it cannot indicate whether the foetus has been damaged. Treatment with spiramycin in pregnancy is safe but of unproven benefit.

Listeria

- Maternal infection may be asymptomatic or associated with fever. The infection carries a risk of miscarriage, stillbirth, or the birth of an infected baby.
- Symptoms in the mother are so nonspecific that the diagnosis is rarely made during the acute illness, especially because the only useful diagnostic test is blood culture.
- Patients with fever for 48 hours who are pregnant and who have no obvious other source of infection should have a blood culture specifying *Listeria*. Treatment is with intravenous ampicillin.

Group B Streptococcal Infection

- Group B streptococcal (GBS) infection is the commonest severe infection in infants in the first 7 days of life (RCOG, 2017).
- Routine screening for GBS is not recommended in the United Kingdom.

- If performed (e.g., in patients considered at high risk), screening should be performed 3 to 5 weeks before the expected delivery.
- Situations in which neonatal GBS infection is more likely are:
  - Neonatal GBS infection in a previous baby
  - Vaginal, urinary, or intestinal GBS present in the patient in this pregnancy
  - Preterm (before 37 weeks) labour
  - Prolonged (>18 hours) rupture of membranes
  - Fever during labour (>38°C)
- Consider patients at risk, as discussed previously, for intravenous antibiotics during labour or the newborn baby for antibiotics until blood cultures show that there is no GBS present.

Hepatitis A

Reassure the mother that the infant will not be harmed, although the infant may be infected if it is occurring shortly before term.

Hepatitis B

- Hepatitis B is not influenced by pregnancy, but if the mother is infected, there is a risk of acute infection of the foetus or neonate.
- Discuss the management of babies born to hepatitis B surface antigen–positive mothers with a specialist in infectious disease.

Herpes Simplex

Genital Herpes

- Primary infection at delivery gives a 20% to 50% risk of neonatal herpes, which is frequently fatal. Recurrent herpes at delivery gives a risk of 0% to 3%. Lower segment caesarian section (LSCS) is therefore only recommended if the patient has her first attack during labour (BASSH & RCOG, 2014).
- Viral shedding is less in subsequent attacks, and maternal IgG crosses the placenta to provide some foetal protection. There is little value in taking viral swabs in the last month of pregnancy in those with a history of infection but without active lesions.
- Acyclovir (400 mg tds) in the last month of pregnancy reduces viral shedding and vertical transmission (Braig et al, 2001).

Labial Herpes

The mother, and indeed any family or friends with labial herpes, should refrain from direct contact with the baby (i.e., kissing) after the infant is born.

Genital Warts

Respiratory papillomatosis in a child is strongly related to maternal genital warts during pregnancy. However, the risk is small (6.9 cases per 1000 live births, against a risk of 0.03 per 1000 live births with no such maternal history) and is not reduced by caesarean section (Silverberg et al, 2003).

Human Immunodeficiency Virus

> **GUIDELINE**
>
> British HIV Association. (2020). *Guidelines for the management of HIV in pregnancy and postpartum.* Retrieved from https://www.bhiva.org/pregnancy-guidelines.

- A mother who is HIV positive has a risk of foetal infection of 15% to 25%, but this can be substantially reduced by delivery by caesarean section, antiretroviral therapy, or both. Vaginal delivery is recommended for those with a low viral load.
- Screening should be offered to all patients. Some babies are HIV antibody positive at birth because of maternal antibody but become negative as maternal antibody is cleared.
- All patients who are HIV positive should receive combination antiretroviral therapy. Changes may need to be made to existing regimens because the effectiveness of some therapies changes during pregnancy. Those who test positive during pregnancy should start treatment as soon as possible.
- Breastfeeding increases the chance of vertical transmission and is not recommended in countries where there is adequate access to alternative nutrition. If a patient must breastfeed, then exclusive breastfeeding rather than mixed feeding should be recommended because neonatal seroconversion may be greatest with the bowel inflammation secondary to artificial feeds. A patient with an undetectable viral load may choose to breastfeed after being counselled about the risks of this.
- Zidovudine as a single agent is usually given to the infant for 2 to 4 weeks to reduce the chance of vertical transmission.
- Pregnancy does not appear to hasten the onset of acquired immunodeficiency virus (AIDS) in patients who are HIV positive.

Parvovirus B19 Infection (Fifth Disease or Slapped Cheek Syndrome)

- This is common in schools and nurseries, especially in April and May. If a patient is exposed in the first 20 weeks of pregnancy, there is an increased risk of intrauterine death (excess risk, 9%), and if infection occurs between 9 and 20 weeks' gestation, foetal anaemia leading to hydrops foetalis (3% of whom die, included in the excess 9%). The consequences usually occur within 3 to 5 weeks of maternal infection.

- Maternal asymptomatic infection is as likely to damage the foetus as symptomatic infection.
- Check antibodies in all patients exposed as soon as possible, informing the laboratory of the clinical details.
  a. If specific IgG is detected and specific IgM is not detected, the patient can be reassured that she has had past infection.
  b. If specific IgM is detected but specific IgG is not, a further sample should be tested immediately. Refer all patients who are positive to an obstetrician.
  c. If specific IgG and IgM are not detected, a further sample should be tested after 1 month.

Pruritis

- Pruritis, without jaundice, is the commonest manifestation of obstetric cholestasis, which in turn is associated with premature birth in 60%, foetal distress in up to 33%, and intrauterine death in up to 2% (Milkiewicz et al, 2002). Although most patients with pruritis in pregnancy do not have obstetric cholestasis, it should be considered in every case because of its serious implications.
- Check liver function tests (LFTs). Transaminases are increased in 60% of cases of obstetric cholestasis, though only 25% have a raised bilirubin.
- Refer all affected patients. Most obstetricians will deliver the baby at 37 weeks.

Excessive Weight Gain

- A patient's BMI should be calculated at the first booking appointment.
- The average weight gain in pregnancy is 10 to 12.5 kg (0.65 kg in the first quarter, 4 kg by midpregnancy, 8.5 kg by the third quarter, and 12.5 kg by term). More than one-quarter of the total gain is caused by fat deposition in the middle two-quarters of pregnancy.
- The ideal weight gain depends on the prepregnancy BMI. A patient with a BMI that is low or normal has fewest obstetric and neonatal adverse outcomes if her weight gain is less than 10 kg. A patient with a BMI of 25 to 30 kg/m^2 does best if her weight gain is less than 9 kg, and an obese patient does best with a weight gain less than 6 kg (Cedergren, 2007). Excessive weight gain may be associated with an increased incidence of preeclampsia. Check blood pressure, urine, and the presence of oedema.
- Despite the above, there is no evidence that the regular weighing of patients is of benefit, and it is not recommended.
- *Obesity.* Obesity is associated with an increase in congenital malformations and first trimester abortions, gestational diabetes, hypertension, macrosomia, stillbirth, prolonged labour, and caesarean birth. All patients with obesity should be seen by an obstetrician and monitored closely for weight gain, blood pressure, and diabetes (Stotland, 2009).

- *Eating disorders* are common in pregnancy; the disorder may worsen or improve as the pregnancy progresses (Ward, 2008). Patients with a recognised eating disorder should be referred to an obstetrician and the eating disorder service early in pregnancy. Suggested screening questions at each antenatal visit are:
  a. What is your current eating pattern? Are you restricting your dietary intake? Do you binge? Do you vomit or take laxatives after eating?
  b. How do you feel about your shape and weight?
  c. What is your weight? Are you gaining weight appropriately?
  d. What is your mood like? Do you feel low or anxious?
  e. What exercise are you taking? Are you exercising too much?

Fundal Height

- At 22 weeks' gestation the fundus should have reached the umbilicus and at 32 weeks' gestation the lower rib border.
- The symphysis-to-fundus height in centimetres should be within 2 of the number of weeks' gestation between 20 and 36 weeks' gestation; after 36 weeks' gestation, it should be within ±3 cm.
- If the fundus is over 3 cm less than dates, refer for exclusion of foetal IUGR or oligohydramnios.
- If the fundus is 3 cm more than dates, refer for assessment for possible multiple pregnancy or hydramnios.

Hypertension

> **GUIDELINE**
>
> National Institute for Health and Clinical Excellence. (2023). *Hypertension in pregnancy: Diagnosis and management. NICE guideline 133*. Retrieved from https://www.nice.org.uk/guidance/ng133.

- Blood pressure decreases early in the first trimester as the decrease in peripheral resistance exceeds the rise in cardiac output. Blood pressure reaches its nadir by 16 weeks, plateaus until 22 weeks, and then increases towards term.
- *Pregnancy-induced hypertension (PIH):* Blood pressure which rises to exceed 90 mm Hg diastolic on more than one occasion in the second half of pregnancy resolves after delivery and is *not* complicated by proteinuria. The International Society for the Study of Hypertension in Pregnancy has chosen this definition rather than one based on a relative increase in diastolic pressure because any increase in pressure varies according to when the baseline was taken and because a relative increase seems to correlate less well with outcomes than the use of an absolute cu-off point.
- *Preeclampsia:* This is defined in the same way as above but is associated with proteinuria greater than 300 mg/24 hours, increased creatinine, abnormal LFT results,

neurologic symptoms, low platelet count, and IUGR. The terms *PIH* and *preeclampsia* should not be used interchangeably because the former is not associated with poor maternal or foetal outcome, but preeclampsia is a leading cause of maternal and foetal morbidity.
- *Antihypertensives* do not lessen the risk of developing PIH or alter its progression, but they do protect against stroke and possibly placental abruption. The antihypertensives of choice in pregnancy include labetalol, nifedipine, and methyldopa.
- *Aspirin* prophylaxis (75–150 mg/day) may prevent the development of preeclampsia and moderate the condition after it has started.
- *Chronic hypertension* predates pregnancy or appears before 20 weeks' gestation. A blood pressure of 140/90 mm Hg or greater before 20 weeks' gestation suggests preexisting hypertension and needs specialist assessment.
- *Action to be taken if new hypertension is discovered after 20 weeks' gestation (gestational hypertension) in the absence of signs of preeclampsia:*
  - Blood pressure of 140/90 to 159/109 mm Hg
    a) Aim for a blood pressure of 135/85 mm Hg.
    b) Check blood pressure once or twice weekly.
    c) Perform dipstick for proteinuria once or twice weekly.
    d) Measure FBC, LFTs, and renal function at presentation and then weekly.
    e) Offer foetal heart auscultation at every appointment.
    f) Liaise with the obstetric team with regards to regular ultrasound assessment.
  - Blood pressure greater than 160/110 mm Hg: Admit.

Preeclampsia

- *Patients with any of the following should be referred for specialist assessment before 20 weeks' gestation:*
  - Previous preeclampsia
  - Multiple pregnancy
  - Underlying medical conditions
    a. Preexisting hypertension or booking diastolic blood pressure of 90 mm Hg or greater
    b. Preexisting renal disease or booking proteinuria (≥ + on more than one occasion or ≥300 mg/24 hours)
    c. Preexisting diabetes
    d. Presence of antiphospholipid antibodies
- *Patients with any two or more of the following should be referred for specialist assessment before 20 weeks' gestation:*
  - First pregnancy
  - More than 10 years since the last baby
  - Age older than 40 years
  - BMI of 35 kg/m^2 or greater
  - Family history of preeclampsia (mother or sister)
  - Booking diastolic blood pressure of 80 mm Hg or greater
- All patients with suspected preeclampsia should be managed in conjunction with specialist advice. This is usually undertaken in a special day assessment centre.

Note: Symptoms associated with preeclampsia include headache, visual disturbance, nausea, vomiting, and epigastric pain.

Long-Term Follow-up

- Continue to monitor blood pressure at home every 1 to 2 days postpartum and consider reducing the dosage of any medication if the blood pressure is less than 140/90 mm Hg.
- Patients who have had preeclampsia are at higher long-term risk of cardiovascular disease (CVD) and at higher risk that the disease may occur earlier.
- Inform them that their risk of CVD when young is still low but that they should concentrate on prevention.
- Counsel all patients who have had preeclampsia about a healthy lifestyle.
- Screen for the emergence of other risk factors for CVD at an earlier stage than usual.

Eclampsia

- This is a medical emergency with a high maternal mortality rate. The patient must be resuscitated and transferred to hospital as fast as possible. The anticonvulsant of choice to prevent further fits is magnesium sulphate.
- *Recurrence and follow-up:* Many patients have posttraumatic stress disorder when their normal physiological pregnancy has been taken from them. It is important to explain what happened and the relatively low chance of recurrence in future pregnancies (20%). Many units offer uterine artery Doppler as a screening test in subsequent pregnancies, with the possibility that aspirin can reduce this rate further.

Proteinuria

A trace of protein is acceptable. It may be caused by contamination with vaginal secretions or to a delay since the urine was passed.

Proteinuria in the Absence of Increased Blood Pressure

- *One plus (+).* Arrange for a midstream urine for culture and microscopy and check urine polymerase chain reaction or albumin:creatinine ratio. Review in 1 week. If culture and microscopy are negative but the protein:creatinine ratio is positive, check the serum creatinine and the 24-hour urinary protein and refer. Continue to look for preeclampsia. Ten percent of patients who develop eclampsia have proteinuria without an increased blood pressure (Douglas & Redman, 1994).
- *More than +* Arrange to be seen in a specialist clinic within 48 hours.
- *At least + with a symptom associated with preeclampsia.* Refer for same-day assessment.

Using the Different Tests for Proteinuria

- *The protein dipstick* is prone to both false-negative and false-positive results (Chappell & Shennan, 2008). Although recommended by NICE for the routine assessment of urinary protein in antenatal care, it is the least useful of the available tests.
- *The urinary spot protein:creatinine ratio* has few false-negative results but rather more false-positive results. It is therefore a good screening test (if the result is negative, the patient almost certainly does not have significant proteinuria), but a more accurate test is required to confirm a positive finding. A positive result is considered to be 30 mg/mmol or greater.
- *Twenty-four-hour urinary protein* remains the most accurate test available, with a cutoff of 300 mg/24 hours. False-negative results occur when the patient forgets to collect every sample, and different laboratories use different assays, so they get different results.

Bacteriuria

- About 2% to 10% of pregnant patients have asymptomatic bacteriuria. If untreated, 30% will develop a urinary tract infection. Antibiotics are very effective in preventing pyelonephritis (Smaill, 2001).
- Treat with ampicillin, amoxicillin, cephalosporin, or nitrofurantoin according to sensitivities.
- Repeat the mid stream urine (MSU) 2 weeks after treatment.

Glycosuria

- This occurs in 70% of pregnant patients.
- If there is 2+ of glucose in urine or + on two occasions, then arrange for a modified glucose tolerance test. If the sugar level is raised (fasting sugar $\geq$5.6 mmol/L or the 2-hour sugar $\geq$7.8 mmol/L), refer the patient urgently.

Gestational Diabetes

> **GUIDELINE**
>
> National Institute for Health and Care Excellence. (2020). *Diabetes in pregnancy: Management from preconception to the postnatal period. NICE guideline 3.* Retrieved from https://www.nice.org.uk/guidance/ng3.

- A patient should be managed intensively if her 2-hour sugar is greater than 9 mmol/L or her fasting glucose is over 6 mmol/L. For most patients, however, diet is sufficient to control blood sugars. Active management with diet; blood glucose monitoring; and, if necessary, metformin or insulin has been shown to reduce the risk of serious perinatal complications (Crowther et al, 2005). Recheck fasting glucose 6 to 13 weeks postpartum to be sure that it has returned to normal.
- Warn the patient of her 20% to 30% chance of developing diabetes in the next 5 years. This risk can be decreased by maintenance of a 'diabetic diet' after pregnancy.

Anaemia

- As the plasma volume increases in pregnancy, the haemoglobin decreases. Only a haemoglobin below 11 g/dL

(WHO) in the first trimester or less than 10.5 g/dL at 28 weeks' gestation is considered to be anaemia.

- Routine iron supplementation is not recommended.
- A low serum ferritin is not a reliable guide to iron deficiency in pregnancy. It may reflect a shift of iron stores to the increased red cell mass rather than a low total body iron. However, there is no better noninvasive test.

Anaemia Developing in Pregnancy

- Check full blood count, film, and serum ferritin. Check vitamin B_{12} and red cell folate if there is macrocytosis.
- Start iron in treatment doses if the haemoglobin is below 10 g/dL or the mean corpuscular volume is below 82 fl (e.g., give ferrous sulphate 200 mg OD and folic acid 5 mg/day). The addition of folate can almost double the rise in haemoglobin regardless of the patient's folate status (Juarez-Vazquez, Bonizzoni, & Scotti, 2002).
- Repeat haemoglobin in 2 weeks. It should increase by about 0.8 g/dL per week.
- If there has been no response:
  a. Exclude occult infection, especially urinary, and either
  b. Consider arranging for parenteral iron or
  c. If the serum ferritin is normal, check the serum B_{12} and red cell folate (if not already checked) and continue combined iron and folate.
- If the haemoglobin remains low, seek expert advice. Consider an haemoglobin electrophoresis regardless of the apparent ethnic origin.

Rhesus-Negative Patients

- Check antibodies at booking and in primigravidas at 28 and 36 weeks; in multigravidas, check antibodies monthly from 24 weeks. If the maternal anti-D levels are 0.5 to 10.0 IU, antibody levels are needed every 2 weeks. A level above 10 IU means that foetal blood sampling is needed, and referral to a foetal medicine unit is indicated. If gestation allows, delivery, rather than intrauterine transfusion, may be the preferred option. It is important to realise (and explain) that subsequent pregnancies may behave similarly.
- Offer routine anti-D immunisation to all rhesus-negative patients at 28 and at 34 weeks if nonsensitised except when the patient:
  a. Is certain she will not have another child after the present pregnancy
  b. Is in a stable relationship with the father of the child and the father is known to be rhesus D negative (NICE, 2002)
- In addition to routine antenatal anti-D immunisation, offer it postnatally and if a sensitising event occurs antenatally, namely:
  a. Abdominal trauma, including external cephalic version
  b. CVB and amniocentesis
  c. Antepartum haemorrhage
  d. Ectopic pregnancy
  e. Termination of pregnancy or evacuation of retained products of conception (ERPC)
  f. Threatened or complete miscarriage after 12 weeks
  g. Intrauterine death
- Use 250 IU up to 20 weeks of pregnancy. Give 500 IU thereafter followed by a Kleihauer test for foetal haemoglobin. If the foetomaternal haemorrhage exceeds 4 mL red cells, a further dose is needed.

Abnormal Lie

- Check the lie from 32 to 34 weeks' gestation onwards. If a transverse lie is found at 32 weeks or later, then either:
  a. Refer or
  b. Arrange a scan and reassess at 36 weeks. Refer if still transverse.
  Note: A breech presentation should be seen at the hospital by 37 to 38 weeks' gestation.

High Head

- A 'high head' is one that lies completely out of the pelvis. Make sure that the bladder and rectum are empty before accepting that the head is high.
- *Primipara:* Refer by 36 weeks' gestation.
- *Multipara:* Refer if still high at 38 weeks' gestation.

Premature Rupture of Membranes

All patients suspected of rupturing membranes should be referred for specialist assessment. After 35 weeks' gestation, the specialist is likely to recommend induction of labour. Before 35 weeks' gestation, a short inpatient stay with antibiotic cover is more likely.

Postmaturity

- If the expected date of delivery was established by USS in early pregnancy, routine induction of labour at 41 weeks reduces perinatal mortality rates (Crowley, 2002), and both NICE and the RCOG recommend induction of labour between 41 and 42 weeks' gestation. Routine induction does not cause an increase in the rate of LSCS, nor in lower maternal satisfaction.
- Patients who have not given birth by 41 weeks' gestation should be offered a pelvic examination and membrane sweep and discussion and information about induction of labour.

Specific Medical Conditions and Pregnancy
Asthma

- Deterioration occurring during pregnancy is usually caused by a reduction in therapy because of a fear that it will harm the foetus.
- Explain that poorly controlled asthma has been linked to IUGR.
- Explain that beta-sympathomimetics, inhaled steroids, and ipratropium are safe, but oral steroids and theophylline have been linked to preterm delivery.

Diabetes (Types 1 And 2)

- Optimum control of blood sugars should be achieved by the time of conception to reduce the risk of congenital malformations.
- The GP should emphasise the importance of good control throughout pregnancy even if the majority of the management will be done by the hospital.
- Because of the higher risk of NTDs, patients with diabetes should take 5 mg (instead of 400 μg) of folate daily before conception until the end of the 12th week.
- Patients should be referred to the diabetes clinic and seen every 2 weeks before 28 weeks' gestation and then weekly.
- NICE now recommend real-time continuous glucose monitoring or intermittently scanned continuous glucose monitoring ('flash' monitoring) for patients with type 1 diabetes.
- The insulin dose may need to be doubled or tripled and needs to be reduced immediately after delivery to the prepregnant dose.
- Patients taking oral hypoglycaemic drugs should be changed to insulin.
- Blood sugar profiles should show the majority of readings (before meals) below 6 mmol/L.
- Aim to keep the HbA_{1c} at 6% (42 mmol/mol) or below.
- Discontinue angiotensin-converting enzyme I and II inhibitors before conception or as soon as pregnancy is confirmed. Substitute with a more suitable drug.
- Discontinue statins before pregnancy or as soon as pregnancy is confirmed.
- Patients should have serial ultrasound scans to exclude macrosomia and placental insufficiency. They should have examination of the foetal heart at 18 to 20 weeks' gestation.

Thyroid Disorders

Preexisting Thyroid Disease

- *Hypothyroidism.* Patients should be advised to delay conception until thyroid function is stable on levothyroxine. Thyroid function should be checked at booking, at least once in each trimester, and after any dose changes. Thyroxine requirements may increase during pregnancy.
- *Hyperthyroidism.* Refer all pregnant patients with hyperthyroidism to an endocrinologist as soon as they present. It is important that they remain euthyroid throughout the pregnancy. Propylthiouracil is the preferred drug during pregnancy, given at the lowest effective dose to reduce the risk of foetal hypothyroidism and goitre (Marx, Amin, & Lazarus, 2008).

Postnatal Thyroiditis

- Up to 10% of patients develop transient autoimmune thyroiditis after delivery. This is usually between 1 and 3 months and may present with features of hyperthyroidism but more commonly with those of hypothyroidism (i.e., fatigue and lethargy) at a time when she is understandably tired anyway. Thyroxine is necessary for 6 months, followed by repeat thyroid function tests (TFTs). Antithyroid drugs are not usually needed for the hyperthyroid state, but beta-blockers may be given to control symptoms.
- Follow the patient with yearly TFTs. Up to 20% develop hypothyroidism in the subsequent 4 years.

Epilepsy

- The association between epilepsy and its treatment with congenital malformations has been discussed. About 20% of patients have an increase of fits during pregnancy caused by either poor compliance or a decrease in serum levels because of the physiological changes of pregnancy. Seizures are more common when patients are tired.
- Do not stop anticonvulsants or reduce their dose if a patient presents already pregnant. Any teratogenic effect will have already occurred. Liaise with her neurologist to plan the rest of the pregnancy. In general, it is not necessary to monitor serum levels of anticonvulsant in pregnancy but to be guided by the clinical condition and only to increase the dose of a drug if the frequency of fits increases.
- Encourage the patient to take her treatment correctly. Poor compliance is the main reason for seizures in pregnancy.
- Ensure that an anomaly ultrasound is performed at 18 to 19 weeks' gestation.
- Recommend folic acid 5 mg/day to all patients with epilepsy until the end of the 12th week. This is particularly important in patients taking sodium valproate or carbamazepine or who have a history of a previous baby with a NTD.
- Prescribe vitamin K 10 mg/day for the last 4 weeks of pregnancy to reduce the risks of maternal and foetal bleeding in those taking enzyme-inducing drugs (i.e., phenytoin, barbiturates, and carbamazepine).
- Reassure patients that the majority have a normal delivery and that epilepsy is not an indication for elective caesarean section.

Inflammatory Bowel Disease

- Inflammatory bowel disease is not worsened by pregnancy and may improve (Fergusson, Mahsu-Dornan, & Patterson 2008). If the disease is quiescent at the time of conception, it remains so in two-thirds of patients. If the disease is active, two-thirds of patients will have ongoing active disease.
- Patients with inactive disease have no increased risk of an adverse outcome. Patients with active disease have up to a 35% miscarriage rate. Patients with Crohn's disease have an increased risk of low birth weight, preterm delivery, and adverse perinatal outcomes.
- Assessment of inflammatory bowel disease in pregnancy is based on clinical factors (e.g., abdominal pain, stool frequency, and bleeding). Pregnancy affects haemoglobin

concentration, erythrocyte sedimentation rate, and serum albumin. C-reactive protein is not altered by pregnancy.

- Reassure the patient that it is most important to achieve the best control of the disease possible and that this seems to give the best outcome. All patients should be seen urgently by the gastroenterology and obstetric team.
- For the safety of commonly used drugs for inflammatory bowel disease, see Caprilli et al (2006).

Depression

GUIDELINE

National Institute for Health and Care Excellence. (2020). *Antenatal and postnatal mental health: Clinical management and service guidance. Clinical guideline 192.* Retrieved from https://www.nice.org.uk/guidance/cg192.

- Rates of depression are higher during pregnancy than at any other point in a female's life.
- About half of postnatal depression starts during pregnancy.
- Two-thirds of patients with recurrent depression will relapse during pregnancy if they stop their antidepressants after conception.
- Depression during pregnancy is associated with poorer outcomes, especially preterm delivery.
- Patients depressed during pregnancy are more likely to drink alcohol and smoke and less likely to attend antenatal appointments.
- If major depression is present and drug treatment is being considered, the following are relevant and should be shared with the patient:
  a. Tricyclic antidepressants (TCAs; amitriptyline, imipramine, and nortriptyline) are safer for foetuses than other antidepressants.
  b. TCAs are more dangerous in overdosage than selective serotonin reuptake inhibitors (SSRIs).
  c Fluoxetine is the SSRI of choice during pregnancy but not when breastfeeding because it is present in breast milk in high concentrations. Familiarity with other SSRIs such as sertraline and citalopram during pregnancy is growing.
  d. SSRIs, when taken after 20 weeks' gestation, are associated with a very small risk of persistent pulmonary hypertension in the neonate.
  e. Paroxetine in the first trimester may be associated with a small increased risk of cardiac abnormalities.
  f. Venlafaxine may cause high blood pressure and greater difficulty in withdrawal in the neonate.
  g. All antidepressants may cause withdrawal symptoms in neonates, though these are usually mild. The possible symptoms are hypotonia, excessive crying, sleeping difficulties, and mild respiratory distress.
  h. The choice of antidepressant is likely to be influenced by what the patient is already taking or what she has responded well to in the past.

PATIENT INFORMATION

Bumps, which is run by the UK Teratology Information Service, has information on many medications both for patients and professionals. Available at http://www.medicinesinpregnancy.org.

Drug Misuse

- Liaise with local substance misuse services.
- *Amphetamines and cocaine.* Stop the drugs immediately.
- *Benzodiazepines.* Withdraw over 4 weeks.
- *Barbiturates.* Arrange admission. If there is any delay, maintain the patient on phenobarbital.
- *Opiates.* Arrange an urgent outpatient appointment. Maintain the patient on oral methadone meanwhile.

Intrapartum Care

POLICY STATEMENT

Royal College of GPs and the British Medical Association. (1997). *General practitioners and intrapartum care: Interim guidance.* Available from BMA House, Tavistock Square, London WC1H 9JP.

This section does not cover the clinical aspects of delivery.
- The guidance above defines three levels of GP involvement in intrapartum care:
  a. The GP provides general medical care only, with the responsibility to refer a patient to another professional to provide intrapartum care if the patient wishes to deliver at home.
  b. The GP attends a patient in labour as nonspecialist backup for the midwife, with the midwife taking responsibility for the delivery.
  c. The GP provides intrapartum care and has the competence, over and above that of the average GP, to do so. The general practice committee (GPC) of the BMA advises GPs that to assume this role, they must be skilled in the identification of abnormalities of labour, in perineal suturing, in the resuscitation of mothers and babies, and the insertion of an intravenous line (GPC, 1999).
- It is the policy of the two relevant Royal Colleges that patients who wish to have a home birth should be able to do so.
- There is growing evidence that the risks of planned home delivery have been overemphasised in the United Kingdom, with a perinatal hazard associated with planned home births of less than 1% (Northern Region Perinatal Mortality Survey Co-ordinating Group, 1996).
- Home delivery is valued by those who choose it, even in those who are transferred to hospital during labour (Davies et al, 1996).

When a Patient Requests a Home Delivery

- Check that there are no medical or obstetric contraindications. Some contraindications (e.g., previous retained placenta) can be dealt with by 'domino', in which most of labour takes place at home with the briefest possible admission for the delivery.
- Refer to the community midwife, who has a statutory duty to provide a service at home, whether or not a GP is willing to provide maternity services.

Postnatal Care

At 6 Weeks

- Does she have any outstanding questions about what happened during labour or birth?
- Is she getting enough sleep? Who is sharing in the work of caring for the baby? How is she feeling in herself? Is she feeling depressed? How is she getting along with her partner (if she has one)? Is she getting any time away from the baby?
- Ask about pain in her breasts, back, and perineum.
- Ask about urinary and faecal incontinence, haemorrhoids, and constipation.
- Ask about sex. Around 90% of patients report having sex by 10 weeks postpartum, and 2% report not attempting sex by 1 year (Glazener, 1997). An explanation that libido is often low in the first year may relieve a couple who are finding that this is the case.
- Perform a vaginal examination only if symptoms dictate or if a smear is due.
- Offer contraceptive advice.
- *Prevention of sudden infant death syndrome.* Reinforce the importance of:
  a. The sleeping position (on the back)
  b. Not smoking
  c. Not giving the baby a duvet

Breastfeeding

Advantages of Breastfeeding

- *Advantages for the baby* include less infection, less chance of atopy or diabetes, and better bonding.
- *Advantages for the mother* include a lower risk of breast and ovarian cancers, weight loss, and less postpartum bleeding. It is also cheaper.

Problems With Breastfeeding

The majority of problems centre round the infant's attempts to remove milk. The baby needs to be in a comfortable position to allow jaw and tongue to drain the milk ducts under the areola.

- Check that the mother and baby are managing the following:
  a. The baby's chest against the mother's chest, with the baby's chin to the breast

  b. The mouth wide open
  c. Both lips curled back
  d. The lower lip at the junction of the areola and breast
  e. Rhythmic movements of jaw muscles

Failing Lactation

- Suckling is the strongest stimulus. Ensure that the baby is suckling well (see earlier).
- Advise the mother to go to bed for 2 days with the baby to feed on demand (mother and baby).
- In general, drugs should not be used, but a short course of domperidone may restore prolactin secretion.

Sore Nipples

> **GUIDANCE**
>
> The Breastfeeding Network. (2019). *Differential diagnosis of nipple pain.* Retrieved from http://www.breastfeedingnetwork.org.uk.

- Sore nipples are usually caused by the baby's tongue rubbing the nipple rather than the areola.
- Check that the nipple is positioned in an upwards direction towards the roof of the baby's mouth.
- Allow breast milk to dry on the nipple when not feeding, or if the skin is broken, use white soft paraffin.

Skin Infection

> **GUIDANCE FOR PATIENTS AND HEALTH PROFESSIONALS**
>
> The Breastfeeding Network. (2020). *Thrush (of the breast/nipple) and breastfeeding.* Retrieved from http://www.breastfeedingnetwork.org.uk.

- This may be caused by *Candida* infection and may present as localised soreness, as pain around the areola and nipple, or as pain in the breast after a feed.
- Treat the mother with miconazole cream and the baby with miconazole oral gel, whether the baby has signs of infection or not. It is unnecessary for the mother to remove the cream before feeding.
- Consider using oral fluconazole if local treatment alone is not working. This use is not licensed, but the WHO recognises fluconazole as compatible with breastfeeding. Download the leaflet mentioned earlier for guidance on dosing. The unlicensed use must be discussed with the mother and documented.

Blocked Duct

- This presents as a hard lump anywhere in the breast.
- Get the mother to massage the breast while feeding the baby from that breast.
- The baby's position should be altered so that the lower lip is nearer the blocked duct.

Breast Engorgement

- The pain of engorgement is one of the commonest reasons for stopping breastfeeding in the first 2 weeks. Treatment is disappointing with cabbage leaves, ultrasound, and cold packs being no better than placebo (Snowden, Renfrew, & Woolridge 2001).
- Give simple analgesia and support.
- Attempt to prevent engorgement by removing any obstacles to easy breastfeeding.

Mastitis

- Early mastitis is inflammatory, not infectious, and may respond to effective emptying of the breast plus a non-steroidal antiinflammatory drug (NSAID).
- Reassess the feeding position of the baby to ensure that milk is removed completely.
- Prescribe an NSAID.
- Treat with flucloxacillin for 10 to 14 days if the patient is unwell or febrile or there is any suspicion of abscess formation. Use erythromycin if the patient is allergic to penicillin. Warn mothers that the milk will change in taste and feeding may be harder initially or that the baby may develop diarrhoea and need to feed more frequently.
- *Breast abscess.* If an abscess forms which is large enough to need draining, admit the patient for incision and drainage.

Suppression of Lactation

This usually takes 4 to 5 days after stopping breastfeeding. It may be very painful and require analgesia and a supportive bra. It is usually not necessary to use drugs. However, after stillbirth or if there is another good reason to stop lactation, use bromocriptine 2.5 mg at night for 2 nights and then 2.5 mg bd for 3 weeks. If used for a shorter period, a number of patients relapse.

Vaginal Bleeding After 24 Hours

- The traditional management of excessive bleeding more than 24 hours after delivery (secondary post partum haemorrhage (PPH)) is surgical. However, ERPC yields placental tissue in fewer than 30% of these cases, so the majority of patients do not benefit.
- *Mild bleeding.* Give both:
  a. Ergometrine 0.5 mg intramuscularly; then 0.5 mg tds orally for 4 days
  b. Antibiotics, such as amoxicillin–erythromycin ± metronidazole for 5 days
- *Severe bleeding* or if the os still admits one finger after 7 days. Admit.

Fever

- *Endometritis.* Patients with fever, pain, and foul-smelling lochia are likely to need admission, but early cases could be treated at home with amoxicillin–erythromycin and metronidazole.
- Be aware that deep vein thrombosis and urinary tract infection can cause fever without localised symptoms.

Depression

GUIDELINES

National Institute for Health and Care Excellence. (2020). *Antenatal and postnatal mental health: Clinical management and service guidance. Clinical guideline 192.* Retrieved from https://www.nice.org.uk/guidance/cg192.
    Royal College of Obstetricians and Gynaecologists. (2011). *Good practice no.14: Management of women with mental health issues during pregnancy and postnatal period.* Retrieved from https://www.rcog.org.uk/guidance/browse-all-guidance/good-practice-papers/management-of-women-with-mental-health-issues-during-pregnancy-and-the-postnatal-period-good-practice-no14/.

- Depression after birth is experienced by one in seven patients in the year after childbirth. It is distinct from the transient 'blues' of the first 10 days and from a puerperal psychosis, which is likely to need admission.
- RCOG recommends starting to screen for depression during the antenatal period by asking the following questions at each appointment:
  1. During the past month, have you often been bothered by feeling down, depressed, or hopeless?
  2. During the past month, have you often been bothered by having little interest or pleasure in doing things?
- The EPDS (see Appendix 19) is recommended by NICE as a screening tool during the postpartum period but with the understanding that it is a screening, not a diagnostic, tool. Clinical assessment is needed to establish the diagnosis. Between 30% and 70% of patients who screen positive with the EPDS are not depressed (Oates, 2003).
- Factors associated with developing depression in the year after childbirth are:
  a. Perceived lack of social, emotional, and practical support, particularly from a partner
  b. Physical health problems
  c. Exhaustion
  d. Infant factors: unsettled or 'difficult' babies
  e. Negative life events
  f. A previous psychiatric history, although this only accounts for a small number of the patients who experience depression
  g. Not breastfeeding
  h. Preterm delivery, infant health issues, or need for neonatal intensive care
- There is little or no evidence of any direct association between depression after birth and hormonal factors.
- During the postnatal visit, every patient should have the opportunity to speak about how she is feeling and how she is coping with the transition to motherhood. Some simple questions that may assist patients to talk about how they are really feeling are (Gunn et al, 2003):
  a. How are you feeling?
  b. How are you sleeping?
  c. How is your relationship going?

d. Who is sharing in the work of caring for the baby?
e. How much time do you get to yourself?
f. How do you find being a mother?

Management of Postnatal Depression

- Antenatal and postnatal interventions offered routinely to all patients in an effort to prevent postnatal depression have been ineffective (Lumley, Austin, & Mitchell, 2004) apart from programmes consisting of a redesigned community midwifery model of care (MacArthur et al, 2002).
- Antenatal and postnatal interventions offered only to patients perceived to be at a higher risk of developing depression have been ineffective (Lumley et al, 2004).
- Interventions offered to patients identified as experiencing depression have been effective, and there is strong evidence that postnatal counselling (from active listening to cognitive-behavioural therapy) reduces depression with a number needed to treat of two to three (Lumley et al, 2004). Simple nondirective counselling by health visitors, weekly for 8 weeks, doubles the recovery rate (Holden et al, 1989).
- Check for physical health problems. Patients experiencing the common postnatal physical problems are more likely to be depressed. Ask about:
  - Tiredness. Consider checking haemoglobin, ferritin, and TFTs
  - Backache
  - Sexual problems
  - Perineal pain
  - Mastitis and feeding problems
  - Urinary and faecal incontinence
  - Constipation and haemorrhoids
- *Offer counselling or psychotherapy.* Cognitive-behavioural therapy is as effective as fluoxetine in reducing postnatal depression. The choice of treatment can be made by the patient herself (Appleby et al, 1997).
- *Offer an antidepressant* to the 3% to 5% of patients whose depression is moderate or severe (Oates, 2003) and for whom an effective form of counselling or psychotherapy is not immediately available or who chooses an antidepressant. SSRIs are first-line treatment with sertraline and paroxetine the drugs of choice in patients who are breast-feeding, although a previous good response to another medication may influence choice. TCAs are used much less commonly; if they are, then doxepin should be avoided and imipramine or nortriptyline used.
- Consider referral if a multidisciplinary mental health team is able to offer more than the primary healthcare team. Ideally, if the patient requires admission, this should be to a mother and baby facility.
- Refer urgently, to be seen within 24 hours, any patient with ideas of suicide or of harming the baby.

PATIENT INFORMATION AND SUPPORT

Association for Postnatal Illness. Helpline: 020 7386 0868. Available at http://www.apni.org.

Exhaustion

- Tiredness is common, even among patients who are not depressed. It is uncommon to find a specific cause, but anaemia, iron deficiency, and thyroid problems should be considered.
- Lack of sleep is one of the commonest causes. Taking note of the baby's sleep patterns, excluding depression, offering time to talk, encouraging time-out from childcare, and encouraging sharing the work of looking after the baby are all simple support strategies.

Common Physical Problems

- Physical problems are common: around 44% of patients will experience backache, 26% sexual problems, 21% haemorrhoids, 21% perineal pain, 17% mastitis, 13% bowel problems, 11% urinary incontinence, and 6% faecal incontinence (Brown & Lumley, 1998; MacArthur, Bick, & Keighley 1997).
- Unfortunately, there is little evidence to guide our management of postpartum incontinence or perineal pain. Three-quarters of patients with urinary incontinence at 3 months postpartum still had the problem 6 years later despite conservative nurse-led pelvic floor and bladder training management of urinary and faecal incontinence (Glazener et al, 2005).

References

Appleby, L., Warner, R., Whitton, A., & Faragher, B. (1997). A controlled study of fluoxetine and cognitive-behavioural counselling in the treatment of postnatal depression. *British Medical Journal, 314,* 932–936.

BASSH & RCOG. (2014). *Management of genital herpes in pregnancy.* Retrieved from https://www.rcog.org.uk/guidance/browse-all-guidance/other-guidelines-and-reports/management-of-genital-herpes-in-pregnancy/.

Bech, B. H., Obel, C., Henriksen, T. B., & Olsen, J. (2007). Effect of reducing caffeine intake on birth weight and length of gestation: Randomised controlled trial. *BMJ, 334,* 409–412.

Best, J. M., O'Shea, S., Tipples, G., Davies, N., Al-Khusaiby, S. M., Krause, A., Hesketh, L. M., Jin, L., & Enders, G. (2002). Interpretation of rubella serology in pregnancy—pitfalls and problems. *BMJ (Clinical research ed.), 325,* 147–148.

Bracken, M. B., Triche, E. W., Belanger, K., Saftlas, A., Beckett, W. S., & Leaderer, B. P. (2003). Asthma symptoms, severity, and drug therapy: A prospective study of effects on 2205 pregnancies. *Obstetrics and Gynecology, 102,* 739–752.

Braig, S., Luton, D., Sibony, O., Edlinger, C., Boissinot, C., Blot, P., & Oury, J. F. (2001). Acyclovir prophylaxis in late pregnancy prevents recurrent genital herpes and viral shedding. *European Journal of Obstetrics, Gynecology, and Reproductive Biology, 96,* 55–58.

Brocklehurst, P. (2000). Interventions aimed at decreasing the risk of mother-to-child transmission of HIV infection. *Cochrane Database of Systematic Reviews, 2002*(2), CD000102. doi:10.1002/14651858. CD000102.

Brown, S., & Lumley, J. (1998). Maternal health after childbirth: Results of an Australian population based survey. *British Journal of Obstetrics and Gynaecology, 105*, 156–161.

Calder, R., Gant, E., Bauld, L., McNeill, A., Robson, D., & Brose, L. (2021). Vaping in pregnancy: A systematic review. *Nicotine & Tobacco Research, 23*(9), 1451–1458.

Caprilli, R., Gassull, M. A., Escher, J. C., Moser, G., Munkholm, P., Forbes, A., Hommes, D. W., Lochs, H., Angelucci, E., Cocco, A., Vucelic, B., Hildebrand, H., Kolacek, S., Riis, L., Lukas, M., de Franchis, R., Hamilton, M., Jantschek, G., Michetti, P., O'Morain, C., ... European Crohn's and Colitis Organisation. (2006). *European evidence based consensus on the diagnosis and management of Crohn's disease: Special situations. Gut, 55*(Suppl. 1), i36–i58.

Cedergren, M. I. (2007). Optimal gestational weight gain for body mass index categories. *Obstetrics and Gynecology, 110*, 759–776.

Chappell, L. C., & Shennan, A. H. (2008). Assessment of proteinuria in pregnancy. *BMJ, 336*, 968–969.

Crowley, P. (2000). Interventions for preventing or improving the outcome of delivery at or beyond term. *Cochrane Database of Systematic Reviews*, (2), CD000170. doi:10.1002/14651858.CD000170.

Crowther, C. A., Hiller, J. E., Moss, J. R., McPhee, A. J., Jeffries, W. S., Robinson, J. S., & Australian Carbohydrate Intolerance Study in Pregnant Women (ACHOIS) Trial Group. (2005). Effect of treatment of gestational diabetes mellitus on pregnancy outcomes. *New England Journal of Medicine, 352*, 2477–2486.

Davies, J., Hey, E., Reid, W., & Young, G. (1996). Prospective regional study of planned home births. Home Birth Study Steering Group. *BMJ (Clinical research ed.), 313*, 1302–1306.

Douglas, K. A., & Redman, C. W. G. (1994). Eclampsia in the United Kingdom. *BMJ (Clinical research ed.), 309*, 1395–1400.

Fairgrieve, S. D., Jackson, M., Jonas, P., Walshaw, D., White, K., Montgomery, T. L., Burn, J., & Lynch, S. A. (2000). Population based, prospective study of the care of women with epilepsy in pregnancy. *BMJ (Clinical research ed.), 321*, 674–675.

Fergusson, C. B., Mahsu-Dornan, S., & Patterson, R. N. (2008). Inflammatory disease in pregnancy. *BMJ (Clinical research ed.), 337*, 170–173.

Glazener, C. (1997). Sexual function after childbirth: Woman's experiences, persistent morbidity and lack of professional recognition. *British Journal of Obstetrics and Gynaecology, 104*, 330–335.

Glazener, C. M., Herbison, G. P., MacArthur, C., Grant, A., & Wilson, P. D. (2005). Randomised controlled trial of conservative management of postnatal urinary and faecal incontinence: six year follow up. *BMJ (Clinical research ed.), 330*(7487), 337. doi:10.1136/bmj.38320.613461.82.

GPC (1999). *The role of the GP involved in intrapartum care*. BMA. Retrieved from www.bma.org.uk; choose 'Committees' then 'GPC Guidance' then 'General Practitioners and maternity medical services'.

Gunn, J., Southern, D., Chondros, P., Thomson, P., & Robertson, K. (2003). Guidelines for assessing postnatal problems: Introducing evidence-based guidelines in Australian general practice. *Family Practice, 20*, 382–389.

Harris, R., Lane, B., Harris, H., Williamson, P., Dodge, J., Modell, B., Ponder, B., Rodeck, C., & Alberman, E. (1999). National confidential enquiry into counselling for genetic disorders by non-geneticists: General recommendations and specific standards for improving care. *British Journal of Obstetrics and Gynaecology, 106*, 658–663.

Holden, J. M., Sagovsky, R., & Cox, J. L. (1989). Counselling in a general practice setting: Controlled study of health visitor intervention in treatment of postnatal depression. *BMJ (Clinical research ed.), 298*, 223–226.

Inskip, H. M., Crozier, S. R., Godfrey, K. M., Borland, S. E., Cooper, C., Robinson, S. M., & Southampton Women's Survey Study Group. (2009). Women's compliance with nutrition and lifestyle recommendations before pregnancy: General population cohort study. *BMJ (Clinical research ed.), 338*, b481.

Jewell, D., & Young, G. (2003). Interventions for nausea and vomiting in early pregnancy. *Cochrane Database of Systematic Reviews*, (4), CD000145. doi:10.1002/14651858.CD000145.

Juarez-Vazquez, J., Bonizzoni, E., & Scotti, A. (2002). Iron plus folate is more effective than iron alone in the treatment of iron deficiency anaemia in pregnancy: A randomised, double blind clinical trial. *BJOG, 109*, 1009–1014.

Leung, J., Grosse, S., Yockey, B., & Lanzieri, T. (2022). Ganciclovir and valganciclovir use among infants with congenital cytomegalovirus: Data from a multicenter electronic health record dataset in the United States. *Journal of the Pediatric Infectious Diseases Society, 11*(8), 379–382. Retrieved from https://doi.org/10.1093/jpids/piac034.

Lilford, R. J. (1991). The rise and fall of chorionic villus sampling. *BMJ (Clinical research ed.), 303*, 936–937.

Luise, C., Jermy, K., May, C., Costello, G., Collins, W. P., & Bourne, T. H. (2002). Outcome of expectant management of spontaneous first trimester miscarriage: Observational study. *BMJ (Clinical research ed.), 324*, 873–875.

Lumley, J., Austin, M. P., Mitchell, C. (2004). Intervening to reduce depression after birth: A systematic review of the randomized trials. *International Journal of Technology Assessment in Health Care, 20*, 128–144.

MacArthur, C., Bick, D., Keighley, M. R. (1997). Faecal incontinence after childbirth. *British Journal of Obstetrics and Gynaecology, 104*, 46–50.

MacArthur, C., Winter, H. R., Bick, D. E., Knowles, H., Lilford, R., Henderson, C., Lancashire, R. J., Braunholtz, D. A., & Gee, H. (2002). Effects of redesigned community postnatal care on womens' health 4 months after birth: A cluster randomised controlled trial. *Lancet, 359*, 378–385.

Martel, M. J., Rey, E., Beauchesne, M. F., Perreault, S., Lefebvre, G., Forget, A., & Blais, L. (2005). Use of inhaled corticosteroids during pregnancy and risk of pregnancy induced hypertension: Nested case-control study. *BMJ (Clinical research ed.), 330*, 230.

Marx, H., Amin, P., & Lazarus, J. H. (2008). Hyperthyroidism and pregnancy. *BMJ (Clinical research ed.), 336*, 663–667.

MBBRACE-UK. (2022). *Saving lives, improving mothers' care: Core report: Lessons learned to inform maternity care from the UK and Ireland confidential enquiries into Maternal deaths and morbidity 2018-20*. Retrieved from https://www.npeu.ox.ac.uk/assets/downloads/mbrrace-uk/reports/maternal-report-2022/MBRRACE-UK_Maternal_CORE_Report_2022_v10.pdf.

Milkiewicz, P., Elias, E., Williamson, C., & Weaver, J. (2002). Obstetric cholestasis. *BMJ (Clinical research ed.), 324*, 123–124.

Nachum, Z., Ben-Shlomo, I., Weiner, E., & Shalev, E. (1999). Twice daily versus four times daily insulin dose regimens for diabetes in pregnancy: Randomised controlled trial. *BMJ (Clinical research ed.), 319*, 1223–1227.

National Institute for Health and Care Excellence. (2002). *Guidance on the use of routine antenatal anti-D prophylaxis for RhD-negative women*. NICE. Retrieved from www.nice.org.uk.

National Institute for Health and Care Excellence. (2014). Antenatal and postnatal mental health: Clinical management and service guidance. Clinical Guideline 45. Retrieved from www.nice.org.uk.

Nielsen, S., & Hahlin, M. (1995). Expectant management of first trimester spontaneous abortion. *Lancet, 345*, 84–86.

Northern Region Perinatal Mortality Survey Co-ordinating Group. (1996). Collaborative survey of perinatal loss in planned and unplanned home births. *BMJ, 313,* 1306–1309.

Oates, M. (2003). Postnatal depression and screening: Too broad a sweep? *British Journal of General Practice, 53,* 596–597.

O'Brien, P. (2007). Is it all right for women to drink small amounts of alcohol in pregnancy? *BMJ (Clinical research ed.), 335,* 856–857.

Olesen, C., Steffensen, F. H., Nielsen, G. L., de Jong-van den Berg, L., Olsen, J., & Sørensen, H. T. (1999). Drug use in first pregnancy and lactation: A population-based survey among Danish women. The EUROMAP group. *European Journal of Clinical Pharmacology, 55,* 139–144.

Palacios, C., Kostiuk, L. K., & Peña-Rosas, J. P. (2019). Vitamin D supplementation for women during pregnancy. Cochrane Database of Systematic Reviews, 7(7), CD008873.

Regan, L., Braude, P. R., & Trembath, P. L. (1989). Influence of past reproductive performance on risk of spontaneous abortion. *BMJ (Clinical research ed.), 299,* 541–545.

Royal College of Obstetricians and Gynaecologists (2001). *Chickenpox in pregnancy.* Clinical Green Top Guideline No. 13. Retrieved from www.rcog.org.uk (choose 'Good practice' then 'Clinical green top guidelines').

Royal College of Obstetricians and Gynaecologists (2017). *Prevention of early onset neonatal group B streptococcal disease.* Clinical Green Top Guideline No. 36. Retrieved from www.rcog.org.uk (choose 'good practice' then 'clinical green top guidelines').

Rush, D. (1994). Periconceptional folate and neural tube defect. *American Journal of Clinical Nutrition, 59*(Suppl. 2), 511S–515S.

Sikorski, J., Wilson, J., Clement, S., Das, S., & Smeeton, N. (1996). A randomised controlled trial comparing two schedules of antenatal visits: The antenatal care project. BMJ (Clinical research ed.), *312,* 546–553.

Silverberg, M. J., Thorsen, P., Lindeberg, H., Grant, L. A., & Shah, K. V. (2003). Condyloma in pregnancy is strongly predictive of juvenile-onset recurrent respiratory papillomatosis. *Obstetrics and Gynecology, 101,* 645–652.

Smaill, F. (2001). Antibiotics for asymptomatic bacteriuria in pregnancy (Cochrane review). In: The Cochrane Library. Update Software, Oxford Issue 4. Retrieved from www.nelh.nhs.uk/cochrane.asp.

Snowden, H. M., Renfrew, M. J., & Woolridge, M. W. (2001). Treatments for breast engorgement during lactation (Cochrane review). In: The Cochrane Library. Update Software, Oxford Issue 4. Retrieved from www.nelh.nhs.uk/cochrane.asp.

Steel, J. M., Johnstone, F. D., Hepburn, D. A., & Smith, A. F. (1990). Can pre-pregnancy care of diabetic women reduce the risk of abnormal babies? *BMJ (Clinical research ed.), 301,* 1070–1074.

Stotland, N. E. (2009). Obesity and pregnancy. *BMJ (Clinical research ed.), 338,* 107–110.

Three Centres Consensus Guidelines on Antenatal Care Project. (2001). *Melbourne: Mercy Hospital for Women, Southern Health.* Melbourne, Australia: Women's and Children's Health.

Villar, J., Carroli, G., Khan-Neelofur, D., et al. (2001). Patterns of antenatal care for low-risk pregnancy (Cochrane review). In: The Cochrane Library. Update Software, Oxford Issue 4. Retrieved from www.nelh.nhs.uk/cochrane.asp.

Ward, V. B. (2008). Eating disorders in pregnancy. *BMJ (Clinical research ed.), 336,* 96.

Weng, X., Odouli, R., Li, & D. K. (2008). Maternal caffeine consumption during pregnancy and the risk of miscarriage: A prospective cohort study. *American Journal of Obstetrics and Gynecology, 279,* e1–e8.

Wisborg, K., Kesmodel, U., Bech, B. H., Hedegaard, M., & Henriksen, T. B. (2003). Maternal consumption of coffee during pregnancy and stillbirth and infant death in first year of life: Prospective study. *BMJ (Clinical research ed.), 326,* 420–422.

Wong, M. K. Y., Crawford, T. J., Gask, L., & Grinyer, A. (2003). A qualitative investigation into women's experiences after a miscarriage: Implications for the primary healthcare team. *British Journal of General Practice, 53,* 697–702.

14

Older People

Maria Panourgia

CHAPTER CONTENTS

Keeping Older People Healthy

Screening and Prevention

- In general, cancer screening programmes continue until older age. There is little evidence that screening is no longer worthwhile as people age, and most programmes recommend continuing to age 75 years, although in the United Kingdom, some *routine* screening ends at 65 years of age. However, the benefits and risks of screening older adults should be assessed on an individual basis, taking into account the patient's estimated remaining life expectancy and comorbidities and the action to be taken as a result of any screening results.

- If older people can tolerate their medications, then treating those with high blood pressure and high cholesterol will prolong life expectancy and reduce the risk of heart disease and stroke. The decision to initiate medications in older adults, and particularly those 80 years and older, should be individualised based on comorbidities and recognition of problems that may arise from polypharmacy in this population (Guasti 2022; Yandrapalli 2019).

- Influenza and pneumococcal vaccinations are recommended in the United Kingdom and elsewhere for all persons aged 65 years and older. More than 90% of deaths from influenza are in the over-60 age group (Nichol et al, 1994).

In the United Kingdom, herpes zoster vaccination is also now offered to those aged 70 years with a catch-up programme for those aged 70 to 79 years based on the evidence of cost-effectiveness and because this age group is likely to have the greatest benefit from vaccination (Immunisation against infectious disease (Green Book) 2006, last update 2023).

Smoking

- Advise smoking cessation for all older people. Ten years after a person stopped smoking, the risk of death by lung cancer falls to half compared to a smoker. Nicotine replacement has not been specifically studied in older adults but can be used (Curb et al, 1996). Simple advice from primary care doctors is effective in smoking cessation (Abdullah & Simon, 2006).

Alcohol

- Although alcohol consumption decreases with age, 17% of males and 7% of older females exceed safe limits. About 1% to 5% of older people who drink more than occasionally report that they are 'problem drinkers', males more so than females (Department for Health and Social Care (DHSC), 1994).
- Simple advice from the general practitioner (GP) may be effective in reducing alcohol consumption (Anderson, 1993).
- Using brief interventions could reduce excessive drinking, but there still appears to be a gap between actual practice and potential for preventive work relating to alcohol problems: primary care doctors report little specific training and a lack of support (Wilson et al, 2011).

The National Institute for Health and Care Excellence (NICE)has specific guidance on the prevention of alcohol and harmful drinking.

Exercise

- A total of 30 to 60 minutes of sustained low-level activity, such as walking, on at least 3 days per week (Manley, 1996) will result in moderate health benefits such as reduced fatigue, weight loss, increased socialisation, improved control of type 2 diabetes, and less shortness of breath on exertion (Rooney, 1993).
- Older people who exercise develop disability at a quarter of the rate of those who do not even though the exercisers have a higher rate of fractures and resultant short-term disability. Even very old people benefit from exercise

because of improvements in muscle strength, gait velocity, and the ability to climb stairs (Elon, 1996).

- Advise regular, safe physical activity as part of daily activities. Simple advice delivered in primary care is effective in increasing activity for older patients (Kerse et al, 1999; Elley et al, 2003).
- Recommend exercise which mimics the activities of daily living (ADLs) such as repetitive sit to stand and walking. This type of exercise is more acceptable and more beneficial for older people.
- Referral to physiotherapy for specific strength and balance training will reduce falls by 40% in females older than age 80 years (Campbell et al, 1997).
- Participation in group based tai chi for older people is associated with health benefits, including improvements in maximal oxygen uptake (VO_2 max), muscular strength, and flexibility, as well as a reduced risk of falls.

Nutrition

Good nutrition is important for a multitude of reasons. Immune function to help fight infections such as influenza; optimal bowel transit time to prevent constipation and resulting risk of urinary tract infection (UTI), acute confusional state, and bowel cancer; adequate vitamin and micronutrient intake to avoid increasing the risk of memory disturbance, osteoporosis, and anaemia; and many more.

- The UK National Diet and Nutrition Survey (1989–2016) indicated that in those older than the age of 65 years:
  a. The average intake of vitamins and minerals was above recommended levels except for some in residential and nursing homes.
  b. Vitamin D status was poor in some, particularly those in residential and nursing homes.
  c. Poor oral health, especially a lack of natural teeth, was associated with poor diet and nutritional status.
  d. The average intake of sugars and saturated fatty acids exceeded recommended levels.
  e. The average fibre intake was lower than recommended.
  f. The diet of older adults is generally better than younger peers.
- However, in the United Kingdom, around 1 in 10 people older than the age of 65 years are affected by malnutrition (Malnutrition Task Force, https://www.malnutritiontaskforce.org.uk).
- Poorer households consume:
  a. Less of the following: fruit and vegetables, salads, wholemeal bread, whole-grain and high-fibre cereals, and oily fish
  b. More of the following: white bread, full-fat milk, table sugar, and processed meat products (which are often high in fat)
- Assess the risk of dietary deficiencies in older patients, especially those with chronic diseases, poor dentition, or poor mobility; with low incomes; and who are housebound.

- Have a low threshold for checking the vitamin B_{12} status of older people, especially if they develop neuropsychiatric symptoms.
- Consider checking a patient's vitamin D status. Vitamin D deficiency is common in older people as the skin decreases in capacity to synthesise the provitamin Calcidol, exacerbated by their low exposure to sunlight. Deficiencies are more common in housebound older adults. Poor muscle strength and weakness are associated with vitamin D deficiency, and this weakness may contribute to the risk of falls.
- Advise patients, no matter their age, to maintain a healthy diet, including at least five portions of fruit and vegetables a day. There is indirect evidence that the modified Mediterranean diet is associated with increased survival among older people (Trichopoulou, 2005). Refer to a dietician if there is concern about dietary intake. Ask the patient to do a food diary for 1 week before being seen.
- Advise isolated patients to contact social services and local nongovernmental organisations (e.g., Age Concern). Eating with others may offer more interaction and reduce loneliness, and there is evidence that family-style meals may improve nutrition in older people (Nijs et al, 2006).
- The involuntary loss of more than 5% to 10% of an older person's usual weight during 1 year is an important clinical sign associated with increased risk of death. Weight loss should thus be treated as a serious symptom and prompt a search for the cause.
- Involuntary weight loss is generally related to one or a combination of four conditions: inadequate dietary intake, appetite loss (anorexia), muscle atrophy (sarcopenia), or inflammatory effects of disease (cachexia).

Managing Frailty

- Frailty is a clinical state in which there is an increase in an individual's vulnerability for developing increased dependency or mortality when exposed to a stressor (Morley et al, 2013).
- General practice, as part of the primary healthcare network, is well placed to detect and treat emerging frailty and prevent further deterioration.
- The Nottingham Extended Activities of Daily Living (EADL; see Appendix 29) scale may be useful in detecting unsuspected functional decline. Electronic indexes are being developed to identify individuals with frailty, but the effectiveness of this type of case finding has not been proved.
- Comprehensive geriatric assessment is associated with improved outcomes for older people, such as reducing hospital admission, readmission, and survival rates as well as improved physical and cognitive functioning (Ellis et al, 2011).
- One specific organ manifestation of frailty is the decline in renal function with age, a decline which has implications for the prescribing of drugs that are renally excreted and

for the management of conditions which, in themselves, impair renal function. An increase in serum creatinine is a late sign of renal impairment and could not be evident to older patients with low muscle mass; estimation of the glomerular filtration rate (eGFR) is more useful.

Early Intervention

- Preventive home visits by health professionals or lay people trained in case finding reduce mortality rates and admission to residential care and may promote independence and improve quality of life for frail older people (Elkan et al, 2001).
- Effective management of minor ailments, such as painful foot problems, may halt declining mobility and improve long-term outcomes.
- Physical therapy aimed at reducing functional impairment in older people with moderate frailty delays functional decline (i.e., in ADL score; Gill et al, 2002).
- Maximising the management of chronic problems and minimising polypharmacy may halt functional decline. The UK National Service Framework recommends an annual review of medication for people aged 75 years and over, with a 6-monthly review for those taking four or more medicines.

Supporting Older People at Home

- There is considerable variation in the availability of services for older people internationally and within countries, both in formal and informal provision. Generally, there is a multitude of services available aimed at staying healthy, either maintaining function or providing rehabilitation.
- Services can be accessed either by direct referral or through specialist geriatric services.
- A comprehensive assessment is recommended before referring to services.
- In general, services are accessed in the United Kingdom through a social worker, in Australia by direct referral or through geriatric assessment services, and in New Zealand through the needs assessment service coordinator.

Difficulty Maintaining Living Arrangements

- Refer to an occupational therapist for assessment of ADL function at home and provision of equipment.
- Refer to a social worker to arrange a home carer for housework.
- Refer to a social worker for Meals-on-Wheels (daily hot food or weekly frozen meal deliveries) where these are available.
- Refer to a podiatrist or chiropodist for foot care.

Isolation

- Refer to Age Concern for provision of a volunteer or befriending service.

- Refer to a social worker for day centre placement.
- Refer to Dial-a-Driver or social worker to access a subsidised taxi service.

Carer Stress

- Ask any carer specifically how they are coping.
- Ascertain the source of any stress.
- Refer for access to respite services, including day and night respite, and residential home placement for short periods.
- Refer for home care for personal assistance.
- Refer to an occupational therapist for assessment of ADL function and equipment.

Functional Deterioration at Home

Refer to:
a. A geriatrician for comprehensive assessment
b. A day hospital, for multidisciplinary assessment and treatment
c. Physiotherapy for musculoskeletal assessment and exercises (Gill et al, 2002)
d. Occupational therapy for ADL functional assessment, provision of equipment, and treatment
e. A social worker for personal home care
f. The district nurses for a bathing service
g. A speech language therapist if the condition affects communication or swallowing
h. A dietician

Poor Recovery After an Acute Episode

- Consider referral to:
  a. The appropriate hospital service
  b. The district nursing service
  c. The occupational therapist or physiotherapist for functional assessment and provision of equipment
  d. The social worker for temporary provision of personal care and housework

Suicide

- Late-life depression often goes undetected and has a significant adverse impact on quality of life, outcomes of medical disease, healthcare utilisation, morbidity, and mortality (O'Connell et al, 2004).
- Suicide rates are almost twice as high in older adults compared with the general population, with the rate highest for White males older than 85 years of age
- The ratio of parasuicide to completed suicide is much lower, suggesting that suicidal behaviour in older people has a much greater degree of intent.
- The main psychological factor associated with suicide in older people is recurrent major depression.
- Poor physical health and disability seem to be associated with the 'wish to die'.

- Consider identifying all those with a known history of depressive disorder and question directly as to whether they have considered suicide. Treat or refer as appropriate.

Delirium, Acute Confusion, Agitation, and Loss of Mobility

- A change in mental or physical status of usually well, independent older people should be taken seriously and treated urgently. Symptoms of serious illness are often masked, and pyrexia may be lower than expected, even in overwhelming infection.
- Acute change can be caused by serious disease without overt symptomatology related to that disease. Confusion can be as simple as 'the patient has suddenly changed, something is wrong, or the level of function has deteriorated'.
- Behaviour change may occur and can be described as verbal, vocal, or motor activity that is not explained by needs. The cause of this may be subtle and may be caused by undiagnosed pain, acute illness, or simply the inability to communicate needs.
- A loss of mobility or 'taken to bed' may be caused by serious illness, particularly when the deterioration is rapid.
- Establishing the onset of deterioration and prior function is essential to identify delirium characterised by a fluctuating level of consciousness, disorientation, and global cognitive deficit. This is almost always from an organic cause, usually infection, which is hard to diagnose with confidence.

Confirmation of the Presence of an Acute Confusional State

- A formal assessment is the Confusion Assessment Method (CAM), which states that the patient has delirium if the following are present:
  - There was an acute onset with a fluctuating course.
  - There is inattention.
  - There is either disorganised thinking or an altered level of consciousness. Consciousness may be depressed, or the patient may be hyperalert.
- The CAM has a sensitivity of at least 94% and a specificity of at least 90% for the diagnosis of delirium when used by nonpsychiatrists (Inouye et al, 1990).

Diagnosis of the Cause of the Confusion

A diagnosis of acute serious illness or medication toxicity should be assumed until proven otherwise. There are many causes for acute confusion, including:
a. Infection, most commonly, pneumonia or UTI
b. Cardiovascular disorder, especially myocardial infarction or congestive heart failure
c. Neurologic disorder, most commonly stroke

d. Medication interaction or toxicity, particularly psychotropic or cardiovascular medications
e. Acute alcohol withdrawal
f. Acute psychiatric disorder, including psychosis
g. Electrolyte disturbance, dehydration, or hyponatraemia
h. Endocrine disorder, thyroid disease, or diabetes
i. Acute change in hearing or vision
j. Faecal impaction or retention of urine
k. Neoplasia
l. Acute surgical emergency, such as peritonitis from appendicitis or gallbladder disease
m. Undiagnosed fracture
n. Hypothermia

Specific Evaluation

A thorough history and physical examination are necessary, including:
a. History of prior functional level, social support, medications, and medical problems. Involving caregivers or family member to get a history may be necessary
b. Examination of the cardiovascular and neurologic systems
c. Musculoskeletal examination, especially for those with reduced mobility. Suspect undiagnosed fracture after apparent minor injury with excessive disability.
d. Abdominal examination to exclude an acute abdomen
e. Rectal examination
f. Investigations will be guided by the history and physical examination (Box 14.1).

Possible Investigations

a) Full blood count (FBC) and erythrocyte sedimentation rate (ESR)
b) Creatinine, eGFR, and electrolytes
c) Liver function tests (LFTs)
d) Vitamin B_{12}
e) Thyroid function tests (TFTs)
f) Midstream specimen of urine (MSU) or dipstick urine test
g) Blood glucose

• BOX 14.1   Abbreviated Mental Test Score

Each question scores 1. A score of 6 or less suggests dementia.
1. Age (exact number of years)
2. Time (to the nearest hour)
3. A simple address, e.g., 42 West Street, to be repeated by the patient at the end of the test
4. Year (the current year)
5. The place (exact address or the name of the surgery or hospital)
6. Recognition of two persons present (by name or role)
7. Date of birth (correct day and month)
8. Year of the First World War (1914 or 1918 is enough)
9. Name of the monarch (must be the current monarch)
10. Count backwards from 20 to 1 (with no mistakes or with mistakes which the patient corrects without prompting)

---

h) Calcium
i) Blood cultures
j) Electrocardiography (ECG)
k) Chest radiography and other radiography as suggested by the examination.

Management

Delirium or Acute Confusion

- Refer for assessment if the diagnosis cannot be clearly identified and the patient cannot initially be managed at home or if a diagnosis is made (e.g., pneumonia or stroke) that requires admission.
  If treating the patient at home:
- Treat any infection with an appropriate antibiotic.
- Stop medications with potential toxicity, especially sedative–hypnotics if they are suspected of causing acute confusion. Check for new medication as a precipitant cause.
- Treat dehydration with fluids with attention to cardiovascular function.
- Be alert to the possibility of an acute kidney injury.
- Deal with faecal impaction in the usual way, with attention to follow-up bowel function. Fluids, exercise, and fibre are all needed for adequate bowel function in older people.

Change in Behaviour With Stress and Distress Behaviour Evident

- Behavioural management is useful for any agitated patient, including:
  a. Allowing wandering in a safe environment
  b. Relocation to alternative living arrangements if agitation becomes a constant problem and cannot be managed in the current living arrangement
  c. Encouraging participation in usual activities
  d. Avoiding confrontation if aggression is a feature
  e. Avoiding physical restraint; it worsens agitation and can cause injury
- Treat the cause as above, especially undiagnosed pain.
- Refer for admission to geriatric or psychogeriatric assessment ward if the patient cannot be managed at home.
- Refer to a psychiatrist for evaluation if psychosis is suspected.
- If no cause is found and the patient has underlying dementia, see later discussion.
- *Medication.* Avoid medication to sedate because this may prolong delirium or shift the patient to a hypoactive delirium instead. Reserve antipsychotics, typical or atypical, for patients who are so agitated that they pose a risk to themselves or to others. Antipsychotics are also associated with increased mortality risk, especially from stroke and sudden cardiac death. Haloperidol may be associated with less risk than the atypicals. Use the smallest dose for the shortest duration possible.
- Avoid benzodiazepines. Even short-acting benzodiazepines accumulate in older persons and worsen the confusion.

They increase the risk of injury from falling, with patients taking higher doses of certain drugs, (oxazepam, flurazepam, and chlordiazepoxide) having the highest risk (Tamblyn et al, 2005).

Loss of Mobility

- Treat acute illness as for acute confusion above.
- If minor injury is the cause, significant disability has resulted, and there is no fracture:
  a. Give adequate pain relief.
  b. Mobilise as soon as possible.
  c. Refer to community physiotherapy or outpatient department or day hospital services for rehabilitation (Forster, Young, & Langhorne, 2002).
- Refer the patient to a day hospital, which can improve overall functional outcome and reduce service utilisation when compared with no comprehensive care (Forster et al, 2002).
- Refer for comprehensive inpatient geriatric assessment and management if the patient's overall function has deteriorated without apparent cause.

Deterioration Over a Longer Period of Time Without Acute Illness, Depression, or Dementia

- Deterioration in mental or physical status can be slow and progressive and not apparently caused by an acute illness (i.e., not delirium).
- If the onset is slow and the workup has not shown a treatable acute cause, then the differential diagnoses of dementia and depression must be considered.

Diagnosis

- The diagnosis of depression is often missed in older people because the prominence of physical symptoms compounds the diagnosis.
- Dementia is of more insidious onset than depression.
- In depression, cognitive and physical deterioration is worse in the mornings.
- In depression, insight is present; in dementia, it is rare.
- Orientation is poor in dementia and preserved in depression.
- Memory loss is characteristically worse for recent events in dementia but can be similar for recent and remote events in depression.

Specific Evaluation

- Ask about a family and personal history of depression.
- Ask about recent significant events. Bereavement and relocation predispose to social isolation and depression.
- Check functional status and independence in ADLs.
- Check the patient's social and financial supports.
- Ask about driving. Specific driving assessment may be necessary later.
- The five-question geriatric depression scale is useful in diagnosing depression in those without severe dementia and works in a variety of settings (Rinaldi et al, 2003).

- Assess the patient's cognitive state formally using one or both of the following tests or use the TYM ('test your memory') test see later:
  - *Clock drawing* is a useful, nonthreatening test of mental function. Simply draw a circle and ask the patient to 'make it into a clock with the time at 10 to 2'. If numbers are not spread throughout all four quadrants, then the test is suggestive of dementia, particularly if short-term recall is reduced for three words (Mini-Cog test).
- A standardised mental test score, such as the Abbreviated Mental Test Score (see box) is only reliable if used precisely (Holmes & Gilbody, 1996). A more well-validated but time-consuming score is the Mini Mental State Examination (MMSE) (see later).

Management

- Treatment of dementia is outlined in the next section.
- Refer for geriatric medical or geriatric psychiatric assessment if the diagnosis is not clear.
- Treat depression, if present, with one or both of the following:
  a. An antidepressant (Wilson et al, 2002)
  b. Psychological therapy, including cognitive-behavioural therapy. Poor access to publicly funded counselling services may limit its availability.
- Follow-up is essential to ensure recovery of function.

Dementia

GUIDELINE

National Institute for Health and Care Excellence (NICE). (2018). *Dementia: Assessment, management and support for people living with dementia and their carers. NICE guideline 97.* https://www.nice.org.uk/guidance/ng97.

- Dementia affects 10% of those older than age 65 years and 20% of those older than age 80 years.
- Absolute numbers of those with dementia will increase exponentially in the next two decades as the world population ages.
- New therapies recently available and currently under investigation mean that identification of early dementia may become important in the future.
- A UK parliamentary committee report (House of Commons, 2008) criticised the whole range of dementia care:
  a. Poor diagnosis – only one-third receive a formal diagnosis
  b. Fragmented home support
  c. Untrained staff in care homes
  d. A failure to recognise and manage dementia in hospitals

Diagnosis

- Suspect dementia when the patient has the following:
  a. Impairment in short- and long-term memory, abstract thinking, judgment, other higher cortical function, or personality change.
  b. The disturbance is severe enough to interfere significantly with work, social activities, or relationships
  c. Delirium is absent (American Psychiatric Association, 1987).
- Confirm it with a formal assessment. NICE mentions:
  a. Six-item cognitive impairment test
  b. The Mini-Cog
  c. 10-point Cognitive Screener
  d. Memory Impairment Screen (MIS)
- A good combination is the Abbreviated Mental Test Score plus the clock drawing test (see earlier). The former tests orientation and memory, and the latter tests praxis and spatial perception.
- Another test is the TYM test (Brown et al, 2009). It has three advantages over other tests currently in use: it tests many different cognitive domains; it is performed by the patient alone, taking less than 1 minute of the doctor's or nurse's time to score it; and it is sensitive for the detection of early Alzheimer disease. Using a score of 42 or less of 50 as positive, it is 93% sensitive and 86% specific for Alzheimer disease. The original article and the test itself are available at http://www.tymtest.com.
- Determine, from the history and examination, whether it is possible to decide on the cause of the dementia (see later). This entails examination of the patient's mental state and cognition, a neurologic and cardiovascular examination, and a screen for depression. However, many patients have atypical or nonspecific presentations.
- Exclude the few cases of reversible cognitive impairment as in Box 14.2, which lists the clinical features of the types of dementia.

Specific Evaluation

- Take a history from a caregiver or a source other than the patient. Objective assessment of change (e.g., from the carer) may help support the diagnosis. Use the Informant Questionnaire on Cognitive Decline in the Elderly (IQCODE) or the informant component of GPCOG.
- Screen for depression.
- Examine the patient's mental state, cognition, and neurologic system.
- Examine the cardiovascular system.
- Investigations:
  a. Vitamin B_{12} level
  b. Thyroid function
  c. FBC, creatinine, eGFR, electrolytes, LFTs, calcium, glucose, and ESR
  d. Chest radiography, MSU
  e. Syphilis screening may no longer be needed unless there is a specific risk factor or the patient is from certain parts of the United States.

> **• BOX 14.2 Types of Dementia Listed in Order of Prevalence**
>
> **Dementia: Alzheimer Type**
> - Accounts for the majority of dementia cases
> - Insidious onset over several years
> - Global deficits
>
> **Vascular Dementia**
> - Accounts for 10% of dementia cases, though 29%–41% of dementia cases autopsied have some vascular pathology
> - Stepwise progression
> - Bilateral neurologic signs
> - A history of cardiovascular disease suggests vascular dementia
> - Risk factors or a history of risk factors for cardiovascular disease makes vascular dementia more likely
>
> **Dementia With Lewy Bodies**
> Dementia plus the following:
> - Balance and gait disorder
> - Prominent hallucinations and delusions
> - Sensitivity to antipsychotics
> - Fluctuations in alertness
>
> **Frontotemporal Dementia**
> - Early loss of personal awareness
> - Early loss of social awareness
> - Hyperorality (putting inappropriate things in the mouth)
> - Stereotyped, perseverative behaviours
>
> **Prion Disease (Creutzfeldt–Jakob Disease)**
> - Rapidly progressive symptoms
> - Characteristic electroencephalographic pattern of periodic sharp wave complexes
> - Pathological brain tissue diagnosis
> - CSF 14-3-3 protein (high sensitivity and specificity for diagnosis of Creutzfeldt–Jakob disease)

- Imaging with computed tomography or magnetic resonance imaging. Availability limits access in some regions.
- Other options are not recommended or not appropriate for primary care. Imaging with single-photon emission computed tomography or positron emission tomography is not recommended for routine use. Genetic testing and genotyping are not currently recommended. The CSF 14-3-3 protein may become available and has overall sensitivity of 92% and a specificity of 80% in diagnosing sporadic Creutzfeldt Jacob disease (Muayqil et all, 2012).

Management
General

- It is widely accepted that patients with dementia should be assessed by a psychogeriatrician or geriatrician.
- Cognition, function, mood, and behaviour as well as general health should be reevaluated every 6 months in patients with dementia.
- *Prognosis.* If the family wishes to know, explain that a diagnosis of Alzheimer disease reduces life expectancy in a way that depends on the person's age. At age 65 years, the

median survival time with Alzheimer disease is 8 years; at 90 years, it is 3 years (Brookmeyer et al, 2002).

- *Driving.* In the United Kingdom, advise the patient to inform the DVLA and their insurance company. If there is reasonable concern about public safety, the GP should inform the Driver and Vehicle Licensing Agency (DVLA) themselves. Download and give to the patient the leaflet *Driving and Dementia* (Breen et al, 2007). Indicate that the maximum time driving might be allowed is 3 years (Breen et al, 2007). Be wary of being too certain; clinical assessment is poorly associated with driving ability. There is no evidence-based information to guide physician assessment of medical fitness to drive (Malnar et al, 2005).

Training the Carers

- Refer for intensive long-term education and support for caregivers (if available) to delay time to residential care placement. A meta-analysis has shown that interventions designed to support carers can improve their mental health and result in the patient with Alzheimer disease staying at home longer (Spijker et al, 2008).
- Explain the principles of reality orientation and how to cope with a person with dementia (see later).
- If the patient is not already too impaired, explain how he or she can reduce the impact of the condition on their life (see later).
- If sleep is a problem, train the carers in sleep hygiene practices, including advice about exercise, sleep at regular times, and avoiding naps. This has been shown to improve sleep patterns with daytime benefits as well. To achieve these benefits, carers need considerable support (McCurry et al, 2003).
- Refer for home support.
- Consider referral for placement in dementia-specific long-term care. This may reduce carer strain.
- Consider whether the patient might be in pain. Many older patients have painful conditions. A patient with dementia may be unable to communicate that pain is a problem. Look out for signs of distress (frowning, looking frightened, aggression, agitation, or withdrawal) and give an analgesic if pain could be the cause (Scherder et al, 2005). Specific assessment and treatment of pain can reduce distress (Husebo et al, 2011).

For Patients in Residential Care

- Offer residential care staff education about the behavioural management of patients with Alzheimer disease.
- Explain that a safe wandering space is essential for older persons with dementia to avoid agitation and unnecessary restraint, although there is no direct evidence of benefit (Price et al, 2002). This is especially useful for 'sundowning' (increased agitation in the late afternoon).
- Scheduled toileting and prompted voiding reduce urinary incontinence.
- Music therapy, simulated natural sounds, and intensive multimodality group training may improve overall function.

- Specific assessment and treatment of pain can reduce distress (Husebo et al, 2011).

Psychosocial Interventions

- The main nonpharmacologic approaches that can play a role are as follows (Gitlin, Kales, & Lyketsos, 2012):
    a. Reality orientation is based on the belief that continual, repetitive reminders will keep the patient stimulated and better orientated. There is some evidence of improved cognition and behaviour in people with dementia (Woods et al, 2012).
    b. Memory enhancement strategies include setting shorter term goals, maintaining a social circle, and the family role.
    c. Present dementia as a disability that can be accommodated and emphasise the person's continuing abilities.

General Principles For Carers

a. Treat the patient with respect and dignity and address the patient as though you expect them to understand.
b. Recognise the patient's level of capability but do not talk down or treat them as a child.
c. Encourage all attempts at personal care and ADLs.
d. When talking, look directly at the person and maintain eye contact.
e. Use short sentences expressing one thing at a time.
f. Do not use implied messages; say exactly what you mean.
g. If not understood, repeat the message a different way. Do not shout and do not rush them.
h. Mention names of familiar people and the date, week, and time in all conversations.
i. Reward the patient's attempts with a smile or compliment. Reality orientation in the patient's home could include:
a. A large clock and a calendar visible at all times
b. Wearing a watch with a date display
c. Having stimulating materials available (e.g., newspapers and magazines)
d. A reality orientation board with a schedule of daily activities and reminders (e.g., appointments, at what time to expect a carer that day, as well a reminder of the day and date)

Medications for Cognitive Symptoms

- The pharmacologic treatment of symptoms is complex and rapidly changing. Each decision should be personalised to the individual's needs rather than an improvement on a 'score'.

Alzheimer Disease

- NICE has issued guidance on the use of donepezil, galantamine, rivastigmine, and memantine for treatment of patients with Alzheimer disease.
- *Cholinesterase inhibitors* have been shown to improve cognition and global functioning in patients with Alzheimer disease. The improvements are small and come at the cost

of an increase in adverse effects. The benefits are greatest for those in whom the disease is moderate or moderately severe:

- Donepezil, galantamine, and rivastigmine are now recommended as options for managing mild as well as moderate Alzheimer disease.
- Memantine is now recommended as an option for managing moderate Alzheimer disease for people who cannot take cholinesterase inhibitors and as an option for managing severe Alzheimer disease.
- Treatment should be continued only when it is considered to be having a worthwhile effect on cognitive, global, functional, or behavioural symptoms.
- The severity of the condition may be assessed using the MMSE, in which 'moderate' to 'moderately severe' are represented by scores of 10 to 20 points (Table 14.1). However, the MMSE should not be used if another condition makes it unreliable (e.g., learning difficulties, sensory impairment, or linguistic problems).
- The drug should be initiated by a specialist in the care of patients with dementia.
- When assessing the severity of Alzheimer disease and the need for treatment, healthcare professionals should not rely solely on cognition scores.
- Families may ask their GP's opinion of various drugs that can be bought over the counter; for instance:
  - *Vitamin E* supplementation might slow functional decline in males with mild to moderate Alzheimer disease, but neither vitamin E nor memantine appears to affect cognitive function or dementia severity.
  - *Gingko biloba.* There is inconsistent evidence of benefit in cognitive function from taking gingko biloba and no evidence of increased harm. 'Over-the-counter' preparations vary considerably in potency compared with the pure product used in randomised controlled trials (RCTs). Relatives can be advised that the chance of benefit is small.

Ischaemic Vascular Dementia and Mixed Dementia
- Evidence-based data supporting pharmacologic efficacy of agents to treat patients with non–Alzheimer disease dementia are less strong than for Alzheimer disease.
- Some research shows that patients with vascular dementia benefit from galantamine (Erkinjuntti et al, 2002).

TABLE 14.1	Grading of Severity in Alzheimer's Disease According to the Mini Mental State Examination (MMSE)
Severity	**MMSE Score**
Mild	21–26
Moderate	15–20
Moderately severe	10–14
Severe	<10

Galantamine 16 to 24 mg/day is associated with improved ADLs and cognition scores.
- Donepezil 5 to 10 mg/day is associated with small improvements in cognitive function (Malouf & Birks, 2004).
- Offer all the measures appropriate for the secondary prevention of cardiovascular disease if the patient's condition and life expectancy warrant it. Blood pressure control with perindopril and indapamide has been shown to slow cognitive decline and reduce disability (Fransen et al, 2003). Blood pressure–lowering strategies have not been specifically tested for treatment or prevention of vascular dementia, and this effect is likely to be due to further stroke prevention.
- Similarly, other interventions (e.g., aspirin) may not halt cognitive decline, although they are likely to reduce the risk of other vascular disease (Rands et al, 2005).
- Based on the observed prevalence of potentially modifiable risk factors (e.g., hypertension, diabetes, inactivity) combined with their associated relative risk for dementia, it has been estimated that risk factor reductions of 10% to 25% could prevent up to half of dementia cases if treated early.

Medication for Behavioural Symptoms
- The treatment of *delirium*, an acute change in mental status characterised by fluctuation in level of consciousness, attention, and cognitive function is more complex than in those with the stable symptoms of dementia (Britton & Russell, 2002).
- Look for an organic cause, most commonly undiagnosed pain, infection, or cardiovascular disorder, as with well older people.
- Use behavioural and environmental modification. 'Reality orientation' (presenting orientation information based on time, place, and person related) has been shown in one systematic review of small RCTs to improve behaviour (Woods et al, 2012).
- Treat stress and distress behaviour and symptoms of psychosis as follows:
  a. Psychotropic medication should be cautiously used for treatment of severe agitation or psychosis with the potential for harm (e.g., low-dose haloperidol, 0.5–1.0 mg orally or intramuscularly) daily dose up to a maximum of 5 mg.. Use the smallest possible dose for the shortest periods of time. In patients with a parkinsonian disorder or Lewy Body dementia, use an 'atypical' antipsychotic instead.
  b. Benzodiazepines should be avoided in patients with delirium except in withdrawal syndromes or when other drugs cannot be used.
- Withdraw an antipsychotic from a patient with dementia unless the need for it is overwhelming. A UK RCT in patients with dementia on antipsychotic treatment found that those whose antipsychotic medication was switched to placebo had a better chance of surviving over 12 months than those in whom the medication was continued (Ballard et al, 2009).

Teaching the Patient to Cope With Cognitive Impairment

- In the early stages of cognitive impairment, the patient can be taught how to minimise the functional disability. A simple analogy, such as 'If you had a limp, you'd use a stick, but since it's your memory that's not so good, you need to learn ways to help it' may help the patient to accept the concept. Another phrase that is readily understood is 'Use it or lose it'.
- Family and carers should be involved in this process from the beginning. This helps to overcome their frustration at living with a cognitively impaired relative and, as the patient becomes more impaired, they can take over some of the tasks.
- Cognitive impairment is embarrassing and frustrating. The natural tendency is to try to cover it up. The approach outlined next depends on the opposite: accepting it and adopting techniques to minimise its effect.
- Advise the patient to:
  a. Do things when you are most alert.
  b. Take rest.
  c. Use relaxation techniques to reduce stress.
  e. Keep active (e.g., household jobs, visiting, reading).
  f. Be involved in sports, music, and other activities that involve coordination.
  g. Keep a regular routine.
  h. Learn to live with pain and not expect all pain to be relieved but use analgesics when necessary, particularly for night pain.
  i. Express feelings.
  j. Eat well-balanced meals.
  k. Reduce alcohol intake.
  l. Consider counselling.

Memory Difficulties

- Memory involves learning, storage, and recall. There is little that can be done to improve the storage of memory, but there are techniques to improve learning and recall.
- Advise the patient to:
  a. Avoid undermining their confidence. Remember 'no one's memory is perfect'! If you forget something, don't get too upset about it.
  b. Reduce alcohol and avoid sedatives,
  c. Try to concentrate in a place free of distractions,
  d. Try to motivate yourself to learn. Make sure you understand and remember all the information,
  e. Improve retention by rehearsing or repeating information and by making associations to improve retention,
  f. Learn one new thing at a time and try to avoid the confusion that comes with information overload.
  g. When learning something, study for short periods and frequently rather than long periods.
  h. Use memory aids, such as dry wipe boards, sticky note pads, diaries, a calendar, and alarms.

Anxiety, Moodiness, and Irritability

- Advise the patient to:
  a. Identify the sources of aggravation and try to come up with a simple solution.
  b. Practise talking to oneself (e.g., stay calm, relax).
  c. Leave the situation explaining that you will need to calm down and go back to it later.
  d. Use relaxation techniques (e.g., recordings, therapy, counting to 10).
  e. Take regular exercise.
  f. Get things 'off your chest' by talking or writing.

Difficulty in Initiating Activities

- Advise the patient to:
  a. Improve their organisational skills (daily routines, use of a diary, avoid putting things off, priority lists, break the task into smaller tasks, use simple methods to achieve things, ask for help or delegate, take time and not to rush, if necessary involve others in decision making).
  b. Involve others so they can help motivate you.
  c. Reward yourself when steps are completed. Do this frequently and make the goals reasonable.
  d. If orientation is a problem use maps, landmarks, planned routes, and written directions.

Reading

- Having to reread something several times is common. This may be a result of concentration or memory problems but may also result from a change in the brain's ability to handle a lot of information.
- Advise the patient to try:
  a. Moving a finger under each word at a comfortable pace
  b. Blocking off the words underneath the sentence with a sheet of paper
  c. Creating a window, in a card, that only allows one line to be read at a time
  d. Taking notes to help focus and concentrate on the important parts
  e. Reading larger print
  f. Testing themselves about what they have read

Problems in Social Situations

- People with dementia may have difficulties in understanding certain social situations and jump to conclusions that are inappropriate.
- Different patterns of cognitive impairment require different specific approaches. See entries under Alzheimer disease, Parkinson disease, and Huntington disease.
- Advise the patient to:
  a. Clarify what was meant.
  b. Explain what they believe was said.
  c. Get feedback from others.
  d. Recognise problem situations or people and plan how to respond beforehand.
  e. Communicate openly and honestly; above all, respect the other person's position.

f. Give the 'benefit of the doubt' to others and assume they mean no harm.

Financial and Legal Aspects (united Kingdom)

- Patients may be eligible for exemption from Council tax.
- Advise that it may be appropriate for someone else to be given power of attorney.

SUPPORT GROUPS

Alzheimer's New Zealand. tel. 0800 004 001. http://www.alzheimers.org.nz.

Alzheimer's Society. Gordon House. Helpline: 0300 222 11 22, http://www.alzheimers.org.uk.

Details of Alzheimer's Associations in other countries can be found on the website of the Alzheimer's Disease International. http://www.alzint.org.

Age Concern. New Zealand, http://www.ageconcern.org.nz.

Age Concern England. http://www.ageconcern.org.uk.

Details of other UK branches of Age Concern can be found on the UK website above.

Falls

GUIDELINES

National Institute for Health and Care Excellence. (2013). *Falls in older people: Assessing risk and prevention*. https://www.nice.org.uk/guidance/cg161.

(2022). Montero-Odasso et al, World guidelines for falls prevention and management for older adults: A global initiative. *Age and Ageing*. 2022 Sep 2;51(9):afac205.

Falls are serious and common for those older than age 75 years. Risk factors and specific interventions proven to reduce falls have been identified.

Risk Factors

a. Age older than 80 years
b. Cognitive impairment
c. History of falls and fall-related injury
d. Arthritis
e. Depression
f. Use of a mobility aid
g. Gait and balance impairment
h. Lower limb muscle weakness
i. Visual deficit
j. Impaired daily functioning or a low score on the Nottingham EADL scale (see earlier)
k. Use of psychotropic medications

Those with multiple risk factors are at a higher risk of falls.

Diagnosis

- Ask older people (aged 75 and older) routinely, once a year, 'Have you had a fall in the past year'?

- Use the 'three key questions':
  a. Have you fallen in the past year?
  b. Do you feel unsteady when standing or walking?
  c. Do you have worries about falling?

Gait or balance disturbances should be assessed following a positive answer to history of fall or any of the three key questions.

- Perform a simple gait assessment (see later).
- Distinguish between 'hot' and 'cold' falls.
  a. 'Hot' falls result from major medical conditions such as stroke, myocardial infarction, or seizure. Treatment of the acute illness usually entails admission to hospital.
  b. 'Cold' falls occur in the absence of serious acute illness. This part of the chapter deals with management of cold falls and those with high risk of falls.
- Refer anyone with a recent 'cold' fall, with recurrent falls in the past year, or with an abnormality of gait or balance for falls risk assessment.
- NICE recommends a multifactorial risk assessment of older people who present for medical attention because of a fall or report recurrent falls in the past year.

Specific Evaluation

A falls risk assessment includes:
a. History of fall circumstances
b. Medication review
c. Review of chronic medical problems, including alcohol misuse
d. Examination of
  - Vision
  - Gait and balance (see later)
  - Lower leg strength
  - Neurologic system, especially proprioceptive and coordination function and including mental status
  - Cardiovascular system, especially heart rate and rhythm, lying and standing blood pressure, and the murmurs of valvular disease
e. The environment where the falls occurred, with attention to:
  - Hazards such as loose mats, cords, and unstable furniture
  - Lighting levels
f. Assessment of the person's fear of falling and the effect it is having on functional ability
g. Investigations including FBC and ECG

SIMPLE GAIT ASSESSMENT

Ask the patient to stand from a chair and without using the arms, walk 3 m, turn around, and return (the 'Get Up and Go' test) (Mathias, Nayak, & Isaacs, 1986). Unsteadiness or difficulty completing this in less than 30 seconds shows a gait and balance deficit, and further evaluation is needed.

Management

- Results of the evaluation should guide specific management. Most patients needing intervention have multiple risk factors.
- Multifactorial intervention is more effective than single intervention in preventing future falls.
- Refer all with a history of unexplained syncope to a physician. Investigations such as a lying and standing blood pressure or multiday ECG may reveal a cause. Carotid sinus hypersensitivity can be detected by carotid sinus massage in controlled conditions, including cardiac monitoring.

Community-Dwelling Older People at High Risk of Recurrent Falls

- Exercise may reduce falls in community-dwelling older persons (Sherrington et al, 2008).
- Review medications and reduce psychotropics. Drugs that are especially likely to cause falls are benzodiazepines, tricyclic antidepressants (TCAs), phenothiazines and butyrophenones, antihypertensives, anticholinergics, and hypoglycaemic agents (American Geriatric Society, 2015).
- Assess vision and refer if necessary. Cataract surgery reduces the risk of falls with hip fracture (Tseng et al, 2012).
- *Home environment.* Assess whether shoes and slippers fit properly. Check whether loose carpets, poor lighting, or general cluttering of furniture is increasing the risk. Refer for modification of other environmental hazards according to the availability of occupational therapy.
- Review all medical conditions. Treat cardiovascular disorders, including postural hypotension and any cardiac arrhythmia.
- *Osteoporosis.* When patients can tolerate it, consider giving vitamin D_3 800 IU daily with calcium co-supplementation to reduce the risk of vertebral fracture. The vitamin D may, in addition, increase muscle strength, particularly for those who are deficient in vitamin D. (Gillespie et al, 2009 and 2012).

Older People in Residential Care and Assisted Living Settings at High Risk of Recurrent Falls

- A systematic review of studies of fall prevention in hospitals and long-term care facilities found inconclusive evidence for the effectiveness of most approaches. These approaches appear less effective in the real world than in research studies (Coussement et al, 2008).
- Refer to physiotherapy for gait and balance training and advice on use of assistive devices. This depends on the availability of physiotherapy services in long-term care.
- Consider giving vitamin D_3 to achieve a level greater than 30 ng/mL.
- It is reasonable for clinicians to consider the use of hip protectors in patients at high risk of hip fractures who are willing to comply with their use. They are only effective if they are actually worn. They do not work at an institutional level (Santesso et al, 2014).

Vestibular Rehabilitation Exercises

a. *In bed*, performed slowly initially and then more rapidly:
   - *Eye movements.* Move the eyes up and down, side to side, focusing on a finger as it moves from 1 m away to 30 cm away.
   - *Head movements.* Move the head forwards then backwards and turning from side to side.
b. *Sitting.* Rotate the head; bend down and stand up with eyes open and closed.
c. *Standing.* Throw a small ball from hand to hand, turning through 360 degrees.
d. *Moving about.* Walk across the room, up and down a slope, and up and down stairs with the eyes open and then closed.

Lower Leg Problems

Night Cramps

Nocturnal leg cramps are common occurrences among older generally healthy adults, 70% of whom experience them at some time (Butler, Mulkerrin, & O'Keeffe, 2002).

Diagnosis

Most are idiopathic, but they are more common in certain conditions:
- Peripheral vascular disease
- Renal failure
- Diabetes
- Thyroid disease.
- Hypomagnesaemia
- Hypocalcaemia
- Hypokalaemia

Possible Investigation

- FBC and ESR
- Creatinine, eGFR, and electrolytes
- LFTs
- Blood glucose
- Calcium and magnesium
- TFTs

Management

- Treat the underlying cause whenever possible.
- Look for a drug cause. Diuretics, nifedipine, beta-agonists, steroids, morphine, cimetidine, penicillamine, statins, and lithium have all been implicated.
- Explain the technique to abort a cramp as it is starting: forcibly stretch the muscle that is in spasm. Thus, for cramp in the calf, the patient should stand up with the leg straight and forcibly dorsiflex the foot by pressing the ball of the foot on the floor.
- Recommend a trial of calf-stretching exercises; they have been found helpful. The technique is to stand 3 feet from a wall, rest against it with the arms outstretched, then tilt towards it, keeping the heels on the floor, until the stretch is felt in the calves, holding the position for

10 seconds. Do this three times a day, with three stretches each time. If after 3 days there is improvement, continue it long term.
- *Drug treatment*
  - Quinine sulphate is not recommended. Quinine carries the risk of a severe sensitivity reaction in 1 in 1000 to 3500, of which the main manifestation is severe thrombocytopenia. Hepatitis and haemolytic uraemic syndrome have also been described. Finally, it is very dangerous in overdose. Because of these risks, the US Food and Drug Administration has banned its marketing for cramps, but it remains licensed for cramps in the United Kingdom.
  - There is limited and inconsistent evidence that calcium channel blockers, vitamins, minerals, and naftidrofuryl reduce the frequency of cramps (Blyton et al, 2012).

Restless Legs Syndrome

REVIEWS

European Federation of Neurological Societies/European Neurological Society/European Sleep Research Society. (2012). Guideline on management of restless legs syndrome. *European Journal of Neurology, 19*(11):1385.
    Leschziner, G., & Gringras, P. (2012). Restless legs syndrome. *British Medical Journal,* 2012 May 23;344:e3056.

- The syndrome is characterised by 'creepy crawly' sensations in the lower limbs. These occur at rest in the evenings or at night and are temporarily relieved by moving the limbs. The minimum diagnostic criteria proposed by International Restless Legs Syndrome Study Group and National Institutes of Health are:
  - The urge to move legs often accompanied by an unpleasant feeling
  - The onset or worsening of symptoms when at rest
  - Partial or complete relief by movement for as long as movement continues
  - Circadian pattern of symptom expression with high frequency of occurrence in evening and at night (often interferes with sleep)
- Evidence is inconsistent for association with iron deficiency, but screening is generally recommended by consensus panels.

Workup
a. FBC
b. Serum ferritin
c. Folic acid
d. Vitamin B_{12}
e. Creatinine, eGFR, and electrolytes
  - Examine to exclude peripheral neuropathy.
  - Review the patient's drugs. Possible causes are neuroleptics, lithium, beta-blockers, calcium channel blockers, TCAs, phenytoin, and H2 blockers.

- Explain what to do during an attack: walk about, stretch the legs, have a bath, do something interesting as a distraction, or massage the legs.
- Nonpharmacologic therapy options for prevention include avoidance of aggravating drugs and substances such as caffeine, mentally alerting activities, exercise, leg massage, and applied heat. In patients with mild or intermittent symptoms, these therapies may be sufficient for symptom relief.
- Consider drug treatment for patients with symptoms that are sufficiently severe and frequent. Be wary of treating mild and infrequent symptoms with indefinite medication duration. Options include:
  a. A dopamine agonist. These classes of drugs have been shown to be effective compared with placebo, but the diagnostic uncertainty and side effects often limit their use.
  b. A calcium channel ligand (e.g., gabapentin), appears to improve symptoms in patients with moderate to severe restless legs syndrome, particularly if neuropathy is present.

PATIENT SUPPORT AND INFORMATION

RLS-UK. http://www.rls-uk.org.

Postural Ankle Oedema

- Many patients are given diuretics inappropriately for postural oedema. Diuretics can cause paradoxical oedema.
- Assess carefully to exclude a cardiac, renal, or hepatic cause.
- Treat postural oedema by advising the patient to:
  a. Keep active.
  b. Elevate the legs when sitting.
  c. Use support hosiery.
- Give a diuretic only where the oedema is too severe to permit the patient to pull on a support stocking, and even then, only give it for a maximum of 3 weeks.
- Consider a trial without diuretics for those already started on them. In one study, 85% of those suitable were successfully withdrawn from diuretics (de Jonge et al, 1994). Be aware that even patients who do not need their diuretics are likely to have an initial increase in oedema as a rebound phenomenon, which may take 6 weeks to settle.

Elder Abuse

- Age UK estimated that 400,000 older people were the victims of abuse in 2022.
- There are no statutory guidelines or legislation; however, abuse is a crime. Intervention should always be interdisciplinary.
- Abuse may take the form of:
  a. *Physical:* hitting, slapping, pushing, kicking, misuse of medication, restraint, or inappropriate sanctions

b. *Psychological,* including emotional abuse, threats of harm or abandonment, deprivation of contact, humiliation, blaming, controlling, intimidation, coercion, harassment, verbal abuse, isolation, or withdrawal from services or supportive networks

c. *Sexual,* including rape and sexual assault or sexual acts to which the vulnerable adult has not consented, could not consent to, or was pressurised into consenting to

d. *Financial or material abuse,* including theft, fraud, exploitation, pressure in connection with wills, property or inheritance or financial transactions, or the misuse or misappropriation of property, possession, or benefits

e. *Neglect and acts of omission,* including ignoring medical or physical care needs; failure to provide access to appropriate health, social care, or educational services; the withholding of the necessities of life, such as medication or adequate nutrition

f. *Discriminatory abuse,* including racist, sexist, based on a person's disability, and other forms of harassment

- Abuse can occur anywhere:
  a. In someone's own home
  b. In a carer's home
  d. In day care
  e. In a residential or nursing home
  f. In hospital
- Abuse may occur for many reasons.
  a. In the home, the causes include poor quality long-term relationships; a carer's inability to provide the level of care needed, or a carer with mental or physical health problems.
  b. In other settings, it may be a symptom of a poorly run establishment, especially when staff are inadequately trained and poorly supervised.
- Suspect abuse when:
  a. There is delay in seeking medical help.
  b. There are differing histories from patient and carer, especially if explanations are implausible.
  c. There are inconsistencies on examination.
  d. There are frequent calls for visits by the GP or Accident and Emergency (A&E) attendances.
  e. The carer does not accompany the patient when it would be expected.
  f. There is abnormal behaviour in the presence of the carer (e.g., fear or withdrawal).
- Discuss the situation with the patient, carer, and involved care agencies. Further action should depend on the wishes and competence of the patient and the nature and severity of the abuse.
- Discuss the case with Action on Elder Abuse (see later box).

PROFESSIONAL AND PATIENT INFORMATION

Hourglass. Information leaflets are available. http://wearehourglass.org.

Sex and Older Adults

- Sexual activity is common in older adults with studies indicating that at least 50% of 60- to 90-year-old people remain sexually active. Although coitus declines in frequency, interest is maintained in different ways (e.g., masturbation, oral sex). There is a shift from genital sex to intimacy.
- In a study looking at the secular trends in health the sexual activity of Swedish 70-year-olds in 1971 was compared with 70-year-olds in 2001. Males and females from the latter group reported higher satisfaction with sexuality, fewer sexual dysfunctions, and more positive attitudes to sexuality in later life (Beckman et al, 2008).
- Medication may cause changes in sexual function, particularly beta-blockers, antidepressants, and antipsychotics (Thomas, 2003).
- Phosphodiesterase 5 inhibitors are used in the treatment of erectile dysfunction. They work in older males but less than in younger males (Müller et al, 2007).
- Males. Explain the 'normal' changes associated with ageing (Masters & Johnson, 1970):
  a. The urgency of sexual interest declines from the late 40s.
  b. Erections are less frequent.
  c. Erections need more stimulation especially tactile.
  d. Erections are is more difficult to sustain.
  e. The turgidity of erections diminishes.
  f. Ejaculation is less forceful.
  g. The refractory period is longer.
  h. There may be periods of difficulty establishing erections, and the frequency of these episodes increases over time. However, the pleasure derived from sex may not be significantly altered.
- *Females.* Explain the 'normal' changes associated with ageing (Masters & Johnson, 1966):
  a. Arousal requires more stimulation.
  b. The lining of the vaginal wall thins, and vaginal lubrication decreases.
  c. There are less vaginal vasocongestion and tensing.
  d. Uterine contractions are fewer.
  e. Clitoral detumescence is rapid.
  f. The capacity to achieve orgasm remains into old age, but the length of time taken to achieve it increases.
- Consider the risk of sexually transmitted infections in older people embarking on new relationships and counsel them on the importance of safe sex.
- Be willing to discuss sexual issues with all but particularly with:
  a. females undergoing gynaecologic operations
  b. Males undergoing prostate treatment
  c. Patients who have severe arthritis (changing position and timing of analgesia may be needed)
  d. Patients who have had a stroke or myocardial infarction

Sexual Activity in Residential and Nursing Homes

- Patients in nursing or residential homes may continue to have an interest in sexual activity. Sexual behaviour is often seen as a problem rather than an expression of a need for love and intimacy. Males with dementia are more likely to exhibit inappropriate sexual behaviour.
- *'Inappropriate behaviour'.* Advise staff about sexuality in older adults and advise them against unintentionally giving cues that may be misinterpreted (e.g., when washing them). In addition, consider:
  a. *Behavioural approaches.* Tell the patient that the behaviour is inappropriate, isolate them from residents of the sex they are subjecting to inappropriate behaviour, or use clothing that opens at the back for males who expose their genitals.
  b. *Drug therapy.* There is little evidence, but consider selective serotonin reuptake inhibitors in very difficult cases:

Legal Aspects

Power of Attorney

- At an early stage of declining mental function, suggest to the family that they consult a solicitor about a lasting power of attorney (LPA) *before* the patient is incapable of signing the form.
- To sign, the patient must be capable of understanding the implications of so doing and may be capable of this even if incapable of managing his or her affairs. If it is left too late, it is then necessary to apply to the Court of Protection to appoint a receiver, and this is much more cumbersome.
- The LPA must be registered before it can be used. Note that this is different from the registration of the older power, the enduring power of attorney, which only becomes necessary when the person who signed it is or is becoming incapable of managing his or her own affairs.

POWER OF ATTORNEY

For more information about enduring power of attorney, lasting power of attorney, Court of Protection, and other relevant legal aspects in the United Kingdom, see http://www.gov.uk and search on 'Office of the Public Guardian'.

Detention of an Older Person

GUIDELINE

United Kingdom, The Mental Capacity Act, 2005.

- In 2005, an amendment was made to the Mental Capacity Act (2005) known as the 'Deprivation of Liberty Safeguards', which took effect in England and Wales. The use of these safeguards should be considered when someone is subject to continuous supervision or control and whether they are free to leave a given environment.

- These safeguards make provision for the use of restrictions and restraint (including, e.g., the use of locks to stop people going to different parts of a building or the use of bed rails). They only apply to hospitals and care homes, but the Court of Protection can authorise the deprivation of liberty in other settings.
- They are applicable to those who lack capacity to consent to the restrictions placed upon them.
- An application for the deprivation of someone's liberty should be made to the local authority, who will then appoint an assessor to adjudicate as to whether the act applies or whether other legislation (e.g., the Mental Health Act) may be more applicable.
- Under the act, those who lack capacity and who do not have the support of family or friends to make decisions, are entitled to have access to an Independent Mental Capacity Advocate who can be appointed by social services.
- In Australia and New Zealand, refer to the local geriatric assessment team if there is a need for legal intervention to ensure patient safety and well-being.

Further Reading

Anonymous. (2003). Managing patients with restless legs. *Drug and Therapeutics Bulletin, 41,* 81–88.

Avenell, A., Gillespie, W. J., Gillespie, L. D., & O'Connell, D. (2009). Vitamin D and vitamin D analogues for preventing fractures associated with involutional and post-menopausal osteoporosis. *Cochrane Database of Systematic Reviews, (2),* CD000227.

Bains, J., Birks, J. S., & Dening, T. R. (2002). The efficacy of antidepressants in the treatment of depression in dementia (Cochrane review). In: The Cochrane Library, Issue 4. Update Software, Oxford.

Becker, C., Kron, M., Lindemann, U., Sturm, E., Eichner, B., Walter-Jung, B., & Nikolaus, T. (2003). Effectiveness of a multifaceted intervention on falls in nursing home residents. *Journal of the American Geriatrics Society, 51,* 306–313.

Brodaty, H., Green, A., & Koschera, A. (2003). Meta-analysis of psychosocial interventions for caregivers of people with dementia. *Journal of the American Geriatrics Society, 51,* 657–664.

Doody, R. S., Stevens, J. C., Beck, C., Dubinsky, R. M., Kaye, J. A., Gwyther, L., Mohs, R. C., Thal, L. J., Whitehouse, P. J., DeKosky, S. T., & Cummings, J. L. (2001). Practice parameter: Management of dementia (an evidence-based review). Report of the Quality Standards Subcommittee of the American Academy of Neurology. *Neurology, 56,* 1154–1166.

Farina, N., Llewellyn, D., Isaac, M. G. E. K. N., & Tabet, N. (2017). Vitamin E for Alzheimer's dementia and mild cognitive impairment. *Cochrane Database of Systematic Reviews, 4(4),* CD002854.

Gillespie, L. D., Robertson, M. C., Gillespie, W. J., Sherrington, C., Gates, S., Clemson, L. M., & Lamb, S. E. (2012). Interventions for preventing falls in older people living in the community. *Cochrane Database of Systematic Reviews, 2012(9),* CD007146.

Immunisation against infectious disease (Green Book). Published 2006, last updated 2023. https://assets.publishing.service.gov.uk/media/6196386dd3bf7f054f43e02d/Greenbook-cover-Nov21.pdf

Jensen, J., Lundin-Olsson, L., Nyberg, L., & Gustafson, Y. (2002). Fall and injury prevention in older people living in residential care facilities. *Annals of Internal Medicine, 136,* 733–741.

Jin, P. T. (1992). Efficacy of tai chi, brisk walking, meditation, and reading in reducing mental and emotional stress. *Journal of Psychosomatic Research, 36,* 361–370.

Lan, C., Lai, J. S., Wong, M. K., & Yu, M. L. (1996). Cardiorespiratory function, flexibility, and body composition among geriatric tai chi chuan practitioners. *Archives of Physical Medicine and Rehabilitation, 77,* 612–616.

Larson, E. B., Wang, L., Bowen, J. D., McCormick, W. C., Teri, L., Crane, P., & Kukull, W. 2006. Exercise is associated with reduced risk for incident dementia among persons 65 years of age and older. *Annals of Internal Medicine, 144,* 73–81.

Li, F., Harmer, P., McAuley, E., Fisher, K. J., Duncan, T. E., & Duncan, S. C. (2001). Tai chi, self-efficacy, and physical function in the elderly. *Prevention Science, 2,* 229–239.

Lord, S. R., Castell, S., Corcoran, J., Dayhew, J., Matters, B., Shan, A., & Williams, P. (2003). The effect of group exercise on physical functioning and falls in frail older people living in retirement villages: A randomized, controlled trial. *Journal of the American Geriatrics Society, 51,* 1685–1692.

Mold, J. (1996). Principles of geriatric care. American Health Consultants. *Primary Care Reports, 2,* 2–9.

Montorio, I., & Izal, M. (1996). The Geriatric Depression Scale: A review of its development and utility. *International Psychogeriatrics, 8,* 103–112.

Morley, J. E., Vellas, B., van Kan, G. A., Anker, S. D., Bauer, J. M., Bernabei, R., Cesari, M., Chumlea, W. C., Doehner, W., Evans, J., Fried, L. P., Guralnik, J. M., Katz, P. R., Malmstrom, T. K., McCarter, R. J., Gutierrez Robledo, L. M., Rockwood, K., von Haehling, S., Vandewoude, M. F., & Walston, J. (2013). Frailty consensus: A call to action. *Journal of the American Medical Directors Association, 14*(6), 392–397.

National Institute for Health and Care Excellence. (2007, September). *Donepezil, galantamine, rivastigmine (review) and memantine for the treatment of Alzheimer's disease (amended).* Technology appraisal guidance 111 (amended).

Nikolaus, T., Specht-Leible, N., Bach, M., Oster, P., & Schlierf, G. (1999). A randomized trial of comprehensive geriatric assessment and home intervention in the care of hospitalized patients. *Age Ageing, 28,* 543–550.

Robertson, M. C., Gardner, M. M., Devlin, N., McGee, R., & Campbell, A. J. (2001). Effectiveness and economic evaluation of a nurse delivered home exercise programme to prevent falls. 2: Controlled trial in multiple centres. *BMJ (Clinical research ed.), 322,* 701–704.

Robinson, J., & Turnock, T. (1998). *Investing in rehabilitation; review findings.* London: King's Fund.

Schneider, L. S., Dagerman, K. S., & Insel, P. (2005). Risk of death with atypical antipsychotic drug treatment for dementia. *JAMA, 294,* 1934–1943.

Venning, G. (2005). Recent developments in vitamin D deficiency and muscle weakness among elderly people. *BMJ (Clinical research ed.), 330,* 524–526.

Vetter, N., & Ford, D. (1990). Smoking prevention among people aged 60 and over: A randomized controlled trial. *Age Ageing, 19,* 164–168.

Walters, A. (1995). Towards a better definition of restless legs syndrome. The International Restless Legs Syndrome Study Group. *Movement Disorders, 10,* 634–642.

Warner, J., Butler, R., & Arya, P. (2005). *Dementia. Clinical Evidence, Issue 12.* London: BMJ Publishing Group.

Wolf, S. L., Barnhart, H. X., Kutner, N. G., McNeely, E., Coogler, C., & Xu, T. (1996). Reducing frailty and falls in older persons: An investigation of Tai Chi and computerized balance training.

Atlanta FICSIT Group. Frailty and Injuries: Cooperative Studies of Intervention Techniques. *Journal of the American Geriatrics Society, 44,* 489–497.

References

American Geriatric Society. (2015). American Geriatrics Society 2015 updated Beers criteria for potentially inappropriate medication use in older adults. *Journal of the American Geriatrics Society, 63*(11):2227–2246

American Psychiatric Association (1987). *Diagnostic and statistical manual of mental disorder* (3rd ed., revised). Washington DC: American Psychiatric Association.

Anderson, P. (1993). Effectiveness of general practice interventions for patients with harmful alcohol consumption. *British Journal of General Practice, 43,* 386–389.

Ballard, C., Hanney, M. L., Theodoulou, M., Douglas, S., McShane, R., Kossakowski, K., Gill, R., Juszczak, E., Yu, L. M., Jacoby, R., & DART-AD investigators. (2009). The dementia antipsychotic withdrawal trial (DART-AD): Long-term follow-up of a randomised placebo-controlled trial. *Lancet Neurology, 8,* 151–157.

Beckman, N., Waern, M., Gustafson, D., & Skoog, I. (2008). Secular trends in self reported sexual activity and satisfaction in Swedish 70 year olds: Cross sectional survey of four populations, 1971–2001. *BMJ 2008;337:*a279.

Blyton, F., Chuter, V., & Burns, J. (2012). Unknotting night-time muscle cramp: a survey of patient experience, help-seeking behaviour and perceived treatment effectiveness. *Journal of foot and ankle research, 5,* 7.

Breen, D. A., Breen, D. P., Moore, J. W., Breen, P. A., & O'Neill, D. (2007). Driving and dementia. *BMJ (Clinical research ed.), 334,* 1365–1369.

Britton, A., & Russell, R. (2002). Multidisciplinary team interventions for delirium in patients with chronic cognitive impairment (Cochrane review). In: The Cochrane Library, Issue 1. Update Software, Oxford.

Brookmeyer, R., Corrada, M. M., Curriero, F. C., & Kawas, C. (2002). Survival following a diagnosis of Alzheimer disease. *Archives of Neurology, 59,* 1764–1767.

Brown, J., Pengas, G., Dawson, K., Brown, L. A., & Clatworthy, P. (2009). Self administered cognitive screening test (TYM) for detection of Alzheimer's disease: Cross sectional study. *BMJ (Clinical research ed.), 338,* b2030.

Butler, J. V., Mulkerrin, E. C., & O'Keeffe, S. T. (2002). Nocturnal leg cramps in older people. *Postgraduate Medical Journal, 78,* 596–598.

Campbell, A. J., Robertson, M. C., Gardner, M. M., Norton, R. N., Tilyard, M. W., & Buchner, D. M. (1997). Randomised controlled trial of a general practice programme of home based exercise to prevent falls in elderly women. *BMJ (Clinical research ed.), 315,* 1065–1069.

Coussement, J., De Paepe, L., Schwendimann, R., Denhaerynck, K., Dejaeger, E., & Milisen, K. (2008). Interventions for preventing falls in acute- and chronic-care hospitals: a systematic review and meta-analysis. *Journal of the American Geriatrics Society, 56*(1), 29–36.

Curb, J. D., Pressel, S. L., Cutler, J. A., Savage, P. J., Applegate, W. B., Black, H., Camel, G., Davis, B. R., Frost, P. H., Gonzalez, N., Guthrie, G., Oberman, A., Rutan, G. H., & Stamler, J. (1996). Effect of diuretic-based antihypertensive treatment on cardiovascular disease risk in older diabetic patients with isolated systolic hypertension. Systolic Hypertension in the Elderly Program Cooperative Research Group. *JAMA, 276,* 1886–1892.

de Jonge, J. W., Knottnerus, J. A., van Zutphen, W. M., de Bruijne, G. A., & Struijker Boudier, H. A. (1994). Short term effect of withdrawal of diuretic drugs prescribed for ankle oedema. *BMJ (Clinical research ed.)*, *308*, 511–513.

Department for Health and Social Care (DHSC). (1994). *Living in Britain: Results from the 1994 General Household Survey*. Norwich: HMSO.

Elkan, R., Kendrick, D., Dewey, M., Hewitt, M., Robinson, J., Blair, M., Williams, D., & Brummell, K. (2001). Effectiveness of home based support for older people: Systematic review and meta-analysis. *BMJ (Clinical research ed.)*, *323*(7315), 719–725.

Elley, C. R., Kerse, N., Arroll, B., & Robinson, E. (2003). Effectiveness of counselling patients on physical activity in general practice: Cluster randomised controlled trial. *BMJ (Clinical research ed.)*, *326*, 793.

Ellis, G., Whitehead, M. A., O'Neill, D., Langhorne, P., & Robinson, D. (2011). Comprehensive geriatric assessment for older adults admitted to hospital. *Cochrane Database of Systematic Reviews*, (7), CD006211.

Elon, R. D. (1996). Geriatric medicine. *BMJ (Clinical research ed.)*, *312*, 561–563.

Erkinjuntti, T., Kurz, A., Gauthier, S., Bullock, R., Lilienfeld, S., & Damaraju, C. V. (2002). Efficacy of galantamine in probable vascular dementia and Alzheimer's disease combined with cerebrovascular disease: A randomised trial. *Lancet (London, England)*, *359*, 1283–1290.

Forster, A., Young, J., & Langhorne, P. (2002). Medical day hospital care for the elderly versus alternative forms of care (Cochrane review). In: The Cochrane Library, Issue 1. Update Software, Oxford.

Fransen, M., Anderson, C., Chalmers, J., Chapman, N., Davis, S., MacMahon, S., Neal, B., Sega, R., Terent, A., Tzourio, C., Woodward, M., & PROGRESS. (2003). Effects of a perindopril-based blood pressure-lowering regimen on disability and dependency in 6105 patients with cerebrovascular disease: A randomized controlled trial. *Stroke*, *34*, 2333–2338.

Gill, T. M., Baker, D. I., Gottschalk, M., Peduzzi, P. N., Allore, H., & Byers, A. (2002). A program to prevent functional decline in physically frail, elderly persons who live at home. *New England Journal of Medicine*, *347*, 1068–1074.

Gillespie, L. D., Robertson, M. C., Gillespie, W.J., Sherrington, C., Gates, S., Clemson, L. M., Lamb, S. E. (2012) Interventions for preventing falls in older people living in the community. *Cochrane Database Syst Rev. 12*, CD007146.

Gitlin, L. N., Kales, H. C., & Lyketsos, C. G. (2012). Nonpharmacologic management of behavioral symptoms in dementia. *JAMA*, *308*(19), 2020–2029.

Guasti, L., Ambrosetti, M., Ferrari, M. et al. Management of Hypertension in the Elderly and Frail Patient. *Drugs Aging 39*, 763–772 (2022).

Holmes, J., & Gilbody, S. (1996). Differences in use of the abbreviated mental test score by geriatricians and psychiatrists. *BMJ (Clinical research ed.)*, *313*, 465.

House of Commons. (2008). *Public Select Committee. Improving services and support for people with dementia*. Sixth report. Retrieved from www.publications.parliament.uk/pa/cm200708/cmselect/cmpubacc/228/228.pdf.

Husebo, B. S., Ballard, C., Sandvik, R., Nilsen, O. B., & Aarsland, D. (2011). Efficacy of treating pain to reduce behavioural disturbances in residents of nursing homes with dementia: Cluster randomised clinical trial. *BMJ (Clinical research ed.)*, *343*, d4065

Inouye, S. K., van Dyck, C. H., Alessi, C. A., Balkin, S., Siegal, A. P., & Horwitz, R. I. (1990). Clarifying confusion: The confusion assessment method. A new method for detection of delirium. *Annals of Internal Medicine*, *113*, 941–948.

Kerse, N. M., Flicker, L., Jolley, D., Arroll, B., & Young, D. (1999). Improving the health behaviours of elderly people: Randomised controlled trial of a general practice education programme. *BMJ (Clinical research ed.)*, *319*(7211), 683–687.

Malnar, F. J., Byszewski, A. M., Marshall, S. C., & Man-Son-Hing, M. (2005). In-office evaluation of medical fitness to drive: Practical approaches for assessing older people. *Canadian Family Physician*, *51*, 372–379.

Malouf, R., & Birks, J. (2004). Donepezil for vascular cognitive impairment (Cochrane review). In: The Cochrane Library, Issue 1. John Wiley, Chichester, UK.

Manley, A. (1996). *Physical activity and health. A report of the Surgeon General*. Pittsburgh, United States: Department of Health and Human Services.

Masters, W. H., & Johnson, V. E. (1966). *Human sexual response*. Several different publishers since 1966.

Masters, W. H., & Johnson, V. E. (1970). *Human sexual inadequacy*. Several different publishers since 1970.

Mathias, S., Nayak, U., & Isaacs, B. (1986). Balance in elderly patients: The 'Get up and Go' test. *Archives of Physical Medicine and Rehabilitation*, *67*, 387–389.

McCurry, S. M., Gibbons, L. E., Logsdon, R. G., Vitiello, M., & Teri, L. (2003). Training caregivers to change the sleep hygiene practices of patients with dementia: The NITE-AD project. *Journal of the American Geriatrics Society*, *51*, 1455–1460.

Morley, J. E., Vellas, B., van Kan, G. A., Anker, S. D., Bauer, J. M., Bernabei, R., Cesari, M., Chumlea, W. C., Doehner, W., Evans, J., Fried, L. P., Guralnik, J. M., Katz, P. R., Malmstrom, T. K., McCarter, R. J., Gutierrez Robledo, L. M., Rockwood, K., von Haehling, S., Vandewoude, M. F., & Walston, J. (2013). Frailty consensus: A call to action. *Journal of the American Medical Directors Association*, *14*(6), 392–397.

Muayqil, T., Gronseth, G., & Camicioli, R. (2012). Evidence-based guideline: Diagnostic accuracy of CSF 14-3-3 protein in sporadic Creutzfeldt-Jakob disease: Report of the guideline development subcommittee of the American Academy of Neurology. *Neurology*, *79*(14), 1499–1506.

Müller, A., Smith, L., Parker, M., & Mulhall, J. P. (2007). Analysis of the efficacy and safety of sildenafil citrate in the geriatric population. *BJU International*, *100*(1), 117–121.

Nichol, K. L., Margolis, K. L., Wuorenma, J., & Von Sternberg, T. (1994). The efficacy and cost effectiveness of vaccination against influenza among elderly persons living in the community. *New England Journal of Medicine*, *331*(12), 778–784.

Nijs, K. A., de Graaf, C., Kok, F. J., & van Staveren, W. A. (2006). Effect of family style mealtimes on quality of life, physical performance, and body weight of nursing home residents: Cluster randomised controlled trial. *BMJ (Clinical research ed.)*, *332*, 1180–1183.

O'Connell, H., Chin, A. V., Cunningham, C., & Lawlor, B. A. (2004). Suicide in older people. *BMJ (Clinical research ed.)*, *329*, 895–899.

Parker, M. J., Gillespie, W. J., & Gillespie, L. D. (2006). Effectiveness of hip protectors for preventing hip fractures in elderly people: Systematic review. *BMJ (Clinical research ed.)*, *332*(7541), 571–574.

Price, J., Hermans, D., & Grimley Evans, J. (2002). Subjective barriers to prevent wandering of cognitively impaired people (Cochrane review). In: The Cochrane Library, Issue 1. Update Software, Oxford.

Rinaldi, P., Mecocci, P., Benedetti, C., Ercolani, S., Bregnocchi, M., Menculini, G., Catani, M., Senin, U., & Cherubini, A. (2003). Validation of the five-item geriatric depression scale in elderly subjects in three different settings. *Journal of the American Geriatrics Society*, *51*(5), 694–698.

Rooney, E. (1993). Exercise for older patients: Why it's worth the effort. *Geriatrics, 48*, 68–72.

Santesso, N., Carrasco-Labra, A., & Brignardello-Petersen, R. (2014). Hip protectors for preventing hip fractures in older people. *Cochrane Database of Systematic Reviews, 2014*(3), CD001255.

Scherder, E., Oosterman, J., Swaab, D., Herr, K., Ooms, M., Ribbe, M., Sergeant, J., Pickering, G., & Benedetti, F. (2005). Recent developments in pain in dementia. *BMJ (Clinical research ed.), 330*, 461–464.

Sherrington, C., Whitney, J. C., Lord, S. R., Herbert, R. D., Cumming, R. G., & Close, J. C. (2008). Effective exercise for the prevention of falls: A systematic review and meta-analysis. *Journal of the American Geriatrics Society, 56*(12), 2234–2243.

Spijker, A., Vernooij-Dassen, M., Vasse, E., Adang, E., Wollersheim, H., Grol, R., & Verhey, F. (2008). Effectiveness of nonpharmacological interventions in delaying the institutionalization of patients with dementia: A meta-analysis. *Journal of the American Geriatrics Society, 56*(6), 1116–1128.

Tamblyn, R., Abrahamowicz, M., du Berger, R., McLeod, P., & Bartlett, G. (2005). A 5-year prospective assessment of the risk associated with individual benzodiazepines and doses in new elderly users. *Journal of the American Geriatrics Society, 53*, 233–241.

The Malnutrition Task Force was set up by Age UK, apetito, Bapen, Nutricia Advanced Medical Nutrition and Royal Voluntary Service in 2012 to reduce malnutrition in later life. https://www.malnutritiontaskforce.org.uk/sites/default/files/inline-files/State%20of%20the%20Nation%202020%20revise2.pdf

Thomas, D. R. (2003). Medications and sexual function. *Clinics in Geriatric Medicine, 19*(3), 553–562.

Trichopoulou, A., Orfanos, P., Norat, T., Bueno-de-Mesquita, B., Ocké, M. C., Peeters, P. H., van der Schouw, Y. T., Boeing, H., Hoffmann, K., Boffetta, P., Nagel, G., Masala, G., Krogh, V., Panico, S., Tumino, R., Vineis, P., Bamia, C., Naska, A., Benetou, V., Ferrari, P., ... Trichopoulos, D. (2005). Modified Mediterranean diet and survival: EPIC-Elderly Prospective Cohort study. *BMJ (Clinical research ed.), 330*, 991–995.

Tseng, V. L., Yu, F., Lum, F., & Coleman, A. L. (2012). Risk of fractures following cataract surgery in Medicare beneficiaries. *JAMA, 308*(5), 493–501.

Williams, P. S., Rands, G., Orrel, M., & Spector, A. (2000). Aspirin for vascular dementia. *Cochrane Database of Systematic Reviews, 2000*(4), CD001296.

Wilson, G. B., Lock, C. A., Heather, N., Cassidy, P., Christie, M. M., & Kaner, E. F. (2011). Intervention against excessive alcohol consumption in primary health care: A survey of GPs' attitudes and practices in England 10 years on. *Alcohol and Alcoholism (Oxford, Oxfordshire), 46*(5), 570–577.

Wilson, K., Mottram, P., Sivanranthan, A., & Nightingale, A. (2001). Antidepressant versus placebo for depressed elderly. *Cochrane Database of Systematic Reviews, 2001*(2), CD000561.

Woods, B., Aguirre, E., Spector, A. E., & Orrell, M. (2012). Cognitive stimulation to improve cognitive functioning in people with dementia. *Cochrane Database of Systematic Reviews*, (2), CD005562.

15

Contraception, Sexual Problems, and Sexually Transmitted Infections

Kate Robinson

CHAPTER CONTENTS

CONTRACEPTION

Information for Professionals

Faculty of Sexual & Reproductive Healthcare. Retrieved from http://www.fsrh.org.

Information for Patients

Family Planning Association. 23-28 Penn Street, London, N1 5DL. Tel: 020 7608 5240; Available at http://www.fpa.org.uk.

- When giving contraceptive advice, it is good practice to back it up with appropriate and accessible written information. The Family Planning Association (FPA) provides a range of leaflets covering all methods, which is regularly revised and is available through the local Health Promotion Unit or from the website (see box).
- These leaflets should be used when a patient is deciding on a method, initiating a method, and from time to time as a refresher. However, leaflets are not a substitute for discussion (Jones, 2008).
- Patients wanting to go to a family planning clinic or who are being referred from general practice in the United Kingdom can get details of a convenient clinic from the FPA. The FPA's website allows a search on a map with details right down to street level.

Hormonal Contraception

Combined Oral Contraceptive Pill

GUIDELINE

Faculty of Sexual & Reproductive Healthcare. (January 2019; amended October 2023). *FRSH clinical guideline: Combined hormonal contraception*. Retrieved from https://www.fsrh.org/standards-and-guidance/documents/combined-hormonal-contraception/.

Effectiveness

With perfect use of the combined oral contraceptive (COC), failure rates are as low as 0.3% in the first year (Trussell, 2007). However, with typical use, this increases to 9%. Drug interactions, malabsorption, and patient weight greater than 90 kg may also impact effectiveness.

Assessment of the Patient

The following are the essential components of the assessment before initiating the COC (Clinical Effectiveness Unit, 2006a):

a. Menstrual and obstetric history.
b. History of migraine and presence of aura.
c. Past or current illnesses which might represent contraindications.
d. Family history of venous thromboembolism (VTE), myocardial infarction (MI), cerebrovascular accident (CVA), hypertension, and breast cancer.
e. Current drug therapy (prescribed and over the counter (OTC)).
f. Allergies.
g. Blood pressure measurement (defer starting the COC until 8 weeks after delivery in women who have had preeclampsia even if the blood pressure is normal).
h. Baseline height and weight: body mass index (BMI; important because it is a risk factor for VTE).
i. No blood tests are necessary before first prescription of a COC without specific clinical indication.
j. In asymptomatic women, breast and pelvic examinations are not recommended before first prescription of a COC (Stewart et al, 2001). Cervical screening is also not a prerequisite, although should be discussed.

Contraindications

UK Medical Eligibility Criteria (UKMEC) give four categories of condition in which use of the COC is (or is not) contraindicated (Clinical Effectiveness Unit, 2009):

- UKMEC1 is a condition for which there is no restriction on use of the method.
- UKMEC2 is when the advantages of the method generally outweigh the theoretical or proven risks.
- UKMEC3 is when the theoretical or proven risks usually outweigh the advantages. Provision of a method requires expert clinical judgement or a referral to a specialist contraceptive provider.
- UKMEC4 is a condition which represents an unacceptable health risk and the method should not be used.

Unacceptable Health Risk (UKMEC4)

a. Postpartum and *breastfeeding:* less than 6 weeks
b. *Postpartum (nonbreastfeeding):* 0 to 3 weeks postpartum with additional risk factors for VTE
c. *Smoking:* aged older than 35 years and smoking more than 15 cigarettes/day
d. *Hypertension:* blood pressure 160 mm Hg or greater systolic or 100 mm Hg or greater diastolic
e. *Vascular disease:* peripheral vascular disease, hypertensive retinopathy, and transient ischaemic attacks (TIAs)
f. *VTE:* current or previous
g. *Major surgery with prolonged immobilisation*
h. *Known thrombogenic mutations* such as Factor V Leiden, prothrombin variant G20210A, protein S, protein C, and antithrombin III deficiencies
i. *Ischaemic heart disease:* current or previous
j. *Stroke disease:* current or previous
k. *Complicated valvular or congenital heart disease:* complicated by pulmonary hypertension, atrial fibrillation, history of infective endocarditis
l. *Atrial fibrillation*
m. *Cardiomyopathy with impaired cardiac function*
n. *Migraine with aura*
o. *Breast cancer:* current
p. *Systemic lupus erythematosus (SLE):* with positive or unknown antiphospholipid antibodies
q. *Cirrhosis:* severe (decompensated)

r. *Liver tumours:* benign (hepatocellular adenoma) or malignant (hepatoma)

Risks Usually Outweigh Benefits (UKMEC3)

a. *Postpartum (non-breastfeeding):* 0-21 days without other risk factors; 21-42 days with other risk factors for VTE
b. *Smoking:* aged 35 years or older and smoking less than 15 cigarettes/day; aged 35 years or older and stopped smoking less than 1 year ago
c. *BMI:* 35 kg/m^2 or greater
d. *Previous bariatric surgery with BMI greater than 35 kg/m^2*
e. *Complicated organ transplant:* graft failure (acute or chronic), rejection, cardiac allograft vasculopathy
f. *Hypertension:* on treatment with blood pressure adequately controlled; elevated blood pressure (140–159 mm Hg systolic or 90–99 mm Hg diastolic)
g. *Family history of VTE:* in a first-degree relative aged younger than 45 years
h. *Immobility:* wheelchair use, debilitating illness
i. *Multiple risk factors for arterial cardiovascular disease (CVD)*
j. *Migraine without aura:* for consideration of continuation
k. *Migraine with aura:* occurring 5 or more years ago
l. *Breast cancer:* past history of and no evidence of recurrence for 5 years; carriers of known mutations associated with breast cancer (e.g., BRCA1)
m. *Undiagnosed breast symptoms:* for consideration of initiation
n. *Diabetes:* neuropathy, nephropathy, retinopathy, or other vascular disease
o. *Gallbladder disease:* current or medically treated
p. *History of cholestasis with past COC use*
q. *Viral hepatitis:* acute or flare (for consideration of initiation)

Arterial and Venous Thrombosis

- The risk factors for VTE and arterial disease should be assessed separately.
- Age is a risk factor common to both conditions. Many of the risk factors can be viewed as being on a sliding scale; for instance, there is not suddenly a problem with age on the 35th birthday.
- Smoking status, weight, and immobility are the only factors that may be changed in the future and the suitability for the COC reviewed.

Choosing a Combined Pill

- Pill formulations contain one of eight progestogens.
- The initial dose of oestrogen should normally be in the range 20 to 35 μg combined with a low or standard dose of progestogen.
- A monophasic COC containing 30 μg of ethinylestradiol with norethisterone or levonorgestrel is a suitable first pill.
- As of June 1999, desogestrel- and gestodene-containing pills were recommended again as first-line COCs, following the pill scare of October 1995 (Anonymous, 1999). However, in view of the apparent increased risk

TABLE 15.1	Risks of Venous Thromboembolism	
Background rate of VTE in healthy non-pregnant women not taking a COC	5/100,000/year	
Healthy women taking levonorgestrel or norethisterone COCs	15/100,000/year	
Healthy women taking gestodene or desogestrel COCs	25/100,000/year	
Pregnancy	60/100,000/year	

COC, Combined oral contraceptive; VTE, venous thromboembolism.

of VTE with these preparations (relative risk (RR), 1.7) compared with levonorgestrel or norethisterone pills (Kemmeren, Algra, & Grobbee, 2001), the slightly increased risk of VTE should be explained to the patient (Table 15.1), and these pills should not be used in those with a risk factor for VTE. Norgestimate-containing pills have similar rates of VTE to levonorgestrel pills (Jick et al, 2006).

- For all COCs, the risk of VTE is greatest in the first year of use. For COCs containing levonorgestrel, for instance, the RR for VTE in the first year is 6.6 compared with women not taking the pill, decreasing to 1.3 after 5 years use (Brechin & Penney, 2004).
- Desogestrel- and gestodene-containing pills are probably best avoided for young first-time users. Their risk of VTE is 3.1 times the risk they would run with a levonorgestrel or norethisterone preparation (Kemmeren et al, 2001). These brands may be useful, however, for those who have side effects, for patients with acne, and for patients with cycle control problems.
- Co-cyprindiol (ethinylestradiol with cyproterone acetate) is licensed as an acne treatment but is an effective contraceptive too. It should be used only in those with significant acne. There is a higher risk of VTE than with levonorgestrel pills: RR 3.9 (Vasilakis-Scaramozza & Jick, 2001).
- Females react individually to the pill; if side effects are experienced, it is well worth trying at least one other brand before abandoning the method.

Higher Doses of Oestrogen

Formulations containing 50 μg of ethinylestradiol should not be used unless specific individual circumstances warrant a higher dose:

a. Long-term use of an enzyme-inducing drug. The National Institute for Health and Care Excellence (NICE) recommends that females taking enzyme-inducing antiepileptic drugs are started on 50 μg; if breakthrough bleeding (BTB) occurs, the dose may be increased to 75 μg or 100 μg/day (Stokes et al, 2004).
b. Persistent BTB on a standard strength COC, provided no other cause is found.

c. Past true COC method failure, suggesting unusually rapid metabolism or malabsorption (an alternative is tricycling and shortening the pill-free interval (PFI) to 4 days; see later).

Special Cases

- Recommend an alternative method when there has been a previous failure of COC or when pill efficacy may be reduced because the patient:
    a. Is on long-term hepatic enzyme-inducing drugs, such as for fungal infection, tuberculosis, epilepsy, daytime sleepiness, or human immunodeficiency virus (HIV) or taking OTC drugs (e.g., St John wort; consult BNF (British National Formulary)) (Clinical Effectiveness Unit. 2005a)
    b. Has severe malabsorption
- If an alternative method is unacceptable, consider one of the following:
    a. Starting a high-dose pill, or two low-dose pills, to give at least 50 µg of ethinylestradiol
    b. Running three packs of pills together (the 'tricycle' regimen) plus reducing the 3-monthly PFI to 4 days
- If BTB still occurs, try 75 µg or 100 µg per day (Stokes et al, 2004).

Phased Preparations

These preparations:

a. Give a better bleeding pattern for a lower monthly dose (has been shown for levonorgestrel preparations) (Rosenberg & Long, 1992)
b. Are more expensive than fixed-dose preparations, not least because these products attract two dispensing fees (biphasics) or three dispensing fees (triphasics) in the United Kingdom
c. Have a reduced margin for error, especially early in the packet
d. May cause premenstrual tension–like symptoms towards the end of the packet
e. Are less flexible when a patient wants to postpone a period

Taking the Pill: Procedure and Advice

Starting the Pill

a. *Days 1 to 5 of the cycle.* If started on or before day 5, then no other precautions are necessary (Clinical Effectiveness Unit, 2006a).
b. *After day 5,* other precautions should be used for the first 7 days.
c. *Changing from a hormonal method.* COC can be started immediately if the previous method has been used consistently and correctly or if it is reasonably certain the patient is not pregnant (Box 15.1). There is no need to wait for the next period.
d. *After childbirth.* If starting at the end of the third week postpartum, no other precautions are needed. A later start necessitates extra precautions for 7 days. Note that the earliest recorded ovulation after delivery is day 30 (Guillebaud, 1989), so waiting until a postnatal examination is not an option unless a female is exclusively breastfeeding.

> **• BOX 15.1**   **How a Clinician Can Be Reasonably Certain a Female Patient Is Not Pregnant**
>
> There should be no symptoms or signs of pregnancy, and any ONE of the following criteria should be met:
> The patient has not had sex since the start of the last normal menstrual period.
> The patient has been correctly and consistently using a reliable[a] method of contraception.
> The patient is within the first 7 days of her cycle.
> The patient is within the first 7 days after an abortion or miscarriage.
> The patient is fully breastfeeding, amenorrhoeic, and <6 months postpartum.
> The patient is not breastfeeding and is <3 weeks postpartum or has had no unprotected sex since delivery.
> A pregnancy test adds weight to the diagnosis, but only if 3 weeks have elapsed since the date of last sex.
>
> [a]The author does not regard condoms, coitus interruptus, or fertility awareness as reliable enough to exclude the possibility of pregnancy.
> From Anonymous. (2005). *Selected practice recommendations for contraceptive use* (2nd ed.). Geneva: World Health Organization; Clinical Effectiveness Unit. (2006a). *First prescription of combined oral contraception.* London: Faculty of Family Planning and Reproductive Healthcare.

---

e. *After miscarriage or TOP (Termination of Pregnancy).* Start within 7 days. If starting later, extra precautions are needed for 7 days. The earliest recorded ovulation after TOP is day 16 (Guillebaud, 1989).

How to Take the Pill

- The standard regimen for any COC involves taking a pill for 21 days followed by a 7-day PFI before the next pill packet is commenced.
- There now exists a number of 'tailored' regimens. All are unlicensed but endorsed by the Faculty for Reproductive and Sexual Health (FRSH). Females should be adequately counselled to make the choice which is most suitable for them and should be signposted to written or digital information in addition. Whichever regimen is used, the PFI should never exceed 7 days because of the risk of ovulation and subsequent contraceptive failure. Females should have their regular contraceptive checks in the same way as for the standard regimen.
    a. Continuous use
        - Back-to-back use of packs can be continued until the patient wishes to stop her contraception or an alternative contraceptive method becomes more suitable because of a change in health or personal circumstances.
        - BTB on 4 or more consecutive days can be treated with taking a 4-day break without compromising contraceptive efficacy.
    b. Extended use
        - Akin to tricycling the packs, but the timing of the PFI can range from 4 to 7 days and can be fixed or flexible to suit the patient.
        - PFI must not exceed 7 days.
    c. Shortened PFI
        - Packs are taken for 21 days as for the standard regimen, but the PFI is reduced to 4 days.

Changing the Pill

- *Same or higher strength oestrogen but the same progestogen.* Start it after the 7-day break. No extra precautions are necessary.
- *Lower strength oestrogen or a different progestogen.* Omit the 7-day break. If the break is not omitted, extra precautions are needed for 7 days.

Postponing a Bleed

This is possible (see later).

Stopping Combined Oral Contraceptives

Alternative methods of contraception are needed from the day of stopping the COC, not the end of the PFI.

Advice

Mode of Action

- The main action of the pill is to suppress the normal cycle so that ovulation does not occur; the 'periods' while on the pill are withdrawal bleeds (WBs).
- Within 7 days of use, the ovaries are fully suppressed.
- Conversely, during the PFI, there is no significant follicular development unless the PFI is lengthened beyond 7 days.

Risks

a. *VTE.* The risk of VTE while using any COC is increased but is less than the risk of VTE during pregnancy (see Table 15.1) (Brechin & Penney, 2004). New research from Denmark has suggested that concomitant use of nonaspirin nonsteroidal antiinflammatory drugs (NSAIDs) and COC increases the risk of VTE (Meaidi et al, 2023). Although the effect is small, the FRSH advise that patients should be appropriately counselled when using OTC medications.

b. *MI.* The risk of MI on a COC is confined to smokers (RR, 9.5 compared with nonsmokers not taking COCs) (Khader et al, 2003) and those with arterial risk factors. Patients who do not smoke, who have their blood pressure checked, and who do not have hypertension or diabetes are at no increased risk of MI on a COC regardless of their age.

c. *Ischaemic stroke.* The risk of ischaemic stroke in COC users is increased (RR, 2.7) (Chan et al, 2004). Among females with no history of migraine, who do not smoke, who have their blood pressure checked, and who do not have hypertension, the risk is less.

d. *Gallstones.* COCs may accelerate the presentation of cholelithiasis in those who are predisposed. Their use should be avoided in those with known gallbladder disease. They can be used after cholecystectomy (UKMEC2) but usually not after medical treatment for gallstones (UKMEC3).

e. *Hypertension.* COCs can induce hypertension, particularly in the early months of use (Poulter, 1996). About 1% of COC users become clinically hypertensive with modern formulations. Pill-induced hypertension should not be treated with antihypertensive drugs, but the pill should be stopped and observation continued.

f. *Cancer.* Overall, the balance of risks and benefits of the COC on cancer is beneficial. There is an increased risk of cancer of the cervix; this is mitigated by a large reduction in risk of cancer of the ovary (RR, 0.73) (Collaborative Group on Epidemiological Studies of Ovarian Cancer, 2008) and the endometrium (Weiderpass et al, 1999) and by a reduction in the risk of cancer of the colon (RR, 0.82) (Fernandez et al, 2001). The COC probably accelerates development of cancer of the cervix caused by chronic infection with oncogenic human papillomavirus (HPV); with 5 years or more of use, the RR is 1.90 (International Collaboration of Epidemiological Studies of Cervical Cancer, 2007). The literature on the COC and breast cancer is conflicting, but some good-quality studies show no increased risk (Clinical Effectiveness Unit, 2010b). Both UK cohort studies show no increased risk: RRs of 1.0 (Vessey & Painter, 2006) and 0.90 (Hannaford et al, 2010) respectively. By the age of 40 to 44 years, however, COC use is associated with 30 extra cancers per 100,000 female patients. A recent study has shown an increased risk of meningioma in high cumulative users of nomegestrol acetate, the progesterone found in Zoely (Nguyen et al, 2021). The FRSH therefore advises against its use in females with previous or current meningioma and for prescribers to be vigilant to the presentation of possible meningioma in all users of Zoely.

g. *Inflammatory bowel disease (IBD).* IBD may be associated with VTE, hepatobiliary disease, and osteoporosis, all of which would need to be taken into consideration when considering suitability for the COC (Clinical Effectiveness Unit, 2009). Also, the efficacy of the COC may be reduced in female patients with Crohn's disease who have small bowel disease and malabsorption.

Side Effects

There are side effects, but most wear off after the first few cycles, especially bloating, nausea, and breast tenderness. Nausea may be reduced by taking the pill at night.

Noncontraceptive Benefits

- The following have all been shown to be beneficial effects of the COC:
  - Lighter, shorter bleeding (less anaemia)
  - Less dysmenorrhoea
  - Less premenstrual syndrome (PMS)
  - Less pelvic inflammatory disease (PID)
  - Fewer ectopic pregnancies
  - Less benign breast disease
  - A bone-sparing effect
  - Fewer functional ovarian cysts
  - Less hospitalisation for fibroid
  - Less symptomatic endometriosis
- The COC tends to improve acne. There is little to choose between COC formulations. COCs need to be taken for

at least 6 months for their full effect on the skin to become apparent. Evidence for the use of co-cyprindiol, if a COC fails to improve acne, is of poor quality (Arowojolu, 2009).

Bleeding

- WBs are usually lighter than periods.
- BTB may occur during the first two or three cycles.
- BTB is not a reason for stopping the pill in the middle of a packet.

Missed Pills

- The riskiest time for pills to be forgotten is on either side of the pill-free week (Clinical Effectiveness Unit, 2006a).
- Forgetting in the middle of a packet is less likely to give rise to breakthrough ovulation or pregnancy.
- *If more than 24 hours late*, this is classed as 'missed pills', and the agreed rules are as in Fig. 15.1.

Diarrhoea or Vomiting

- This requires extra precautions for the period of illness and for 7 days afterwards, as discussed earlier.
- If this would run into the PFI, the PFI should be omitted.
- However, it is known that diarrhoea has to be of dysenteric proportions to reduce pill absorption.

Drugs for Infections

- The Faculty of Sexual & Reproductive Healthcare (FSRH) no longer recommends the need to use barrier methods of contraception for non–enzyme-inducing antibiotics (Clinical Effectiveness Unit, 2005a, 2011).
- Rifampicin, rifabutin, griseofulvin, and some antiretroviral drugs (ART; notably ritonavir-boosted protease inhibitors) induce liver enzymes.
- Oral antifungal agents have also been associated with anecdotal reports of COC failure.
- Extra precautions should be taken during the treatment and for 7 days thereafter. If this runs into the PFI, the next packet should be started without a break. Rifampicin and rifabutin are such powerful enzyme inducers that extra precautions should be taken for 4 weeks even after a 2-day course and elimination of PFIs during this time (Clinical Effectiveness Unit, 2006a).

Surgery

The COC should be stopped from 4 weeks before until 2 weeks after any major surgery, varicose vein surgery or sclerotherapy, or any operation likely to be followed by immobilisation (e.g., leg surgery) (Clinical Effectiveness Unit, 2009). It is otherwise not necessary to stop the COC.

Postponing or Avoiding Bleeds

Monophasic Pills

Patients on a fixed-dose combined pill can postpone the next WB by starting the next packet immediately, omitting the PFI.

Phased Preparations

- If the patient is taking Synphase, another packet can be taken immediately after the first.
- If the patient is taking other phased preparations, there would be an abrupt decrease in progestogen levels if the above regimen were followed, leading to a risk of bleeding. Advise one of the following:
  a. Tablets from the last phase of a spare packet can be taken, to give 7 (TriNovum) or 10 (Logynon, Triadene) or 14 (Binovum) days' postponement
  b. A packet can be started of the next higher dose monophasic pill, omitting the PFI. With Qlaira, the 17 highest dose tablets should be used.
- *If postponement by a few days* is needed (e.g., to avoid a bleed at weekends), the necessary number of pills from a fresh pack should be taken and the rest of that pack thrown away. If on phased preparations, they should follow the principles above.
- *Note: ED (every day) preparations.* In all the above advice, the seven inactive pills in ED preparations should be discarded.
- Extended use of the COC has become widespread; running several or all packets together reduces bleeding days and menstrual cycle–related symptoms (Archer, 2006). When used continuously for 1 year, 18% of patients achieve amenorrhoea by 3 months of use and 88% by 10 months (Miller & Hughes, 2003). Extended use can be at the personal preference of the patient according to how often she wishes to bleed or recommended on medical grounds (e.g., for low bone density, endometriosis, PMS, or withdrawal headaches).

Follow-up

- The patient should be seen again at 3 months or earlier if side effects occur. Do not give repeat prescriptions without someone seeing the patient and at least checking the blood pressure.
- After being established on the pill, review the patient annually. This can be done face to face or virtually where means allow. Make sure to:
  a. Assess whether there are any new risk factors, including migraine.
  b. Check whether the patient is smoking.
  c. Ask about side effects.
  d. Check blood pressure (discontinue if blood pressure increases to and remains at 160/95 mm Hg). If the blood pressure is satisfactory 2 years after commencement of the COC, blood pressure checks can be extended to annually in females without risk factors or relevant diseases.
  e. Check BMI.

Changing the Pill Because of Side Effects

When changing a pill because of side effects, the choice lies between changing oestrogen or progestogen dominance and changing to a pill with a different progestogen (see later).

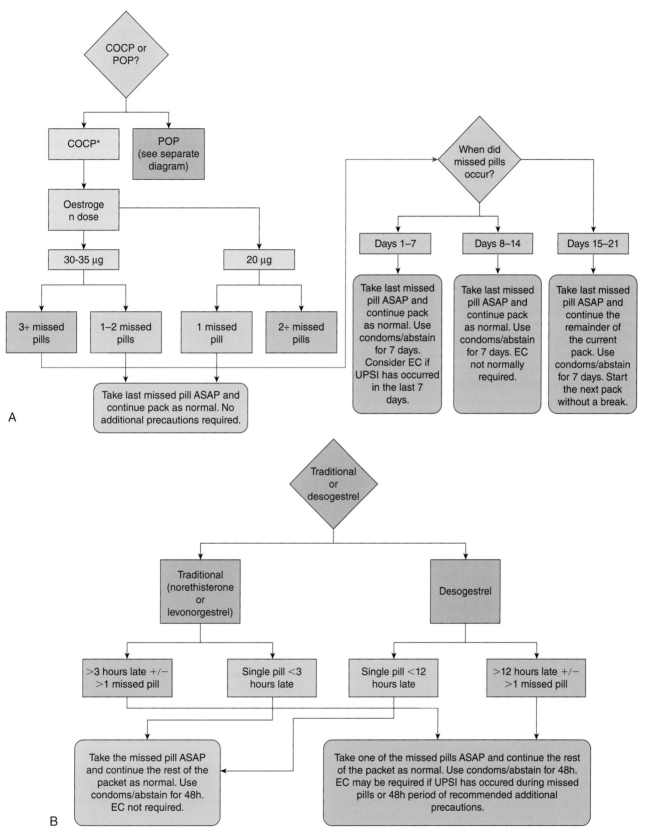

A

B

*Except Zoely and Qlaira, please refer to the manufacturers' patient advice leaflet) *UPSI* - unprotected sexual intercourse; *EC* - emergency contraception; *POP* - Progesterone only pill; *COCP* - Combined oral contraceptive pill.

• **Fig. 15.1** Missed pill rules. (Faculty of Sexual and Reproductive Healthcare clinical guidance. Missed pill recommendations. 2011. Oxfordshire County Council "What should I do if I miss a pill (progesterone only pill)?" found at https://fisd.oxfordshire.gov.uk/kb5/oxfordshire/directory/advice.page?id=DwljeKXaTXo)

Breakthrough Bleeding

- BTB occurs in up to 30% of users in the first few cycles but tends to settle by the third cycle. Unless prior warning of this is given, discontinuation rates will be high, especially in young patients.
- *If BTB occurs in the first 3 months*, ask whether pills have been missed; encourage the patient to persevere.
- *If BTB continues beyond 3 months*, exclude lesions of the cervix and problems with taking the pill (e.g., vomiting). Also encourage smokers to quit because smokers are more likely to have BTB (Rosenberg, Waugh, & Stevens 1996). Give a pill with a higher progestogen dose, change to a progestogen with better cycle control (e.g., gestodene), or change to a triphasic formulation of the same progestogen. If this fails, consider increasing the oestrogen content as well.
- *If BTB occurs when previous control had been good*, exclude lesions of the cervix, chlamydia infection, interacting drugs, gastrointestinal disorder, and a change to a vegetarian diet.
- *Absent WB*
  a. Explain that this is not unsafe and does not signify overdosage.
  b. Missing one WB does not need any action. If two are missed, exclude pregnancy.
  c. If the patient is concerned despite reassurance, consider a switch to a triphasic pill.

Oestrogen Withdrawal Headache During the Pill-Free Interval

- Consider advising the patient to use either a tricycle or tailored regimen.

Combined Transdermal Patch

- At present, there is only one combined transdermal patch, Evra (Clinical Effectiveness Unit, 2004b). This patch releases norelgestromin 150 μg/day and ethinylestradiol 20 μg/day into the circulation. The patch is applied weekly for 21 days, and the fourth week is patch free; a tailored regimen can be used if preferred following the principles described above for COC use. Suitable sites are the upper outer arm, upper torso (excluding breast), buttock, or lower abdomen.
- The effectiveness is similar to that of the COC. The same contraindications apply as for the COC. The same drug interactions as for the COC must be presumed. BTB, spotting, and breast tenderness are more common than with the COC in the first two cycles.
- *If a patch is partly detached for less than 24 hours*, it should be reapplied to the same site or replaced with a new patch immediately. No additional contraception is needed, and the next patch should be applied on the usual change day.
- *If a patch remains detached for more than 24 hours* or if the user is not aware when the patch became detached, she should stop the current contraceptive cycle and start a new cycle by applying a new patch, giving a new 'day 1'; additional precautions must be used concurrently for the first 7 days of the new cycle.
- *If application of a new patch at the start of a new cycle is delayed*, contraceptive protection is lost. A new patch should be applied as soon as remembered giving a new 'day 1'; additional nonhormonal methods of contraception should be used for the first 7 days of the new cycle. If intercourse has occurred during this extended patch-free interval, the possibility of fertilisation should be considered.
- If applications of a patch in the middle of the cycle is delayed (i.e., the patch is not changed on day 8 or day 15):
  a. For up to 48 hours, apply a new patch immediately; the next patch change day remains the same and no additional precautions are required.
  b. For more than 48 hours, contraceptive protection may have been lost. Stop the current cycle and start a new 4-week cycle immediately by applying a new patch, giving a new 'day 1'. Additional precautions should be used for the first 7 days of the new cycle.
- *If the patch is not removed at the end of the cycle* (day 22), remove it as soon as possible and start the next cycle on the usual change day, after day 28. No extra precautions are required.

Combined Vaginal Ring

- NuvaRing was launched in 2009. It releases 120 μg of etonogestrel and 15 μg of ethinylestradiol per day from an ethylene vinyl acetate copolymer ring with an outer diameter of 54 mm. The same contraindications and drug interactions apply as for the COC.
- Tampon use has no effect on the systemic absorption of the hormones released from NuvaRing.
- A ring can be removed (e.g., for sex) for up to 3 hours.
- Before dispensing, NuvaRing is stored at 2° to 8°C. After it has been dispensed, storage is at room temperature, and the shelf life is 4 months.
- Females use a ring for 3 weeks followed by a ring-free week during which time they have a WB. A new ring is needed for each 4-week cycle. A tailored regimen can be used if preferred following the principles described earlier for COC use.
- NuvaRing has high effectiveness no different from the combined pill, especially when adherence is good (Oddsson et al, 2005; Ahrendt et al, 2006).
- Cycle control is better than with the combined pill (Bjarnadóttir, Tuppurainen, & Killick 2002; Roumen, op ten Berg, & Hoomans, 2006; Merki-Feld & Hund, 2007).
- The ring can, however, cause leucorrhoea, vaginal discomfort, vaginitis, and ring-related events, including foreign body sensation, coital problems, and expulsion (Oddsson et al, 2005; Ahrendt et al, 2006).
- *If the ring-free interval is extended beyond 7 days*, the patient should insert a new ring as soon as she remembers.

Extra precautions should be used for the next 7 days. If unprotected sex took place during the ring-free interval, the use of emergency contraception can be considered or a pregnancy test done after 3 weeks.

- *If the ring was temporarily outside the vagina*, it should be rinsed in lukewarm water and reinserted. If the ring was outside the vagina for less than 3 hours, no further action is necessary. If the ring was outside the vagina for more than 3 hours, extra precautions should be used for the next 7 days. If the loss in continuity of use of the ring for more than 3 hours occurs in the third week of use, a new ring should be inserted without the ring-free interval.
- *If the ring is left in place for more than 3 weeks*, this is acceptable up to a total of 4 weeks even if there is then a ring-free week. If the ring has been left in the vagina for longer than 4 weeks, pregnancy should be excluded before another ring is inserted.

Progestogen-Only Pill

GUIDELINE

Faculty of Sexual & Reproductive Healthcare. (August 2022; amended July 2023). *FSRH clinical guideline: Progestogen-only pills*. Retrieved from https://www.fsrh.org/documents/cec-guideline-pop/.

There are four different progestogen-only pills (POPs) available in the United Kingdom: desogestrel; drospirenone; and the two 'traditional' POPs, levonorgestrel and norethisterone. Desogestrel (Cerazette) is much more likely than traditional POPs to inhibit ovulation, but comparative data on efficacy are lacking. Available data show that its effectiveness is similar to that of the COC (Trussell, 2007), but traditional POPs are probably less effective than COCs.

Patients for Whom the Progestogen-Only Pill Is Particularly Indicated

a. *Older females:* those older than 45 years old without risk factors and those older than 35 years old who smoke. POP can be taken until age 55 years, in comparison with COC, which is recommended only until age 50 years (without other factors prohibiting its use).
b. *Those with medical contraindications to oestrogen*, including a personal history of VTE.
c. *Those with risk factors for arterial disease*, including hypertension, diabetes mellitus, migraine with aura and smokers aged older than 35 years.
d. *Lactating mothers.* Progestogen in the breast milk has no adverse effect on the baby (Clinical Effectiveness Unit, 2009).
e. *Those who choose it*, especially those aged older than 25 or 30 years, and who accept that it may be less reliable than the COC.

Unacceptable Health Risk (UKMEC4)

a. Breast cancer: current

Risks Usually Outweigh Benefits (UKMEC3)

a. *Ischaemic heart disease:* current or previous history if occurred when taking POP
b. *Stroke:* history of CVA, if occurred when taking POP
c. *Breast cancer:* past and no evidence of current disease for 5 years
d. *Cirrhosis:* severe (decompensated)
e. *Liver tumours:* benign (hepatocellular adenoma) and malignant (hepatoma)

Other Risk Considerations

- Drospirenone is an aldosterone agonist and therefore should be avoided in those with severe renal insufficiency and acute renal failure because of the risk of hyperkalaemia.
- Those with known hyperkalaemia or untreated hypoaldosteronism or who are taking potassium-sparing diuretics or potassium supplements should have their blood pressure and urea and electrolytes closely monitored unless the decision has been made to stop drospirenone POP.

Taking the Progestogen-Only Pill: Procedure and Advice

Starting the POP:
a. *Days 1–5 of the cycle.* If started on or before day 5, then no other precautions need be taken.
b. *After day 5.* Extra precautions should be taken for the first 2 days.
c. *Switch from COC.* If changing from a COC, go straight on to the POP without a 7-day break. Extra precautions are not necessary, but it may be necessary to take the pill at a different time of day.
d. *Postpartum.* Start at 3 weeks postpartum. Extra precautions are only needed for the next 2 days if starting later than that.
Note: Time of day. Traditional POPs must be taken regularly at the same time each day (ideally at least 4 hours before the most frequent time of intercourse to ensure maximal mucus-thickening effect).

Advice

a. *Efficacy.* Efficacy is lowest in females with no alteration in cycle activity and is greatest in those with complete suppression of cycles and consequent amenorrhoea. Roughly 40% of females continue to ovulate; in 40%, there is variable interference with the follicular and luteal phase; and in 20%, ovulation is inhibited completely.
b. *Bleeding pattern.* From above, it follows that 40% have similar cycles to their normal pattern, 40% have shorter cycles (which may gradually lengthen towards normal over time) with episodes of spotting or BTB, and 20% have long cycles or amenorrhoea.
c. *Safety.* There is no evidence of increased cardiovascular risk (Heinemann et al, 1999). However, there is emerging evidence that all progesterone-only methods may confer a similar increased risk of breast cancer to COC in current or recent users (Fitzpatrick et al, 2023). No

changes have been made to FRSH guidelines, but this should be discussed with the individual female.

d. *Antibiotics.* The POP is not affected by antibiotics, except rifampicin, rifabutin, and griseofulvin (see h).

e. *Missed pills.* If one or more pills are missed or delayed for more than 3 hours, then take one pill as soon as remembered; take the next pill at the usual time (this may mean taking two pills in one day); and continue taking pills, one daily. Extra precautions need to be taken for 2 days. For Cerazette, the instructions are the same except the window is 12 hours instead of 3 hours. Emergency contraception can be considered if unprotected sex occurs during this 2-day period.

f. *Diarrhoea or vomiting.* If vomiting or diarrhoea occur, continue to take the pill regularly but take extra precautions during the attack and for the next 2 days.

g. *Obesity.* There is no evidence that the efficacy of POPs is reduced in female patients weighing more than 70 kg; the licensed use of one pill per day is recommended.

h. *Enzyme-inducing drugs.* Patients taking enzyme-inducing drugs are best advised not to rely on POPs (Clinical Effectiveness Unit, 2005a, 2008a).

Side Effects

Nonmenstrual

These are the usual progestogenic ones such as headaches, tender breasts, acne, depression, weight gain, and loss of sexual drive. But because the dose of progestogen is so low, these side effects are not that common and often not severe.

Irregular Bleeding

- Examine to exclude a pathological cause.
- Do not change to another POP. There is no suggestion that with traditional POPs, changing brand will improve menstrual or nonmenstrual side effects.
- Suggest a change to another method.

Abdominal Pain of Gynaecological Origin

- Consider ectopic pregnancy. If it can be excluded, then refer for ultrasound examination. It may be attributable to a functional ovarian cyst. Such a cyst usually resolves without treatment.

Amenorrhoea When Cycles Have Been Present

- Exclude pregnancy before assuming that it is caused by the POP.
- Encourage the patient to persevere with the POP. She is in the group least likely to become pregnant with it.

Injectable Progestogens

GUIDELINE

Faculty of Sexual & Reproductive Healthcare. (December 2014; amended July 2023). *FSRH clinical guideline: Progesterone-only injectable contraception. Clinical Effectiveness Unit.* Retrieved from https://www.fsrh.org/documents/cec-ceu-guidance-injectables-dec-2014/.

Preparations

- Depot medroxyprogesterone acetate (DMPA)
  - Depo-Provera: 150 mg in 1 mL via deep intramuscular (IM) injection administered by a healthcare professional
  - Sayana Press: 104 mg in 0.65 mL via self-administered subcutaneous (SC) injection
- Norethisterone enantate (NE)
  - Noristerat: 200 mg in 1 mL via IM injection administered by a healthcare professional

Note: NE is not licensed for long-term use. When used for longer than 16 weeks, this use outside the licence must be discussed with the patient.

Indications

The indications are similar to those for the POP. Patients for whom injectable progestogens are especially indicated are females:

a. *Likely to forget* (or to worry about forgetting) to take daily pills

b. *For whom higher dose long-term progestogens are beneficial* (e.g., those with fibroids or endometriosis)

c. *With sickle-cell disease.* DMPA improves the blood picture and reduces the number of crises (Westhoff, 2003).

Unacceptable Health Risk (UKMEC4)

a. *Breast cancer:* current

Risks Outweigh Benefits (World Health Organization (WHO) 3)

a. *Vascular disease:* ischaemic heart disease, peripheral vascular disease, hypertensive retinopathy, or TIAs. Injectables have hypooestrogenic effects and reduce high-density lipoprotein levels.

b. *Stroke:* history of CVA.

c. *Unexplained vaginal bleeding:* before evaluation.

d. *Breast cancer:* past and no evidence of current disease for 5 years.

e. *Diabetes:* with nephropathy, retinopathy, neuropathy, other vascular disease.

f. *Cirrhosis:* severe (decompensated).

g. *Liver tumours:* benign (hepatocellular adenoma) or malignant (hepatoma).

h. *SLE:* with positive or unknown antiphospholipid antibodies.

Before Starting

Discuss with the patient the following.

Advantages

- Injectables are effective and independent of coitus, with no oestrogenic side effects.
- They are 'invisible', which may be important to some female patients (e.g., those in controlling or abusive relationships).
- They decrease the risk of endometrial cancer, PID, ectopic pregnancy, fibroids, and iron-deficiency anaemia (Westhoff, 2003).

- They may enhance lactation and relieve premenstrual and menstrual symptoms.
- Seizure control has been reported to be improved in some patients with epilepsy.

Effectiveness

- Injectables are a very effective means of contraception. Perfect use failure rates are less than 0.7% for DMPA in the first year and less than 1.0% for NE. Typical use failure rates are 6%.
- Blood levels of DMPA are not affected by drugs, including enzyme inducers; there is no justification for increasing the dose or reducing injection intervals for this reason (Clinical Effectiveness Unit, 2005a). With NE, care is needed with concurrent ART, certain antiepileptics, and rifampicin and rifabutin (UKMEC2).

Side Effects

- *Erratic bleeding.* This occurs in most female patients initially. Prolonged episodes of bleeding may occur but are rarely heavy and decrease over time (WHO, 1987).
  - Examine (especially the cervix).
  - Give one of the following
    a. The next injection early (but not earlier than 4 weeks after the last one)
    b. A short course of oestrogen (e.g., the COC, if no contraindication)
    c. A course of mefenamic acid
  - Refer if the above do not control the bleeding.
  - Alternatively, the patient may prefer to discontinue the method.
- *Amenorrhoea.* This is likely, more so the longer the method is used. The amenorrhoea rate with DMPA is around 70% at 12 months (Canto De Cetina, Canto, & Ordoñez Luna 2001). With NE, episodes of bleeding are the more usual pattern and the amenorrhoea rate at 12 months is 25%. Explain that these methods make the lining of the womb so thin that there is no monthly shedding. Many females find the amenorrhoea a very acceptable side effect.
  - Exclude pregnancy (beware of weight gain at successive visits with nausea or breast symptoms).
  - Discuss other concerns. There is concern that injectables can lower ovarian oestradiol production; see the later discussion of bone mineral density (BMD). There is a lack of consensus on any action to be taken with continuous amenorrhoea for more than 5 years. Some authorities have recommended checking serum oestradiol, but this is not a useful proxy indicator for BMD. Bone densitometry is the test of choice but is expensive and not always freely available.
- *Weight gain.* Weight gain is possible, through appetite stimulation, although some studies show no effect on weight (Westhoff, 2003). Weight gain of more than 5% at 6 months of use is a predictor of continued weight gain. The weight gain is not generally the result of fluid retention. Modifications of diet and behaviour tend to counteract the weight gain. Any weight gain is less likely with NE.
- *Return of fertility.* This may be delayed, with a mean time to ovulation of 18 weeks from the expiry of the last dose of DMPA (maximum, 49 weeks). Return of fertility is much faster with NE, with a mean of 4 weeks and a maximum of 26 weeks (Fotherby & Howard, 1986).

Risks

- *Reduced BMD.* DMPA reduces BMD in many female patients who use it. However, so far, no studies have shown an increased risk of osteoporosis or fractures. When a reduction in BMD occurs, it takes place over the first 2 to 3 years and then tends to level off. The reduction is generally less than 1 standard deviation (i.e., not into the osteopenic range; Curtis & Martins, 2006). After discontinuation of DMPA, BMD consistently returns towards, or to, baseline values in females of all ages (Kaunitz, Arias, & McClung, 2008). Patterns of BMD recovery are similar to those seen after cessation of lactation. Available evidence does not justify the requirement of a limit to the duration of DMPA use, even in adolescents, although initiation of DMPA in those younger than 18 years should only occur if all other methods have been explored. Care is needed in high-risk groups, including smokers and patients with BMIs less than 19 kg/m^2, thyroid disease, taking long-term antiepileptic therapy, and a family history of osteoporosis. Avoid in those taking oral steroids.
- *Cancer.* There is some evidence of an increased risk of breast cancer for current or recent users (RR, 1.18) but no increase 10 or more years after stopping (Collaborative Group on Hormonal Factors in Breast Cancer, 1996). DMPA has a strong protective effect against endometrial cancer (RR, 0.21) (WHO, 1991).

Initiating Treatment and Follow-up

Schedule for the Injections

- Give the first injection within 5 days of the onset of menstruation, within 3 weeks of delivery, or 1 to 5 days after miscarriage or termination. The patient should use additional precautions for 7 days after the first injection unless it was given as above.
- Use the upper outer quadrant of the buttock or the lateral thigh for IM Depo-Provera and Noristerat. The deltoid can be used for IM Depo-Provera when the patient is obese because it is important the drug reaches muscle. Warn the patient not to massage the site because doing so may speed up drug release.
- Advise females to inject SC DMPA into either the anterior thigh or the abdomen. The vial should be at room temperature and thoroughly mixed.
- Give subsequent injections as follows: Depo-Provera 150 mg every 12 weeks, Sayana Press 104 mg every 13 weeks, or Noristerat 200 mg every 8 weeks.
- If the patient returns late for the next injection of DMPA or NE, proceed as in Table 15.2.

TABLE 15.2 Management of Late Injections of Injectable Progestogens

Timing of Injection	Has Unprotected Sex Occurred?	Can the Injection Be Given?	Is Emergency Contraception Indicated?[a]	Is Additional Contraception or Abstinence Advised?	Should a Pregnancy Test Be Performed?
Up to 14 weeks since last DMPA injection or up to 10 weeks since last NET-EN injection	Not applicable as long as next injection is given 14 weeks since the last DMPA injection or 10 weeks since the last NET-EN injection or before	Yes	No	No	No
When an injection is overdue: 14 weeks + 1 day or more since last	No (abstained or used barrier methods)	Yes	No	Yes, for the next 7 days	No, if abstained Yes, if used barrier methods but at
DMPA injection or 10 weeks + 1 day or more since last NET-EN injection	Yes, but only in the past 3 days[b]	Yes	Yes, should offer Levonelle 1500 or a copper IUD	Yes, for the next 7 days	least 21 days later Yes, at least 21 days later
	Yes, but only in the past 4–5 days[b]	Yes	Yes, should offer a copper IUD	No, if opts for copper IUD	Yes, at least 21 days later
	Yes, more than 5 days ago[b]	No	No	Yes, for 21 days until the result of a pregnancy test is confirmed negative and for a further 7 days after giving the injection	Yes, at the initial presentation and at least 21 days later

[a]If Emergency contraception (EC) is declined, decisions about ongoing use of depot medroxyprogesterone acetate (DMPA) or Norethisterone enanthate (NET-EN) should be tailored to the individual female patient. Alternative methods if required should then be considered.
[b]Not applicable if unprotected sex occurred within 14 weeks of the last DMPA injection or 10 weeks of last NET-EN injection.
EC, Emergency contraception; IUD, intrauterine device; NET-EN, norethisterone enanthate..
Clinical Effectiveness Unit, 2008. Reproduced with permission of the Faculty of Sexual & Reproductive Healthcare.
Source: https://www.fsrh.org/documents/cec-ceu-guidance-injectables-dec-2014/

Etonogestrel-Releasing Implant: Nexplanon

GUIDELINE

Faculty of Sexual & Reproductive Healthcare. (February 2021; amended July 2023). *FRSH guidelines: Progestogen-only implant.* Retrieved from https://www.fsrh.org/documents/cec-ceu-guidance-implants-feb-2014/.

- Nexplanon releases a mean etonogestrel dose of 60 to 70 μg/day.
- Subdermal implants should only be inserted and removed if specific practical training has been obtained and a minimum number of implants are inserted and removed to keep up the necessary skills.
- Nexplanon has the advantage that it lasts for 3 years but is reversible should the need arise. It has a high effectiveness, 0.05% in the first year, higher even than vasectomy (Trussell, 2007). Pregnancies in females using Nexplanon are generally caused by noninsertion and drug interactions (Harrison-Woolrych & Hill, 2005).
- The return of fertility after removal of Nexplanon is immediate; ovulation occurs mostly within 3 weeks of removal. Nexplanon has a beneficial effect on dysmenorrhoea. Nexplanon is more cost-effective than the COC (National Collaborating Centre for Women's and Children's Health, 2005).
- Disadvantages are the discomfort of insertion and removal.
- *Practicalities.* If it is implanted other than on days 1 to 5 of the menstrual cycle, extra precautions are needed for the first 7 days if there is no previous method providing cover. For postpartum females, including those who are breastfeeding, insert at up to 3 weeks postpartum. After abortion or miscarriage, insert at up to 5 days. The patient should use additional precautions for 7 days after insertion unless timed as discussed earlier.

Unacceptable Health Risk (UKMEC4)

a. *Breast cancer:* current

Risks Outweigh Benefits (UKMEC3)

a. *Ischaemic heart disease:* current or previous history if occurred when using implant
b. *Stroke:* current or previous if occurred when using implant
c. *Unexplained vaginal bleeding:* before evaluation
d. *Breast cancer:* previous history and no evidence of current disease for 5 years
e. *Cirrhosis:* severe (decompensated)
f. *Liver tumours* benign (hepatocellular adenoma) or malignant (hepatoma)
g. *SLE:* with positive or unknown antiphospholipid antibodies

Monitoring

- There is no reason to check weight and blood pressure.
- There is no reason to do any routine follow-up.

Problems With the Implant

Menstrual

- Bleeding patterns are variable even in an individual over time. Frequent irregular bleeding, spotting, and prolonged bleeding are all possible. Heavy bleeding is rare.
- Amenorrhoea occurs in 21% of users.
- Those who discontinue tend to be from the groups with less favourable patterns: prolonged bleeding (17%) and frequent bleeding (6%).
- Problematic bleeding can be treated as per that which occurs with injectable progesterone. Some clinicians add a progestogen such as Cerazette or norethisterone; there are no data to support this.

Nonmenstrual

Issues include acne, mastalgia, headache, weight gain, abdominal pain, emotional lability, and depression.

Levonorgestrel Intrauterine Device

GUIDELINE

Faculty of Sexual & Reproductive Healthcare. (March 2023; amended July 2023). *FRSH guidelines: Intrauterine contraception.* Retrieved from https://www.fsrh.org/standards-and-guidance/fsrh-guidelines-and-statements/method-specific/intrauterine-contraception/.

- Preparations include:
  - *Mirena:* contains 52 mg of levonorgestrel. Licensed for contraception and menorrhagia (for 5 years) and for endometrial protection (4 years). It is more cost-effective than the COC (National Collaborating Centre for Women's and Children's Health, 2005).
  - *Levosert:* contains 52 mg of levonorgestrel. Licensed for contraception and menorrhagia (for 6 years).
  - *Benilexa:* contains 52 mg of levonorgestrel. Licensed for contraception and menorrhagia (for 6 years).
  - *Kyleena:* contains 19.5 mg of levonorgestrel. Licensed for contraception only (5 years). It is smaller in size than Mirena and a good choice for those who suffer mechanical pain with the larger devices.
  - *Jaydess:* contains 13.5 mg of levonorgestrel. Licensed for contraception only (3 years). Same dimensions as for Kyleena.
- *Protection after insertion.* The levonorgestrel intrauterine device (LNG-IUD) takes 7 days to provide effective contraceptive protection. Unless it is inserted within the first 7 days of the cycle, extra precautions are advised for the next 7 days. If there has been a risk of conception it would be inappropriate to insert an LNG-IUD that cycle.
- *The LNG-IUD in older females.* Females who have the Mirena inserted at the age of 45 years or older for contraception can retain the device until the menopause is confirmed or until contraception is no longer required.

Advantages of the Levonorgestrel Intrauterine Device Over the Copper Intrauterine Devices

a. LNG-IUDs reduce blood loss instead of increasing it and are a form of therapy for menorrhagia (although Kyleena and Jaydess are not licensed for this) even in the presence of fibroids.
b. LNG-IUDs reduce dysmenorrhoea.
c. LNG-IUDs are more reliable as a contraceptive, with a failure rate of 0.2% in the first year compared with 0.8% for Cu-IUDs. LNG-IUDs are approximate in effectiveness to female sterilisation.
d. It has a very low rate of ectopic pregnancy.

Disadvantages of the Levonorgestrel Intrauterine Device

a. The initial cost is much more than the Cu-IUD.
b. It is slightly more difficult to insert than a Cu-IUD because of a wider insertion diameter (although this is less of an issue with Kyleena and Jaydess).
c. The patient may have irregular slight bleeding in the first 3 months of use.
d. Progestogenic side effects (headache, breast tenderness, nausea, mood changes, acne) are possible, especially to begin with, because there is some systemic absorption; the rate of occurrence is no different from Cu-IUDs after 5 years.

Patients for Whom the Levonorgestrel Intrauterine Device Is Particularly Indicated

- As an alternative to sterilisation when the family is complete
- Those with menorrhagia; LNG-IUD is more likely to be effective than other medical treatments
- Those in whom the COC is contraindicated
- Those with learning disabilities or physical disabilities needing long-term contraception

Unacceptable Health Risk (UKMEC4)

a. *Postpartum sepsis*
b. *Postabortion sepsis*

c. *Gestational trophoblastic disease with persistently elevated human chorionic gonadotropin (hCG) or malignant disease*

d. *Sexually transmitted infection (STI) (current purulent cervicitis, chlamydial infection, or gonorrhoea) or PID: current*

Risks Usually Outweigh Benefits (UKMEC3)

a. *Postpartum: from 48 hours to 4 weeks;* Considered safe before 48 hours but with a higher expulsion rate

b. *Complicated organ transplant* (initiation)

c. *Gestational trophoblastic disease with decreasing hCG levels*

d. *Distortion of the uterine cavity:* congenital malformation, submucous fibroids

e. *Ischaemic heart disease:* current or previous (continuation)

f. *Stroke disease* (continuation)

g. *Long QT syndrome* (initiation)

Nonhormonal Methods of Contraception

Copper Intrauterine Devices

> **GUIDELINE**
>
> Faculty of Sexual & Reproductive Healthcare. (March 2023; amended July 2023). *FRSH guidelines: Intrauterine contraception.* Retrieved from https://www.fsrh.org/standards-and-guidance/fsrh-guidelines-and-statements/method-specific/intrauterine-contaception/.

- The typical use failure rate for Cu-IUDs is 0.8% in the first year (Trussell, 2007).
- Cu-IUDs should only be fitted if specific practical training has been obtained and a minimum number of devices are fitted to keep up the necessary skills.
- All Cu-IUDs with frames have copper on the stem, the arms, or both. GyneFix is a frameless device with six copper cylinders on a thread. Modern copper-containing IUDs are clinically effective and safe for at least 5 years. The TT380 Slimline and TCu380A QuickLoad are effective for 10 years.
- The risk of perforation associated with insertion of Cu-IUDs is 1 in 1000.
- IUDs do not offer any protection against STIs, but previous studies that purported to show an increased risk of PID have now been shown to be flawed (Grimes, 2000). There is no evidence that prophylactic use of antibiotics for IUD insertion is of significant benefit in healthy females (Grimes, Schulz, & Stanwood, 2004).
- The currently available high-load IUDs protect against ectopic pregnancy compared with using no contraception.
- Cumulative expulsion rates at 5 years for copper IUDs are around 5%. Expulsion may occur at any time after insertion but is most likely in the early cycles, especially during menstruation. Patients who are older and of higher parity are less likely to expel their devices.

Unacceptable Health Risk (UKMEC4)

a. Pregnancy

b. Puerperal sepsis

c. Immediately after septic abortion

d. Insertion before evaluation of unexplained vaginal bleeding

e. Gestational trophoblastic disease with persistently elevated β-hCG levels or malignant disease

f. Cervical or endometrial cancer: current

g. STI (current purulent cervicitis, chlamydial infection, or gonorrhoea) or PID: current

h. Pelvic tuberculosis (TB)

Risks Usually Outweigh Benefits (UKMEC3)

a. Postpartum insertion between 48 hours and 4 weeks postpartum in females who are breast feeding or not breast feeding or after caesarean section

b. Distortion of the uterine cavity (e.g., congenital malformation, submucous fibroids)

c. Ovarian cancer

d. Gestational trophoblastic disease with decreasing hCG levels

e. Long QT syndrome (initiation)

Adverse Effects

Heavier Periods, Intermenstrual Bleeding, and Dysmenorrhoea

- Warn the patient that these are common in the first few cycles after insertion.
- Examine for infection or malposition of the device.
- Prescribe NSAIDs, which may reduce pain and bleeding.
- Remove the IUD if it appears to be associated with a change in bleeding pattern. If the pattern does not return to normal, refer for gynaecologic assessment.

Pelvic Infection

- Symptoms of infection require examination and endocervical swabs for STIs.
- Treat with antibiotics.
- If the symptoms settle, the IUD can be left in place.
- *Actinomyces-like organisms* may be found on a cervical smear:
  a. If the patient is asymptomatic, leave the IUD in place.
  b. If the patient has symptoms (i.e., pain or discharge), remove the IUD and investigate the patient for pelvic pain and STIs, treat with antibiotics as appropriate, and consider referral to a genitourinary (GUM) or gynaecology specialist.

Pregnancy

- If symptoms suggest an ectopic pregnancy, admit to hospital; 6% of pregnancies that occur with an IUD in place are ectopic.
- If a scan indicates that the pregnancy is intrauterine, gently remove the IUD if the threads are visible and the pregnancy is less than 12 weeks' gestation. This will halve the miscarriage rate. If the pregnancy is greater than 12 weeks' gestation or no threads are seen, refer early for antenatal assessment.

Lost Threads

- Teach the patient to feel for the threads after each period, or on the first of the month if there is amenorrhoea with the LNG-IUD.
- If the threads are not palpable, warn the patient temporarily to use other precautions and arrange for USS (Ultrasound scan).
- If USS confirms that the device is in situ, leave it in place until it is due to be changed. Repeat vaginal examination yearly, and only repeat USS if there is reason to suspect expulsion.

Timing of Insertion

- Insertion can be at any time during the menstrual cycle if it is reasonably certain that the patient is not pregnant (see Box 15.1).
- Do not insert between 48 hours and 4 weeks postpartum.
- An IUD can be safely fitted immediately after a first trimester abortion (spontaneous or therapeutic), although this carries an increased risk of expulsion (Grimes et al, 2004).
- All fitters should have up-to-date resuscitation training.

Removal or Refit

- *Females aged 40 years and older:* An IUD fitted after the age of 40 years can be left as the only means of contraception until menopause. When there has been 6 months of amenorrhoea, it should be removed; later removal may be difficult because of cervical stenosis. If a female presents more than 6 months after menopause with a device in situ, attempt to remove it. If difficulty is encountered, try again after a short course of treatment with topical oestrogen.

Timing of Removal

- *If pregnancy is desired*, the IUD may be removed at any time.
- *If pregnancy is not desired*, remove the IUD when the patient is established on a hormonal method or when barrier methods have been used carefully since the last period.
- *Emergency contraception* may be necessary if intercourse has occurred within the previous 5 days and removal of the IUD is urgent.

Prophylactic Antibiotics for Cardiac Disease

For females with previous endocarditis or with a prosthetic heart valve, it is no longer recommended to give antibiotic prophylaxis during IUD insertion or removal (NICE, 2008).

Follow-up

- Review after 6 weeks. Thereafter follow-up is not necessary.
- Ask about menstrual blood loss, pelvic pain, vaginal discharge, and discomfort to the partner.
- Do a pelvic examination and check the presence of the threads.

Barrier Methods

> **GUIDELINE**
>
> Faculty of Sexual & Reproductive Healthcare. (August 2012; updated October 2015). *FRSH guidelines: Barrier methods for contraception and STI prevention. Clinical Effectiveness Unit.* Retrieved from https://www.fsrh.org/standards-and-guidance/documents/ceuguidancebarriermethodscontraceptionsdi/.

- These have the advantage of protecting against STIs and HPV, as well as pregnancy.
- However, efficacy is utterly dependent on consistent use before or during sex; there is considerable potential for user failure, especially among young people.
- Condoms and diaphragms made of latex rubber, as well as newer condoms brands made from polyisoprene (Skyn) or lamb intestine (Naturalamb), can be damaged by oil-based products such as:
  - Baby oil, bath oil, body oil, and Vaseline
  - Suntan oil and massage oil
  - Cream, ice cream, and salad cream
  - Lipstick and hair conditioner
  - Many antithrush preparations
  - Progesterone pessaries
- Latex condoms, diaphragms, and caps should not be used in people with latex allergy (UKMEC3).
- Diaphragms, cervical caps, and sponges should not be used if the female has a history of toxic shock syndrome (UKMEC3).

Male Condoms

- Male condoms give a pregnancy rate of 2% to 15% in the first year.
- There is no evidence that lubrication with nonoxynol-9 (N-9) spermicide conveys any additional contraceptive benefit, and its use is not recommended by the FRSH.
- Use of appropriate lubricant does reduce the chances of condom breakage during anal sex and is recommended, but the thickness of the condom has no bearing.
- Ensure the couple knows to use condoms bearing the CE mark and preferably also the British Standards Institution Kitemark.
- Advise the couple about use of emergency contraception in the event of a mishap.

Female Condom

- There are several available brands in the United Kingdom:
  - Femidom is a loose-fitting polyurethane sheath with two flexible rings which is inserted into the vagina. It is prelubricated with dimethicone, an odourless, nonspermicidal lubricant.
  - Domica is made of natural latex.
  - Pasante female condoms are latex free. They are prelubricated with a nitrile- and silicone oil–based lubricant.

- It lines the vagina and covers some of the vulva. It is disposable and comes in one size. Its failure rate is 5% to 21% in the first year.

Diaphragms

- Diaphragms are more effective than condoms and have the advantage that they do not need to be inserted and removed at the time of intercourse.
- They are not, however, as effective a protector as condoms against STIs.
- They have a failure rate of 6% to 16% in the first year.
- They come in sizes rising in steps of 5 mm and in the form of coiled spring, arcing spring, or flat spring. Coil spring and arcing diaphragms are also available in silicone. The correct size and type are determined on vaginal examination.
- Use:
  a. The diaphragm should be inserted before sex and left in place for at least 6 hours after the last act of sex.
  b. A strip of spermicide about 5 cm long should be placed on the upper side of the diaphragm before insertion. If sex takes place more than 3 hours later, more spermicide should be inserted, either as a pessary or as cream with an applicator.
  c. The diaphragm must be washed in warm soapy water, dried after use, and stored in a cool place in its container to maintain its shape.
- Check the fit and comfort after 1 week and discuss again the routine for its use.
- See after 3 months and then annually but more frequently if there are difficulties or if there is a weight change of more than 3 kg.
- Prescribe a new diaphragm annually.

Cervical Caps

- FemCap is made of silicone (Clinical Effectiveness Unit, 2004c). Failure rates are 10% to 18% in the first year. Before starting, sizing is needed by a doctor or nurse. FemCap comes in three sizes and is reusable.

Fertility Awareness

> **GUIDELINE**
>
> Faculty of Sexual & Reproductive Healthcare. (June 2015; updated November 2015). *FRSH guidelines: Fertility awareness methods. Clinical Effectiveness Unit.* Retrieved from https://www.fsrh.org/standards-and-guidance/documents/ceuguidancefertilityawarenessmethods/.

- Fertility awareness or natural family planning (NFP) relies on avoidance of intercourse around the time of ovulation.
- Failure rates can be as low as 2.6% in the first year when multiple indicators are used in combination to define the beginning and the end of the fertile period (European Natural Family Planning Study Groups, 1993), but this high efficacy rate is only achieved by highly motivated and well-trained couples.
- Expert training is essential; advise the patient to contact Fertility UK (see box) for information about local classes. Computerised thermometers and saliva testing kits are on sale, but they are unevaluated and cannot be recommended.

> **PATIENT INFORMATION**
>
> Fertility UK. Bury Knowle Health Centre, 207 London Road, Headington, Oxford, OX3 9JA. Available at http://www.fertilityuk.org.

- Recognised indicators are
  a. (Waking) basal body temperature changes
  b. Changes in cervical secretions (presence or absence)
  c. Cervical changes (firmness, height, and dilatation)
  d. Calculation based on cycle length
  e. Minor changes, e.g., Mittelschmerz (midcycle pain)
- Combining indicators is best; the combination of temperature and cervical secretions (symptothermal) is commonly used.
- Suitability for natural family planning may be affected by females who have menstrual irregularities, have recently stopped a hormonal method, are postpartum, take known teratogenic medications, or have medical conditions for which pregnancy is high risk.
- *Persona* is a fertility monitor that measures estrone-3-glucuronide and luteinising hormone (LH) in the urine and predicts fertile days for an individual by storing information on the female's biochemistry and cycle length. It requires eight urine tests per cycle. A red light indicates fertile days, and a green light indicates nonfertile days. A yellow light indicates that a urine test is required. It must be realised that when this device is used by the non-NFP (Natural Family Planning) fraternity without combining indicators, failure rates will be higher. Nevertheless, a failure rate of 6.2% in the first year is predicted in such a population (Bonnar et al, 1999).

Emergency Contraception

> **GUIDELINE**
>
> Faculty of Sexual & Reproductive Healthcare. (March 2017; amended July 2023). *FRSH clinical guideline: Emergency contraception.* Retrieved from https://www.fsrh.org/documents/ceu-clinical-guidance-emergency-contraception-march-2017/.

Hormonal Preparations

- Levonorgestrel 1500 μcg (Levonelle) is a progestogen. It is licensed to be taken within 72 hours of (the first episode of) unprotected intercourse.

- Ulipristal acetate 30 mg (ellaOne) is a progesterone receptor modulator. It is licensed to be taken within 120 hours of (the first episode of) unprotected intercourse and is considered to be significantly more effective than levonorgestrel.

Both are available from general practitioner (GP) surgeries, sexual health clinics, and community pharmacies. There may be a charge when obtained via the latter. In some circumstances, they may also be available via online pharmacies, school nurses, young people's services, and NHS walk-in services.

Intrauterine Device Insertion

- *Insertion of a Cu-IUD* can be considered if either of the following is present:
  a. The patient presents within 5 days of unprotected intercourse
  b. Within 5 days of the calculated time of ovulation if intercourse took place more than 5 days before presentation, whether or not further intercourse has taken place in the last 5 days
- Patients who have failed to take oral contraception correctly
  a. *COC.* Either method can be considered for a patient who misses three or more pills (see Fig. 15.1).
  b. *POP.* Either method can be considered for a patient who has unprotected sex during the 48-hour window after regular pill taking has been reestablished after missed pills.

Contraindications

a. Established pregnancy.
b. *IUD.* Contraindications to the insertion of an IUD apply except that, in an emergency, an IUD can be inserted with antibiotic cover in a patient at risk of PID. Contraindications to the long-term use of an IUD do not apply because the IUD can be removed after the next period.
c. Ulipristal should not be used in those needing oral steroids such as asthma or in those taking drugs which increase gastric pH (e.g., antacids, H2-receptor antagonists, proton pump inhibitors).

Special Situations

a. *Enzyme-inducing drugs.* These may be prescribed or bought OTC. Patients taking enzyme-inducing drugs should take two Levonelle 1500 pills instead of one. Ulipristal should not be used in those taking enzyme inducers.
b. *Previous ectopic pregnancy.* Patients should understand that neither method will protect against a further ectopic pregnancy.
c. Patients who want the most reliable method or in whom there has been multiple exposure should use an IUD.
d. Women administered Levonelle EC who wish to start ongoing hormonal contraception should be offered it via the quick-start method – beginning the hormonal contraception of choice whilst using condoms or abstinence for 7 days (COC) or 2 days (POP). Those administered Ulipristal EC who wish to start ongoing hormonal contraception should wait 5 days before starting their chosen COC or POP, but should use condoms or abstinence to cover those 5 days plus 7 days (COC) or 2 days (POP).
e. *Weight.* Females who weigh more than 70 kg or have a BMI greater than 26 kg/m² should be offered a choice of Cu-IUD or Ulipristal as the most effective options, with double-dose (3 mg) Levonelle as a second-line choice.
f. *Breastfeeding.* Insertion of an IUD during lactation has a higher (but still small) risk of uterine perforation. Ulipristal is expressed in breastmilk, so females should be advised to discard their milk for 1 week after treatment.

Management

- The treatment of choice is usually with oral preparations; however, patients should be informed about the Cu-IUD method and its greater effectiveness.
- Establish from the consultation:
  a. Date of last menstrual period (LMP)
  b. Whether the LMP was normal
  c. The normal menstrual cycle length and probable date of ovulation
  d. *All* the occasions of unprotected sexual intercourse (UPSI) in the last cycle
  e. The number of hours since the first episode of UPSI
  f. The method of contraception normally used
- Warn patients that the maximum risk of pregnancy after midcycle UPSI is about 9% (Wilcox et al, 2001), but it depends on the inherent fertility of the couple.
- Explain to the patient that:
  a. The method is not guaranteed. The average risk of pregnancy from a single episode of coitus is 3% (Wilcox et al, 2001). The progestogen-only method and ulipristal reduce this risk by around 85%. The IUD is more effective, reducing the risk by 99% (Liying & Bilian, 2001).
  b. If the hormonal method is given and ongoing hormonal contracpetion is not being initiated via the quick-start method, then barrier methods must be used until the next period, which may be a little earlier or later than expected. Choice of ongoing contraception may then be started.
  c. She should reattend if the next period does not come or she has any other worries.
  d. If vomiting occurs within 2 hours of taking the dose, she should reattend urgently.

Follow-up

- If a normal period has not occurred, exclude pregnancy and bear in mind the possibility of ectopic pregnancy.
- Discuss the long-term need for contraception. Use the opportunity to counsel young and inexperienced patients. Consider whether a supply of Levonelle 1500 in advance might be appropriate for patients who do not

wish planned contraception but who anticipate the need for occasional emergency contraception after unplanned sex. In a US study, it increased the use of emergency contraception without reducing the use of routine contraception (Jackson et al, 2003).

Contraception in Special Cases

Contraception and Young People

(Clinical Effectiveness Unit, 2010a)

> **GUIDELINE**
>
> Faculty of Sexual & Reproductive Healthcare. (March 2010). FRSH guidelines: Contraceptive choices for young people. Found at: https://www.fsrh.org/standards-and-guidance/documents/cec-ceu-guidance-young-people-mar-2010/

> **INFORMATION AND ADVICE**
>
> Brook Free (confidential counselling service for young people). Available at http://www.brook.org.uk.
>   Sexwise (for patients younger than 18 years of age with problems with sex, relationships, and contraception). Available at https://www.sexwise.org.uk/

- In England and Wales, provision of contraceptive advice and treatment by health professionals to those aged younger than 16 years of age is governed by a health circular issued on 29 July 2004 (Anonymous, 2004a). Advice and treatment may be given, according to the Fraser guidelines, without parental knowledge when the young person:
  a. Has sufficient maturity to understand the moral, social, and emotional implications of the treatment
  b. Cannot be persuaded to inform the parents or allow them to be informed
  c. Is very likely to begin, or to continue, sexual intercourse with or without contraception
  d. Would be likely to suffer in terms of physical or mental health if no contraceptive advice or treatment is given
  e. Has their best interests served by being given contraceptive advice or treatment without parental consent
- Young people continue to have concerns about the possibility of breaches of confidentiality. Improving young people's trust in the confidentiality of their practice should help remove one of the main obstacles that deter some teenagers from seeking early sexual health advice (Donovan et al, 2000). Every practice should develop its own confidentiality policy.
- *Legal aspects.* Inform the patient (and, if she gives her consent, her parents) of the legal situation. It is an offence for a person to have sexual contact with a girl younger than the age of 16 years even if the girl consents (Sexual Offences Act, 2003).

- *Smoking.* Discuss the importance of not smoking, especially if the COC is to be used.
- Raise the advantages, both psychological and physical, of not having sex at a young age.
- Stress the value of using the condom in addition to any other method to reduce the risk of STIs including HIV (dual protection). Young people should be shown how to use condoms.

Contraception and Older Female Patients

> **GUIDELINE**
>
> Faculty of Sexual & Reproductive Healthcare. (August 2017; amended July 2023). *FRSH guideline: Contraception for women aged over 40 years.* Retrieved from https://www.fsrh.org/documents/fsrh-guidance-contraception-for-women-aged-over-40-years-2017/.

- Females older than 40 years of age are more likely to have irregular cycles, but ovulation still occurs in around 35% of these cycles, and there is still need for contraception.
- Current advice is for contraception to be continued in females aged 40 to 50 years of age until there has been 2 years' amenorrhoea and in females older than 50 years until there has been 1 year's amenorrhoea.
  - Until age 50 years, age itself is not a barrier to any one form of contraception. From 50 years of age on, females should be advised against the use of all forms of combined hormonal contraception because of their increased risk profile, as well as use of DMPA because of its adverse effect on BMD.
  - When amenorrhoea occurs in those who have been having periods, menopause may be diagnosed after 2 years if aged younger than 50 years or 1 year if aged older than 50 years. For those aged older than 50 years who have been amenorrhoeic on progesterone-only contraceptives, follicle-stimulating hormone (FSH) may be checked to help determine menopausal status if desired.

Hormone Replacement Therapy

- Hormone replacement therapy (HRT) is not contraceptive because the natural oestrogens do not necessarily inhibit ovulation.
- LNG-IUD is the only progesterone which is licensed for both contraception and endometrial protection as part of a combined HRT regimen.
- All forms of progesterone-only contraception may be used alongside HRT when required.
- Females taking the COC do not need HRT until the COC is stopped.
- *Females started on HRT before menopause* should continue contraception (barrier or IUD, possibly the POP) until there is reason to think that they have reached menopause (e.g., at age 50 years). It is impossible to assess the timing of the natural menopause in females

using HRT. If a female is unwilling to discontinue HRT for 3 to 4 months to allow accurate assessment of FSH levels, then barrier contraception, an IUD, or the POP can be used until the age of 55 years, at which time loss of natural fertility can be assumed.

Contraception and Learning Disability

Contraception is most likely to be considered in females with learning disability who (Cooper, 2000):

a. Are entering a sexual relationship. There is a 40% chance of learning disability in children born to a couple in which both parents have learning disability.
b. Are in danger of being exploited
- *Consent.* Consult a consultant psychiatrist if there is doubt about the ability to give consent. The majority of patients with moderate and mild learning disability are able to give consent.
- *Sex education.* Refer to the local community learning disability team, social services department, education department, or voluntary organisation.
- *Epilepsy.* If patients are on enzyme-inducing antiepileptics, the dose of the COC needs to be higher. Those on the POP should change method.

Sterilisation

When counselling for sterilisation the following should be borne in mind (Anonymous, 2004b; Brechin & Bigrigg, 2006):

a. Both partners should ideally be seen together.
b. Patients should be made aware of the high efficacy of alternative long-acting reversible contraceptive methods (National Collaborating Centre for Women's and Children's Health, 2005).
c. The possibility of death of a partner or child should be covered.
d. The possibility of relationship breakdown should be discussed.
e. The pros and cons of male versus female sterilisation should be explained.

Which Partner Should Be Sterilised?

Sometimes it is not the partner who presents themself who is subsequently sterilised. Points to be raised here are:

a. Vasectomy is more effective than tubal occlusion: 1 in 2000 lifetime pregnancy risk (when postoperative semen analysis is adhered to) compared with 1 in 200 for tubal occlusion (all varieties of technique). The effectiveness of the Filshie clip is a little more favourable, but the data are less robust.
b. Vasectomy is a more minor operation.
c. Vasectomy is safer as it is usually performed under local anaesthesia.
d. Males have a longer reproductive span to lose.
e. Males are more likely to feel threatened (fear of loss of sexual drive and sexual prowess).

Reversal

- If a patient wants a reversal of sterilisation, patency rates of around 90% can be achieved with microsurgical techniques, but fertility is lower: 31% to 92% in females and 9% to 82% in males (rates tend to be at the low end of this range when the vasectomy was performed more than 10 years previously).
- When counselling a patient, be aware that risk factors for subsequent regret about sterilisation include:
  a. Age younger than 30 years
  b. No children
  c. Not in a relationship
  d. Association in time with pregnancy (full term or abortion)
  e. Crisis in the relationship or not in a mutually faithful relationship
  f. Coercion by a partner or health professional
  g. Psychological or psychosocial issues

Termination of Pregnancy

- Laws around the termination of pregnancy (TOP) are highly variable in different countries (Anonymous, 2004c). Local legislation should be adhered to.
- In the United Kingdom, the Abortion Act 1967, as amended by the Human Fertilisation and Embryology Act 1990, allows TOP if two doctors agree that one of the following is present:
  a. The continuance of the pregnancy would involve risk to the life of the pregnant female patient greater than if the pregnancy were terminated.
  b. The termination is necessary to prevent grave permanent injury to the physical or mental health of the pregnant female patient.
  c. The pregnancy has not exceeded its 24th week, and the continuance of the pregnancy would involve risk, greater than if the pregnancy were terminated, of injury to the physical or mental health of the pregnant female patient.
  d. The pregnancy has not exceeded its 24th week, and the continuance of the pregnancy would involve risk, greater than if the pregnancy were terminated, of injury to the physical or mental health of any existing child(ren) of the family of the pregnant female patient.
  e. There is a substantial risk that if the child were born, they would suffer from such physical or mental abnormalities as to be seriously disabled.
  Note: There is no time limit for grounds a, b, and e.
- The mortality rate for a TOP is 0.2 per 100,000 compared with 6 per 100,000 for death in childbirth.
- The risk of serious complications and death increases with advancing gestation, so do not be responsible for delays in referral.
- TOP is not associated with an increase in breast cancer risk.
- There are no proven associations between TOP and subsequent ectopic pregnancy, placenta praevia, or infertility.

- TOP may be associated with a small increase in the risk of subsequent miscarriage or preterm delivery.
- Higher quality studies show no higher risk of mental health sequelae in those who have TOPs compared with females with unintended pregnancies who continue (Charles et al, 2008).
- Counsel the patient to help her come to her own informed decision about TOP that she will not regret and to lessen the risk of emotional disturbance, whatever decision is reached.
- Ensure that she is aware of the alternative of continuing the pregnancy and keeping the baby or giving it up for adoption.
- Check she is not under pressure from partner or parent.
- Discuss the need for and, if possible, plan future contraception, including information about emergency contraception if not already known about.
- Arrange a follow-up appointment 2 weeks after the termination to check for medical and psychological sequelae.
- Early medical TOP with mifepristone and misoprostol up to 9 weeks' gestation (Fiala & Gemzell-Danielsson, 2006) is now widely available. Check that the patient does not have any contraindications (e.g., severe asthma not controlled by therapy, chronic adrenal failure). As of August 2022 and in response to the COVID-19 pandemic, at-home early medical abortions have been made available for females before 10 weeks' gestation in England and Wales.

Patients Younger Than 16 Years Old

- Involve the parents or guardians, with the patient's consent. They will be needed to sign the consent form as well as to support the patient before and after the termination (Anonymous, 2004a).
- If the patient refuses to inform a parent or guardian, she has the right in the United Kingdom, under the Family Law Reform Act 1969, to consent to treatment herself, provided she understands the nature of the procedure, including its risks and complications.
- If a competent child consents to treatment, a parent cannot override that consent.

INFORMATION FOR PATIENTS

Faculty of Sexual & Reproductive Healthcare & Royal College of Obstetricians and Gynaecologists. (n.d.). *Abortion and abortion care factsheet: To support relationships and sex education in secondary schools*. Retrieved from https://www.fsrh.org/documents/abortion-and-abortion-care-factsheet-2021/#:~:text=This%20is%20a%20factsheet%20for,abortion%20care%20in%20the%20UK.

Infertility

GUIDELINE

National Institute for Health and Clinical Excellence. (February 2013; updated 2017). *Fertility problems: Assessment and treatment. NICE clinical guideline 156* Retrieved from http://www.nice.org.uk.

- Reassure the couple that 75% of couples achieve conception within 6 months and 84% by 12 months. If the female is aged 35 years, the success rate is 94% over 3 years. If the female is aged 38 years, the success rate is 77% over 3 years.
- Start investigations as soon as the couple voices anxiety about conceiving. Explain that in 30% of cases, the problem lies with the male alone; in 30% with the female alone; and in the remainder, it is mixed or unexplained.
- Aim to consider referral after 1 year or sooner if there is good reason to predict difficulties (e.g., oligo- or amenorrhoea, abnormal sperm count, a history of PID, or maternal age 36 years or older). Refer the couple direct to a tertiary centre holding the contract for the treatment of subfertility, not to a general gynaecology clinic.

Investigations

Assessment of the Female Patient

a. The history should include details of menstrual cycle, previous pregnancies, and pelvic infections or operations. Regular periods are a reliable guide to the fact that the patient is ovulating. Check that they are having intercourse at the female's most fertile time (as well as throughout the cycle). Do not bother with temperature charts.

b. Check that the female is rubella immune and taking folic acid.

c. Screen for *Chlamydia* infection.

d. Examine for evidence of pelvic pathology.

e. *Progesterone level.* Take blood 7 days before menstruation is due. A level greater than 16 nmol/L suggests ovulation, and a level greater than 30 nmol/L confirms it. Borderline levels may be caused by a deficient luteal phase or mistimed sampling. Levels below 16 nmol/L confirm that the cycle was anovulatory.

f. *Measure FSH and LH* in a female with irregular cycles in whom it is impossible to predict when to check the blood progesterone.

Note: There is no value in measuring thyroid function tests (TFTs) or prolactin in females with regular menses in the absence of galactorrhoea or symptoms of thyroid disease.

Assessment of the Male Patient

a. The medical history should include operations on or infections of the testes and operations on the prostate.

b. Drug history. Sulfasalazine, tetracyclines, allopurinol, anabolic steroids, cannabis, and cocaine have all been shown to interfere with male reproductive function.

c. Examine the male patient, including genitals and secondary sexual characteristics.

d. Screen for *Chlamydia* infection.

e. Arrange for semen analysis. Semen should be produced by masturbation 3 days after the last ejaculation and examined within 1 hour.

f. If the count is low, repeat after 3 months and refer to a specialist fertility clinic if it is still low. However, if the count is severely low, refer after a single count.

g. Warn the patient that even a 'normal' sperm count does not mean that there is not some sperm dysfunction which can only be detected on more sophisticated tests.

Normal Values for Semen

Normal Values include (WHO 2021)
a. Volume: 1.4 mL or greater
b. PH: 7.2 or higher
c. Concentration: 16×10^6 per mL or greater
d. Total sperm number: 39×10^6 per ejaculate or greater
e. Motility: 42% with 30% showing progressive motility
f. Vitality: more than 54% live
g. Morphology: more than 4% normal forms
h. White blood cells: less than 1×10^6 cells per mL

Advice

Advice to the couple should routinely be:
a. Both should stop smoking.
b. The female should drink no more than 1 or 2 units of alcohol once or twice weekly while trying to conceive.
c. Males who drink heavily should cut their drinking to no more than 3 to 4 units in any day.
d. Females and males with BMIs greater than 30 kg/m² should lose weight whether or not ovulation is a problem.
e. Males should avoid soaking in hot baths, wearing tight underwear, and remaining seated for many hours at a time.
f. Couples should be advised to have regular sex throughout the cycle, every 2 to 3 days. There is no evidence that use of temperature charts and LH detection tests to time sex improve pregnancy rates.
- Use of clomiphene in general cannot be justified in general practice in view of the increased risk of multiple pregnancy and ovarian cancer. An exception to this is if a female who previously conceived using it presents again with anovulatory cycles.

The Role of the General Practitioner After Referral

- Administer the drugs for assisted conception according to a protocol agreed with the specialist clinic.
- Support the couple throughout the drawn-out process of investigation and treatment.

Infertility Network UK (a self-help organisation which supplies literature and runs support networks). Tel: 01424 732361; Available at http://www.infertilitynetworkuk.com.
  The Human Fertilization and Embryology Authority (books and videos about assisted conception). 10 Spring Gardens, London, SW1A 2BU. Tel: 020 7291 8200. Available at http://www.hfea.gov.uk.

Sexual Problems

- Sexual problems may have a physical or psychological origin, but often they are mixed.
- All patients with sexual problems develop 'performance anxiety', in which they are not relaxed and spontaneous in love making, are alert to further failure, and become spectators of their own sexual performance.
- In about 30% of patients, the partner also has a problem.
- In any consultation about sexual problems, it is important to ascertain:
  a. What is the real complaint?
  b. Why is the problem being presented now?
  c. Is the desire for change real?
  d. Who is really complaining, the patient or the partner?
  e. What are the expectations of the patient?
- Consider the following psychological aspects in any patient presenting with a problem:
  a. *Ignorance and misunderstanding.* These include faulty sex education and technique, inability to communicate sexual needs, and unrealistic expectations caused by stereotyped views of expected behaviour and performance.
  b. *Anger and resentment.* These often remain unresolved, with the couple unable to communicate their feelings to each other clearly. They often arise when the partners were unable to express their feelings as children because of excessive unresolved anger in their parents. It may occur in response to relationship difficulties, financial difficulties, children, in-laws, or stress at work.
  c. *Shame, embarrassment, and guilt.* These may be caused by a negative sexual attitude laid down in childhood, in which the parents looked upon sexuality as 'bad'. Traumatic sexual experiences may add to these fears.
  d. *Anxiety or fear about sex.* Fear of closeness, vulnerability, letting go, and failure may lead to a self-perpetuating cycle of anxiety.
  e. *Poor self-image* may contribute to lack of interest in sex and sexual response. Changes in females may occur after operations, especially mastectomy or hysterectomy, postmenopausally, and after childbirth. Both sexes commonly suffer after redundancy and when depressed.

INFORMATION FOR PATIENTS

Netdoctor. (n.d.). *Self-help material on the internet: 'Sex and relationships').* Retrieved from https://www.relate.org.uk/get-help.

Erectile Dysfunction

GUIDELINE

National Institute for Health and Clinical Excellence. (2023). *CKS erectile dysfunction.* Available at https://cks.nice.org.uk/topics/erectile-dysfunction/.

- Erectile dysfunction (ED) occurs in 10% to 15% of males but varies with age, with some degree of dysfunction being experienced by 40% of males at age 40 years and by 70% at age 70 years. ED in an otherwise asymptomatic male may be a marker for underlying CVD. Although at least 50% of the patients referred to specialist clinics have an organic component, anxiety about the situation makes things worse.
- From the history, assess particularly whether either of the following is present:
  a. The ED has arisen suddenly, with a precipitating cause, and is variable, with erections occurring in the early morning but not during intercourse. These patients are likely to have a psychological cause for the problem.
  b. The onset was gradual and is constant, with partial or poorly sustained erections and no full early morning erections. These patients are likely to have a physical cause, although a psychological component is frequently superimposed.
- Consider the psychological aspects discussed earlier (under the section on sexual problems).
- Be alert to psychiatric problems including generalised anxiety states (excessive adrenergic constrictor tone), depression, psychosis, body dysmorphic disorder, gender identity problems, and alcoholism.
- Be aware of the possibility of relative energy deficiency in sport (RED-S) in both recreational and professional athletes.
- Check for the cause being an adverse drug reaction to beta-blockers, thiazides, spironolactone, cimetidine, antidepressants, phenothiazine antipsychotics, and especially, alcohol.
- Examine:
  a. Blood pressure, heart rate, waist circumference, and weight
  b. For signs of testosterone deficiency (gynaecomastia, sparse body hair, reduced muscle mass)
  c. Genitalia (including testicular size, fibrosis in the shaft of the penis, and retractibility of the foreskin)
- Further examination may sometimes be indicated by age or findings in the history especially cardiovascular, neurologic, endocrine, and urinary systems.

Workup

a. Haemoglobin A1c (or fasting blood glucose) and lipids.
b. Testosterone (if history or examination, suggest possible hypogonadism or if required to reassure patient). Take blood between 9 and 11 AM and not within 3 months of serious illness, which can depress the testosterone level.
c. Consider testing prostate-specific antigen, TFT, and liver and renal function based on the individual and clinical judgement.

Erectile Dysfunction as a Risk Factor for Cardiovascular Disease

- Observational studies show that factors associated with ED are similar to those associated with CVD (sedentary lifestyle, obesity, smoking, hypercholesterolaemia, and the metabolic syndrome).
- ED seems to carry an independent risk for CVD of 1.46, making it as powerful a predictor of CVD as smoking.
- When a male presents with ED which appears to be vascular in origin, assess his risk of CVD.

Treatment in General Practice

- *Exercise and weight loss.* In the Massachusetts Male Aging Study, males who started exercise in midlife had a 70% reduced risk for ED later in life. There is some evidence that exercise and weight loss in those with established ED leads to a significant reduction in ED. Be mindful in those who may have RED-S that a reduction in exercise or an increase in caloric intake may be required.
- *Other lifestyle advice.* Males should be advised to stop smoking and reduce alcohol when applicable. In those who cycle for more than 3 hours per week, a trial of reduced time in the saddle may be advisable.

Phosphodiesterase Type 5 Inhibitors

- These are facilitators rather than initiators of erections and require sexual stimulation to facilitate an erection; they have a slower onset of action than injected or transurethral alprostadil (see later). Sildenafil and vardenafil are relatively short-acting phosphodiesterase type 5 (PDE5) inhibitors, having a half-life of about 4 hours (suitable for occasional use); tadalafil has a longer half-life of 17.5 hours (suitable for longer periods, e.g., over a weekend).
- In the United Kingdom, generic sildenafil is available on the NHS for all males with ED. It is also available OTC as 'Viagra Connect'. Other PDE5 inhibitors can only be prescribed at NHS expense to males who have not responded to sildenafil and who have any of the conditions approved by the Department of Health (see the BNF), marking the prescription SLS (selected list scheme), and giving enough (usually) for one treatment 1 week. A private prescription can be issued to any patient who does not come within the Department of Health guidelines.
- Studies have shown that patients often take PDE5 inhibitors incorrectly and that almost half of previous nonresponders respond if the drugs are taken correctly.
- Instruct the patient to:
  a. Take sildenafil or vardenafil 30–60 minutes before intercourse and tadalafil several hours before intercourse.
  b. Avoid excessive food or alcohol, hough absorption is less of a problem with tadalafil.
- Beware the drug interaction with nitrates and nicorandil in those with cardiovascular comorbidity.

Nonresponders

- Patients should use the drug eight times at maximal dosage before being classified as nonresponders.
- Recheck testosterone and prolactin levels in nonresponders. PDE5 inhibitors are less effective in those with low or

low-normal testosterone levels, and there is some evidence of improved response with testosterone replacement.

- *Counselling* may be successful in psychogenic impotence and is appropriate for couples that do not wish to be referred:
  a. See the couple together.
  b. Recommend a manual such as *The Relate Guide to Sex in Loving Relationships* (see earlier box).
  c. Instruct the couple on the sensate focus programme. Instructions can be downloaded at https://counselling-matters.org.uk/sites/counselling-matters/files/SensateFocus.pdf).
  d. Set 'homework' assignments for the couple; these can be tailored to meet specific needs.

Referral

- Refer those not responding for sex therapy via the local family planning clinic or Relate. The outcome is successful in 50% to 80% of cases.
- Refer for relationship counselling those whom you sense have larger relationship or personality problems.
- Refer to a cardiologist before prescribing a PDE5 inhibitor if the male is at high cardiovascular risk from sexual activity.
- Refer to an endocrinologist if hypogonadism is suspected or testosterone replacement is being considered.
- Refer to a urologist those with physical causes, those who have not responded to PDE5 inhibitors or who have contraindications to it, and those with psychological causes that are proving intractable. Possible treatments are:
  a. HRT in those with hypogonadism
  b. Alprostadil as injections into the corpus cavernosum or transurethrally
  c. Vacuum devices
  d. Penile prostheses

> **DETAILS OF THERAPISTS**
>
> British Association for Sexual and Relationship Therapy. Tel: 020 8543 2707. Available at http://www.basrt.org.uk.
> Institute of Psychosexual Medicine. Building 3, Chiswick Park, 566 Chiswick High Road, Chiswick, London, W4 5YA, Tel: 020 7580 0631. Available at http://www.ipm.org.uk.

Lack of Sexual Desire

- This is the commonest presenting female sexual dysfunction (Basson, 2006).
- A low level of sexual desire is usually accompanied by low levels of arousal and sexual excitement and infrequent orgasms and is frequently associated with sexual dissatisfaction.
- Underlying psychological difficulties are frequent. These may relate specifically to sex (e.g., previous sexual abuse), or they may relate to a more widespread psychological disorder. Physical illness and drugs or substances are also possible causes.

- Females specifically lose sexual desire:
  a. Postpartum
  b. Because of pain
  c. When their partner's performance repeatedly leads to frustration, as in premature ejaculation or ED
- In general, psychological interventions and sex therapy are of greater benefit than drugs.
- Check for the presence of depression and anxiety.
- Reassure the patient that sexual desire varies at different times of life and that loss of desire is not necessarily abnormal.
- Enquire whether she wants to improve her sexual desire or whether it is her partner's wish.
- Consider factors that may be contributing (see earlier).
- Recommend the website of the College of Sexual and Relationship Therapists (https://www.cosrt.org.uk), which discusses the problem of lack of desire.
- Offer counselling along the lines described under the section on ED.

Dyspareunia

- This may be primary or secondary to a physical cause, and considerable skill may be needed to unravel the problem (Weijmar et al, 2005).
- Distinguish from the history and examination between:
  a. Lack of lubrication because of lack of interest.
  b. Vaginismus, which usually becomes apparent at vaginal examination (see later).
  c. Vulval or vaginal causes: infections, vulvar vestibulitis syndrome, lichen sclerosus, lichen planus, urethral caruncle, postmenopausal vaginitis, or postepisiotomy syndrome. Those for whom there is no specific treatment may benefit from 5% lidocaine ointment applied 20 minutes before sexual intercourse; they can also be referred to specialist physiotherapists.
  d. Pelvic causes with tenderness on rocking the cervix or palpating the fornices (e.g., endometriosis, pelvic infection, ovarian pathology).
  e. Psychogenic causes, in which vulval burning or pain is caused by somatisation of other difficulties.
- When a physical cause is not found, cognitive-behavioural therapy and selective serotonin reuptake inhibitors have been found to be beneficial.

> **INFORMATION FOR PATIENTS AND THEIR PARTNERS**
>
> Vulval Pain Society. PO Box 7804, Nottingham NG3 5ZQ. Available at http://www.vulvalpainsociety.org.

Vaginismus

- This consists of a phobia of penetration and involuntary spasm of the pubococcygeal and associated muscles surrounding the lower third of the vagina. Such females may avoid having cervical smears and sometimes present with infertility.

- Explore the root cause. It may be:
  a. Fear of the unknown or the patient's ignorance of her own anatomy
  b. A past history of unpleasant experiences such as rape, sexual abuse, or severe emotional trauma or previous dyspareunia
  c. A defence mechanism against growing up and becoming a female adult. (A common pattern is for the patient to live close to her parents, remaining the daughter and marrying an unassertive male.)
- Desensitise simple cases by encouraging the female to examine herself and encourage her to be confident enough to insert a finger into the vagina. Some females may prefer to use vaginal trainers.
- Refer to a sex therapist if this simple approach fails. Hypnotherapy may be helpful (McGuire & Hawton, 2003).

Disorders of Orgasm

Anxiety tends to delay a female's orgasm but accelerates a male's.

Premature Ejaculation

- This is present when ejaculation occurs sooner than either partner would wish, usually before penetration or soon after. Interest in sex may be reduced in both partners (Waldinger, 2007).
- Advise the patient that with practice, he can learn to delay ejaculation. The stop–start technique can be taught by therapists or learnt from the book cited earlier. In essence, when during caressing or during intercourse, a male feels he is close to climax, he should stop being stimulated and relax for 30 seconds. Stimulation can then recommence until he is close to climax again, and the relaxation is repeated. If this fails, the female should squeeze the penis at the base of the glans between her finger and thumb during relaxation phases.
- Paroxetine 20 mg or clomipramine 25 mg each evening are both effective in delaying ejaculation, but are off-label.

Retarded Ejaculation

- This is usually a sign of long-standing sexual inhibition. Often the patient can ejaculate by masturbation but not intravaginally.
- Explore any feelings of anxiety and guilt.
- Start a sensate focus programme (see earlier).
- If 'home therapy' fails, refer for psychosexual counselling.

Orgasmic Problems in Females

- A female who has never achieved an orgasm may have deep-seated psychological reasons for being afraid to let go. She may need 'permission' to investigate her body's own responses further, either by masturbation or vibrator. When she has learnt how to relax, she should be encouraged to tell her partner and incorporate caressing into their usual lovemaking (Meston et al, 2004).

- Females who have lost the ability to achieve orgasm may need counselling, especially about their current relationship or a recent loss of self-image.
- Check that the patient is not taking drugs that inhibit orgasm (e.g., clonidine) and that her failure to achieve orgasm is not from neurologic disease or pelvic surgery. Total hysterectomy does not impair the ability to achieve orgasm (Farrell & Kieser, 2000).

Sexually Transmitted Infections and Human Immunodeficiency Virus

REFERENCE

British Association for Sexual Health and HIV. (2023). *BASHH Summary Guidance on Testing for Sexually Transmitted Infections*. Retrieved from https://www.bashh.org/_userfiles/pages/files/resources/bashh_summary_guidance_on_stis_testing_2023.pdf.

- STIs frequently coexist, so patients diagnosed with one STI generally need further investigation to exclude other infections.
- GUM or sexual health clinics provide full screening, immediate microscopy, and assistance for patients in the treating and informing of partners (partner notification or contact tracing). This is important in limiting the spread of disease, and patients diagnosed with an STI should be routinely referred to a GUM clinic for further management.
- The frequency of testing depends on the individual circumstance:
  - At the start of a long-term mutually exclusive relationship
  - Annually and then after each partner change for those who are sexually active and in relationships which are not long-term or exclusive
  - Every 3 months for those at high risk of STIs (including >10 partners/year, preexposure prophylaxis users, those having multiple or anonymous partners, and those with sexualised drug use)
- Late diagnosis of HIV is a major cause of avoidable death in infected individuals, and GPs have an important role in making earlier diagnoses, which improves prognosis and can limit ongoing transmission.

Patients Requiring Investigation by a General Practitioner

a. Those who are eligible for a local or national screening programme (e.g., for chlamydia)
b. Those who require treatment urgently and cannot attend a GUM clinic immediately (e.g., symptomatic PID out of hours)
c. Those who are unwilling or unable to attend a GUM clinic after discussion and recommendation, and require testing for STIs or HIV

d. Those presenting with a possible STI-related problem in a primary care setting which has training and experience in managing STIs, including partner notification (e.g., through locally enhanced service schemes or GPs with a special interest)

Patients Requiring Management by a General Practitioner

a. Those who have tested positive for an STI at the surgery and wish to be managed in primary care or cannot attend GUM clinic immediately
b. Those who present as contacts of an STI and decline to attend a GUM clinic for testing, treatment, and partner notification advice after discussion and recommendation of this course of action

Contact Tracing (Partner Notification)

- This is usually best done by GUM clinic or at least with their support and advice.
- As a minimum, screening of all contacts of acute STIs over the previous 3 months should be attempted. For syphilis and HIV, there is no arbitrary limit, and partner notification will depend on who is contactable, and the earliest likely time of infection.
- If the patient is diagnosed with nonspecific urethritis, chlamydia, syphilis, *Trichomonas vaginalis* infection, or gonorrhoea, the partner should be treated even if test results are negative.

Principles of Treatment

- Give appropriate antibiotics, bearing in mind any recent travel history.
- Advise complete abstinence from all sexual contacts until both the patient and partner are treated.
- Follow up after completion of antibiotics for compliance and possibly retesting (which is indicated only in pregnancy or when symptoms persist).

Workup for Cases to Be Managed in Primary Care

- Take a full sexual history, focusing on the previous two partners (irrespective of time interval) or all partners in the previous 3 months (if more than two).
- Current practice is moving towards testing asymptomatic individuals without examination and reserving examination for those who are symptomatic.
- When examination is indicated, examine the genitalia for discharge, ulcers, and warts (including the vagina and cervix in females) and the mouth for ulcers and perform proctoscopy if there are anal symptoms or a history of anal intercourse.

Diagnostic Tests in Females
- *Gonorrhoea:* cervical and urethral swabs; also oropharyngeal and rectal swabs if symptomatic at those sites, if a partner has gonorrhoea, or if suggested by the sexual history.

- *Chlamydia:* endocervical chlamydia swab (rotate well) (unless first-catch urine or self-taken vulvovaginal swab is being used for screening).
- T. vaginalis, *bacterial vaginosis, and* Candida *spp.:* high vaginal swabs may detect candidal infection but are only useful in the diagnosis of *T. vaginalis* if inoculated into a trichomonal culture medium. Swabs without immediate microscopy are of limited use for diagnosing bacterial vaginosis.
- Check that cervical smears are up to date.

Diagnostic Tests in Males
- *Gonorrhoea and chlamydia:* urethral swabs (insert 1–4 cm and rotate) and a slide for the laboratory if there will be a delay in swab transport. Oral and rectal swabs may be indicated by the sexual history.

Tests to Be Done in All Patients Suspected of Having Sexually Transmitted Infections
- Check syphilis serology and repeat it 3 months after exposure if there has been a significant risk.
- Check hepatitis B serology in patients who have been exposed in countries with high incidence, if a sexual partner comes from an endemic area, in homosexual males, and when the patient and partner have a history of injecting drug use. Consider the need for immediate hepatitis B immunisation.
- Discuss and offer HIV testing to all patients. Where a patient does not wish to attend a GUM clinic, consideration should be given to testing in primary care.

Specific Management of Sexually Transmitted Infections

> **GUIDELINE AND REVIEW**
>
> British Association for Sexual Health and HIV. *National guideline on the management of* Trichomonas vaginalis. Retrieved from http://www.bashh.org (search on 'Guidelines')

See also entries on PID, bacterial vaginosis, and candidiasis.

Gonorrhoea

Genital Gonorrhoea (Uncomplicated)
- Gonorrhoea is strongly concentrated among individuals with high-risk sexual behaviours and their partners. Referral to or, at the least, advice from GUM is therefore strongly recommended, and screening for other STIs should be routinely undertaken.
- Antibiotic resistance patterns are changing rapidly, and it is advisable to check with the GUM clinic for current recommendations.
- One of the following:
  - Ceftriaxone 1 g IM as a single dose with 2 g of azithromycin oral as a single dose

- Cefixime 400 mg oral as a single dose with 2 g of azithromycin oral as a single dose
- Spectinomycin 2 g IM as a single dose with 2 g of azithromycin oral as a single dose
- Treat all patients for chlamydia infection. The coinfection rate is 40%.
- Seek advice for all pregnant females.
- Treat those with HIV the same as those without.
- Trace and treat contacts over the previous 3 months.
- Follow up at least once to confirm compliance, resolution of symptoms, and partner notification. Test of cure is advised.

Chlamydia Infection (Uncomplicated)

- Nucleic acid amplification tests (NAATs) are now standard for swab or urine samples. Their sensitivity is greater than 95%.
- Treatment and partner notification should be undertaken on strong suspicion (e.g., mucopurulent cervicitis or PID) before the result is back. Endocervical swabs should be rotated firmly, and male urethral swabs should be rotated 1 to 4 cm inside the urethra.
- Give one of the following:
  a. Doxycycline 100 mg bd for 7 days; or
  b. Azithromycin 1 g as a single oral dose then 500 mg once daily for 2 days; or
  c. Alternative regimens if both of the above are contraindicated. One of the following:
  Erythromycin 500 mg bd for 14 days
  Ofloxacin 200 mg bd or 400 mg od for 7 days
- In pregnancy, give one of the following along with a test of cure performed 3 weeks after completing therapy:
  a. Azithromycin 1 g as a single oral dose; then 500 mg once daily for 2 days
  b. Erythromycin 500 mg bd for 14 days or 500 mg qds (four times daily) for 7 days
  c. Amoxicillin 500 mg tds (three times daily) for 7 days
- Patients should be referred to a GUM clinic to discuss partner notification with a trained health adviser. The UK chlamydia pilots suggest that this is acceptable to patients diagnosed in primary care. A cut-off for 4 weeks is used for symptomatic males. For all others, the look-back should be for 6 months or to the last partner (whichever is the longer).

Screening for Chlamydia *Infection*

- A screening programme for genital chlamydia has been implemented in England aimed at covering 17% of people younger than 25 years old every year (NHS, 2009).
- Screening is particularly important for:
  - Females seeking TOP and their partners
  - Sexually active females and males younger than 25 years old, especially teenagers
  - Males and females aged 25 years and older with a new sexual partner or two or more partners in 1 year

- Offer screening with an endocervical swab because it is slightly more sensitive and stable but agree to urine testing (where available) by a NAAT if the female patient prefers it.
- Repeat the screen if the female patient changes her partner.

Nonspecific Urethritis

- Test all patients who have urethritis for gonorrhoea and chlamydia.
- The most commonly implicated organisms are *Chlamydia trachomatis and Mycoplasma genitalium*; however, these are not detected in up to 80% of cases.
- First-line treatment, if test results for chlamydia and gonorrhoea are negative, is doxycycline 100 mg twice a day for 7 days. Alternative regimens are azithromycin 1 g orally stat; then 500 mg od (once daily) for 2 days, or ofloxacin either 200 mg bd or 400 mg od for 7 days. Follow up at 2 weeks. For symptomatic patients, all partners during the previous 4 weeks should be treated, and treatment of the regular partner is recommended in all cases.
- Patients should abstain from sexual intercourse until they and their sexual partner have completed treatment.
- Refer unresolving cases and all cases in which you are unable to complete partner notification to a GUM clinic. Some males have recurring urethritis because of noninfectious causes, in these cases, specialist advice and diagnostics followed by reassurance are important.

Trichomonas Vaginalis

- *T. vaginalis* infection is almost exclusively sexually transmitted through urethral or vaginal inoculation. It is sometimes diagnosed on cervical cytology, with which there is a false-positive rate of about 30%, so tests should be repeated.
- *Trichomonas* infection is strongly associated with other STIs, and full screening should be undertaken.
- Metronidazole 400 mg bd for 5 to 7 days clears 95% of infections. An alternative regimen is metronidazole 2 g orally stat. There is an increased risk of treatment failure with the stat dose (Howe & Kissinger, 2017), and it is more likely to be associated with adverse effects (Forna & Gulmezoglu, 2000). Test of cure is required only if symptoms persist, in which case the patient should attend a GUM clinic. Alcohol should be avoided during and for 48 hours after treatment.
- Symptomatic disease in early pregnancy can be controlled with clotrimazole pessaries 100 mg/day for 7 days or Aci Gel [AciGel] before systemic treatment with metronidazole 400 mg bd for 7 days in the second trimester.
- Current partners should be screened for STIs.

Anogenital Warts

- Most anogenital warts cause minor irritation or are simply cosmetic. However, they cause a good deal of psychological distress. Patients should be given an explanation of their condition, emphasising that the majority of anogenital warts are caused by HPV types 6 and 11, which are not associated with cervical neoplasia.

- Many carriers of HPV have no visible lesions.
- Condom use may prevent transmission of warts to uninfected partners. Their use with regular partners, however, has not been shown to affect the outcome of treatment in patients with visible warts.
- Perianal warts are associated with anal sex (although they can occur without) and should suggest the need for anorectal samples for other STIs and GUM referral.
- None of the existing treatments is satisfactory, and all have high recurrence rates. Patients should be made aware of this. The evidence base for distinguishing first- and second-line treatments is weak. Smokers may respond less well than nonsmokers.
- *Pregnancy*: Pregnant females can be treated using cryotherapy, trichloroacetic acid, or other ablative therapies in a specialist setting. However, warts often worsen during pregnancy and improve afterwards. The risk of transmitting warts or laryngeal papillomata to neonates is small, and caesarean section is indicated only in rare cases of giant vulval warts or gross cervical warts.

Soft, Nonkeratinised Warts

- Prescribe podophyllotoxin 0.5% (twice daily for 3 consecutive days, repeated weekly for up to a total maximum of 5 weeks). Patients using podophyllotoxin at home must take great care to follow the instructions to avoid chemical burns. It should not be used in pregnancy and is not licensed for extragenital lesions, such as anal warts.
- Imiquimod 5% cream is an immune response modifier which can be used three times weekly for up to 16 weeks. It should not be used in pregnancy.

Keratinised Warts

- Use ablative therapy such as cryotherapy, which is available at GUM clinics.

Genital Herpes

- New diagnoses of primary herpes may be caused by HSV type 1 or type 2. After childhood, HSV type 1 is equally likely to be acquired in the genital or oral areas (Langenberg et al, 1999).
- Many cases of genital herpes are caused by orogenital contact and can therefore occur in patients who may not consider themselves 'sexually active'.
- Primary herpes is often asymptomatic, and patients often present many years later with symptoms, which are caused by recurrence.
- Autoinoculation (e.g., from labial herpes) can only occur during primary episodes. Patients who have developed herpes for the first time but had no recent sexual contact should be referred to a consultant in GUM who will be familiar with such cases and able to advise patients at a time of considerable distress and uncertainty.

- Genital herpes can be acquired from asymptomatic partners, sometimes in a long-term relationship. Some patients never develop symptoms, although those with HSV type2 usually develop symptoms at some point (Langenberg et al, 1999).
- Initial episodes are typically far more severe and of longer duration than recurrences. Recurrences tend to decrease over time but are more frequent with HSV type 2 (Benedetti, Zeh, &Corey 1999).
- Diagnosis is by culture or polymerase chain reaction testing and typing of the virus using a swab from the base of an ulcer, sent rapidly to the laboratory in special transport media.
- In primary episodes, patients can benefit from practical counselling in relation to the natural history and issues in relationships (including risk to the partner). This can be provided at the GUM clinic. Psychological stress does not increase recurrences (Green & Kocsis, 1997).
- Partner notification is guided by the individual case and history of symptoms in the partner. Health advisers in the GUM clinic are experienced in this issue and can help with this.

Management of a First Symptomatic Episode

- *Oral antiviral therapy*, commenced within 5 days of the episode or while new lesions are forming, reduces the severity and duration of the first episode. Options are acyclovir 400 mg three times daily or valaciclovir 500 mg bd, both for 5 days (preferred). Alternatives include acyclovir 200 mg five times daily or famciclovir 250 mg three times daily, both for 5 days.
- *Offer analgesia* and recommend saline bathing. Topical anaesthetics can be used, although they occasionally cause sensitisation. It may be easier to pass urine in a tepid bath.
- *Admit* patients with urinary retention, meningism, or severe systemic symptoms.
- *Offer counselling*, including a discussion of the risk of asymptomatic shedding and its implications for relationships and the need to inform healthcare workers in the case of later pregnancy. Health advisers at the GUM clinic are experienced in this area.

All above options may be extended beyond 5 days if new lesions appear or healing is incomplete.

Management of Recurrences

- Most recurrences cause minor symptoms of a few days' duration.
- Severe recurrences may be shortened by oral antiviral agents as discussed earlier. There is no evidence that topical antiviral creams are effective. Saline bathing, Vaseline, or lidocaine gel may aid symptoms.
- *Episodic antiviral treatment* may reduce episodes by a median of 1 to 2 days. Patient-initiated courses with standby prescriptions is most effective because of early treatment. See BNF for regimens.
- *Suppressive therapy*. Depending on patient preference, relationship status, and severity of symptoms, it may be

appropriate to offer systemic antiviral treatment to reduce the duration and severity of attacks and frequency. This can reduce anxiety, help in adjustment, and improve quality of life, usually in patients with six or more recurrences a year. Suppressive therapy should be undertaken for a defined period of time before review and is best undertaken by or in collaboration with the GUM clinic. See BNF for regimens.

> **PATIENT SUPPORT GROUP**
>
> The Herpes Viruses Association. 41 North Road, London N7 9DP. Tel: 0845 123 2305. info@herpes.org.uk. Available at http://www.herpes.org.uk.

Syphilis

- Like gonorrhoea, syphilis is concentrated among individuals at high behavioural risk and their partners, and untreated syphilis also has major long-term sequelae.
- Patients with suspected or diagnosed syphilis must be referred to the GUM clinic, where further investigation, treatment, and partner notification will be undertaken.
- Long-term partner notification is required, and these patients may be at very high risk for other STIs and bloodborne viruses.

Human Immunodeficiency Virus and Acquired Immunodeficiency Virus

Prevention and Early Diagnosis

- Prevention of HIV is an essential part of contraceptive care, travel care, and well-person clinics. Testing for HIV should now be universally offered as part of antenatal care, so that females avoid vertical transmission and access services.

Advising on Safer Sex and Avoiding High-Risk Activities

- Hugging, kissing, and mutual masturbation are safe.
- HIV has been transmitted through oral sex, but this is rare. A condom can be used for receptive oral sex to improve protection. Condoms can be lubricated with KY Jelly or similar lubricants but *not* oils or Vaseline, which reduce their strength by 95%.
- High-risk sexual activities include penetrative vaginal or anal sex without a condom.
- Other high-risk activities include sharing needles or syringes for intravenous drug use.
- Sex with local residents in high-prevalence areas of the world (e.g., Africa, Thailand, parts of South America) or with people otherwise at high risk (e.g., males who have sex with males (MSMs)) increases the risks in the event of condom breakage or unprotected sex.
- By the end of 2015, an estimated 101,200 people were living with HIV in the United Kingdom, of whom 13%

remained unaware of their infection. HIV incidence is increasing among MSMs. In 2015, 2800 MSMs were diagnosed with HIV in the United Kingdom, of whom most probably became infected in the United Kingdom. In 2015, there were 2360 cases of new heterosexually acquired HIV, and this was the first year since the 1990s that the number of new heterosexual diagnoses of people born within the United Kingdom exceeded the number of those born outside the United Kingdom.

- MSMs, migrants from countries with high HIV incidence, and injecting drug users remain the populations at greatest risk of HIV infection.
- A high proportion of deaths are now avoidable and attributable to late diagnosis, and early diagnosis is now recognised as a mainstay both of transmission prevention and of clinical care.
- HIV testing is now recommended on GP registration in high-prevalence areas and for a range of 'indicator diseases' in which HIV is much more likely than in the general population. These indicator diseases include all STIs, as well as many other conditions likely to present to GPs, such as severe psoriasis or seborrhoeic dermatitis, chronic diarrhoea, unexplained weight loss or lymphadenopathy, bacterial pneumonia, recurrent herpes zoster, unexplained blood dyscrasia, peripheral neuropathy, pyrexia of unknown origin, aseptic meningitis, mononucleosis-like syndrome, and dementia (British Association for HIV, British Association for Sexual Health and HIV, & British Infection Society, 2008).

Note regarding insurance reports: The British Medical Association and Royal College of General Practitioners advise doctors *not* to answer the lifestyle questions on insurance reports even with consent. These questions allocate a person to an at-risk group, which is discriminatory, but only high-risk behaviour is relevant.

The Human Immunodeficiency Virus Antibody Test

- The HIV test is 99.9% sensitive and specific 3 months after exposure to the virus (Sloand et al, 1991), although the 'window period' before becoming positive can occasionally be longer (e.g., after postexposure antiretroviral prophylaxis).
- If HIV primary infection is suspected, P24 antigen and plasma proviral DNA or HIV RNA testing may be appropriate because the prognosis may be improved by antiretroviral therapy at this time. GUM specialist advice should be sought.
- A positive antibody test result should be repeated to exclude identification errors.

Human Immunodeficiency Virus Testing

- HIV testing is now more accepted as part of good clinical care and in the United Kingdom is offered to all pregnant females and patients with TB. Primary care practitioners and emergency departments are now encouraged to undertake HIV testing, particularly when it is unlikely to occur in another setting or where the prevalence is high.

- Patients who do not wish to have the result recorded in their primary care notes should be referred to the GUM clinic.
- The patient should understand that having the test is entirely voluntary.
- Written information about the test and its pros and cons is available at http://www.tht.org.uk (choose 'HIV Testing').

Pretest Discussion

- Patients should have an HIV test only with their informed consent and normally need to come back in person for the result.
- Issues to be covered in pretest discussion for HIV include:
  a. The difference between HIV infection and AIDS, how the virus is transmitted, and whether the patient has any misapprehensions.
  b. The latency between transmission and seroconversion. Ensure that the patient is not in the 3-month 'window period' (occasionally longer). If so, discuss the need to postpone or repeat the test.
  c. The importance of screening for other STIs and of making plans for safer sex whatever the test result.

  Advantages of the Test
  1. Effective therapies are available which extend life expectancy to near normal.
  2. Knowing the result means that partners can be protected if the result is positive or make decision to move to safer sex if negative.
  3. Decisions about pregnancy can be made.
  4. Anxiety caused by uncertainty about HIV status is ended.
  5. Informed decisions about medical issues, such as live vaccines, can be made.

  Other Considerations
  1. If the result is positive, the patient will need to cope with a difficult diagnosis. They need to consider whom to tell.
  2. A positive (but not a negative) result may affect insurance and possibly employment prospects.

Posttest Discussion

Negative Results
- Discuss any concerns that have given rise to the test and how the patient plans to protect themselves in future. Discuss the window period and whether further testing will be needed for full reassurance.

Positive Results
- Ensure that you have time and there will be no interruptions to the interview. Tell the patient early in the interview to allow time for reflection and questions.
- Establish what the patient knows and expects to happen and ensure that they understand the difference between HIV infection and AIDS. Ensure the patient understands that there are now many very effective therapies that dramatically improve prognosis.

- Explain that the virus is not passed on by normal domestic or work contact.
- Refer to a specialist clinic, which may be the GUM service or the infectious diseases unit, for specialist follow-up and support. Clinics will fit in a newly diagnosed patient urgently.
- Discuss and advise on concerns about transmission to others (see 'Advising on Safer Sex and Avoiding High-Risk Activities') and the need for protected sex.
- Find out what the patient's plans are for the rest of the day and ensure that they arrange to meet someone for support.
- Arrange to see the patient again in a few days. Do not overload with information and issues at this initial interview.
- Give information on patient helplines.

PATIENT INFORMATION

Terrence Higgins Trust. 314-320 Gray's Inn Road, London, WC1X 8DP. Tel: 080 8802 1221. Available at http://www.tht.org.uk.

The National AIDS Helpline (NAH) on 0800 567 123 for free and confidential advice and information about HIV/AIDS, other sexually transmitted infections, and sexual health matters. A 24-hour, 7 days a week telephone service, NAH can also give details about local services, including sexual health clinics and support agencies for people with HIV/AIDS and their partners, families, and friends.

Managing Patients with Human Papillomavirus in the Community

GUIDELINE

BHIVA (British HIV Association). (2023 interim update). *BHIVA guidelines on antiretroviral treatment for adults living with HIV-1 2022.* https://www.bhiva.org/HIV-1-treatment-guidelines.

- In the past few years, communication between specialist HIV clinicians and primary care has improved, and patients are often managed in collaboration. This allows GPs to gain experience in the condition while encouraging patients to access care for unrelated conditions and to use out of hours care and community nursing appropriately.
- Following publication of the Standards for HIV Clinical Care (BHIVA, RCP, BASHH, BIS, 2009), there has been an emphasis on provision of HIV care within a managed service network, which will be expected to support primary care and others in providing nonspecialist HIV services.

Routine Care

- All HIV-positive patients should be offered the chance to start ART within 2 to 4 weeks of diagnosis.
- The aim is to suppress the viral load to less than 50 copies/mL.

- Syphilis serology, baseline hepatitis B and C serology, full blood count, and liver function tests should be repeated yearly. Cytomegalovirus (CMV) antibodies and toxoplasma antibodies should be assessed at baseline.
- Lipids, blood sugar, calcium and phosphate, and possibly other monitoring tests are needed if the patient is on therapy. Females should have yearly cervical smears because of the increased incidence of carcinoma.
- Advise patients which symptoms should be treated seriously, including fever, weight loss, diarrhoea, lymphadenopathy, shortness of breath or cough, paraesthesiae, headache, mouth ulceration, and visual disturbances.
- Avoid bacille Calmette–Guerin and yellow fever vaccines. Seek specialist advice for other live vaccines but otherwise vaccinate as usual. Hepatitis B vaccination should be offered if the patient is seronegative.
- Advise the patient to avoid exposure to toxoplasmosis (uncooked meat and unwashed salads) and to *Cryptosporidium* if they are severely immunosuppressed (unboiled tap water).
- Encourage patients with a CD4 count less than 200 Cells/mm^3 to take prophylaxis against *Pneumocystis carinii* pneumonia (PCP) in the form of co-trimoxazole 960 mg/day or thrice weekly, dapsone 100 mg/day, or nebulised pentamidine 300 mg every 4 weeks.
- Ensure the patient has adequate psychological support in adjusting to their diagnosis.
- The issue of pregnancy and contraception, together with safe sex, needs to be discussed with females on an ongoing basis. Effective interventions are now available which can reduce the risk of transmission to the baby to less than 1%. Specialist advice should be sought at an early stage.
- Risk reduction in relation to sexual partners needs to be regularly reviewed. Transmission of HIV to uninfected partners or transmission of resistant strains is possible, and safe sex must be practised.

Symptoms Needing Special Consideration

- *Cough*, especially dry cough with breathlessness in a patient with minimal chest signs, and (initially) a normal chest radiograph can indicate PCP. This requires urgent specialist care. Patients are also at increased risk of community-acquired pneumonia, TB, and bacterial chest infection.
- *Headaches* can suggest cerebral toxoplasmosis; non-Hodgkin lymphoma; tuberculoma; or, importantly, cryptococcal meningitis, which may *not* be accompanied by neck stiffness or headache.
- *Diarrhoea* can indicate opportunistic bowel infection, including *Cryptosporidium* or *Microsporidium*, although often no cause is found, and symptomatic treatment is required.
- *Dysphagia* can indicate oesophageal candidiasis, treatable with fluconazole 100 mg od for 14 to 21 days or (in the severely immunocompromised) CMV ulceration.
- *Visual disturbances,* including flashes and floaters, can suggest CMV retinitis. This should be referred urgently.

Venepuncture

- The same universal precautions should be taken as with patients of unknown serostatus (gloves, avoid resheathing needles, place in appropriately sealed packaging, and transport in safe containers). Avoidance of resheathing needles should be standard practice.
- Some laboratories require 'high-risk' stickers. This depends on local policy. 'High risk' does not require stating the diagnosis of HIV for transport purposes, which is unnecessary for routine tests and can generally be avoided in other cases. This practice is an unnecessary risk to patient confidentiality.
- Spills should be mopped up with hypochlorite (10 parts water to 1 part household bleach) or undiluted Milton.

Postexposure Prophylaxis for Healthcare Workers (Including Needlestick Injuries)

> **GUIDELINE**
>
> Department of Health. (2008). *HIV post-exposure prophylaxis: Guidance from the UK Chief Medical Officer's Expert Advisory Group on AIDS.* Retrieved from https://www.gov.uk/government/uploads/system/uploads/attachment_data/file/203139/HIV_post-exposure_prophylaxis.pdf.

- The risk of acquiring HIV infection after percutaneous exposure to HIV-infected blood is on average around 3 per 1000 and less than 1 in 1000 after mucocutaneous exposure.
- The risk is increased in cases of deep injury, visible blood on the device causing the injury, a needle which had entered an artery or vein, or terminal illness in the source patient.
- An 80% reduction in the transmission rate can be achieved by appropriate prophylaxis, and all districts should have an arrangement for 24-hour access to such supplies for exposed healthcare workers.
- The risk of acquiring hepatitis is, in most parts of the world, greater than that of HIV.

Management

- After *any* exposure to blood (whether or not the source patient is known to be HIV or hepatitis B or C positive), wash the wound liberally with soap and water but do not scrub. Antiseptics should not be used.
- Telephone for advice on local arrangements for 24-hour access to HIV prophylaxis and specialist advice on risk assessment, based on the nature of the exposure, the risk posed by the source, and the immune status of the contact. The local consultant in communicable disease control (via the Public Health Department), consultant microbiologist or virologist, or consultant in genitourinary medicine will be able to advise if you do not have information to hand. Drug starter packs are usually held at the local accident and emergency department.

- Take blood for baseline HIV and hepatitis B and C serology.
- If the risk is assessed as potentially significant, antiretroviral drugs should be commenced as soon as possible, preferably within 1 hour. Medication should be continued for a total of 4 weeks if subsequent risk assessment confirms this is appropriate. The contents of starter packs are under constant review.
- Unless the source is already known to be negative for hepatitis B, or the contact known to be fully immunised, give active immunisation against hepatitis B. Passive immunisation with hepatitis B immunoglobulin (HBIG) can be given within 48 hours but may still be worthwhile up to 7 days after exposure. However, HBIG is expensive, in short supply, and only available for immunocompromised or pregnant patients exposed to known hepatitis B. Patients already immunised against hepatitis B need a booster of active immunisation.
- If the source patient is of unknown status, they should routinely be approached (by someone other than the exposed patient) to ask for consent for testing.
- Arrange follow-up, by occupational health, the GUM department, or another appropriate department, for the exposed worker to consider testing for HIV and hepatitis B and C in confidence at a later stage.

Summary of Postexposure Prophylaxis
1. Clean the wound.
2. Get advice. If significant risk exists, offer
   a. Antiretroviral drugs within 1 hour
   b. Active immunisation with hepatitis B vaccine
   c. Passive immunisation with HBIG if donor is hepatitis B virus positive and recipient immunocompromised or pregnant
3. Take blood for baseline serology of contact and source (with consent).
4. Arrange follow-up

Further Reading

BHIVA guidelines on antiretroviral treatment for adults living with HIV-1 2022 (2023 interim update). Retrieved from https://www.bhiva.org/HIV-1-treatment-guidelines.

British Association for Sexual Health and HIV. (2023). *Summary guidance on testing for sexually transmitted infections*. British Ass for Sex Health & HIV 2023. https://www.bashh.org/_userfiles/pages/files/resources/bashh_summary_guidance_on_stis_testing_2023.pdf

Clinical Effectiveness Unit. (2003). Desogestrel-only pill (Cerazette). *The Journal of Family Planning and Reproductive Health Care, 29*, 162–164.

Clinical Effectiveness Unit. (2007a). *Male and female condoms*. London: Faculty of Family Planning & Reproductive Healthcare.

Clinical Effectiveness Unit. (2007b). *Female barrier methods*. London: Faculty of Family Planning & Reproductive Healthcare.

Clinical Effectiveness Unit. (2008b). *Progestogen-only injectable contraception*. London: Faculty of Sexual & Reproductive Healthcare.

Clinical Effectiveness Unit. (2008c). *Progestogen-only implants*. London: Faculty of Sexual & Reproductive Healthcare.

Postexposure Prophylaxis Following Sexual or other Nonoccupational Exposure

- Postexposure prophylaxis for HIV may be required after sexual exposure. Examples may include some cases of sexual assault and condom failure between HIV-discordant couples or unprotected anal sex in MSMs. In these circumstances, prophylaxis against hepatitis B should also be considered.
- Policies and regimens for HIV postexposure prophylaxis, including indications for use after sexual exposure, can be found on the BASHH's website (http://www.bashh.org/documents/58/58.pdf). The consultant at the local GUM clinic should be able to give immediate advice and assist in risk assessment. Prophylaxis, if required, should be started as soon as possible and certainly within 72 hours.

Notification and Surveillance

Microbiology laboratories voluntarily notify positive HIV results (confidentially and anonymously) to the Communicable Disease Surveillance Centre, Centre for Infections, 61 Colindale Avenue, London NW9 5EQ, or Health Protection Scotland (http://www.hps.scot.nhs.uk). These establishments then write to the clinician concerned asking for further clinical details.

- Doctors may also notify cases directly. If the patient has not been referred on for further specialist management, the GP who receives a positive test result may be invited to provide information for the voluntary, confidential, anonymised database.
- Details of HIV and AIDS surveillance, together with recent data, can be seen at http://www.gov.uk.

Clinical Effectiveness Unit. (2016a). *UK Medical Eligibility Criteria*. London: Faculty of Sexual and Reproductive Healthcare.

Clinical Effectiveness Unit. (2016b). *Postnatal sexual and reproductive health*. London: Faculty of Sexual and Reproductive Healthcare.

Clinical Effectiveness Unit. (2017). *FSRH guideline: Emergency contraception*. London: Faculty of Sexual & Reproductive Healthcare. Retrieved from http://www.fsrh.org.

Department of Health. (2003). Online. Retrieved from http://www.doh.gov.uk (search on 'Keep Safe').

FSRH Guideline (January 2019, amended October 2023) Combined hormonal contraception. (2019). *BMJ Sexual & Reproductive Health, 45*(Suppl. 1). http://dx.doi.org/10.1136/bmjsrh-2018-CHC.

FSRH Guideline (August 2022) Progestogen-only pills. (2022). *BMJ Sexual & Reproductive Health, 48*(Suppl. 1). Retrieved from http://dx.doi.org/10.1136/bmjsrh-2022-PoP.

Gallo, M. F., Grimes, D. A., Lopez, L. M., & Schulz, K. F. (2006). Non-latex versus latex male condoms for contraception. *The Cochrane Database of Systematic Reviews*, (1), CD003550.

Glasier, A. F., Cameron, S. T., Fine, P. M., Logan, S. J., Casale, W., Van Horn, J., Sogor, L., Blithe, D. L., Scherrer, B., Mathe, H.,

Jaspart, A., Ulmann, A., & Gainer, E. (2010). Ulipristal acetate versus levonorgestrel for emergency contraception: A randomised non-inferiority trial and meta-analysis. *Lancet, 375*, 555–562.

Grimes, D. A., & Schulz, K. F. (1999). Antibiotic prophylaxis for intrauterine contraceptive device insertion. *Cochrane Database of Systematic Reviews, (3)*, CD001327.

MacGregor, E. A. (2007). Migraine and use of combined hormonal contraceptives: A clinical review. *The Journal of Family Planning and Reproductive Health Care, 33*, 159–169.

Mansour, D., Korver, T., Marintcheva-Petrova, M., & Fraser, I. S. (2008). The effects of Implanon® on menstrual bleeding patterns. *The European Journal of Contraception & Reproductive Health Care, 13*(Suppl. 1), 13–28.

Marchbanks, P. A., McDonald, J. A., Wilson, H. G., Folger, S. G., Mandel, M. G., Daling, J. R., Bernstein, L., Malone, K. E., Ursin, G., Strom, B. L., Norman, S. A., Wingo, P. A., Burkman, R. T., Berlin, J. A., Simon, M. S., Spirtas, R., & Weiss, L. K. (2002). Oral contraceptives and the risk of breast cancer. *NEJM, 346*, 2025–2032.

Narla, A., Kaiser, K., & Tannock, L. R. (2018). Extremely low testosterone due to relative energy deficiency in sport: A case report. *AACE Clinical Case Reports, 5*(2), e129–e131.

National Institute for Health and Care Excellence. (2023). *CKS erectile dysfunction*. NIfor HaCE 2023. https://cks.nice.org.uk/topics/erectile-dysfunction/.

von Hertzen, H., Piaggio, G., Ding, J., Chen, J., Song, S., Bártfai, G., Ng, E., Gemzell-Danielsson, K., Oyunbileg, A., Wu, S., Cheng, W., Lüdicke, F., Pretnar-Darovec, A., Kirkman, R., Mittal, S., Khomassuridze, A., Apter, D., Peregoudov, A., & WHO Research Group on Post-ovulatory Methods of Fertility Regulation (2002). Low dose mifepristone and two regimens of levonorgestrel for emergency contraception: A WHO multicentre randomised trial. *Lancet (London, England), 360*(9348), 1803–1810.

Wingo, P. A., Austin, H., Marchbanks, P. A., Whiteman, M. K., Hsia, J., Mandel, M. G., Peterson, H. B., & Ory, H. W. (2007). Oral contraceptives and the risk of death from breast cancer. *Obstetrics and Gynecology, 110*(4), 793–800.

References

Ahrendt, H. J., Nisand, I., Bastianelli, C., Gómez, M. A., Gemzell-Danielsson, K., Urdl, W., Karskov, B., Oeyen, L., Bitzer, J., Page, G., & Milsom, I. (2006). Efficacy, acceptability and tolerability of the combined contraceptive ring, NuvaRing, compared with an oral contraceptive containing 30 microg of ethinyl estradiol and 3 mg of drospirenone. *Contraception, 74*(6), 451–457.

Anonymous (1999) Medicines Commission, 1999. Combined oral contraceptives containing desogestrel or gestodene and the risk of venous thromboembolism. *Current Problems in Pharmacovigilance*, 25, p.12.

Anonymous. (2004a). *Best practice guidance for doctors and other health professionals on the provision of advice and treatment to young people under 16 on contraception, sexual and reproductive health.* London: Department of Health.

Anonymous. (2004b). *Male and female sterilisation. Evidence-based guideline no. 4* (2nd ed.). London: Royal College of Obstetricians & Gynaecologists.

Anonymous. (2004c). *The care of women requesting induced abortion. Evidence-based guideline no. 7* (2nd ed.). London: Royal College of Obstetricians & Gynaecologists.

Anonymous. (2005). *Selected practice recommendations for contraceptive use* (2nd ed.). Geneva: World Health Organization.

Archer, D. F. (2006). Menstrual-cycle-related symptoms: A review of the rationale for continuous use of oral contraceptives. *Contraception, 74*, 359–366.

Arowojolu, A. O., Gallo, M. F., Grimes, D. A., & Garner, S. E. (2009). Combined oral contraceptive pills for treatment of acne. *Cochrane Database of Systematic Reviews, (7)*, CD004425.

Basson, R. (2006). Sexual desire and arousal disorders in women. *NEJM, 354*, 1497–1506.

Benedetti, J. K., Zeh, J., & Corey, L. (1999). Clinical reactivation of genital herpes simplex infection decreases in frequency over time. *Annals of Internal Medicine, 131*, 14–20.

BHIVA, BASHH, BIA, BPS, CHIVA, DHIVA, FPH, HPA, HIVPA, LGA, NHIVNA, RHIVA, RCGP, RCN, RCP & SCIE (2013). *Standards of Care for people living with HIV*. https://www.bhiva.org/file/ZAjcrEFgMNHkz/BHIVAStandardsA5.pdf

Bjarnadóttir, R. I., Tuppurainen, M., & Killick, S. R. (2002). Comparison of cycle control with a combined contraceptive vaginal ring and oral levonorgestrel/ethinyl estradiol. *American Journal of Obstetrics and Gynecology, 186*(3), 389–395.

Bonnar, J., Flynn, A., Freundl, G., Kirkman, R., Royston, R., & Snowden, R. (1999). Personal hormone monitoring for contraception. *The British Journal of Family Planning, 24*(4), 128–134.

Brechin, S., & Bigrigg, A. (2006). Male and female sterilisation. *Current Obstetrics and Gynaecology, 16*, 39–46.

Brechin, S., & Penney, G. C. (2004). *Venous thromboembolism and hormonal contraception. Guideline no. 40* (pp. 1–13). London: Royal College of Obstetricians & Gynaecologists.

British Association for HIV, British Association for Sexual Health and HIV, British Infection Society. (2008). *UK national guidelines for HIV testing*. British Ass for HIV 2008.

Canto De Cetina, T. E., Canto, P., & Ordoñez Luna, M. (2001). Effect of counseling to improve compliance in Mexican women receiving depot-medroxyprogesterone acetate. *Contraception, 63*(3), 143–146.

Chan, W. S., Ray, J., Wai, E. K., Ginsburg, S., Hannah, M. E., Corey, P. N., & Ginsberg, J. S. (2004). Risk of stroke in women exposed to low-dose oral contraceptives: A critical evaluation of the evidence. *Archives of Internal Medicine, 164*(7), 741–747.

Charles, V. E., Polis, C. B., Sridhara, S. K., & Blum, R. W. (2008). Abortion and long-term mental health outcomes: A systematic review of the evidence. *Contraception, 78*, 436–450.

Clinical Effectiveness Unit. (2004b). Norelgestromin/ethinyloestradiol transdermal contraceptive system (Evra®). *The Journal of Family Planning and Reproductive Health Care, 30*(1), 43–45.

Clinical Effectiveness Unit. (2004c). *FemCap*. London: Faculty of Family Planning & Reproductive Healthcare.

Clinical Effectiveness Unit. (2005a). Drug interactions with hormonal contraception. *The Journal of Family Planning and Reproductive Health Care, 31*(4), 335–336.

Clinical Effectiveness Unit. (2006a). *First prescription of combined oral contraception*. London: Faculty of Family Planning and Reproductive Healthcare.

Clinical Effectiveness Unit. (2015). *Intrauterine contraception*. London: Faculty of Sexual & Reproductive Healthcare. Retrieved from http://www.fsrh.org.

Clinical Effectiveness Unit. (2008a). *Progestogen-only pills*. London: Faculty of Sexual & Reproductive Healthcare.

Clinical Effectiveness Unit. (2009). *Sexual and reproductive health for individuals with inflammatory bowel disease*. London: Faculty of Sexual and Reproductive Healthcare.

Clinical Effectiveness Unit. (2010a). *Contraceptive choices for young people*. London: Faculty of Sexual and Reproductive Healthcare.

Clinical Effectiveness Unit. (2010b). *Contraceptive choices for women aged over 40 years*. London: Faculty of Sexual and Reproductive Healthcare.

Clinical Effectiveness Unit. (2010c). *Antiepileptic drugs and contraception*. London: Faculty of Sexual and Reproductive Healthcare.

Clinical Effectiveness Unit. (2011). *Drug interactions with hormonal contraception*. London: Faculty of Sexual and Reproductive Healthcare.

Collaborative Group on Epidemiological Studies of Ovarian Cancer. (2008). Ovarian cancer and oral contraceptives: Collaborative reanalysis of data from 45 epidemiological studies including 23 257 women with ovarian cancer and 87 303 controls. *Lancet, 371*, 303–314.

Collaborative Group on Hormonal Factors in Breast Cancer. (1996). Breast cancer and hormonal contraceptives: Collaborative reanalysis of individual data on 53 297 women with breast cancer and 100 239 women without breast cancer from 54 epidemiological studies. *Lancet, 347*, 1713–1727.

Cooper, E. (2000). Couples with learning disabilities. In S. Killick (Ed.), *Contraception in practice* (pp. 229–240). London: Martin Dunitz.

Curtis, K. M., & Martins, S. L. (2006). Progestogen-only contraception and bone mineral density: A systematic review. *Contraception, 73*, 470–487.

Donovan, C., Hadley, A., Jones, M., et al. (2000). *Confidentiality and young people*. London: Royal College of General Practitioners and Brook.

European Natural Family Planning Study Groups. (1993). Prospective European multicenter study of natural family planning (1989–1992): Interim results. *Advances in Contraception, 9*, 269–283.

Farrell, S. A., & Kieser, K. (2000). Sexuality after hysterectomy. *Obstetrics and Gynecology, 95*, 1045–1051.

Fernandez, E., La Vecchia, C., Balducci, A., Chatenoud, L., Franceschi, S., & Negri, E. (2001). Oral contraceptives and colorectal cancer risk: A meta-analysis. *British Journal of Cancer, 84*(5), 722–727.

Fiala, C., & Gemzell-Danielsson, K. (2006). Review of medical abortion using mifepristone in combination with a prostaglandin analogue. *Contraception, 74*, 66–86.

Fitzpatrick, D., Pirie, K., Reeves, G., Green, J., & Beral, V. (2023). Combined and progestagen-only hormonal contraceptives and breast cancer risk: A UK nested case–control study and meta-analysis. *PLoS Medicine, 20*(3), e1004188.

Forna, F., & Gulmezoglu, A. M. (2000). Interventions for treating trichomonas in women (Cochrane review). In *The Cochrane Library*, Issue 3. Oxford: Update Software.

Fotherby, K., & Howard, G. (1986). Return of fertility in women discontinuing injectable contraceptives. *Journal of Obstetrics and Gynaecology, 6*, S110–S115.

Green, J., & Kocsis, A. (1997). Psychological factors in recurrent genital herpes. *Genitourinary Medicine, 73*, 253–259.

Grimes, D. (2000). Intrauterine device and upper-genital-tract infection. *Lancet, 356*, 1013–1019.

Grimes, D. A., Lopez, L. M., Schulz, K. F., & Stanwood, N. L. (2004). Immediate post-abortal insertion of intrauterine device. *Cochrane Database of Systematic Reviews*, (4), CD001777.

Guillebaud, J. (1989). Contraception and sterilization. In A. Turnbull & G. Chamberlain (Eds.), *Obstetrics* (pp. 1135–1152). Edinburgh: Churchill Livingstone.

Hannaford, P. C., Iversen, L., Macfarlane, T. V., Elliott, A. M., Angus, V., & Lee, A. J. (2010). Mortality among contraceptive pill users: Cohort evidence from Royal College of General Practitioners' Oral Contraception Study. *BMJ (Clinical research ed.), 340*, c927.

Harrison-Woolrych, M., & Hill, R. (2005). Unintended pregnancies with the etonogestrel implant (Implanon): A case series from post-marketing experience in Australia. *Contraception, 71*, 306–308.

Heinemann, L. A., Assmann, A., DoMinh, T., & Garbe, E. (1999). Oral progestogen-only contraceptives and cardiovascular risk: results from the Transnational Study on Oral Contraceptives and the Health of Young Women. *The European Journal of Contraception & Reproductive Health Care, 4*, 67–73.

Howe, K., & Kissinger, P. J. (2017). Single-Dose Compared With Multidose Metronidazole for the Treatment of Trichomoniasis in Women: A Meta-Analysis. *Sexually Transmitted Diseases, 44*(1), 29–34.

International Collaboration of Epidemiological Studies of Cervical Cancer. (2007). Cervical cancer and hormonal contraceptives: Collaborative reanalysis of individual data for 16 573 women with cervical cancer and 35 509 women without cervical cancer from 24 epidemiological studies. *Lancet, 370*, 1609–1621.

Jackson, R. A., Bimla Schwarz, E., Freedman, L., & Darney, P. (2003). Advance supply of emergency contraception: Effect on use and usual contraception - a randomized trial. *Obstetrics and Gynecology, 102*, 8–16.

Jick, S. S., Kaye, J. A., Russmann, S., & Jick, H. (2006). Risk of nonfatal venous thromboembolism with oral contraceptives containing norgestimate or desogestrel compared with oral contraceptives containing levonorgestrel. *Contraception, 73*, 566–570.

Jones, S. (2008). Legal aspects of family planning. In A. Glasier & A. Gebbie (Eds.), *Handbook of family planning and reproductive healthcare* (5th ed., pp. 249–267). Edinburgh: Churchill Livingstone.

Kaunitz, A. M., Arias, R., & McClung, M. (2008). Bone density recovery after depot medroxyprogesterone acetate injectable contraception use. *Contraception, 77*, 67–76.

Kemmeren, J. M., Algra, A., & Grobbee, D. E. (2001). Third generation oral contraceptives and risk of venous thrombosis: Meta-analysis. *BMJ (Clinical research ed.), 323*, 131–134.

Khader, Y. S., Rice, J., John, L., & Abueita, O. (2003). Oral contraceptive use and risk of myocardial infarction: A meta-analysis. *Contraception, 68*, 11–17.

Langenberg, A. G., Corey, L., Ashley, R. L., Leong, W. P., & Straus, S. E. (1999). A prospective study of new infections with herpes simplex virus type 1 and type 2. *The New England Journal of Medicine, 341*(19), 1432–1438.

Liying, Z., & Bilian, X. (2001). Emergency contraception with Multiload Cu-375SL IUD: A multicentre clinical trial. *Contraception, 64*, 107–112.

McGuire, H., & Hawton, K. (2003). Interventions for vaginismus. *The Cochrane Database of Systematic Reviews*, (1), CD001760.

Meaidi, A., Mascolo, A., Sessa, M., Toft-Petersen, A. P., Skals, R., Gerds, T. A., Wessel Skovlund, C., Morch, L. S., Rossi, F., Capuano, A., Lidegaard, O., & Torp-Pedersen, C. (2023). Venous thromboembolism with use of hormonal contraception and non-steroidal anti-inflammatory drugs: nationwide cohort study. *BMJ (Clinical research ed.), 382*, e074450. doi:10.1136/bmj-2022-074450.

Merki-Feld, G. S., & Hund, M. (2007). Clinical experience with NuvaRing in daily practice in Switzerland: Cycle control and acceptability among women of all reproductive ages. *The European Journal of Contraception & Reproductive Health Care, 12*(3), 240–247.

Meston, C. M., Hull, E., Levin, R. J., & Sipski, M. (2004). Disorders of orgasm in women. *The Journal of Sexual Medicine, 1*, 66–68.

Miller, L., & Hughes, J. P. (2003). Continuous combination oral contraceptive pills to eliminate withdrawal bleeding: A randomized trial. *Obstetrics and Gynecology, 101*, 653–661.

National Collaborating Centre for Women's and Children's Health. (2005). *Long-acting reversible contraception (NICE guideline)*. London: RCOG. Retrieved from http://www.nice.org.uk.

National Institute for Health and Care Excellence. (2008). *Prophylaxis against infective endocarditis. NICE clinical guideline 64*. London: National Institute for Health and Clinical Excellence.

Nguyen, P., Hoisnard, L., Neumann, A., Zureik, M., & Weill, A. (2021). *Utilisation prolongée de l'acétate de nomégestrol et risque de méningiome intracrânien: Une étude de cohorte à partir des données du SNDS*. Saint-Denis, le: Groupement d'intérêt scientifique (GIS) EPIPHARE-ANSM-CNAM. Rapport, 20.

NHS. (2009). *National Chlamydia screening programme*. https://www.nao.org.uk/wp-content/uploads/2009/11/0809963.pdf.

Oddsson, K., Leifels-Fischer, B., Wiel-Masson, D., de Melo, N. R., Benedetto, C., Verhoeven, C. H., & Dieben, T. O. (2005a). Superior cycle control with a contraceptive vaginal ring compared with an oral contraceptive containing 30 microg ethinylestradiol and 150 microg levonorgestrel: A randomized trial. *Human reproduction (Oxford, England), 20*(2), 557–562.

Oddsson, K., Leifels-Fischer, B., de Melo, N. R., Wiel-Masson, D., Benedetto, C., Verhoeven, C. H., & Dieben, T. O. (2005b). Efficacy and safety of a contraceptive vaginal ring (NuvaRing) compared with a combined oral contraceptive: a 1-year randomized trial. *Contraception, 71*(3), 176–182.

Poulter, N. R. (1996). Oral contraceptives and blood pressure. In P. C. Hannaford, & A. M. C. Webb (Eds.), *Evidence-guided prescribing of the pill* (pp. 77–88). Carnforth: Parthenon.

Rosenberg, M. J., & Long, S. C. (1992). Oral contraceptives and cycle control: A critical review of the literature. *Advances in Contraception, 8*(Suppl. 1), 35–45.

Rosenberg, M. J., Waugh, M. S., & Stevens, C. M. (1996). Smoking and cycle control among oral contraceptive users. *American Journal of Obstetrics and Gynecology, 174*, 628–632.

Roumen, F. J. M. E., op ten Berg, M. M. T., & Hoomans, E. H. M. (2006). The combined contraceptive ring (NuvaRing): First experience in daily clinical practice in the Netherlands. *The European Journal of Contraception & Reproductive Health Care, 11*, 14–22.

Sexual Offences Act, 2003. https://www.legislation.gov.uk/ukpga/2003/42/contents

Sloand, E. M., Pitt, E., Chiarello, R. J., & Nemo, G. J. (1991). HIV testing. State of the art. *Journal of the American Medical Association, 266*(20), 2861–2866.

South Yorkshire NHS Integrated Care Board, Doncaster CCG *"Primary Care guidance for prescribing SSRIs for premature ejaculation"* 2022. Found at: https://medicinesmanagement.doncasterccg.nhs.uk/wp-content/uploads/2022/09/Primary-Care-guidance-for-premature-ejaculationV1.0-Sept-2022-review-Sept-2025.pdf

Stewart, F. H., Harper, C. C., Ellertson, C. E., Grimes, D. A., Sawaya, G. F., & Trussell, J. (2001). Clinical breast and pelvic examination requirements for hormonal contraception. *JAMA, 285*, 2232–2239.

Stokes, T., Shaw, E. J., Juarez-Garcia, A., Camosso-Stefinovic, J., Baker, R., et al. (2004). *Clinical guidelines and evidence review for the epilepsies: Diagnosis and management in adults and children in primary and secondary care*. London: Royal College of General Practitioners.

Trussell, J. (2007). Contraceptive efficacy. In R. A. Hatcher, J. Trussell, J. A. L. Nelson, W. Cates, F. H. Stewart, & D. Kowal, (Eds.), *Contraceptive technology* (19th ed., pp. 747–826). New York: Ardent Media.

Vasilakis-Scaramozza, C., & Jick, H. (2001). Risk of venous thromboembolism with cyproterone or levonorgestrel contraceptives. *Lancet, 358*, 1427–1429.

Vessey, M., & Painter, R. (2006). Oral contraceptive use and cancer. Findings in a large cohort study, 1968–2004. *British Journal of Cancer, 95*, 385–389.

Waldinger, M. D. (2007). Premature ejaculation: State of the art. *The Urologic Clinics of North America, 34*, 591–599.

Weiderpass, E., Adami, H. O., Baron, J. A., Magnusson, C., Lindgren, A., & Persson, I. (1999). Use of oral contraceptives and endometrial cancer risk (Sweden). *Cancer Causes & Control, 10*(4), 277–284.

Weijmar Schultz, W., Basson, R., Binik, Y., schenbach, D., Wesselmann, U., & Van Lankveld, J. (2005). Women's sexual pain and its management. *The Journal of Sexual Medicine, 2*, 301–316.

Westhoff, C. (2003). Depot-medroxyprogesterone acetate injection (Depo-Provera®): A highly effective contraceptive option with proven long-term safety. *Contraception, 68*, 75–87.

Wilcox, A. J., Dunson, D. B., Weinberg, C. R., Trussell, J., & Baird, D. D. (2001). Likelihood of conception with a single act of intercourse: Providing benchmark rates for assessment of postcoital contraceptives. *Contraception, 63*, 211–215.

World Health Organization. (1987). A multicentred phase III comparative trial of depotmedroxyprogesterone acetate given three-monthly at doses of 100mg or 150mg: II. The comparison of bleeding patterns. *Contraception, 35*, 591–610.

World Health Organization. (1991). Collaborative study of neoplasia and steroid contraceptives. Depot medroxyprogesterone acetate (DMPA) and risk of endometrial cancer. *International Journal of Cancer, 49*, 186–190.

Wylie, K. (Ed.). (2015). *ABC of sexual health* (3rd ed.). Malden: Blackwell.

16

Psychiatric Problems

Sarah Henry & Soumyajit Sanyal

CHAPTER CONTENTS

Depression

- About 25% to 40% of general practitioner (GP) consultations have a significant psychological component (Goldberg & Lecrubier, 1995). Of these, only about 5% are referred to specialist services.
- Recent research has shown how the use of specific questions can help to elicit crucial information about the patient's mental state.
- Qualitative research has shown the importance of the patient's relationship with the GP in such situations. Patients value an empathetic, interested doctor with whom they have a continuing relationship (Buszewicz et al, 2006).

GUIDELINES

National Institute for Health and Clinical Excellence. (2022a). *Depression in adults: treatment and management. NICE clinical guideline 222.* Retrieved from http://www.nice.org.uk.
  Cleare, A., Pariante, C. M., Young, A. H., Anderson, I. M., Christmas, D., Cowen, P. J., Dickens, C., Ferrier, I. N., Geddes, J., Gilbody, S., Haddad, P. M., Katona, C., Lewis, G., Malizia, A., McAllister-Williams, R. H., Ramchandani, P., Scott, J., Taylor, D., Uher, R., & Members of the Consensus Meeting. (2015). Evidence-based guidelines for treating depressive disorders with antidepressants: A revision of the 2008 British Association for Psychopharmacology guidelines *Journal of Psychopharmacology, 29*(5), 459–525.

- GPs fail to diagnose up to half of their patients with a major depressive illness and often fail to treat adequately those whom they do recognise (Freeling et al, 1985; Anderson, Nutt, & Deakin, 2000).
- Depression in people from the African–Caribbean, Asian, refugee, and asylum-seeking communities is often overlooked, although the prevalence is 60% higher than in the White population (NCCMH, 2023). People from Black and minority ethnic communities are much less likely to be referred to psychological therapies.
- Patients whose depression is most likely to be missed are those with somatic complaints or with physical illness, those with long-standing depression, those who do not look depressed, and those who do not realise they are depressed (Freeling et al, 1985; Gill & Hatcher, 2002).
- Depression is often accompanied and masked by anxiety (Goldberg & Bridges, 1987), yet treatment of the anxiety alone is insufficient and may appear to worsen the depression.

Presenting Complaints

- Look for depression in patients with a past history of depression, with chronic physical illness with functional impairment, or with other mental illnesses such as anxiety or dementia. Ask two specific questions: during the past month, have you felt:
  a. Low, depressed, or hopeless?
  b. Little interest or pleasure in doing things (Whooley et al, 1997)?
- If the answer to either question is yes, confirm the diagnosis of depression using the International Classification of Diseases, 11th revision (ICD-11), criteria. Use of a validated measure (e.g., Patient Health Questionnaire-9 (PHQ-9)) when assessing a person with suspected depression is recommended by the National Institute for Health and Clinical Excellence (NICE).
- In the ICD-11, depression is defined as the presence of depressed mood or diminished interest in activities occurring most of the day, nearly every day, for at least 2 weeks, accompanied by five other symptoms such as:
  - Reduced ability to concentrate and sustain attention or marked indecisiveness
  - Beliefs of low self-worth or excessive or inappropriate guilt
  - Hopelessness about the future
  - Recurrent thoughts of death or suicidal ideation or evidence of attempted suicide
  - Significantly disrupted sleep or excessive sleep
  - Significant changes in appetite or weight
  - Psychomotor agitation or retardation
  - Reduced energy or fatigue
- Depression severity is now considered on a spectrum, consisting of the frequency and intensity of symptoms, duration, and impact on functioning. NICE recommends moving away from grouped categories of mild, moderate, and severe episodes into defining depression

into less severe or more severe depression with a score of 16 on PHQ-9 dividing the two (NICE, 2022a).
Cautions:
- In people reacting appropriately to a severe adverse life events and problems, depressive symptoms may be present. However, if they meet the above diagnostic threshold, a depressive episode should be considered.
- A depressive episode should not be considered if the individual is exhibiting normal grief symptoms, including some depressive symptoms. However, the presence of a history of mood disorder, persistent depressive symptoms for more than 1 month, severe depressive symptoms such as extreme beliefs of low self-worth and guilt not related to the lost loved one, the presence of psychotic symptoms, suicidal ideation, or psychomotor retardation should all prompt consideration of a diagnosis of depression (ICD-11).
- Symptoms of anxiety are common in depression, particularly in older people. The focus should be on treating the depression first (NICE, 2022a).

Differential Diagnosis

- *Bipolar affective disorder.* Ask about a history of a manic episode or hypomania. Antidepressants can precipitate a hypomanic, manic, or mixed episode and destabilise the course of bipolar disorder.
- *Mixed episode.* Depressive symptoms in a mixed episode may appear similar to those of a depressive episode, but in a mixed episode, they occur simultaneously or alternate rapidly with several prominent manic symptoms such as irritability, racing thoughts, or increased activity (ICD-11).
- *Attention-deficit hyperactivity disorder.* Symptoms are chronic rather than episodic, and other core features of depression are not present. There is significant comorbidity between the two, and this requires full diagnostic assessment (ICD-11).
- *Neurocognitive disorders.* Cognitive symptoms may be present in older adults with depression, which may be hard to distinguish from dementia. Cognitive decline in dementia does not have all associated features of depression, including thoughts of guilt or hopelessness. There is, however, significant comorbidity between the two, and depressive symptoms often precede the onset of dementia or and start after the diagnosis (ICD-11).

Management of Depression

The GP can manage 90% of depressed patients without referral to a specialised mental health service. The following steps are common to almost all severities of depression.
- Explore the impact of the depression on behaviour and relationships at home and work.
- Explain the nature of the illness, its treatment, and its good prognosis.
- Discuss the link between physical symptoms and mood.
- Encourage the patient not to make major or irreversible decisions about work or family until their mental state improves.

- Check their preference and expectations from treatment and make a shared decision with the person.
- Discuss drug therapy and psychological or psychosocial options depending on severity and patient preference severity (NICE, 2022a).
- *Follow-up.* Explain the need for and frequency of follow-up.
- *Patient information.* Provide one of the leaflets listed in the box and give the patient the details of sources of information and support.

Referral

Refer to a specialist mental health service if:

a. Psychotic features are present or the depression is severe.
b. The history suggests a bipolar illness.
c. There is a significant risk of suicide or severe neglect.
d. Specialised forms of treatment are needed (e.g., cognitive-behavioural therapy (CBT)) if they are not available in primary care.
e. The patient is a child or adolescent with major depressive illness.
f. There has been a poor response to an appropriate antidepressant at the maximum dosage, with good compliance, taken for an adequate period of time.
g. There is social isolation, little family support, or poor compliance.
h. Combination or augmentation treatment is needed.
i. The patient has depression and a diagnosis of personality disorder.

Specific Treatment of Less Severe Depression (PHQ <16)

- Explain the possible options:
  a. *'Watchful waiting'.* The patient may choose to return in, for example, 2 to 4 weeks without treatment. Arrange further assessment and make contact if patient does not attend the follow-up appointment.
  b. *Guided self-help.* The patient works through a written or computer programme which is usually designed along cognitive-behavioural lines (see the 'Information for Patients' box).
  c. *Psychological therapies.* There is evidence to suggest group CBT, group behavioural activation, individual CBT, individual behavioural activation, group exercise, group mindfulness and meditation, interpersonal therapy, problem-solving therapy, and other forms of counselling are beneficial. The choice is based on patient's preference and resources locally available.
- Explain that antidepressants are usually not recommended in patients with subclinical depression unless it has lasted for 2 years (i.e., dysthymia). Any possible benefit is likely to be outweighed by the adverse effects. However, a patient with a past history of more severe depression who presents with subclinical depression may choose to take an antidepressant at this stage.

- Complementary therapies such as St John's Wort are not recommended by NICE because of uncertainty about dose, effect, and variation in preparations and potency.

Specific Treatment of More Severe Depression (PHQ ≥16)

- Antidepressants are one of various choices available as treatment. The choice should be a shared decision based on clinical needs, preferences, and resources available.
- NICE recommends the following options: individual CBT plus antidepressants, individual CBT, individual behavioural activation, antidepressants, individual problem-solving therapy, counselling, short-term psychodynamic psychotherapy, group exercise, group therapy, interpersonal therapy, behavioural couples therapy, and guided self-help (description in resources later).
- *Offering an antidepressant.* The NICE guideline recommends a selective serotonin reuptake inhibitor (SSRI) or serotonin–norepinephrine reuptake inhibitor (SNRI) because they are as effective as tricyclic antidepressants (TCAs) but with a 10% less chance of being discontinued because of adverse effects. Cost-effectiveness studies, in which doctors' time is costed as well as drug expenditure, favour SSRIs or are at least neutral (Stewart, 1998; Simon et al, 1999). However, both drug types have considerable, but different, adverse effects. Attempt to make a choice that is the best for the particular patient (see later).
- Explain to the patient that:
  a. Even if their depression is a reaction to life events, they are as likely to benefit from an antidepressant as if it was endogenous.
  b. They will not notice any improvement for the first 10 days to 3 weeks, but adverse effects are most likely to occur in this period and then lessen.
  c. Antidepressants are not addictive. They will not develop craving or tolerance, but there is the possibility of a discontinuation reaction, especially if stopped abruptly.
  d. Stopping the drug early increases the risk of relapse. All patients should take the drug for 6 months after recovery. Anyone with a recent previous episode of severe depression should take it for 2 years, as should other people at high risk of relapse (e.g., older adults; see later discussion).
- *Drug dosage*
  a. If choosing a TCA, start at the equivalent of amitriptyline start at 50mg/day. A much-criticised meta-analysis (Furukawa, McGuire, & Barbui, 2002) has suggested that the lower doses may be adequate. Such studies and their critics inevitably examine the mean response of a large number of patients. In clinical practice, what matters is the response of the individual. Assess the effect of the lower dose and increase the dose monthly if the response is inadequate.
  b. If choosing an SSRI or SNRI, start at the standard dose. Evidence that subsequent dose increases are beneficial is poor (although higher doses are effective in other conditions).

- *Follow-up.* See the patient 1 week after starting a drug to discuss any adverse effects (e.g., agitation, concern about suicide risk) and to check on compliance. A quarter of patients either never cash in their prescription or only do so once (Boardman & Walters, 2009). If an SSRI is causing agitation, a 2-week course of a benzodiazepine is an alternative to stopping the drug. Slowly increase the time between consultations as the patient responds.
- *Response.* Do not be disappointed by a partial response. Studies of published and unpublished studies combined show that the effect size of all antidepressants is 'small' (number needed to treat (NNT) = 6) (Boardman & Walters, 2009) and certainly less than the claims of manufacturers based on published studies alone (Turner & Rosenthal, 2008).
- *Maintenance.* Continue the drug for at least 6 months after remission. This reduces the relapse rate from 50% to 20%. A reduction in dose should only be made if side effects are a problem. Consider treatment for 1 to 2 years if there has been a previous episode in the recent past or the patient is at high risk because of age, family history, or other features (see later).

Factors That Influence the Choice of an Antidepressant

a. *Older adults.* Avoid highly anticholinergic drugs (e.g., amitriptyline, clomipramine, dosulepin, imipramine).
b. *Young people.* The CSM (Committee on Safety of Medicines) has previously concluded that the majority of SSRIs are contraindicated in children and adolescents up to the age of 18 years because of poor efficacy and a possible increase in the risk of self-harm and suicide. Fluoxetine seems to be an exception to this. The CSM also cautions that very young adults may be at similar risk, even though such a risk has not been detected in trials (CSM Expert Working Group, 2004). The evidence base for antidepressant prescribing in children is considerably smaller than for adults, and more recent evidence suggests that the risks associated with SSRI use in young people may have been overstated (Dwyer & Bloch, 2019). However, prescribing antidepressants for people younger than age 18 years should remain the preserve of specialist services in which experience of their use is growing.
c. *Pregnancy.* Treat only if the benefit outweighs the risks. Consider seeking specialist advice before starting antidepressants or switching the antidepressant of a female who is already being treated for depression when she falls pregnant.
d. *Prostatism or glaucoma.* Avoid all anticholinergic drugs.
e. *Cardiac disease.* Avoid TCAs and venlafaxine; the best evidence for use in ischaemic heart disease is for sertraline.
f. *Suicide risk.* There is no evidence that one class of drugs poses a greater risk of suicide (Cipriani, Barbui, & Geddes 2005), but intuitively, doctors avoid the more toxic TCAs.
g. *Lethargy.* Avoid sedative drugs (e.g., amitriptyline, clomipramine, dosulepin, mianserin, mirtazapine, and trazodone).
h. *Anxiety or insomnia.* Consider the use of a drug with sedative properties.
i. *Obesity.* Use an SSRI.
j. *Epilepsy.* Use SSRIs as first choice. Consider seeking specialist advice (Specialist Pharmacy Service, 2022).
k. *Other drugs.* All classes of antidepressants show considerable interaction with other drugs, but any one interaction rarely applies to all classes and may not be seen with all members of one class. Choose an antidepressant tailored to the patient's other medication.

Management of a Poor Response to Drug Therapy

- Check that the patient was taking the drug correctly. An apparent relapse could be caused by a discontinuation reaction in a patient who has omitted one or more doses.
- When there is evidence that an increased dose may be associated with an improved response and there are no adverse effects, consider increasing the dose gradually, waiting for 4 weeks each time before deciding that the response is inadequate.
- If a dosage increase is not a possibility, assess whether referral is needed or whether the patient's condition allows the trial of another drug. Make a choice, according to any adverse effects experienced with the first drug, between another SSRI, a TCA (but not dosulepin), or a member of a different class (e.g., moclobemide, mirtazapine, or reboxetine). Because it is a reversible inhibitor of monoamine oxidase A, moclobemide cannot be started until the previous antidepressant has washed out of the system. For a TCA, this is 1 week, but for fluoxetine, it is 5 weeks. The STAR* D (Sequenced Treatment Alternatives to Relieve Depression) study found that putting nonresponders through four steps of antidepressant treatment (either increased dosage or a change of drug) increased the rate of remission from 37% with step 1 to 67% by step 4 in those who adhered to treatment (Rush et al, 2006). Against these impressive-sounding results is the fact that drop-out rates were high, and the percentage remitting fell with each step.
- Consider combining psychotherapy with drug treatment. Response is greater than with either alone even if this is just because patients who also receive psychotherapy are more likely to take their drugs (Pampallona, Bollini, & Tibaldi, 2004).

Stopping Maintenance Therapy and Managing Discontinuation Reactions

- Explain tapering to people who want to stop antidepressants successfully.
- Taper slowly in a stepwise fashion, 50% of previous dose, for example. Use smaller reductions (e.g., 25%) at lower doses. At very low doses, liquid preparations can be used. A long-acting drug (e.g., fluoxetine or sertraline) may be given at the same dose but every other day and then every third day. A short-acting drug (e.g., paroxetine or citalopram) should be given daily at decreasing dosage. Tablets may be cut in half, or a liquid form prescribed.

- Warn the patient that a discontinuation reaction is possible on stopping an antidepressant. The incidence is unclear. Estimates based on reports of adverse drug reactions suggest that it is uncommon (5% with paroxetine, <1% with other SSRIs; Price et al, 1996), but such reports rely on the reporting doctor making the diagnosis. A retrospective analysis of patients discontinuing antidepressants found that a reaction occurred in 31% who had taken clomipramine, in 17% who had taken a short-acting SSRI (paroxetine or fluvoxamine), and in only 1.5% who had taken a long-acting SSRI (fluoxetine or sertraline) (Coupland, Bell, & Potokar, 1996). Even if half of these are caused by a placebo effect (Haddad, Lejoyeux, & Young, 1998), the study suggests that the reaction is more common with the shorter acting drugs.
- Explain that a discontinuation reaction is unlikely to feel like a recurrence of depression. Dizziness, paraesthesia, tremor, anxiety, nausea, and palpitations are the commonest symptoms. They occur within days of stopping the drug and last for 10 days on average.
- If a discontinuation reaction occurs:
  - A mild reaction: Explain what is happening and continue the planned reduction if the patient agrees.
  - A more severe reaction: either:
    a. Increase the dose to the last dose that gave no reaction or
    b. Change the patient to a longer acting drug of the same class and
    c. Prepare to tail off over a longer period (e.g., 3–6 months)
- Monitor and review patients regularly during the taper and after finally stopping the drug to ensure they remain well. Advise them to return at the earliest sign of a recurrence.

How to Distinguish an Antidepressant Discontinuation Reaction From a Return of the Underlying Disorder

a. Its onset is within days (compared with weeks for a recurrence of depression).
b. It resolves with 24 hours of restarting the antidepressant.
c. Although the patient may report mood disturbance (low mood, irritability, anxiety) there are likely to be somatic symptoms as well (numbness, paraesthesia, dizziness, headache, myalgia, fatigue, insomnia with vivid dreams).

Cognitive-Behavioural Therapy, Counselling, and Other Psychotherapies

- Ensure patients are aware of the waiting lists. Self-help materials and social support can be provided with regular reviews in the interim.
- In patients at the mild to moderate end of the spectrum of severe depression, cognitive and interpersonal therapies can be as effective as antidepressants and may prevent relapse (Gloaguen et al, 1998). In a meta-analysis, antidepressants and psychotherapy both resulted in remission at a mean of 16 weeks in 46% of patients compared with 24% of control participants (Casacalenda, Perry, & Looper, 2002).
- More patients would choose counselling than drugs if given the choice (Chilvers et al, 2001).
- In severe depression, a combination of antidepressants and CBT can be more effective than either alone (Timonen & Liukkonen, 2008). Other psychotherapies have not shown a benefit from being combined with drugs.
- Most of the evidence for the benefit of psychological therapies in depression lies with certain techniques only, mainly cognitive-behavioural, interpersonal, and problem-solving ones (Mynors-Wallis et al, 2000), and cannot be assumed to exist for all forms of counselling (DoH, 2001).
- A 6-year follow-up study suggests that a course of CBT, in addition to drug therapy, leads to fewer subsequent relapses than drug therapy alone (40% vs 90% in a study of 40 patients; Fava, Ruini, & Rafanelli, 2004).

Prevention of Recurrence

- The continuing nature of the condition and the benefit to be gained from early intervention argue strongly for depression to be managed as a chronic disease, with a systematic approach to follow-up by a dedicated team following agreed protocols (Scott, 2006).
  - Discuss the risk of relapse if a patient wants to stop treatment after remission. The risk of relapse is based on various factors such as history of recurrent episodes; previous incomplete response; history of severe depression; coexisting physical or mental health problems; unhelpful coping styles (e.g., avoidance, rumination); or personal, social, or environmental factors that are contributing to depression.
  - Seventy-five percent of patients with a first episode of major depression have a recurrence within the next 10 years (Angst, 1997). A second episode during the next 4 years requires full initial treatment followed by psychiatric referral to consider prophylaxis with long-term antidepressant medication. In the first 3 years, this reduces the rate of recurrence from 41% to 18%. Only slightly more patients withdraw from treatment on an antidepressant than on placebo (odds ratio, 1.3) (95% confidence interval (CI). 1.07–1.59) (Geddes et al, 2003).
  * As a minimum, consider a 6-month review by a doctor or nurse over the 2 years after treatment is stopped. In a US study, it increased remission over 2 years by 33% (95% CI, 7%–46%) (Rost et al, 2002).

INFORMATION FOR PATIENTS

The Samaritans. Tel: 116 123.jo@samaritans.org. Available at http://www.samaritans.org.
  The Mental Health Foundation has fact sheets for patients as well as other resources at http://www.mentalhealth.org.uk.

Postnatal Depression

GUIDELINE

National Institute of Health and Care Excellence. (2014a; updated 2020). *Antenatal and postnatal mental health: Clinical management and service guidance. NICE clinical guideline 192.* Retrieved from https://www.nice.org.uk/guidance/cg192.

- Postnatal depression occurs in 10% to 15% of females in the first year after delivery, usually in the first 6 months. The symptoms are almost always present at 6 weeks. It is distinct from the transient 'blues' of the first 10 days and from a puerperal psychosis, which is likely to need admission.
- Those most at risk are those with:
  a. Previous psychological disturbance in pregnancy
  b. Poor social support
  c. A poor marital relationship
  d. Recent stressful events
  e. An episode of the 'baby blues'
- The strongest risk factors for puerperal psychosis are a personal or family history of an affective psychosis. A female patient who has one episode of puerperal psychosis has a 25% to 57% risk of a recurrence in a subsequent pregnancy. The risk of nonpuerperal affective psychosis at some stage is even greater.
- Every practice should be aware of the need to identify 'at-risk' patients during the antenatal period and should ensure that they receive more intensive help after birth. Risk factors should be identified during pregnancy and the primary care team need to decide:
  a. What extra care this group should receive
  b. Who is responsible for identifying this condition as early as possible
- Patients often do not realise that they are depressed, and doctors recognise it even less frequently. Females often present with a feeling of not coping rather than with classic symptoms of depression.
- The NICE guideline recommends that every female should be screened for depression and anxiety in the early postnatal period using depression identification questions and 2-item Generalised Anxiety Disorder scale as screening. The Edinburgh Postnatal Depression Scale (Cox, Holden, & Sagovsky, 1987) may be administered by a trained professional (see Appendix 19) as part of the screening process but with the understanding that it is a screening, not a diagnostic, tool. Clinical assessment is needed to establish the diagnosis.

If Depression Is Found

- Check thyroid function tests in those complaining mainly of tiredness.
- *Counsel.* Simple, nondirective counselling by health visitors, weekly for 8 weeks, doubles the recovery rate (Holden, Sagovsky, & Cox, 1989).
- Explain to the patient that she is ill; it is not her fault and does not mean that she is a poor mother.
- *Literature.* Recommend one of the sources of information listed in the Patient Organisations box or print it for the patient.
- *Antidepressants.* NICE advises before starting any treatment in pregnancy and the postnatal period, there is a need to discuss the higher threshold for pharmacologic interventions because of the changing risk-to-benefit ratio. Offer drug treatment at the lowest possible dose and use a single drug when possible. Some females may wish to continue to breastfeed, and this should be supported by the choice of medication and a careful discussion of risks and benefits. Equally, some may choose not to, and this decision should also be supported. Avoid the use of benzodiazepines except in short-term use for severe anxiety and agitation. The baby may experience a discontinuation reaction. Use a long-acting drug and tail off breastfeeding (or the drug if still breastfeeding) slowly.
- Consider obtaining advice from local specialist teams or referral if a multidisciplinary mental health team can offer more than the primary healthcare team.
- Refer immediately for urgent psychiatric assessment any female with ideas of suicide or of harming the baby or with symptoms of puerperal psychosis.

PATIENT ORGANISATIONS

Association for Post Natal Illness. 1st Floor Offices, Fulham Park House, 1a Chesilton Road, London, SW6 5AA. Tel: 020 7386 0868. Available at http://www.apni.org.
  Mental Health Foundation. Available at http://www.mentalhealth.org.uk.
  National Childbirth Trust. Tel: 0300 330 0700. Available at http:// www.nct.org.uk (search 'depression').

Suicide and Suicidal Risk

- Two-thirds of successful suicides are mentally ill (Owens, Lloyd, & Campbell, 2004), mostly with undiagnosed depression. In older adults, the prevalence of mental illness in suicides increases to up to 95% (O'Connell et al, 2004).
- The risk of completed suicide in the first 9 days of drug treatment is 38 times that of the risk in a patient who has been on treatment for at least 3 months (Jick, Kaye, & Jick, 2004). This is independent of the type of antidepressant used.
- There is no evidence that SSRIs increase the risk of suicide in adults, though they may do so in children and adolescents. On the contrary, it seems likely that effective treatment of depression offers the most hope of reducing the risk of suicide. Even in adolescents, the risk of suicide is greater in the month before starting antidepressants than in the first month on therapy (Brent, 2007).
- Suicide is uncommon even in major depressive illness. One study found that only 4% of patients admitted because of depression killed themselves (Bostwick & Pankratz, 2000). Furthermore, this 4% is hard to detect, though an attempt should be made.

- In all patients with depression, assess the risk. For instance, ask a series of questions, only stopping when the answer is no:
  1. Have you thought how nice it would be if you did not wake up one morning?
  2. Have you thought of killing yourself?
  3. Have you decided how to do it?
  4. Have you decided when to do it?
- Judge the risk according to the following risk factors:
  a. A history of previous attempts, especially if determined or violent methods were used, or if a suicide note was left.
  b. Intense feelings of hopelessness and worthlessness.
  c. Major mental illness, including depression.
  d. Suicidal ideation or evidence of planning (e.g., if the patient has decided when to do it and if a sudden and infallible method has been chosen; Boardman & Walters, 2009).
  e. Chronic physical illness or pain.
  f. Recent bereavement or other significant loss, including job loss.
  g. Males. The male:female ratio for suicide is 4:1.
  h. Old age. The risk in those aged older than 75 years is three times that of those aged 15 to 24 years.
  i. Alcohol or other substance misuse.
  j. Previous inpatient psychiatric treatment.
  k. Family history of mental illness, suicide, or alcoholism.
  l. Patients who are positive for acquired immunodeficiency virus or human immunodeficiency virus.
  m. Unmarried, separated, or divorced people, especially if living alone.

Management of Suicidal Patients

Low Risk

- Manage at home patients who have thoughts of suicide but who have:
  a. No clear suicidal plans or past history of a serious suicidal attempt
  b. Good rapport with their GP or local psychiatric services
  c. 24-hour home support
  d. A stable personality
  e. No psychotic illness, chronic physical illness, or drug or alcohol misuse
- *Drugs.* If prescribing, initially give small quantities of medication.

High Risk

- Refer urgently to the mental health team or Crisis service. Check that the patient meets the previously agreed-upon local criteria for same-day referral. A domiciliary visit by a psychiatrist may be indicated (even if a patient refuses all offers of help).
- If the GP and psychiatrist cannot visit together, make sure that the GP is notified immediately of the outcome of the visit.

- Ensure that the carers can provide observation for 24 hours a day until the risk diminishes. The family may need help to provide this level of care. If drug treatment is started, a relative or carer should be asked to supervise the medication.

Follow-up After Attempted Suicide

Often the first time a GP hears about a suicidal patient is when a hospital discharge report is received. When this occurs, the doctor should:
a. Review the records to see if the patient has recently attended.
b. Discuss the management with the mental healthcare team if the patient has a severe long-standing mental illness.
c. Identify anything that might indicate the patient was a suicide risk.
d. Enter suicide attempt on the notes.
e. Ask the patient to make an appointment to see the GP for review.
f. Follow up to:
  - Identify depression or other precipitating life events.
  - Assess the need for treatment including counselling.
  - Make a care plan to review outcome and prevent recurrence.
g. Start treatment (discussed later) if indicated.

SUPPORT ORGANISATIONS

The Samaritans. Tel: 116 123. jo@samaritans.org. Available at http://www.samaritans.org.
PAPYRUS (Prevention of Young Suicide). Helpline: 08000 684141. Available at http://www.papyrus-uk.org.

Helping Those Bereaved by Suicide

- Grief after suicide seems to be particularly intense and often associated with shame and guilt. On average, six people have intense grief for every suicide (Hawton, 2003). Identify the people most likely to be affected and give them a chance to talk about their feelings.
- If their grief is intense, refer for counselling or recommend self-help literature or self-help groups, according to its severity.

SUPPORT ORGANISATIONS

Survivors of Bereavement by Suicide (SOBS). National helpline: 0300 111 5065. Available at http://www.uk-sobs.org.uk.
Winston's Wish is specifically for children bereaved by suicide. Helpline: 08088 020 021. Available at http://www.winstonswish.org.uk.
CRUSE offers support to all those who are bereaved. Day by Day helpline: 0844 4779400. Young person's helpline: 0808 808 1677. Available at http://www.cruse.org.uk.
The Compassionate Friends helps parents and siblings who have lost a child, including from suicide. Helpline: 0345 123 2304. Available at http://www.tcf.org.uk.

Stress Reactions

- Stress reactions may be one of the following:
  a. Acute and brief
  b. An adjustment reaction which may last a few months
  c. Posttraumatic stress disorder (PTSD), with a delay between the stress and the onset of symptoms
- Stress may be a reaction to loss or trauma. Symptoms may be those of anxiety, depression, abnormal behaviour, or an inability to cope with normal events. Symptoms may have been present for a long time before help is sought.
- Stressful events include:
  a. Crime or accidents involving psychological or physical trauma
  b. Bereavement, including siblings in a family in which a child has died
  c. Termination of pregnancy or miscarriage
  d. Redundancy, loss of job, or occupational stress
  e. Divorce, separation, or relationship difficulties
  f. Housing or financial problems
  g. Surviving a disaster
  h. Having to perform in front of an audience or having a work appraisal
  i. Seeking asylum
  j. Drug or alcohol withdrawal

Management

- Identify underlying precipitating events and the steps taken by the patient to modify or cope with the situation.
- Exclude a physical or drug cause for the symptoms (drug or alcohol withdrawal, sudden stopping of a beta-blocker, hyperthyroidism).
- Identify others who might help (e.g., Relate, Citizens' Advice Bureau, Victim Support, union representative, local police domestic violence unit).
- Review what support can be obtained from family, friends, work colleagues, and sources of community support.
- Discuss coping strategies.
- Assess the need for counselling.
- Decide if short-term time off work might be helpful.
- Consider prescribing a beta-blocker if somatic symptoms (shaking and tachycardia) are prominent. Avoid anxiolytic drugs, but if the symptoms are very severe, give them for a maximum of 2 weeks.

Posttraumatic Stress Disorder

- The risk of developing PTSD varies according to the nature of the trauma and the susceptibility of the patient, ranging from 10% after a road traffic accident, 32% after a myocardial infarct (Jones et al, 2007), to 57% after rape (Hull, 2004).
- A study from the Netherlands suggests that nontraumatic life events (e.g., divorce or unemployment) may be more frequently the cause of PTSD than trauma (Mol et al, 2005).
- The presentation may be delayed for several months after the event. In the United States, the lifetime prevalence is 8% (American Psychiatric Association, 2013). An Israeli study found that only 2.4% of patients with PTSD had been detected by their GPs (Munro, Freeman, & Law 2004).
- Look for PTSD specifically in patients who have had an extremely traumatic incident in their lives. The cues to the diagnosis are when, at least 1 month after the event, the patient's life is disturbed by the following:
  - Intrusive symptoms; memories, flashbacks, and nightmares
  - Avoidance of thoughts, activities, and situations associated with the event, as well as emotional numbing
  - Symptoms of autonomic arousal (e.g., hypervigilance, insomnia, irritability, excessive anger, d impaired concentration or memory)
- Check whether the patient has taken refuge in drug or alcohol misuse.
- In severe cases, assess the risk of suicide.

Management

- *Debriefing.* Do not routinely offer debriefing after a traumatic event. It appears to be useless and may be harmful (Bisson, 2004). A follow-up appointment 1 to 2 months after the event is more likely to be useful. Even then, beware of overdiagnosing it in a patient who is recovering spontaneously from a traumatic event.
- Provide information for patient and family (see box).
- Encourage discussion of the precipitator event after PTSD has developed.
- Encourage the patient to discuss their feelings and fears.
- Explain how avoiding things that remind the patient of the trauma prolongs the syndrome.
- Draw up a gradual plan to face avoided activities and situations.
- *Alcohol.* Warn about the need to avoid excess use of alcohol. If the patient is already misusing alcohol or other drugs, treatment of the misuse must come before treatment of the PTSD.
- *Psychological therapy.* Refer for trauma-focused CBT if symptoms are present 3 months after the event. Refer at 1 month if symptoms are severe (NICE, 2018).
- *Antidepressants.* SSRIs reduce all symptoms of PTSD and treat any associated anxiety and depression. Sertraline has been shown to increase the response rate from one-third (with placebo) to half, although the reduction in symptoms was small (Jick et al, 2004). It may take 8 weeks before effects are seen, and high doses may be needed. If effective, continue for at least 6 months in total or at least 12 months if the PTSD has lasted more than 3 months to avoid relapse. There is an impression that patients do better if the drugs are started early in the course of the condition. NICE recommends paroxetine and mirtazapine for general use and other antidepressants for use by mental health specialists (NICE, 2018).
- *Other drugs.* Consider a beta-blocker for a patient disabled by startle and hyperarousal symptoms. The evidence for benzodiazepines is poor. However, consider a nighttime short-acting benzodiazepine for a patient exhausted by

poor sleep. Explain the disadvantages (dependence and tolerance) and obtain the patient's agreement that it will only be used, at the most, twice a week, while waiting for the SSRI to take effect.

- Inform the patient about the resources listed in the Patient Organisations box.

PATIENT ORGANISATIONS

Victim Support: emotional and practical support for victims of crime. Support line: 0808 1689 111. support@victimsupport.org.uk. Available at http://www.victimsupport.org.uk.

The Refugee Council. Tel: 020 7346 6700. Available at http://www.refugeecouncil.org.uk

Combat Stress (Ex-Services Mental Welfare Society) supports ex-service people with PTSD. Tel: 0800 138 1619. contactus@combatstress.org.uk. Available at http://www.combatstress.org.uk.

MIND has an excellent information. Call the Mindinfoline at 0845 766 0163 or download it from http://www.mind.org.uk (search on 'post-traumatic stress disorder').

Insomnia

- Insomnia may be short term (<3 months) or chronic (≥3 nights per week for 3 months or more). Primary insomnia (insomnia not attributable to an underlying cause) and secondary insomnia (insomnia caused by a comorbid condition) are no longer included in classification systems because insomnia is considered to be a disorder in its own right (NICE, 2024). Sleep difficulties without functional impairment do not meet the diagnostic criteria for insomnia. Common causes of chronic insomnia are depression, anxiety, menopausal symptoms, restless legs syndrome, pain, and drugs. Bidirectional or interactive effects often exist between chronic insomnia and comorbid conditions (NICE, 2022).
- Patients with insomnia need treatment of both the underlying condition and of the insomnia. A study of patients with rheumatoid arthritis found that treating insomnia with a short-acting benzodiazepine improved morning stiffness and improved sleep (Walsh et al, 1996).
- Sedatives do significantly increase sleep duration and quality but at the risk of adverse effects, especially cognitive impairment the next day and daytime sleepiness (Glass et al, 2005). They also have addictive potential.
- Check that the insomnia is not caused by an underlying disorder which needs treatment in its own right. Drugs which can cause insomnia include SSRIs, venlafaxine, and high-dose steroids.
- Explain that failing to sleep is a natural part of a reaction to stress and not harmful and that worrying about not sleeping makes sleep harder to achieve.
- Check that the patient is not using alcohol to sleep. In nondependent drinkers, it does improve sleep in the first part of the night but at the expense of early morning rebound awakening. Dependent drinkers lose even this early benefit.
- Explain that simple rules will help (see later) and offer a leaflet (e.g., http://www.patient.co.uk; search 'insomnia'). Behavioural techniques can be more effective than drug treatment, with longer lasting benefit, but they take longer to administer (Sivertsen et al, 2006).
- Offer sleep hygiene for both short-term and chronic insomnia. Consider referral to a sleep clinic if another sleep disorder is present (NICE, 2024). For short-term insomnia, use a nonbenzodiazepine hypnotic (z drug) for 3 to 7 days. Do not prescribe hypnotics to older people or females who are pregnant or breastfeeding. For chronic insomnia, offer CBT for insomnia as first-line treatment. A short course of a hypnotic drug (preferably <1 week) may be considered as an adjunct for severe symptoms or an acute exacerbation (NICE, 2022).
- Consider TCAs in those for whom all other approaches have failed or are inappropriate. Dependence is not a problem, but daytime drowsiness and other adverse effects are. Consider it an option of last resort. An early resort to drugs will distract the patient from the changes in lifestyle and in their mental attitude to insomnia that are necessary.
- Do not prescribe melatonin for most types of insomnia. A meta-analysis has shown that it is ineffective both in secondary insomnia and in jet lag (Buscemi et al, 2006). It may be useful in people with delayed sleep phase syndrome (in which the patient's circadian rhythm is off kilter) (Buscemi et al, 2004). For people older than 55 years of age with persistent insomnia, treatment with a modified-release melatonin may be considered for 3 weeks and a further 10 weeks if there is a beneficial response.

Simple Rules for Sleep Hygiene and to Reduce Insomnia

a. Go to bed and get up at the same time even at weekends. It helps set your 'internal clock'.

b. Prepare for sleep by doing something restful in the half hour before bed. Avoid exercise in the 3 hours before bed. Refuse to discuss exciting or worrying things in bed; keep the bed for sleep and sex.

c. Make sure the room is dark and quiet. Use earplugs if you have to.

d. Avoid caffeine from about 4 PM. This may include chocolate and tea as well as coffee and cola.

e. If you find yourself worrying, write down what the problem is and when you are going to think about it properly. Worrying about something at night magnifies a problem that may seem perfectly solvable in the day.

f. Distract yourself with thoughts of something pleasant.

g. If you still can't sleep, don't lie there fretting. Get up, sit somewhere warm, do something restful, and go back to bed when you feel sleepy.

h. However tired you feel in the day, don't nap. It will mean you sleep even less well at night.

i. If you've slept badly, accept it and lead a full day. Most people can function on less sleep than they think they need.

Anxiety Disorders

- Anxiety disorders are more common than depression, rarely present as pure anxiety, and are even less frequently diagnosed, yet the majority of patients respond to treatment, usually an SSRI or CBT (Table 16.1).
- Detection of an anxiety disorder is improved if the GP uses a few screening questions (Katon & Roy-Byrne, 2007).
- There are few conditions in which a positive, persistent, and supportive stance by the doctor is more important. The patient's instincts will be to avoid facing up to situations that provoke anxiety while treatment relies on facing up to them.
- Almost all anxiety disorders can be managed in primary care, especially if a member of the team is trained in CBT. However, any patient sufficiently distressed by an anxiety disorder who has not responded to primary care management should be offered referral to a specialist mental health service.
- Individual SSRIs and related drugs are licensed in the United Kingdom for one or more types of anxiety but not for all types. There is every reason to think that this is a quirk of licensing and that the benefits are common to all drugs of this class.
- Do not lead the patient to expect a cure; they are likely to be disappointed. Most, however, can expect significant improvement with treatment.
- Anxiety disorders rarely start in midlife or later. Such a presentation suggests another underlying disorder, especially depression or alcohol misuse.

TABLE 16.1	Lifetime Prevalence of Anxiety Disorders in the General Population	
Disorder		**%Population Prevalence**
Panic Disorder		1.6-5.2
GAD		2.8-6.2
Agoraphobia		0.8-2.6
SAD		2.8-13.0
Specific Phobias		8.3-13.8
All Anxiety Disorders		14.5-33.7

Borwin Bandelow & Sophie Michaelis (2015) Epidemiology of anxiety disorders in the 21st century, Dialogues in Clinical Neuroscience, 17:3, 327-335.

Generalised Anxiety

- Check whether the patient also has other mental conditions which need treatment in their own right such as, panic disorder, obsessive-compulsive disorder (OCD), phobia, depression, PTSD, or the misuse of alcohol or drugs.
- Check that there is no physical condition which is mimicking the symptoms of anxiety (e.g., thyrotoxicosis or asthma).

Management of a Crisis

- It may take a crisis to bring the patient to seek help. Immediate treatment is needed to tide the patient over and gain the confidence of the patient and family.
- Give a brief but clear explanation of what is happening and that effective help is available.
- Consider prescribing anxiolytics for 2 to 4 weeks with the clear understanding that this is crisis management only. Use a benzodiazepine, although, in a patient who has misused a benzodiazepine in the past, a sedating antihistamine or an antipsychotic may be preferred (but NICE does not recommend this in primary care). Warn of the risks of dependence, sedation, industrial accidents, and road traffic accidents (Gale & Oakley-Browne, 2004a). Outside the United Kingdom, a longer term role for benzodiazepines is accepted, with the view that dependence and tolerance are rare when they are prescribed for anxiety (Ballenger & Tylee, 2003).
- Arrange an early appointment to begin definitive treatment for the condition.

Long-Term Treatment

- Explain how anxiety causes physical symptoms and how they in turn increase anxiety. Offer a leaflet (see later).
- Assess the patient's disability. How does it affect family relationships, sex, work, and physical and mental state? Is a job at risk? Is alcohol or caffeine intake excessive?
- Explain the options:
  a. *CBT.* CBT has the strongest evidence of benefit (Gale & Oakley-Browne, 2004b). A 1- to 2-hour weekly session is needed for a total of 8 to 20 hours with a trained professional. Briefly, it involves training the patient to act and think differently from their usual manner until a new response to life becomes natural to them. However, do not 'oversell' it to the patient. Even in randomised controlled trials, only half have recovered at 6-month follow-up (Fisher & Durham, 1999). Those who do show some response continue to improve for at least 2 years after

treatment has ended (Dugas, Ladouceur, & Leger, 2003). Anxiety management, without cognitive restructuring, can achieve similar benefit (Gale & Davidson, 2007).

b. *An SSRI.* Almost half of patients show significant improvement with follow-up periods of up to 6 months. However, this yields an NNT of only 5 (because a number improve on placebo) (Kapczinski, Lima, & Souza, 2003). Although this seems an easier option than CBT, there are disadvantages: benefit may not be seen for some weeks and maximum benefit not for 6 months; anxiety may worsen in the first few weeks; at least 6 months treatment will be needed; and although not addictive, there is the possibility that the patient will notice a discontinuation reaction, especially if the drug is stopped suddenly. NICE recommends sertraline as first-line treatment. In patients who cannot take an SSRI, use a TCA.

c. *Self-help* using a written approach with supportive visits to the doctor or nurse. This is also CBT but without a personal therapist. The patient needs to find the motivation to succeed and be comfortable with reading and acting on the written word.

- *Recommend a self-help group*, whichever treatment the patient chooses. Some can assist the patient in a CBT approach, but all provide support and help the patient realise that they are not the only one with this problem.
- *Follow-up.* Unless the patient will be seeing a therapist within 2 weeks, arrange for follow-up along the following lines: at 2, 4 and 6, weeks and then at 3 and 6 months. This applies whether the patient decides on an SSRI or self-help or is waiting to see a CBT therapist.

Practical Details When Prescribing a Selective Serotonin Reuptake Inhibitor for Anxiety

1. Start with a low dose to minimise the increase in anxiety seen with standard doses.
2. If the response at 4 weeks is inadequate, increase slowly to the maximum recommended dose.
3. Treat for a minimum of 6 months after a response is achieved. Patients who show some response at 2 months may continue to improve over the subsequent 6 months.
4. Decide, with the patient, how long to continue to prevent relapse. Treatment for 1 to 2 years is likely to be needed if the condition is longstanding.
5. With prolonged use, sexual dysfunction becomes the most significant adverse effect. For males with erectile dysfunction, sildenafil and related drugs can be used.
6. When stopping the drug, tail it off in fortnightly steps over 1 to 2 months according to what dose was used. If

a discontinuation reaction occurs, go back a step and tail off more slowly.

Special Situations

- *The patient who fails to respond to an SSRI* or in whom it is contraindicated or not tolerated. An alternative is pregabalin, originally used in partial seizure epilepsy. Give it twice daily (Pohl et al, 2005).
- *The patient whose anxiety returns when the SSRI is stopped.* It can be hard to distinguish a discontinuation reaction from the return of anxiety. The symptoms (dizziness, numbness, tingling, nausea, headache, sweating, insomnia, and feeling anxious) are common to both. Sometimes the patient is clear that the symptoms feel different from the original anxiety. If in doubt, restart the SSRI and taper the dose more slowly.
- *The patient whose physical symptoms of anxiety are crippling.* Consider a beta-blocker, although there is a dearth of evidence (Gale & Oakley-Browne, 2004c). A long-acting preparation is needed.

INFORMATION FOR PATIENTS

Self-Help Group

No Panic is a charity that provides information, written treatment programmes, and telephone support for those with anxiety, phobias, and obsessive-compulsive disorders. Helpline: 0300 772 9844. Available at http://www.nopanic.org.uk.

Leaflets

Royal College of Psychiatrists' leaflet 'anxiety, panic and phobias'. Available at http://www.rcpsych.ac.uk.

Panic Disorder

- Follow the management outlined under the discussion of generalised anxiety but without the offer of a benzodiazepine. It is even more important to explain the link between the feeling of panic and the physical symptoms it produces because patients often see it as a physical illness.
- Offer the same triad of behavioural therapy or CBT, an SSRI or SNRI, or self-help.
- If there has been no response after 12 weeks taking an SSRI or SNRI, consider a TCA.
- The details in the Information for Patients box are the same as for generalised anxiety.
- Teach the patient 'first aid' for a panic attack (see later).
- Do not offer a benzodiazepine or another anxiolytic. They are less effective than SSRIs, and they are inappropriate in a disorder that usually lasts more than 4 weeks and in which dependence can occur. They do not treat the depression that is often coexistent or that may emerge as the panic disorder is treated.
- Consider a long-acting beta-blocker. It will abolish some of the somatic symptoms of panic and may help the

subjective terror as well (Mol et al, 2005). However, it will not lead to a lasting cure and may distract the patient from the need to enter more definitive therapy (i.e., CBT).

- Monitor progress with two questions:
  - How many panic attacks have you had since I last saw you?
  - How severe were they, on a scale of 1 to 5, in which 1 is very mild and 5 is extremely severe?
- Prepare yourself, if not the patient, for a relatively poor response to treatment. A Cochrane review (Furukawa, Watanabe, & Churchill, 2007) found that 2 years after the start of treatment, 60% of patients had not achieved a sustained response. Combining psychotherapy with an antidepressant was more likely to achieve a response in the short term than either alone, with an NNT of 10. In other words, if 10 patients are treated with both treatments, one more will respond than if treated with one *or* the other. However, follow-up of 1 or 2 years found that the combination of psychotherapy and antidepressant was better than antidepressant alone (NNT, 6) but no better than psychotherapy alone.

'First Aid' for a Panic Attack: Instructions for the Patient

a. Panic always subsides even if it takes an hour.
b. If some situation has triggered the attack, try to stay in the situation. Leaving can make it harder to go back later.
c. Breathe slowly but not deeply. Deep breathing can mean you hyperventilate and develop more symptoms.
d. Check your watch. What seems like an hour may only be 5 minutes.
e. Distract yourself (e.g., read every detail of the label on something on the supermarket shelf).
f. Have something you say to yourself during the attack, such as, 'It's only a panic attack. I'm not going to faint or vomit (or whatever you most fear), and so, what if I do?'
g. Don't use alcohol. Attacks are more likely as the alcohol wears off.
h. Check whether caffeine has played a part in triggering the attack.

Social Anxiety and Social Phobia

- Patients with social anxiety often think they are excessively shy rather than having a treatable mental disorder.
- Take even more care than usual to explain the nature of the condition. The concept of 'an overactive circuit deep in the brain' may be acceptable to a patient who already understands the concept of, for instance, an overactive thyroid.
- Follow the management outlined under *generalised anxiety* but without the offer of a benzodiazepine. An SSRI or SNRI, exposure therapy, and a combination of the two are all effective during treatment. A large study suggests that those treated with exposure therapy alone

continue to improve in the 6 months after treatment, whereas those treated with sertraline, with or without exposure, show some loss of benefit (Haug et al, 2003). If the SSRI is continued long term, the benefit is sustained, and a treatment course of a minimum of 6 months after remission is needed (Schneier, 2003).
- Offer a beta-blocker to a patient with a circumscribed social anxiety which is disabling and when the somatic symptoms (tremor, palpitations) are preventing the patient from functioning. Performing musicians are the prime example. Warn the patient that they will find it hard not to become psychologically reliant on the drug. However, they may prefer this to the loss of their chosen career.

Phobias

- Phobias require energetic management if they present early to prevent them from becoming fixed. Even those presenting late are amenable to treatment if the patient is willing to undergo therapy. All patients with phobias need treatment.
- Many patients who are phobic do not present with the phobia but with a consequence of it: alcohol or drug misuse, truancy, failure to attend appointments at the surgery, anxiety, or depression. Failure to discover the underlying phobia will result in a failure of treatment.
- Offer referral for CBT, an SSRI, or a self-help programme along CBT lines (see the discussion of generalised anxiety).
- In patients who choose to be treated without referral, use the following programme, with or without treatment with an SSRI:
  a. Urge the patient not to avoid the phobic situation. Avoidance increases the strength of the phobia.
  b. Teach the patient the rules of 'first aid' during an attack of panic.
  c. Plan a programme of gently increasing exposure to the phobia. Do this with imaginary exposure if real exposure is not possible. Exposure must be daily, and the patient must stay in the phobic situation until the panic has subsided. Ask the patient to keep a diary to discuss at each appointment.
  d. Ask what would be 'the worst possible scenario'. Often it turns out to be unpleasant but acceptable. Usually it is that other people will see that the patient is being phobic. Being prepared to 'own up' to a phobia is often a great step forward.
- *Drug treatment at the time of the phobic event.* Avoid giving benzodiazepines for a phobia that poses a problem more than occasionally. The patient is likely to become even less able to face the situation without drugs than before treatment began. Consider a beta-blocker (e.g., propranolol 40 mg) 1 to 2 hours before exposure to the phobic situation in those who cannot tolerate the physical symptoms of panic.

Specific Phobias

- *Fear of flying.* Exposure therapy, either using a computer stimulation or just sitting in an aircraft and imagining that it is flying, show marked short-term benefits, with more than half of patients who previously refused to fly now managing to fly. However, the effect does not last and is almost completely lost after 6 months (Maltby et al, 2002). It is therefore most suitable for someone who has to make a one-off flight. Several organisations offer exposure therapy, including major airlines such as British Airways and Virgin Atlantic.

- *Fear of medical or dental procedures.* CBT is the most effective treatment, but most patients present too late, when the need for help is urgent. Diazepam 10 mg 1 to 2 hours before the event has been shown to reduce anxiety significantly more than placebo, although the placebo effect is also marked (Wilner et al, 2002).
- *Patients with agoraphobia* are likely to find themselves unable to attend primary care clinics and even more likely to have difficulty attending specialist centres. Treatment in primary care using an SSRI and a simple CBT approach (see earlier) will be successful in some and allow others to improve enough to participate in more definitive therapy.

INFORMATION FOR PATIENTS

Self-Help Group

Triumph over Phobia has details of local groups. Available at http://www.triumphoverphobia.com.

Leaflets

Royal College of Psychiatrists. Search on: anxiety, panic, and phobias. Available at http://www.rcpsych.ac.uk.

Obsessive-Compulsive Disorder

- Be on the alert for the diagnosis. Patients are often reluctant to admit to the disorder. In patients whose symptoms raise the possibility of OCD, ask specific questions such as: 'Do you find yourself doing things repeatedly in a way you can't control?' and 'Do you find yourself bothered by certain thoughts that you can't get out of your mind?'. Conditions which raise the possibility of OCD include depression, anxiety, eating disorders, fear of illness, fear of causing others harm, and skin disorders that suggest repeated hand washing.
- After OCD is diagnosed, check for depression. One-third of patients with OCD are currently depressed, and two-thirds will become depressed at some stage (Ballenger & Tylee, 2003).
- Assess the risk of self-harm and suicide.
- The NICE guideline (NICE, 2005) suggests a stepped-care approach, with the starting point being the recognition of the disorder and the offer of information about the condition and the support groups that are available (see box). Later steps involve the provision of self-help material, referral for CBT, and the offer of an SSRI (see later).
- Involve the family or carers in the process of finding out about the disease and its treatment.

- When functional impairment is at least moderate, offer an SSRI as described under the discussion of generalised anxiety. Expect the response to take even longer (≤ 12 weeks) than with other forms of anxiety. Expect to continue it for at least 1 year.
- If the patient cannot take an SSRI, consider clomipramine (Ballenger & Tylee, 2003). NICE advises against other TCAs.
- Offer CBT if it is available. It involves gradual exposure of the patient to situations which provoke anxiety while not allowing the patient the relief of using a ritual to relieve that anxiety. At the same time, the therapist retrains the patient in different patterns of thought. Patients who refuse CBT at first because it sounds too threatening may accept it after partial remission with drug treatment. CBT appears to offer most hope for lasting remission.
- If the patient responds and then relapses after discharge, refer back urgently before the pattern of behaviour becomes firmly established.

PATIENT INFORMATION

Pedrick, C., & Hyman, B. (2010). *The OCD workbook: Your guide to breaking free from obsessive-compulsive disorder* (3rd ed.) New Harbinger, California, USA.
    NICE (2005). *Obsessive-compulsive disorder and body dysmorphic disorder: treatment.* Clinical Guideline no. 31. National Institute for Clinical Excellence. Retrieved from www.nice.org.uk/guidance/cg31.

Patient Support

OCD Action's website includes aids to self-diagnosis, blogs by people with the condition, and information about support groups. Helpline: 0300 636 5478. Available at http://www.ocdaction.org.uk.

Self-Harm

GUIDELINE

National Institute for Health and Clinical Excellence. (2004; updated 2022b). *Self-harm: Assessment, management and preventing recurrence. NICE guideline NG225.* Retrieved from http://www.nice.org.uk/guidance/ng225.

- In the United Kingdom, 1 in 10 teenagers deliberately self-harms. In the years 2015 to 2016 in England and Wales, nearly 19,000 required admissions to hospital (NSPCC, 2016). Seven of eight are female.
- It is the strongest single predictor of successful suicide, being found in 40% to 60% of suicides (Hawton, Zahl, & Weatherall, 2003). However, this does not make it a useful predictor of suicide. Of self-harmers in the United Kingdom, only 0.7% kill themselves within 1 year and 3% in 15 years.

- Two of three self-harmers consult their GP in the subsequent 3 months (Bennewith et al, 2002). One in six harm themselves again within 1 year. However, attempting to assess the risk of repeated self-harm is unlikely to be successful (Kapur et al, 2005).
- A large study of an intervention in which patients were sent an invitation to consult after an episode of self-harm failed to show any benefit in terms of reducing repeated episodes (Bennewith et al, 2002). Indeed, systematic review has failed to identify benefit from any treatment (Soomro, 2004).
- Ask what the patient did, what precipitated it, and whether the problem is still present. Assume it is evidence of serious emotional distress.
- Provide information to patient and carers about support and treatments available self-care, how to deal with injuries, how to manage scars, care plans and safety plans and what they involve, the impact of encountering stigma around self-harm, who will be involved in their care and how to get in touch with them, and what do to in an emergency.
- Assess the current mental state and the suicidal risk and capacity about treatment and decisions to share information.
- Look for other problems, including medical illness, social problems, and past or present physical or sexual abuse, and complete a psychosocial assessment to identify static and dynamic risk factors, hazards, and protective factors.
- Do not use risk assessment tools to predict self-harm risk (NICE, 2022b).
- Manage according to what is found. Make and agree on a collaborative safety plan with the patient. The underlying problem may be trivial (an impulsive act, immediately regretted) or grave (a psychotic illness). Among those who are not mentally ill, being unclear about the reason for the self-harm is a bad prognostic sign, as are male sex and being an older rather than a younger adolescent (Royal College of Psychiatrists, 1998). Self-harm in people older than 65 years of age is especially associated with depression and suicide (NICE, 2022b).
- Teach the patient ways of reducing the risk of serious harm while the underlying problem is being attended to (Mental Health Foundation, 2004):
  - *Harm minimisation* (e.g., make a small cut rather than a large one, take aspirin rather than paracetamol and never more than four at once)
  - *Distraction* (e.g., have a plan of something to do once the urge to self-harm starts to build up such as go for a run or play music very loudly)
  - *Identify someone* you can talk to when you feel in danger.
- Refer to mental health service if the patient's levels of concern or distress are rising or the frequency or degree of self-harm or suicidal intent is increasing. If managed in primary care, ensure they have regular appointments with their GP for self-harm review.

Acute Psychotic Disorders

The possibility of acute psychosis is raised by the following:
- Hallucinations
- Delusions
- Disorganised or strange speech
- Agitation or bizarre behaviour
- Extreme and labile emotional states
- Family concern about recent changes in personality, behaviour or function

Initial Assessment

- Obtain a careful history from family or friends of recent events and changes in the patient's behaviour.
- Ask about drug or alcohol misuse.
- Assess the mental state, including the risk of suicide and of harm to others.
- Make a differential diagnosis if this is a first episode. Consider the possibilities of acute confusional state, drug-induced psychosis, and epilepsy. An episode that is related to cannabis use probably signifies an underlying psychosis triggered by the cannabis.
- If this is a relapse, review past management and outcomes.
- Decide if admission or referral is necessary.
- Explain to the family what you think is wrong and what action is needed. If feasible, give the patient the same information and obtain consent.

When There is a Risk of Violence

GUIDELINES

National Institute of Heath and Care Excellence. (2015). *Violence and aggression: Short-term management in mental health, health and community settings. NICE guideline 10.* Retrieved from https://www.nice.org.uk/guidance/ng10.
    National Institute of Heath and Care Excellence. (2014c). *Psychosis and schizophrenia in adults: Prevention and management. NICE clinical guideline 178.* Retrieved from https://www.nice.org.uk/guidance/cg178/.

- First, try to calm the patient (see guidance earlier).
- Appoint one member of staff to relate to the patient. Others should move away.
- Encourage the patient to move to a safe place.
- If there is a weapon, ask the patient to put it in a neutral place, not to hand it over.
- Explain to the patient throughout, in a calm manner, what you are doing.
- Ask the patient open questions (e.g., 'Tell me what's going on').

Drug Treatment

- NICE advise against starting antipsychotics in primary care, particularly for a first episode. Treatment decisions should be made in conjunction with local mental health services.
- For relapses, follow the treatment care plan, if one is available, and refer to specialist mental health services for

further management. Treatment decisions should be based on patient preference, previous response to medications, and medical history.

- *If a patient initially refuses medication that is urgently needed*, spending time, in a calm manner, can often win the patient's confidence. Do not deny the patient's delusions or hallucinations but say something like: 'I can see you are pretty upset about all this, and I can help with that'.
- *Rarely, an agitated or aggressive patient needs rapid tranquillisation.* Tranquillisation makes subsequent assessment difficult; it is traumatic for the patient; and sedated patients need observation, including pulse, blood pressure and respiratory rate, which may not be possible. If there is no alternative this should be completed only with the support of police and mental health staff.
- *Options for rapid tranquilisation:*
  a. Lorazepam 2 to 4 mg orally or, preferably, sublingually or
  b. Haloperidol 5 to 10 mg orally; or if refused,
  c. Lorazepam 1 to 2 mg intramuscular (IM); have flumazenil available for use if oversedated; or haloperidol 5–10 mg IM combined with promethazine 25 mg IM
  If two drugs are needed, combine lorazepam and haloperidol (with promethazine).
- After rapid tranquillisation, check the patient's pulse, blood pressure, and respiratory rate while waiting for the ambulance to arrive. Ask the crew to continue monitoring with pulse oximetry in the ambulance.

Precautions When Visiting a Disturbed Patient at Home

- Ensure there is no past history of violence or delusions focused on the GP.
- If necessary, organise support and do not go alone.
- Try to ensure that a relative or friend is present.
- Tell someone in the practice whom you are visiting and when.
- Arrange for the practice staff to phone you after a specified time.
- Have an action plan if you do not respond to the phone call.

Referral and Admission

- *Refer all patients with acute psychosis to the psychiatrist or specialist mental health team.* The specialist services will usually decide whether the patient needs admission or can be managed at home.
- *Admission* is usually required in acute psychosis especially if one of the following is present:
  a. It is the first episode.
  b. There is a significant risk of suicide, violence, or neglect.
  c. The patient is noncompliant or has serious side effects.
  d. There is coexisting alcohol or drug misuse.

- *Management at home can be considered* in a patient with a relapse of a known mental illness with a previous good response to treatment when the patient agrees to restart treatment, is at low risk, when home care is safe, and when community support available.
- *Driving.* A patient with an acute psychosis or relapse of bipolar affective disorder should not drive and, in the United Kingdom, the DVLA (Driver and Vehicle Licensing Agency) must be informed.

Compulsory Admission

Indications for Use of the Mental Health Act (England and Wales, 1983)

This account includes amendments made to the Mental Health Act up to 2015. It focuses on sections of the Act most relevant to general practice.

- The Mental Health Act can only be used if the following conditions are met:
  a. The patient has a mental disorder of a nature or degree which warrants detention in a hospital for assessment (or assessment followed by medical treatment) for at least a limited period.
  b. The patient should be detained in the interests of his or her own health or safety or with a view to the protection of others.
  c. There is no alternative management other than compulsory admission to hospital.
- 'Mental disorders' are mental illness, psychopathic disorder, mental impairment, and severe mental impairment. The latter two disorders refer to patients with learning difficulties associated with abnormally aggressive or seriously irresponsible conduct.
- Although often called by relatives or neighbours, the doctor's role is to safeguard the patient's welfare and not that of the relatives or neighbours unless they are in danger.
- A patient can be admitted compulsorily even when they pose no danger, provided that they are sufficiently ill (e.g., acutely psychotic) to need compulsory admission because treatment is urgently needed for the sake of the patient's health.
- An approved mental health professional (AMHP) is responsible for making the application for compulsory admission, coordinating the medical assessment of the patient, providing the forms, and arranging for the transport of the patient to hospital.
- Every practice and integrated care board should have agreed on a procedure for the management of psychiatric crises. Appendix 20 is an example.

Assessment Under the Act

- Obtain all available information from the patient's records and from available friends and family. Try to find out who is the nearest relative (note that this is not necessarily the same person as the next of kin): they have the right to be informed, to object to detention, and to insist that a detained patient be discharged unless that patient poses a danger.

- Telephone the AMHP and agree on a plan. This should include whether to involve a second doctor or the police at this stage.
- If admission looks likely, contact the duty psychiatrist to discuss the availability of a bed and the need for his or her attendance.
- If the decision is made not to admit the patient, work out a care plan. Essential features are that family members know whom to call in an emergency and that intensive follow-up arrangements are put in place.

Which Section of the Act Should Be Used?

How Desperate Is the Situation?

- *The patient is about to injure themself or others.* The doctor may restrain the patient or give emergency treatment knowing that under common law such action is defensible if done in good faith. Such action would normally be followed by an admission under the Act using Section 2 (28 days), though if the emergency continues, Section 4 (72 hours) might be needed.
- *Admission is needed and is so urgent that both of the following are present:*
  a. The doctor cannot leave the patient.
  b. Waiting for an approved clinician (usually an approved psychiatrist) would cause 'undesirable delay'.
  Use Section 4 (detention for 72 hours). This requires assessment by a doctor and an AMHP. Admission must take place within 24 hours of the assessment or the application, whichever is earlier. The fact that attendance by the approved clinician is inconvenient is not grounds for the use of this section.
- *Admission is needed, but there is time to wait for an approved clinician.* Use Section 2 (28 days). This is the preferred section and is used in almost all cases. It requires assessment by a mental health professional approved under Section 12 of the Act (the 'first' doctor) and by a doctor with previous knowledge of the patient (the 'second' doctor) and an AMHP. Admission must take place within 5 days, or the application is void. Arrange to see the patient together if possible, although the Act allows the two doctors to examine the patient up to 5 days apart.

Further Clarifications

- The 'second' doctor should be one with previous knowledge of the patient. However, if no such doctor is available, any doctor may sign provided they do not work in the same hospital as the 'first' doctor.
- In theory, the application for compulsory admission may be made by the nearest relative. In practice, this is rarely wise: an AMHP is needed to ensure that the formalities

are observed, that a full assessment is made, and to avoid later recriminations within the family if the nearest relative made such a decision.

- It is occasionally possible to commit a patient to hospital under the Act even if they agree to informal admission. A psychiatrist may recommend this course of action if, from previous knowledge of the patient, a judgement is made that an apparent agreement to informal admission is not likely to be sustained. If taking this line of action, the reasons for doing so must be stated on the form.
- After an application has been signed, decide how to escort the patient into an ambulance. Given time and patience, it is usually possible to achieve it without force. If force is needed, it is the role of the police rather than the ambulance crew.
- Drug or alcohol dependency is not in itself grounds for compulsory admission. This is only possible if the person also has a mental disorder as defined in the Act. If a patient is under the influence of drugs or alcohol so that a proper assessment cannot be made, it should be postponed until such assessment is possible.
- Learning difficulty is not grounds for compulsory admission under Sections 3 or 4 unless associated with 'abnormally aggressive or seriously irresponsible conduct'. However, the other relevant sections, including Section 2, can be used.
- Psychopathic disorder is defined as 'a persistent disorder or disability of mind (whether or not including significant impairment of intelligence) that results in abnormally aggressive or seriously irresponsible conduct on the part of the person concerned'. It is grounds for compulsory admission regardless of whether it is treatable, provided that the other criteria are met. Only in using Section 3 is it necessary that the psychopathy should be 'treatable' (i.e., that treatment should be necessary to alleviate or prevent deterioration in the patient's condition).

Other Sections of Value

- *Section 3* allows for detention for 6 months. It is occasionally used in the community instead of Section 4 if the patient is already known to the psychiatric services. In practice, it is almost always used after the patient is in hospital and before Section 2 or 4 has expired.
- *Section 7* allows the appointment of a guardian for up to 6 months. The guardian has the power to insist that the patient live at a specified place and attend for work, training, or medical appointments.
- *Section 136* allows the police to remove a person from a public place to a hospital or police station, for a maximum period of 72 hours, if both of the following apply:
  a. They have a mental disorder.
  b. They are in immediate need of care and control.
- *Section 135* allows a magistrate to authorise a police officer (with a doctor and AMHP) to enter any premises

to which access has been denied and remove the patient to a place of safety if there is reasonable cause to suspect that the person is:

a. Suffering from a mental disorder; and

b. Being ill-treated or neglected or not kept under proper control; or

c. Unable to care for themselves and lives alone.

The GP can usually gain entry legally without using Section 135, for instance, by asking the neighbours to open the door or by using his or her relationship with the patient to get the door open.

- *A Community Treatment Order* ensures that assessment and treatment are carried out in the community with the responsible clinician having the power to recall the patient to hospital if necessary.

Regulations for Scotland and Northern Ireland

These follow similar principles to those for England and Wales, but the brief details of the Acts are as follows (Tables 16.2 and 16.3):

- *For emergency detention, the following must apply*:

    a. The person has a mental disorder which causes his or her decision making to be 'significantly impaired'.

    b. It is necessary as a matter of urgency to detain the person for assessment.

    c. The person's health, safety, or welfare or the safety of another person would be at significant risk if they were not detained.

    d. Making arrangements for the possible granting of a short-term detention certificate (see later) would involve an 'undesirable delay'.

- *For short-term detention,* the same four criteria must apply except that it need not be a matter of urgency, and detention is for assessment or treatment.

TABLE 16.2 Mental Health (Care and Treatment) (Scotland) Act of 2003[a]

Type of Compulsion	Professionals	Duration
Emergency detention	GP and MHO if practicable	72 hours
Short-term detention	GP and MHO	28 days
Compulsory treatment order	MHO, AMP, and patient's GP or another AMP	6 months
Power of entry	MHO obtains from sheriff or JP	Single event

[a]For more information, see NHS Education for Scotland (https://www.mwcscot.org.uk/law-and-rights/mental-health-act).
AMP, Approved medical practitioner; *GP,* general practitioner; *JP,* justice of the peace; *MHO,* mental health officer.

TABLE 16.3 Mental Health (Northern Ireland) Order of 1986[a]

Situation	Section	Professionals	Duration
Emergency	4	GP and ASW or relative	7 days
Power of entry	129	ASW obtains from JP; GP and police enter	Single event

[a]For more details, see Guidelines on the Use of the Mental Health (Northern Ireland) Order 1986 (http://www.rqia.org.uk/RQIA/files/4e/4ee9f634-be47-4398-afc9-906a20ff3198.pdf).
ASW, Approved social worker; *GP,* general practitioner; *JP,* justice of the peace.

- *For a compulsory treatment* order, the following must apply:

    a. The patient has a mental disorder.

    b. Medical treatment is available which would be likely to prevent the disorder worsening or would be likely to alleviate the symptoms or effects of the disorder.

    c. There would be a significant risk to the patient or to any other person if the patient was not provided with such treatment.

    d. The patient's ability to make decisions about the provision of medical treatment is significantly impaired because of his or her mental disorder.

    e. The making of the compulsory treatment order is necessary.

A compulsory treatment order may authorise detention in hospital or impose certain requirements on the patient in the community (a community-based compulsory treatment order).

- The Act also allows for the removal to a place of safety of a person who is exposed to ill treatment or neglect or who is unable to look after themself or property or financial affairs. It further allows for a person to be removed from a public place to a place of safety when it is in the interests of that person or when it is necessary to protect other people (NHS Education for Scotland, 2004).

ADVICE FOR PATIENTS AND PROFESSIONALS

MIND provides a leaflet on the Act available at http://www.mind.org.uk (search on 'Mental Health Act').

Chronic Schizophrenia

GUIDELINE

National Institute of Heath and Care Excellence. (2014). *Psychosis and schizophrenia in adults: Prevention and management. NICE clinical guideline 178.* Retrieved from https://www.nice.org.uk/guidance/cg178/.

- About 1% of a practice population will suffer from schizophrenia at some time in their lives, more in cities and in immigrant communities. Between 25% and 40% will lose contact with secondary services while still chronically ill (Anonymous, 1994).
- Structured care offers a chance of improving the management of such patients.
- In the United Kingdom, the average GP will look after 12 patients with schizophrenia, half of them without current involvement of the specialist mental health services (Picchioni & Murray, 2007).

Structured Care

This entails:

a. Establishing a register of patients with severe and enduring mental illness. This can be done from existing clinical codes, from repeat prescriptions for psychotropic drugs, from addresses of hostels and homes catering for the mentally ill, and opportunistically.

b. Using the register to ensure that patients are seen at least annually and actively seeking out patients who default from follow-up. See later for details of the annual review.

c. Developing a care plan that is individualised for patients, taking into account psychiatric, medical, social, and occupational or educational issues. Ideally, this care plan should be shared with carers.

d. Working with local mental health teams to identify agreed policies and guidelines for treatment, referral, and the management of relapse.

e. Adapting existing computer templates to record long-term follow-up and undertaking practice audit of the above goals.

Referral

- Arrange for urgent assessment of the following:
  - Those presenting for the first time
  - Those posing a risk to themselves or to others
  - Those relapsing, or showing the prodrome of a relapse
  - Those at risk of relapse because of one of the following:
    a. A deterioration in their home circumstances
    b. Poor compliance
    c. Abuse of drugs or alcohol
- Those with side effects of medication or who are not taking it.

  Such an assessment is better done at home than in the outpatient department if possible.
- Patients will also need to be referred, although not necessarily urgently if one of the following is present:
- They are becoming increasingly disabled by their illness.
- A care plan needs to be drawn up, as when a patient moves to a new area.
- The patient or family request referral or the therapeutic relationship has broken down.

General Management

- *Education.* The patient and the family need to know:
  (a) About 85% to 90% recover from the first episode in the following 2 years (World Health Organization, 1979). In the 5 years after the first episode, half do not relapse, or they relapse but recover completely between episodes. Twenty percent will never have another episode (Picchioni & Murray, 2007).
  (b) How to identify early signs of relapse. Looking for early warning signs can prevent relapse or reduce its severity (Falloon et al, 1993). The Early Warning Signs Form (see Appendix 22) can be used to help with this.
  (c) How to obtain early treatment.
  (d) That avoiding extremes of expressed emotion by family members, whether hostility or overprotectiveness, can reduce the risk of relapse.
- *Advance directives.* Discuss the use of advance directives with patient and family. These indicate what the patient wants to happen if a relapse occurs. If one is drawn up, the patient and primary and secondary care all need copies.
- Check that the patient has been offered the benefits of case management. In the United Kingdom, this takes the form of the care programme approach, in which a specialist team assists the patient with daily living, in the understanding of the condition and in its management.
- If fit for sheltered work, liaise with the mental health team for advice.
- Assess the patient's housing needs.
- Help the patient to claim the disability living allowance if eligible.

Drug Treatment

- Early drug treatment seems to lead to better medium- and long-term outcomes (Loebel et al, 1992).
- Without drugs, 60% of patients relapse in the 9 months after an acute attack. Maintenance with antipsychotics reduces this by more than 50%.
- Atypical antipsychotics are now first-line drugs in the United Kingdom; however, if a patient is successfully treated with a conventional antipsychotic, it should not be changed. Atypical antipsychotics are chosen because of the lower incidence of extrapyramidal adverse effects and possibly greater effect on cognition and on negative symptoms. However, they are no more effective than typical antipsychotics, and overall, they have as many, but different, adverse effects (Picchioni & Murray, 2007). The exceptions to this are clozapine and olanzapine, which may be more effective than other drugs (Citrone & Stroup, 2006).
- The choice of long-term medication should be made by the psychiatrist and patient together. It will be needed for at least 1 to 2 years after a relapse, and monitoring will be needed for 2 years after that.

- All antipsychotics are associated with an increased risk of sudden cardiac death as well as of stroke. A baseline electrocardiogram (ECG) is recommended if the manufacturer advises one is necessary, if the patient has a personal history of cardiovascular disease, if the physical examination identifies a cardiovascular risk factor (e.g., high blood pressure), or if the patient is being admitted (NICE, 2014c).

Relapse

Ascertain whether the relapse is caused by the patient's discontinuing medication. If it is:
- Assess the reason for stopping treatment (e.g., the presence of side effects, failure to obtain a prescription).
- Decide if restarting previous medication is appropriate and acceptable.
- Review the need for urgent psychiatric assessment.
- If assessment is needed but will be delayed and there is concern about medication, phone for advice from the psychiatrist.
- Inform the patient's care coordinator or the lead clinician identified in their care plan if this is available.

Medication Review

- Patients need a medication review at least annually (NICE, 2014c). The repeat prescription slip should indicate when a medication review is due.
- Someone in the practice needs to be responsible for ensuring such patients have attended for this review and to know what action to take if the patient defaults. The medication review should include:
  a. Assessment of mental state and compliance.
  b. The presence of adverse effects or drug interactions. Adverse effects with conventional antipsychotics are likely to be extrapyramidal; with atypical antipsychotics, they are likely to be weight gain and hyperprolactinaemia.
  c. Existence of drug or alcohol problems.
  d. Whether the patient has been admitted in the past 6 months.
  e. Patients taking clozapine need monitoring for agranulocytosis, weekly for 6 months and then monthly in the United Kingdom. Organising this is the responsibility of the prescriber. If delegated to primary care, a written protocol is needed.

Side Effects of Medication

Conventional Antipsychotics
- *Extrapyramidal adverse effects*. If they occur, discuss management with the specialist. The main options are:
  a. Reduce the dose of the antipsychotic.
  b. Add an anticholinergic drug. Avoid procyclidine, which is a stimulant and can be abused. Try to withdraw an anticholinergic after 3 months without symptoms. Tetrabenazine may help in tardive dyskinesia.

  c. Change to an atypical antipsychotic. Clozapine is the treatment of choice.
- Neuroleptic malignant syndrome occurs in 0.5%.

Atypical Antipsychotics
- Weight gain
- Dizziness and postural hypotension in the early stages
- Diabetes
- Extrapyramidal adverse effects, but they are uncommon and usually respond to dose reduction

All Antipsychotics
- *Palpitations*. Repeat the ECG. If the QT interval is prolonged but is 500 ms or less, reduce the dose. If it is greater than 500 ms, stop the drug (MHRA (Medicines and Healthcare products Regulatory Agency), 2006).

Psychotherapy

Good evidence exists for both CBT and family therapy, and NICE recommends that both forms of therapy be offered to patients and to the family of patients with psychosis. A minimum course of 6 months of either is needed. If they are available, they should be offered as well as medication.

Annual Review

The annual review is likely to be more comprehensive if a checklist or computer template is used. Topics to cover are:
a. Current mental state, including the presence of depression, delusional thoughts, anxiety, hallucinations, and signs of self-neglect. Half of patients with schizophrenia develop depression at some stage. It carries a higher risk of suicide than depression in other patients (Jones & Buckley, 2003)
b. Problems, crises, or admissions since last seen
c. Daily activities, employment, training, income, and disability benefits
d. Substance misuse, which is likely in half of patients
e. Accommodation needs
f. Carers, relationships, dependants (children), and home support
g. Assessment of physical health, including weight, blood pressure, cervical screening, smoking status, family planning needs, fasting sugar, haemoglobin A1C, lipids, and assessment of cardiovascular disease risk. Smoking cessation should be offered when appropriate, and coexisting cardiovascular disease and diabetes should be treated. An annual ECG is recommended in those taking an antipsychotic which can prolong the QT interval
h. Medication review and monitoring blood tests if necessary
i. Whether care is GP only or shared with psychiatrist, Community Psychiatric Nurse (CPN), or social worker
j. Assessment of the carer's needs

Carers' Needs

- People who care for someone with severe and enduring mental illness should have:
  a. A needs assessment at regular intervals
  b. A care plan which is reviewed annually
  c. Links with local carer support groups
- Carers need to be identified, and this information should be put on their summary card or computer problem list. The practice should have a carers' register and a practice policy on whom to assess, when, and by whom. Social services should record each carer's needs and draw up an agreed care plan, which includes:
  a. Information about the mental health needs of the patient
  b. How to identify a relapse and what action to take
  c. Advice on benefits, housing, and employment
  d. Arrangements for short-term breaks
  e. Social support including access to carers' support groups
  f. Information about appeals or complaints procedures

The plan should be confirmed in writing and communicated to the primary care team. The GP is the professional most likely to identify signs of stress or the deteriorating health of a carer. The plan should indicate who should review the carer's needs at such times, and the GP can initiate this.

PATIENT ORGANISATIONS

Rethink Severe Mental Illness, 28 Albert Embankment, London SE1 7GR. National advice line: 0808 801 0525. Available at http://www.rethink.org.

MIND. Mind Infoline: 0300 123 3393. Available at http://www.mind.org.uk.

SANE. Saneline tel: 0300 304 7000; email support at http://www.sane.org.uk.

Bipolar Affective Disorder

GUIDELINE

National Institute of Health and Care Excellence. (2014b; updated 2020). *Bipolar disorder: Assessment and management. NICE clinical guideline 185.* Retrieved from https://www.nice.org.uk/guidance/cg185.

General Management

- All suspected new diagnoses of bipolar disorder should be assessed by a specialist, a treatment plan commenced, and a care plan agreed with the patient.
- In a new presentation of an existing bipolar condition, check that the patient has had a recent assessment by a specialist and that everyone is clear who the key worker is in case of difficulties.
- Explain the nature of the condition to the patient and family.

- Agree on what the warning signs of relapse are for that individual (see Appendix 22).
- Review the plan of action for when relapse occurs. This will depend on the form the relapse takes and the action needed to minimise the potential risks involved; in hypomania, it may mean removing debit and credit cards from the patient; in depression, it may mean intensifying social support. In mania, it may involve supplying medication (an antipsychotic or a benzodiazepine) to be taken at the first sign of relapse. Patients may need to be advised to stop driving during an acute episode of illness.
- Explore whether stressors seem to trigger a relapse such as irregular hours, lack of sleep, or use of alcohol or drugs.
- Enter the patient on the practice register of patients with severe mental illness.
- Ensure recall for annual reviews.
- Offer information about the local and national support that is available (see box).

During Episodes of Depression

- Arrange for specialist assessment and discuss any medication changes with the specialist before assessment if there will be a delay.
- NICE recommend fluoxetine combined with olanzapine or quetiapine alone as first-line treatment, with olanzapine or lamotrigine alone as further options depending on patient preference and previous treatment response.
- If the patient is already taking lithium, then check lithium levels and titrate to the therapeutic range. Fluoxetine and olanzapine or quetiapine alone can be added to lithium and, if this fails, then lamotrigine can be added to lithium in place of fluoxetine with olanzapine.
- Similarly, if the patient is taking valproate, then titrate this to the maximum tolerated dose and then fluoxetine with olanzapine or quetiapine alone can be added.
- Consider offering psychological interventions if available.

During Episodes of Mania or Hypomania

- Avoid unnecessary confrontation.
- Check if there was a trigger for the relapse and whether it can be rectified.
- Assess the risk of impulsive behaviour (e.g., financial or business recklessness).
- Assess the need for admission, including compulsory admission, or for referral to the community mental health team.
- Tell the family who to contact if the patient becomes very agitated or severely disruptive.
- Identify the carer's needs. In chronic illness, consider respite care.

Medication

- Discuss the options with the patient's specialist. They are likely to involve:
  a. An oral antipsychotic (usually haloperidol, olanzapine, quetiapine, or risperidone)
  b. Increasing lithium while keeping the blood level within the therapeutic range

c. Short-term use of a benzodiazepine for night sedation
d. Tailing off an antidepressant if one is being taken
- Do not expect dramatic improvement. Even in the ideal setting of clinical trials, only about half the patients have a 50% improvement of symptoms over 3 to 4 weeks (Keck, 2003).
- Prepare to taper off the antipsychotic over at least 2 weeks when in full remission. Continued use can precipitate depression.

Prevention of Relapse

- The choice of medication to prevent relapse should be based on patient preference and what has previously been effective.
- Lithium is the first-line drug as it is most effective.
- Alternatives are valproate (which can also be added to lithium if lithium alone is ineffective but should be avoided in females of childbearing age) or olanzapine. Quetiapine can also be used especially if it has been effective in previous relapses.

Lithium

The GP needs to:
a. Ensure clear agreement on who is responsible for monitoring lithium treatment.
b. Have an agreed protocol for monitoring blood levels, identifying side effects, and taking appropriate action. Put the patient on the recall register for monitoring blood levels.
c. Provide the patient with a written description of drug side effects and what to do if these develop. Mind (http://www.mind.org.uk) has useful online resources.
d. Check the patient knows to maintain adequate fluid intake and avoid dehydration and nonsteroidal antiinflammatory drugs.
e. Check that the patient understands that the lithium should not be stopped unless toxicity occurs because relapse may occur.
f. *Lithium levels.* Check lithium levels every 3 months. Take blood 12 hours after the last dose. Levels of 0.4 to 0.8 mmol/L are adequate for maintenance, but in acute mania, a level of 0.8 to 1 mmol/L is necessary.
g. *Change in dose.* If the dose is changed, check levels weekly for 4 weeks, then monthly for 3 months, and then every 3 months.
h. Check thyroid and renal function annually.
i. Warn females of reproductive age that lithium is an enzyme inducer which reduces the efficacy of the combined oral contraceptive and that it carries a risk of teratogenicity as well.

Management of Suspected Lithium Toxicity

- Symptoms of toxicity include muscle weakness, shaking, trembling, fasciculation, nausea, vomiting or diarrhoea, ataxia, confusion, slurred speech, toxic psychosis, convulsions, coma, and cardiac arrhythmias.
- Check the lithium level and urea and electrolytes.
- Stop lithium. Levels usually decrease to safety within 24 hours. If the lithium level is more than 1.5 mmol/L

or there is diarrhoea and vomiting, stop lithium immediately and seek urgent specialist advice.
- Identify the cause of the toxicity before restarting lithium.
- If no cause is found, restart at a lower dose.
- Monitor levels monthly for 3 months after toxicity for which there was no obvious reason.

Dealing With Violence

Every practice needs a policy for dealing with violent patients. Many of these patients have a past history of violent or threatening behaviour. A typical policy would include:
a. A notice in the waiting room stating that physical or verbal abuse, racism, threats, and violence to staff will result in removal from the practice
b. Panic buttons in consulting rooms and a clear procedure to follow if one is set off
c. Clear guidelines on who should deal with an aggressive, abusive, or violent patient in the waiting room
d. How risks will be assessed and what action will be taken (Shaw, 2000)
e. A protocol for the management of a patient whose delusions are focused on a specific doctor or nurse
f. Written indications on when to call the police and who should do so
g. Guidance on how to deal with home visit requests of a potentially violent patient
h. Sympathetic support for staff exposed to violent situations
i. A policy of informing other local GPs that a violent patient who has been removed from the practice list and may want to register with them
j. A record kept of all such incidents
k. A way to report these incidents as 'significant events' so that lessons can be learnt by others

Eating Disorders

- Approximately 1.25 million people are thought to have eating disorders in the United Kingdom, according to Beat, a national eating disorders charity.
- Beat estimates that 10% have anorexia nervosa, 40% have bulimia nervosa, and the rest fall into the OSFED (other specified feeding and eating disorders) category, including binge eating disorder.
- Although eating disorders can develop at any age, the risk is highest for young males and females between 13 and 17 years of age.
- Twenty percent of people with eating disorders die prematurely from their illness, either by suicide or from physical complications (Herzog et al, 2000).
- Anorexia nervosa has the highest mortality rate of all the mental health conditions, with one in five of anorexia patients dying by suicide (Arcelus, 2011).
- In 2007, it was estimated through the Adult Psychiatric Morbidity Survey that 6.4% of all adults (older than 16 years of age) in England showed signs of an eating disorder, up to 25% of whom were male (NHS Information Centre for Health and Social Care, 2007).
- Anorexia is characterised by low weight, a fear of gaining weight, a desire to be thin, and a distorted body image; patients believe themselves to be overweight when often they are underweight. Body mass index (BMI) is usually lower end of normal or below normal.
- Bulimia is characterised by episodes of binge eating (described as eating a significant amount at one time to the point of being uncomfortably overfull) followed by episodes of compensatory behaviour such as vomiting (purging), excessive exercise, or use of laxatives or diuretics. The BMI may be normal or slightly above normal.
- Binge eating disorder is similar to bulimia without the compensatory behaviours, and the BMI is usually high.

Assessment in Primary Care

- All patients with a suspected eating disorder should be referred immediately to an age-appropriate eating disorder service. Urgency of referral depends on the clinical situation; seek advice from local specialist services if required.
- The following should be asked about or noted during history taking for eating disorders:
  a. An unusually low or high BMI or body weight for their age
  b. Rapid weight loss
  c. Dieting or restrictive eating practices (e.g., dieting when they are underweight) that are worrying them, their family members or carers, or professionals
  d. Family members or carers reporting a change in eating behaviour
  e. Social withdrawal, particularly from situations that involve food
  f. Other mental health problems, including depression, anxiety, self-harm, and OCD, as well as suicidal ideation
  g. The possibility of alcohol or substance misuse
  h. A disproportionate concern about their weight or shape (e.g., concerns about weight gain as a side effect of contraceptive medication)
  i. Problems managing a chronic illness that affects diet, such as diabetes or coeliac disease
  j. Menstrual or other endocrine disturbances or unexplained gastrointestinal symptoms
  k. Physical signs of:
     i. Malnutrition, including poor circulation, dizziness, palpitations, fainting, or pallor
     ii. Fractures
     iii. Compensatory behaviours, including laxative or diet pill misuse, vomiting, or excessive exercise
  l. Abdominal pain that is associated with vomiting or restrictions in diet and that cannot be fully explained by a medical condition
  m. Unexplained electrolyte imbalance or hypoglycaemia
  n. Atypical dental wear (e.g., erosion)
  o. Whether they take part in activities associated with a high risk of eating disorders (e.g., professional sport, fashion, dance, modelling).
  p. Risk factors for boys and males include nonheterosexuality, previous dieting, previous obesity and participation in sports that emphasise thinness, and body building (Thompson, 2017).
- Be aware that children and young people with an eating disorder may also present with faltering growth (e.g., a low weight or height for their age) or delayed puberty.
- Do not use single measures such as BMI or duration of illness to determine whether to offer referral or treatment for an eating disorder.
- Do not use screening tools as the sole method to determine whether or not people have an eating disorder.
- Good questions to screen for eating disorders (Cotton, Ball, & Robinson, 2003) include:
  a. Do you worry that you have lost control over how much you eat?
  b. Do you make yourself sick when you feel uncomfortably full?
  c. Do you ever eat in secret?
  d. Does your weight affect the way you feel about yourself?
  e. Are you satisfied with your eating patterns? (if the answer is 'no' and 'yes', respectively, to the latter two questions, then an eating disorder is much less likely).

Investigation and Monitoring

- When first assessing a person with an eating disorder, it is likely that blood monitoring will be required, at least once but possibly more frequently if BMI is low or there is ongoing purging, laxative use, or diuretic use. Recommended tests include full blood count, renal function, liver function, glucose, creatine kinase (and thyroid function and C-reactive protein at the first appointment only to rule out other causes of weight change).

- Other investigations should include blood pressure, pulse, BMI, muscle strength using the sit up or squat test (see box), and skin conditions.

TESTS FOR MUSCLE STRENGTH

1. Squat test. The patient is asked to squat down on their haunches and is asked to stand up without using their arms as levers if at all possible.
2. Sit-up test. The patient lies flat on a firm surface such as the floor and has to sit up without using their hands.

- It is important to obtain a BMI, but this can be challenging because many patients are reluctant to be weighed. It may require building of trust before they will agree to stepping onto the scales, but a potential option can be to ask them to step onto the scales *backwards* so that they cannot see the result, but you can note it discreetly. With time, they may then agree to step on forwards because you will have demonstrated sensitivity to their concerns and anxieties.
- Assess whether ECG monitoring is needed in people with eating disorders based on the following risk factors:
  a. Rapid weight loss
  b. Excessive exercise
  c. Severe purging behaviours, such as laxative or diuretic use or vomiting
  d. Bradycardia
  e. Hypotension
  f. Excessive caffeine (including from energy drinks)
  g. Prescribed or nonprescribed medications
  h. Muscular weakness
  i. Electrolyte imbalance
  j. Previous abnormal heart rhythm.
- Advise those who are taking laxatives or diuretics that these will not help weight loss and should be stopped gradually.
- Advise those who are exercising excessively or obsessively to stop doing so.
- Advise those who are vomiting regularly to have regular dental check-ups and avoid brushing their teeth immediately after purging.
- GPs should offer a physical and mental health review at least annually to people with anorexia nervosa who are not receiving ongoing secondary care treatment for their eating disorder. The review should include:
  a. Weight or BMI (adjusted for age if appropriate)
  b. Blood pressure
  c. Relevant blood tests
  d. Any problems with daily functioning
  e. Assessment of risk (related to both physical and mental health)
  f. An ECG, for people with purging behaviours or significant weight changes
  g. A discussion of treatment options
- Monitor growth and development in children and young people with anorexia nervosa who have not completed puberty (e.g., not reached menarche or final height).

- Consider a bone mineral density (BMD) scan:
  a. After 1 year of underweight in children and young people or earlier if they have bone pain or recurrent fractures
  b. After 2 years of underweight in adults or earlier if they have bone pain or recurrent fractures.
- Do not routinely offer oral or transdermal oestrogen therapy to treat low BMD in children or young people with anorexia nervosa.
- Seek specialist paediatric or endocrinologic advice before starting any hormonal treatment for low BMD. Coordinate any treatment with the eating disorders team.

Medication

- Medication should never be the sole treatment for eating disorders, but antidepressants or antianxiety medication may be helpful if there are comorbidities.
- Encourage people with anorexia nervosa to take an age-appropriate oral multivitamin and multimineral supplement until their diets include enough to meet their dietary reference values.
- When prescribing medication for people with eating disorders and comorbid mental or physical health conditions, take into account the impact malnutrition and compensatory behaviours (e.g., vomiting) can have on medication effectiveness and the risk of side effects.
- When prescribing for people with eating disorders and comorbidities, assess how the eating disorder will affect medication adherence (e.g., for medication that can affect body weight). Patients may decline to take any medication which they are concerned may cause them to gain weight, for example.
- When prescribing for people with eating disorders, take into account the risks of medication that can compromise physical health because of preexisting medical complications (e.g., hypokalaemia secondary to vomiting).
- Offer ECG monitoring for people with eating disorders who are taking medications that could compromise cardiac functioning (including medications that could cause electrolyte imbalance, bradycardia <40 beats/min, hypokalaemia, or a prolonged QT interval).

Referral

- If an eating disorder is suspected after an initial assessment, refer immediately to a community-based, age-appropriate (specialist) eating disorder service for further assessment or treatment.
- The aim of treatment is to reach healthy weight, BMI, and psychological well-being.
- It is vital not to delay referral because evidence shows that people have on average already had symptoms of an eating disorder for almost 3 years (Beat, 2017) before they seek help and then wait up to 6 months between first GP visit and starting treatment. It takes on

average 21 months for a person to recognise that they have an eating disorder and then another year before they seek help from a healthcare professional. This leads to a cycle of relapse and recovery of, on average, 6 years in duration. The same report showed that males had to wait over twice as long as females before being referred by their GP. In other words, GPs are not yet recognising eating disorders rapidly enough in males.

- It is important to take patient and family and carer concerns seriously and to avoid potentially dismissive comments implying that the behaviour is 'a phase' or that they will 'grow out of it'.
- Dietary advice (and dietician referral) should only be offered as part of a multidisciplinary approach.
- The mainstay of all eating disorders treatment is psychological therapy. This should be provided by a specialist trained in the appropriate evidence-based modalities.
- For those with eating disorders who have another condition such as diabetes, the secondary care teams will need to collaborate closely to minimise risk and optimise monitoring and treatment.
- Pregnant females with eating disorders require coordinated care from both obstetric and eating disorders specialist teams.
- Admit people with eating disorders whose physical health is severely compromised to a medical inpatient or day patient service for medical stabilisation and to initiate refeeding if these cannot be done in an outpatient setting.
- For people with eating disorders and acute mental health risk (e.g., significant suicide risk), consider psychiatric crisis care or psychiatric inpatient care.
- If a person's physical health is at serious risk because of their eating disorder, they do not consent to treatment, and they can only be treated safely in an inpatient setting, follow the legal framework for compulsory treatment in the Mental Health Act of 1983.

RESOURCES FOR PATIENTS AND CARERS

Websites

Beat Charity. Available at http://www.beateatingdisorders.org.uk.
  Anorexia Bulimia Care (ABC) Charity. Available at http://www.anorexiabulimiacare.org.uk.
  Talk-ED. Available at http://www.talk-ed.org.uk.
  National Centre for Eating Disorders. Available at http://www.eating-disorders.org.uk.

Books

Green, K. (2013). *Lighter than my shadow*. London: Jonathan Cape.
  Hamilton, F. (2016). *Bite sized: A mother's journey alongside anorexia*. London: Jessica Kingsley.
  Smith, J. (2011). *The parent's guide to eating disorders*. Oxford: Lion Books.

Further Reading

American Psychiatric Association. (2013). *Diagnostic and statistical manual of mental disorders* (5th ed., text revision). Washington DC: American Psychiatric Association.

Cleare, A., Pariante, C. M., Young, A. H., Anderson, I. M., Christmas, D., Cowen, P. J., Dickens, C., Ferrier, I. N., Geddes, J., Gilbody, S., & Haddad, P. M. (2015). Evidence-based guidelines for treating depressive disorders with antidepressants: A revision of the 2008 British Association for Psychopharmacology guidelines. *Journal of Psychopharmacology, 29*(5), 459–525.

National Institute for Health and Clinical Excellence. (2004). *Zaleplon, zolpidem and zopiclone for the short-term management of insomnia*. National Institute for Clinical Excellence. Technology Appraisal Guidance 77. Available www.nice.org.uk.

National Institute for Health and Clinical Excellence. (2015). *Violence and aggression: Short-term management in mental health, health and community settings*. NICE clinical guideline 10. Retrieved from www.nice.org.uk.

National Institute for Health and Clinical Excellence. (2017). *Eating disorders: Recognition and treatment*. London: NICE.

Royal College of Psychiatrists. (2022). *Medical emergencies in eating disorders: Guidance on recognition and management*. College Report CR233. London: Royal College of Psychiatrists.

WHO. (2019). *International Classification of Diseases, eleventh revision (ICD-11)*. World Health Organization (WHO) 2019. Retrieved from https://icd.who.int/browse11.

References

American Psychiatric Association. (2013). Post traumatic stress disorder. *Diagnostic and Statistical Manual of Mental Disorders* (5th ed., text revision). Washington DC: American Psychiatric Association.

Anderson, I., Nutt, D., & Deakin, J. (2000). Evidence-based guidelines for treating depressive disorders with antidepressants: A revision of the 1993 British Association for Psychopharmacology guidelines. *Journal of psychopharmacology (Oxford, England), 14*, 3–20.

Angst, J. (1997). A regular review of the long-term follow-up of depression. *BMJ (Clinical research ed.), 315*, 1143–1146.

Anonymous. (1994). Long-term management of people with psychotic disorders in the community. *Drug and Therapeutics Bulletin, 32*, 73–77.

Arcelus, J. (2011). Mortality rates in patients with anorexia nervosa and other eating disorders. *Archives of General Psychiatry, 68*(7), 724.

Ballenger, J., & Tylee, A. (2003). *Anxiety*. Mosby.

Beat. (2017). *Delaying for years, denied for months*. [online] B-eat. Retrieved from https://www.beateatingdisorders.org.uk/about-beat/policy-work/policy-and-best-practice-reports/delaying-for-years-denied-for-months/. Accessed November 29, 2023.

Bennewith, O., Stocks, N., Gunnell, D., Peters, T. J., Evans, M. O., & Sharp, D. J. (2002). General practice-based intervention to prevent repeat episodes of deliberate self harm; cluster randomised controlled trial. *BMJ (Clinical research ed.), 324*, 1254–1257.

Bisson, J. (2004). *Post-traumatic stress disorder: What are the effects of preventive psychological interventions?* Clinical Evidence. Retrieved from www.clinicalevidence.com.

Boardman, J., & Walters, P. (2009). Managing depression in primary care: It's not only what you do it's the way that you do it. *The British Journal of General Practice, 59*, 76–78.

Bostwick, J., & Pankratz, V. (2000). Affective disorders and suicide risk: A reexamination. *The American Journal of Psychiatry, 157*, 1925–1932.

Brent, D. (2007). Antidepressants and suicidal behavior: Cause or cure? *The American Journal of Psychiatry, 164*, 989–991.

Buscemi, N., Vandermeer, B., Hooton, N., Pandya, R., Tjosvold, L., Hartling, L., Baker, G., Vohra, S., & Klassen, T. (2004). *Melatonin for treatment of sleep disorders*. Rockville, MD: Agency for Healthcare Research and Quality. Evidence report/technology assessment No. 108.

Buscemi, N., Vandermeer, B., Hooton, N., Pandya, R., Tjosvold, L., Hartling, L., Vohra, S., Klassen, T. P., & Baker, G. (2006). Efficacy and safety of exogenous melatonin for secondary sleep disorders and sleep disorders accompanying sleep restriction: Meta-analysis. *BMJ (Clinical research ed.), 332*, 385–388.

Buszewicz, M., Pistrang, N., Barker, C., Cape, J., & Martin, J. (2006). Patients experiences of GP consultations for psychological problems: A qualitative study. *The British Journal of General Practice, 56*, 496–503.

Casacalenda, N., Perry, J., & Looper, K. (2002). Remission in major depressive disorder: A comparison of pharmacotherapy, psychotherapy, and control conditions. *The American Journal of Psychiatry, 159*, 1354–1360.

Chilvers, C., Dewey, M., Fielding, K., Gretton, V., Miller, P., Palmer, B., Weller, D., Churchill, R., Williams, I., Bedi, N., Duggan, C., Lee, A., Harrison, G., & Counselling versus Antidepressants in Primary Care Study Group. (2001). Antidepressant drugs and generic counselling for treatment of major depression in primary care: Randomised trial with patient preference arms. *BMJ (Clinical research ed.), 322*, 772–775.

Cipriani, A., Barbui, C., & Geddes, J. (2005). Suicide, depression, and antidepressants. *BMJ (Clinical research ed.), 330*, 373–374.

Citrone, L., & Stroup, T. (2006). Schizophrenia, clinical antipsychotic trials of intervention effectiveness (CATIE) and number needed to treat: How can CATIE inform clinicians? *International Journal of Clinical Practice, 60*, 933–940.

Cotton, M., Ball, C., & Robinson, P. (2003). Four simple questions can help screen for eating disorders. *Journal of General Internal Medicine, 18*(1), 53–56.

Coupland, N., Bell, C., & Potokar, J. (1996). Serotonin reuptake inhibitor withdrawal. *Journal of Clinical Psychopharmacology, 16*, 356–362.

Cox, J. L., Holden, J. M., & Sagovsky, R. (1987). Detection of postnatal depression. *The British Journal of Psychiatry, 150*, 782–786.

CSM Expert Working Group. (2004). *Safety of selective serotonin reuptake inhibitor antidepressants*. London: Committee on Safety of Medicines. Retrieved from https://study329.org/wp-content/uploads/2015/01/CSMReportonSSRISafety1.pdf.

DoH. (2001). *Treatment choice in psychological therapies and counselling: Evidence based clinical practice guideline*. London: Department of Health. Retrieved from www.dh.gov.uk.

Dwyer, J. B., & Bloch, M. H. (2019). Antidepressants for pediatric patients. *Current Psychiatry, 18*(9), 26–42F.

Dugas, M., Ladouceur, R., & Leger, E. (2003). Group cognitive-behavioral therapy for generalized anxiety disorder: Treatment outcome and long-term follow-up. *Journal of Consulting and Clinical Psychology, 71*, 821–825.

Falloon, I., Laporta, M., Fadden, G., & Graham-Hole, V. (1993). *Managing stress in families: Cognitive and behavioural strategies for enhancing coping skills*. London: Routledge.

Fava, G., Ruini, C., & Rafanelli, C. (2004). Six-year outcome of cognitive behavior therapy for prevention of recurrent depression. *The American Journal of Psychiatry, 161*, 1872–1876.

Fisher, P., & Durham, R. (1999). Recovery rates in generalized anxiety disorder following psychological therapy: An analysis of clinically significant change in the STAI-T across outcome studies since 1990. *Psychological Medicine, 29*, 1425–1434.

Freeling, P., Rao, B., Paykel, E., Sireling, L. I., & Burton, R. H. (1985). Unrecognised depression in general practice. *BMJ (Clinical research ed.), 290*, 1880–1883.

Furukawa, T., McGuire, H., & Barbui, C. (2002). Meta-analysis of effects and side effects of low dosage tricyclic antidepressants in depression: Systematic review. *BMJ (Clinical research ed.), 325*, 991–995.

Furukawa, T., Watanabe, N., & Churchill, R. (2007). Combined psychotherapy plus antidepressants for panic disorder with or without agoraphobia. *The Cochrane Database of Systematic Reviews*, (1), CD004364.

Gale, C., & Davidson, O. (2007). Generalised anxiety disorder. *BMJ (Clinical research ed.), 334*, 579–581.

Gale, C., & Oakley-Browne, M. (2004a). *Generalised anxiety disorder: What are the effects of drug treatments? Benzodiazepines*. Clinical Evidence. Retrieved from www.clinicalevidence.com.

Gale, C., & Oakley-Browne, M. (2004b). *Generalised anxiety disorder: What are the effects of cognitive therapy?* Clinical Evidence. Retrieved from www.clinicalevidence.com.

Gale, C., & Oakley-Browne, M. (2004c). *Generalised anxiety disorder: What are the effects of drug treatments? Beta-blockers*. Clinical Evidence. Retrieved from www.clinicalevidence.com.

Geddes, J., Carney, S., Davies, C., Furukawa, T. A., Kupfer, D. J., Frank, E., & Goodwin, G. M. (2003). Relapse prevention with antidepressant drug treatment in depressive disorders: A systematic review. *Lancet (London, England), 361*, 653–661.

Gill, D., & Hatcher, S. (2002). Antidepressants for depression in medical illness (Cochrane review). In: The Cochrane Library. Issue 1. Update Software, Oxford.

Glass, J., Lanctot, K., Herrmann, N., Sproule, B. A., & Busto, U. E. (2005). Sedative hypnotics in older people with insomnia: Meta-analysis of risks and benefits. *BMJ (Clinical research ed.), 331*, 1169–1173.

Gloaguen, V., Cottraux, J., Cucherat, M., & Blackburn, I. M. (1998). A meta-analysis of the effects of cognitive therapy in depressed patients. *Journal of Affective Disorders, 49*, 59–72.

Goldberg, D., & Bridges, K. (1987). Screening for psychiatric illness in general practice: The general practitioner versus the screening questionnaire. *The Journal of the Royal College of General Practitioners, 37*, 15–18.

Goldberg, D., & Lecrubier, Y. (1995). Form and frequency of mental disorders across centres. In B. Ustun & N. Sartorius (Eds.), *Mental illness in general health care: An international study* (pp. 323–334). WHO, John Wiley, Chichester.

Haddad, P., Lejoyeux, M., & Young, A. (1998). Antidepressant discontinuation reactions. *BMJ (Clinical research ed.), 316*, 1105–1106.

Haug, T., Blomhoff, S., Hellstrom, K., et al. (2003). Exposure therapy and sertraline in social phobia: 1 year follow-up of a randomised controlled trial. *The British Journal of Psychiatry, 182*, 312–318.

Hawton, K., Zahl, D., & Weatherall, R. (2003). Suicide following deliberate self-harm: Long-term follow-up of patients who presented to a general hospital. *The British Journal of Psychiatry, 182*, 537–542.

Hawton, K. (2003). Helping people bereaved by suicide. *BMJ (Clinical research ed.), 327*, 177–178.

Herzog, D., Greenwood, D., Dorer, D., Flores, A., Ekeblad, E., Richards, A., Blais, M., (2000). Mortality in eating disorders: a descriptive study. *The International Journal of Eating Disorders, 28*(1), 20-26.

Holden, J., Sagovsky, R., & Cox, J. (1989). Counselling in a general practice setting: Controlled study of health visitor intervention in treatment of postnatal depression. *BMJ (Clinical research ed.)*, *298*, 223–226.

Hull, A. (2004, April). Primary care management of post-traumatic stress disorder. *Prescriber*, pp. 1940–1948.

Jick, H., Kaye, J., & Jick, S. (2004). Antidepressants and the risk of suicidal behaviors. *JAMA*, *292*, 338–343.

Jones, P., & Buckley, P. (2003). *Schizophrenia*. Mosby.

Jones, R., Chung, M., Berger, Z., & Campbell, J. L. (2007). Prevalence of post-traumatic stress disorder in patients with previous myocardial infarction consulting in general practice. *The British Journal of General Practice*, *57*, 808–810.

Kapczinski, F., Lima, M., Souza, J., & Schmitt, R. (2003). Antidepressants for generalized anxiety disorder. *The Cochrane Database of Systematic Reviews*, (2), CD003592.

Kapur, N., Cooper, J., Rodway, C., Kelly, J., Guthrie, E., & Mackway-Jones, K. (2005). Predicting the risk of repetition of self harm: Cohort study. *BMJ (Clinical research ed.)*, *330*, 394–395.

Katon, W., & Roy-Byrne, P. (2007). Anxiety disorders: Efficient screening is the first step in improving outcomes. *Annals of Internal Medicine*, *146*, 390–392.

Keck, P. (2003). The management of acute mania. *BMJ (Clinical research ed.)*, *327*, 1002–1003.

Loebel, A., Lieberman, J., Alvir, J., Mayerhoff, D. I., Geisler, S. H., & Szymanski, S. R. (1992). Duration of psychosis and outcome in first-episode schizophrenia. *The American Journal of Psychiatry*, *149*, 1183–1188.

Maltby, N., Kirsch, I., Mayers, M., & Allen, G. J. (2002). Virtual reality exposure therapy for the treatment of fear of flying: A controlled investigation. *Journal of Consulting and Clinical Psychiatry*, *70*, 1112–1118.

Mental Health Foundation. (2004). *Self harm*. Mental Health Foundation. Retrieved from www.mentalhealth.org.uk.

Medicines and Healthcare products Regulatory Agency. (2006). Cardiac arrhythmias associated with antipsychotic drugs. Curr Prob Pharmacovigilance, *31*, 9.

Mol, S., Arntz, A., Metsemakers, J., Dinant, G. J., Vilters-van Montfort, P. A., & Knottnerus, J. A. (2005). Symptoms of post-traumatic stress disorder after non-traumatic events: Evidence from an open population study. *The British Journal of Psychiatry*, *186*, 494–499.

Munro, C., Freeman, C., & Law, R. (2004). General practitioners' knowledge of post-traumatic stress disorder: A controlled study. *The British Journal of General Practice*, *54*, 843–847.

Mynors-Wallis, L., Gath, D., Day, A., & Baker, F. (2000). Controlled trial of problem solving treatment, antidepressant medication, and combined treatment for major depression in primary care. *BMJ (Clinical research ed.)*, *320*, 26–30.

NICE. (2005). *Obsessive-compulsive disorder and body dysmorphic disorder: treatment* Clinical Guideline no. 31. National Institute for Clinical Excellence. Retrieved from www.nice.org.uk/guidance/cg31.

National Collaboration Centre for Mental Health. (2023). Ethnic Inequalities in Improving Access to Psychological Therapies. NHS Race and Health Observatory. Available: https://www.nhsrho.org/wp-content/uploads/2023/10/Ethnic-Inequalities-in-Improving-Access-to-Psychological-Therapies-IAPT.Full-report.pdf.

National Institute for Health and Clinical Excellence. (2014a). *Antenatal and postnatal mental health: Clinical management and service guidance*. NICE clinical guideline 192. Retrieved from www.nice.org.

National Institute for Health and Clinical Excellence. (2014b). *Bipolar disorder: Assessment and management*. NICE Clinical Guideline 185. https://www.nice.org.uk/guidance/cg185 (2014b). https://www.nice.org.uk/guidance/cg192 (2014a)

National Institute for Health and Clinical Excellence. (2014c). *Psychosis and schizophrenia in adults: Prevention and management*. Clinical Guideline 178.

National Institute for Health and Clinical Excellence. (2018). *Post-traumatic stress disorder*. NICE clinical guideline 116. Retrieved from www.nice.org.uk.

National Institute for Health and Clinical Excellence. (2022a). *Depression in adults: treatment and management*. NICE clinical guideline 222. Retrieved from www.nice.org.uk.

NICE. (2022b). *Self-harm: assessment, management and preventing recurrence*. Guideline no. 225. National Institute for Clinical Excellence. Retrieved from www.nice.org.uk.

NHS Education for Scotland. (2004). *Education for frontline staff*. Mental Health (Care and Treatment) (Scotland) Act. Retrieved from www.nes.scot.nhs.uk/mha.

NHS Information Centre for Health and Social Care. (2007). *Adult psychiatric morbidity in England, 2007: Results of a household survey*. [online] Retrieved from https://digital.nhs.uk/data-and-information/publications/statistical/adult-psychiatric-morbidity-survey/adult-psychiatric-morbidity-in-england-2007-results-of-a-household-survey. Accessed November 29, 2023.

NSPCC. (2016). *Rise in children hospitalised for self-harm as thousands contact Childline*. Retrieved from https://www.nspcc.org.uk/what-we-do/news-opinion/rise-children-hospitalised-self-harm-thousands-contact-childline/.

O'Connell, H., Chin, A.V., Cunningham, C., & Lawlor, B. (2004). Recent developments: Suicide in older people. *BMJ (Clinical research ed.)*, *329*, 895–899.

Owens, C., Lloyd, K., & Campbell, J. (2004). Access to health care prior to suicide: Findings from a psychological autopsy study. *The British Journal of General Practice*, *54*, 279–281.

Pampallona, S., Bollini, P., & Tibaldi, G. (2004). Combined pharmacotherapy and psychological treatment for depression: A systematic review. *Archives of General Psychiatry 61*, 714–719.

Picchioni, M., & Murray, R. (2007). Schizophrenia. *BMJ (Clinical research ed.)*, *335*, 91–95.

Pohl, R., Feltner, D., Fieve, R., & Pande, A. C. (2005). Efficacy of pregabalin in the treatment of generalized anxiety disorder: Double-blind, placebo-controlled comparison of BD versus TID dosing. *Journal of Clinical Psychopharmacology*, *25*, 151–158.

Price, J., Waller, P., Wood, S., & MacKay, A. V. (1996). A comparison of the postmarketing safety of four selective serotonin re-uptake inhibitors including the investigation of symptoms occurring on withdrawal. *British Journal of Clinical Pharmacology*, *42*, 757–763.

Rost, K., Nutting, P., Smith, J., Elliott, C. E., & Dickinson, M. (2002). Managing depression as a chronic disease: A randomised trial of ongoing treatment in primary care. *BMJ (Clinical research ed.)*, *325*, 934–937.

Royal College of Psychiatrists. (1998). *Managing deliberate self-harm in young people*. Council Report CR64. London: Royal College of Psychiatrists.

Rush, A., Trivedi, M., Wisniewski, S., Nierenberg, A. A., Stewart, J. W., Warden, D., Niederehe, G., Thase, M. E., Lavori, P. W., Lebowitz, B. D., McGrath, P. J., Rosenbaum, J. F., Sackeim, H. A., Kupfer, D. J., Luther, J., & Fava, M. (2006). Acute and longer-term outcomes in depressed outpatients requiring one or several treatment steps: A STAR* D report. *American Journal of Psychiatry*, *163*, 1905–1917.

Schneier, F. (2003). Social anxiety disorder. *BMJ (Clinical research ed.)*, *327*, 515–516.

Scott, J. (2006). Depression should be managed like a chronic disease. *BMJ (Clinical research ed.), 332,* 985–986.

Shaw, J. (2000). Assessing the risk of violence in patients. *BMJ (Clinical research ed.), 320,* 1088–1089.

Simon, G., Heiligenstein, J., Revicki, D., VonKorff, M., Katon, W. J., Ludman, E., Grothaus, L., & Wagner, E. (1999). Long-term outcomes of initial antidepressant drug choice in a 'real world' randomized trial. *Archives of Family Medicine, 8,* 319–325.

Sivertsen, B., Omvik, S., Pallesen, S., Bjorvatn, B., Havik, O. E., Kvale, G., Nielsen, G. H., & Nordhus, I. H. (2006). Cognitive behavioral therapy vs zopiclone for treatment of chronic primary insomnia in older adults: A randomized controlled trial. *JAMA, 295,* 2851–2858.

Soomro, G. (2004). Deliberate self-harm. In: *Clinical evidence.* BMJ Publishing Group, London.

Specialist Pharmacy Service. (2022). *Using antidepressants for depression in people with epilepsy.* Retrieved from https://www.sps.nhs.uk/.

Stewart, A. (1998). Choosing an anti-depressant: Effectiveness based pharmacoeconomics. *Journal of Affective Disorders, 48,* 125–133.

Thompson, D. (2017). Boys and men get eating disorders too. *Trends in Urology & Men's Health, 8*(2), 9–12.

Timonen, M., & Liukkonen, T. (2008). Management of depression in adults. *BMJ (Clinical research ed.), 336,* 435–439.

Turner, E., & Rosenthal, R. (2008). Efficacy of antidepressants. *BMJ (Clinical research ed.), 336,* 516–517.

Walsh, J., Muehlbach, M., Lauter, S., Hilliker, N. A., & Schweitzer, P. K. (1996). Effects of triazolam on sleep, daytime sleepiness, and morning stiffness in patients with rheumatoid arthritis. *The Journal of Rheumatology, 23,* 245–252.

Whooley, M. A., Avins, A. L., Miranda, J., & Browner, W. S. (1997). Case-finding instruments for depression: two questions are as good as many. *Journal of General Internal Medicine, 12,* 439–445.

Wilner, K., Anziano, R., Johnson, A., Miceli, J. J., Fricke, J. R., & Titus, C. K. (2002). The anxiolytic effect of the novel antipsychotic ziprasidone compared with diazepam in subjects anxious before dental surgery. *Journal of Clinical Psychopharmacology, 22,* 206–210.

World Health Organization. (1979). *Schizophrenia: An international follow-up study.* Chichester: John Wiley & Sons.

17
Urinary and Renal Problems

Adam Staten

CHAPTER CONTENTS

Urinary Tract Infections

Uncomplicated Lower Urinary Tract Infections in Nonpregnant Females of Childbearing Age

GUIDELINES

National Institute for Health and Care Excellence. (2023). *Urinary tract infection (lower)—in women. NICE clinical knowledge summaries*. Retrieved from http://cks.nice.org.uk/urinary-tract-infection-lower-women.
Health Protection Agency. (2020). *Diagnosis of urinary tract infection—quick reference guide*. Retrieved from http://www.hpa.org.uk/webc/hpawebfile/hpaweb_c/1194947404720.
Scottish Intercollegiate Guidelines Network. (2020). *Management of suspected bacterial urinary tract infection in adults. SIGN clinical guideline 160*. Retrieved from https://www.sign.ac.uk/our-guidelines/management-of-suspected-bacterial-lower-urinary-tract-infection-in-adult-women/

Cystitis and Uncomplicated Lower Urinary Tract Infections

- Half of females who present with frequency and dysuria do not have bacterial infection. Half of bacterial infections resolve within 3 days without antibiotics (Brumfitt et al, 1994). The key to management is in distinguishing an uncomplicated from a complicated urinary tract infection (UTI) (acute pyelonephritis, unusual organism, structural predisposition, refractory, recurrent, or systemic symptoms) and in avoiding unnecessary antibiotics in those without infection or in older adults with asymptomatic bacteriuria.
- It is now advised that asymptomatic bacteriuria is left untreated in all nonpregnant female patients.
  - Exclude other possible causes by considering:
    - Vaginal discharge

- Sexual history: Could it be sexually transmitted infection (STI)?
- Genitourinary syndrome of menopause (vulvovaginal atrophy)
- The management of uncomplicated lower UTI in females can be as effective *over the telephone* as if the patients are seen in person, although this must be done with caution, given General Medical Council advice on prescribing antibiotics in this manner. Females with moderate or severe typical cystitis symptoms can be treated based on history alone, but when there is doubt or if the symptoms are mild, refractory, or relapse, then it is better to do a urine dipstick test and consider the need for a midstream specimen of urine (MSU) test.
- If *positive for nitrites or leukocytes*, assume that it is an infection and treat with antibiotics without sending an MSU. When positive for leukocytes but not nitrites, remember that the symptoms may represent urethral syndrome (see upcoming discussion).
- If *positive for protein or blood only*, then consider the diagnosis and differentials further.
- If *negative for all four tests*, send an MSU for microscopy and culture without starting antibiotics; 95% will have a negative MSU and do not require antibiotics at this stage (MeReC (Medicines Resource Centre), 1995). Urethral syndrome is still possible with these results.
- *If treating, give antibiotics for 3 days.* This is as effective as a 7-day course. A 7-day course, however, is appropriate when treating the older adults, males, pregnant females, and catheterised patients. A single dose is less effective than a 3-day course but may be justified when compliance is likely to be a problem. Follow local guidelines where available. When not available, for the 3-day course, use trimethoprim 200 mg twice a day, although resistance can be above 25% in some areas. Nitrofurantoin 50 mg four times a day or 100 mg modified-release twice daily is an alternative where renal function is normal.
- For patients with mild symptoms and no systemic upset, you can consider treatment with nonsteroidal antiinflammatory drugs (NSAIDs) alone. Many patients will improve with this treatment alone.
- Patients with resistant organisms may need a change of antibiotics. Females who are infected with unusual organisms (e.g., *Proteus* or *Pseudomonas* spp.) need a repeat MSU and further investigation if the organisms are still present.
- Explain to the patient that symptoms should clear within 7 days (i.e., may persist after the 3 days of antibiotics). Advise the patient to return if symptoms are still severe after 3 days or persist after 7 days.
- *Prevention.* In females with recurrent infection, offer self-help advice, as discussed later in the chapter.

Which Midstream Specimen of Urine Results are Abnormal?

- Bacterial counts of 10^5/mL are significant and reported on MSU results, but lower counts may be found with organisms that are difficult to culture (e.g., *Staphylococcus saprophyticus*, *Chlamydia* spp., *Gardnerella* spp.). Counts of 10^3 and 10^4/mL should be repeated if the symptoms suggest infection.
- Organisms without cells can be ignored except in pregnant females and young children. Cells without organisms need further investigation unless the MSU was taken after antibiotics had been started.
- Repeat the MSU and refer if cells are still present.
- Females aged older than 40 years old with refractory UTIs with haematuria or recurrent UTIs with haematuria need a referral to a urologist.

Recurrence of Symptoms
- Repeat the MSU (or do one for the first time) and assess whether the patient has:
  - Relapse—the organism is the same
  - Reinfection—a different organism is present
  - The urethral syndrome (see upcoming discussion)

Relapse
- Treat with an antibiotic to which the original organism was sensitive for 7 days.
- Look for a reason for the failure to clear the original infection. Consider stones and chronic retention. Repeat the dipstick test for protein and haematuria.

Reinfection(s)
- Consider using a different antibiotic; the new organisms are likely to be resistant to the one originally used.

Frequent Reinfection
- *Investigations.* After more than three infections in a short period of time, consider an ultrasound scan (USS). Consider radiography or computed tomography (CT) of the kidneys, urethra, and bladder (according to local protocols) if there is a strong suspicion of calculi and urea, electrolytes, and creatinine to rule out underlying abnormalities. If normal, there is no need for specialist referral, but consider prophylaxis.
- *Prophylaxis.* Consider low-dose prophylaxis in patients with at least four attacks per year. Use nitrofurantoin (immediate release) 50 to 100 mg at night or trimethoprim 100 mg at night and arrange review in 3 to 6 months. They will more than halve the number of attacks. If an infection occurs while on prophylaxis, use a different drug as treatment.
  - Evidence for use of cranberry products is conflicting, and the Scottish Intercollegiate Guidelines Network (SIGN) guidelines state that it is not possible to make a recommendation about their use. Similarly, SIGN make no recommendation with regards to methenamine hippurate.

Infections Occurring After Intercourse
- Advise emptying the bladder after intercourse.
- Give a single dose of antibiotics to be taken within 2 hours of intercourse (e.g., trimethoprim 200 mg, off-licence use).

Asymptomatic Bacteriuria
- Asymptomatic bacteriuria in nonpregnant females requires no treatment but does in pregnancy.

Self-Help

- Recommend that patients:
  - Increase fluids.
  - Increase the frequency of micturition (practise double voiding, i.e., attempting to pass urine a second time immediately after the first).
  - Empty the bladder before sleep and after sexual intercourse.
  - Wear loose-fitting cotton underwear and avoid tights.
  - Avoid external sanitary towels.
  - Make sure a diaphragm, if worn, fits comfortably (or change contraceptive method).
  - Use a lubricant (e.g., K-Y jelly) if vaginal dryness makes intercourse painful.
  - Wipe from front to back (should be routine) and wash the vulva with soapy water.

Urethral Syndrome (Abacterial Cystitis)

- The diagnosis of urethral syndrome (abacterial cystitis) is made on the basis of repeated attacks of frequency and dysuria with repeatedly sterile MSUs. There are no clear diagnostic criteria, and it overlaps with other diagnoses such as painful bladder syndrome (previously known as interstitial cystitis).
- Examine to exclude:
  - Vaginal infection, especially *Candida, Chlamydia, Trichomonas,* and *Gardnerella* spp. and gonorrhoea
  - Urethral herpes or warts
  - Significant anterior prolapse
  - Atrophic vaginitis
- Ask the patient to keep a diary of input, output, and symptoms for 1 week and consider managing as for detrusor instability (see the section on urge incontinence).
- *Self-help.* Patients should:
  - Alkalinize the urine (e.g., with potassium citrate mixture).
  - Avoid coloured toilet paper, scented soaps, bubble baths, douches, antiseptics, talcum powder, vaginal deodorants, and deodorised tampons.
  - Ensure that sexual intercourse is not traumatic because, for instance, of lack of lubrication.
- Do not treat with antibiotics because overgrowth with lactobacilli and *Candida* spp. may be encouraged.
- *If symptoms are disabling*, refer to a urologist for consideration of cystoscopy and further investigation. Urethral dilation is now only used when true urethral stenosis is found because of little evidence for its effectiveness otherwise and potential for dilation to cause periurethral fibrosis, leading to strictures.

Lower Urinary Tract Infection in Males

Initial Assessment and Management

- Consider possible causes, including prostate problems, congenital urinary tract problems, phimosis, previous urinary tract surgery, immunodeficiency, or anal intercourse.
- Examine the abdomen (for a palpable bladder), the testes and epididymis to assess the extent of infection, the prostate, and the urethral meatus for discharge.
- Exclude diabetes with a fasting glucose.
- Arrange for an MSU before and 7 to 14 days after finishing antibiotics.
- Treat with antibiotics for 7 days in the first instance (trimethoprim or nitrofurantoin) and review the MSU results.
- If the patient is ill, admit.

Further Management

- If infection recurs, refer and consider low-dose prophylaxis until the patient is seen by a urologist.
- Consider the possibility of a urinary tract cancer in males with recurrent or persistent UTIs.

  Note: Most episodes of dysuria in young males are caused by urethritis. Consider referral to a genitourinary medicine (GUM) clinic.

Acute Prostatitis

- Send an MSU as well as urethral swabs if there is any suggestion of a STI or refer to the GUM clinic.
- Start treatment with a quinolone antibiotic (ciprofloxacin 500 mg twice a day or ofloxacin 200 mg twice a day) for 28 days. If these cannot be taken, then trimethoprim 200 mg twice a day for 28 days is recommended.
- Give analgesics (e.g., paracetamol) or an NSAID for symptomatic relief.
- If defecation is painful, offer a stool softener such as lactulose.
- Reassess after 48 hours.
- Admit patients who are ill or in whom rectal examination suggests a prostatic abscess.
- After recovery, refer for investigation to exclude an underlying urinary tract abnormality.

Chronic Prostatitis

> **GUIDELINE**
>
> National Institute for Health and Care Excellence. (2022). *Prostatitis—chronic. NICE clinical knowledge summaries.* Retrieved from https://cks.nice.org.uk/prostatitis-chronic.

- Patients present with at least a 3-month history of pain in the perineum or pelvic floor and lower urinary tract symptoms (LUTS). This diagnosis is made after other conditions have been excluded (e.g., UTI; benign prostatic hyperplasia (BPH); cancer of the prostate, bladder, or colon; urethral stricture; calculus; pudendal neuralgia). Only 5% to 10% of patients with this symptom complex (perineal pain, LUTS, variable dipstick, and MSU results) have bacterial infections.

- Establish the diagnosis. Order microscopy and culture on the *first part of the stream of the first urine passed in the morning.* Threads of white cells suggest prostatitis. Prostatic massage is not usually done in primary care.
- *If culture results are positive:* Treat with a quinolone (e.g., ciprofloxacin 500 mg twice a day for 4–8 weeks). Repeat the MSU at 4 weeks and advise an early review if symptoms return. If a sexual infection was implicated, check that the partner has been adequately assessed and treated.
- *If culture results are negative:* No treatment has been clearly shown to aid resolution. Offer a trial of NSAIDs for symptomatic relief and referral to a urologist if symptoms are not resolving. The values of referral are to confirm the diagnosis and assist in explaining it to the patient.
- If there are significant LUTS, then consider a 4- to 6-week trial of an alpha-blocker (e.g., tamsulosin).

Lower Urinary Tract Infection in Other Situations

Children
See Chapter 5, Children's Health.

Pregnancy
- All female patients are screened for bacteriuria at the first antenatal visit.
- If asymptomatic bacteriuria is found, then the female patient should be treated for 7 days with an antibiotic to which the organism is sensitive.
  - If local guidelines are not available, options when sensitivities are known (in order of preference) include:
  - Nitrofurantoin 50 mg four times a day or 100 mg (modified release) twice a day
  - Amoxicillin 500 mg three times a day (only if culture results confirm susceptibility)
  - Cefalexin 500 mg twice a day or 250 mg four times a day
- Repeat an MSU 7 days after completion of treatment and then at every antenatal visit until delivery.
- *Acute pyelonephritis:* Admit.
- *Second UTI during pregnancy:* Refer to an obstetrician.

Postmenopausal Females
- Recurrent UTIs are common after the menopause, affecting more than 10% of females. This is in addition to symptoms caused by urogenital atrophy.
- *Oestrogen therapy.* Prescribe low-dose oestrogen therapy in those with no contraindications. It has been shown to change the colonisation of the vagina and decrease infections. Topical treatment may be sufficient.
- *Culture-negative cystitis.* Organise a further culture if symptoms persist, asking specifically for *Ureaplasma urealyticum* and *Mycoplasma hominis.* Consider treating with tetracycline or erythromycin for 3 months, if present.

- Refer for urodynamic investigation females not responding to these measures or unsuitable for oestrogen.
- *Painful bladder syndrome (interstitial cystitis).* Treatment is palliative and should be decided by the urologist. The options are:
  - Oral therapy with, for example, a tricyclic antidepressant, oxybutynin, or gabapentin
  Or
  - Intravesicular with, for example, botulinum toxin injections

Catheterised Patients
- Of patients with an indwelling catheter, 90% have bacteriuria after 17 days (Anonymous, 1998). Dipsticks are of little value when the patient is catheterised, and asymptomatic bacteriuria does not usually need treatment.
- Infection cannot be prevented by topical antimicrobials applied to the meatus, nor by irrigation with antimicrobials or antiseptics. The best defence against infection is to open the closed drainage system as infrequently as possible.
- *Give antibiotics* for 7 days only if the patient is clearly symptomatic, if the infection is systemic (i.e., the patient is febrile), or if the causative organism is *Proteus* spp. *Proteus* spp. may give rise to triple-phosphate stones and are worth eradicating with antibiotics.
- *If giving antibiotics,* remove the catheter if the patient can manage without it for a few days. Insert a new one after the urine is sterile.
- Consider whether intermittent catheterisation by the patient or a suprapubic catheter might be a better option.
- Wash the meatus daily with soap and water.
- Only give antibiotics prophylactically if they are needed to prevent endocarditis or if patients do badly with UTIs (e.g., many patients with multiple sclerosis are catheterised).

Acute Pyelonephritis
- Admit if the patient is too ill to take oral fluids and medication, if the patient shows signs of sepsis, or if the patient is pregnant. Otherwise:
  a. Arrange an MSU.
  b. Prescribe a broad-spectrum antibiotic (e.g., ciprofloxacin 500 mg twice daily for 7 days or co-amoxiclav 625 mg three times daily for 14 days).
  c. Consider the need for analgesics.

d. Review the patient and the MSU result and confirm that the antibiotic was appropriate.

e. Repeat the MSU 7 days after the antibiotics are finished.

f. *Follow-up:* Consider a USS of the urinary tract.

Urinary Incontinence

GUIDELINE

National Institute for Health and Care Excellence. (2019). *Urinary incontinence and pelvic organ prolapse in women: Management. NICE clinical guideline 123.* Retrieved from https://www.nice.org.uk/guidance/ng123.

- Urinary incontinence effects both males and females across the spectrum of ages and can have a significant physical and psychological impact on those with the condition.
- Many patients do not volunteer the problem to their general practitioners (GPs).

History

- Be ready to ask anyone about incontinence if they have a condition that puts them at risk. A question such as, 'Do you ever have trouble holding your water?' is less threatening than using the word *incontinence.*
- Check, from the history, for other urinary symptoms. Incontinence is usually part of a larger problem. Consider BPH in older males and perform an International Prostate Symptom (IPS) score if indicated (see Appendix 23).
- Identify the type of incontinence from the history: stress, urge, overflow, continuous, or a mixture. Many patients have at least two types.
- Ask about precipitating events such as excess fluids or alcohol, behavioural or cognitive problems, and poor mobility or access to a toilet.
- Check for other underlying conditions. Constipation and UTIs are leading causes of incontinence in older adults. Neurogenic incontinence may present with a mixture of symptoms. Cauda equina syndrome is a surgical emergency, and results are poor when surgery is undertaken more than 48 hours after first presentation.

Examination

- Examine the abdomen, genitals, and prostate in males, with a pelvic examination in females and a rectal examination in both sexes for constipation and for the integrity of the anal reflex.
- Proceed to the BPH guidance for further evaluation (see later discussion) in males in whom this is the suspected cause of the incontinence and perform the upcoming investigations.

Investigations

- Dip the urine for sugar and evidence of infection. Consider an MSU.
- Have the patient keep a frequency and volume diary.
- Consider the use of a validated questionnaire for incontinence severity and quality of life (e.g., the King's Health Questionnaire).
- Consider a urinary USS to assess residual volume, especially if there is a possibility that overflow incontinence is present or if the patient does not respond promptly to the upcoming measures. A residual volume of 200 mL or more is abnormal. In males, a residual volume above 100 mL is associated with other problems relating to BPH.
- Consider referral for urodynamic studies if the type of incontinence is not clear or if a trial of treatment fails.
- *Refer to a urologist or gynaecologist,* as appropriate, at this stage if there is:
  - A severe vaginal or uterine prolapse
  - A pelvic mass (to be seen within 2 weeks in the United Kingdom as a suspected cancer)
  - A vesical fistula
  - Persistent or recurrent infection
  - Evidence of bladder outflow obstruction
  - Evidence of a large residual urine
- Refer to a neurologist if there appears to be a neurologic cause. The possibility of cauda equina syndrome or myelopathy needs urgent discussion with the neurosurgeons (or orthopaedic surgeons).

Management of Primarily Stress Incontinence (Males and Females)

- *Reduce intraabdominal pressure* by weight loss, the avoidance of constipation, and reducing cough by stopping smoking.
- Increase external sphincter tone:
  - By pelvic floor exercises for male and female patients. Teach the patient to practise stopping the flow of urine momentarily midstream and then continue tensing those same muscles for 4 seconds at a time with 4 seconds of rest for a total of 1 hour a day in 10 tightening bursts. Short, repeated bouts of exercises are the most useful. Continue for 3 months before deciding that exercises have not helped.
  - By using intravaginal weighted cones for females (available through urologists or local chemists). The patient inserts the lowest weight cone, with the pointed end downwards, and learns to retain the cone. The weight of the cones is steadily increased to 100 g.
  - By referral to an appropriate physiotherapist.
- *Postmenopausal females with atrophic vaginas.* A Cochrane review demonstrated that oral oestrogen, with or without progestogen, can significantly *worsen* continence. It found that continence may be improved with local oestrogen (Cody et al, 2012).

- *Referral.* Refer patients with troublesome symptoms that do not respond to these measures. Surgery cures or improves 85% of those operated on. Operations include the older open abdominal retropubic suspension procedures as well as the newer and less invasive suburethral sling procedures (including those using transvaginal tape).
- *Duloxetine can be considered as a second-line treatment* in patients not responding to other treatments and who do not wish or who are not suitable for surgery. It should be prescribed alongside advice about pelvic floor exercises. Side effects may limit adherence.

Management of Primarily Urge Incontinence (Males and Females)

- Reduce excessive fluid intake and try avoiding caffeine.
- *Bladder retraining* (also known as bladder drill) results in improvement in many patients.
- Instruct the patient to:
  - Keep a frequency and volume chart for 1 week.
  - Return for discussion of the pattern the diary reveals. In addition, check that the total volume of urine passed does not suggest that the patient is drinking too much.
  - Practise holding the urine when the urge to pass it is there.
  - Slowly increase the interval between voiding up to 2 to 3 hours.
- *Anticholinergic drugs* are helpful in many but are limited by side effects. Undertake a trial for 6 weeks and, if working, review again after 6 months. Use oxybutynin, tolterodine, or darifenacin as first-line treatment. Consider mirabegron if the patient does not respond to these.
- *Desmopressin* given as a single evening dose can be considered when nocturia is a particular problem (off-label use). Be cautious with using desmopressin in patients older than 65 years who are at higher risk of hyponatraemia.
- *Referral.* Refer to a urologist patients who do not respond to these measures.

Management of Primarily Overflow Incontinence

- Refer for assessment by a urologist, neurologist, or other specialist, according to the cause.

Management of Incontinence in Frail Older Adults and Cognitively Impaired Patients

- Assess:
  - *Is it caused by infection?* Older people often do not experience the typical symptoms of urinary infection. Send an MSU when possible.
  - *Is it a symptom of another physical illness or of dementia?*
  - *Are drugs causing or exacerbating the situation?* Diuretics or sedatives, for example, may do this.
  - *Are there issues of practicality and mobility?* How easy is it to get to the toilet? Can mobility be improved? Can clothing be made easier to unfasten?
- Encourage the patient to pass urine regularly to try to preempt the incontinence.

Coping With Incontinence: Conservative Containment Advice for All

- When the situation does not respond to any of these measures, a continence adviser will be able to advise the patient on appliances, some of which are prescribable. Others may be available through social services (including bath and laundry allowance).

Bedding Protection

- *Plastic mattress covers and one-way sheets* can be bought if not available from the community nursing service. They not only increase comfort but also reduce bedsores.

Pads and Appliances

- *Inco pads* may be available from the community nursing service.
- *Cellulose wadding* can be prescribed.
- *Body-worn pads and waterproof pants* usually have to be bought (e.g., Urocare, Kanga, and Kanga pouch).
- *Collecting devices* such as commodes, pans, and urinals can be bought from pharmacists or may be obtained via social services in the United Kingdom.
- *Penile sheaths* are available on prescription. Conveen provides a free sizing kit and sheaths from 17 to 35 mm.

Urinary Drainage Bags

- *Assess the patient's requirements*, including the length of tubing (short for wearing on the thigh or long on the calf), the type of tap (selection should depend on the patient's dexterity), and the capacity needed (350, 500, 750 mL).
- Night bags hold 2 L and should only be used for bedbound patients or overnight.

Urinary Catheters and Problem Solving

GUIDELINE

National Institute for Clinical Excellence. (2012; updated 2017). *Healthcare-associated infections: Prevention and control in primary and community care. NICE clinical guideline 139.* Retrieved from https://www.nice.org.uk/guidance/cg139k.

- Infection makes catheterisation an unattractive solution but one that is likely to be necessary in those with retention or neurogenic bladder dysfunction, with severe pressure ulcers, who are terminally ill, or who cannot cope with less invasive appliances.
- Choose intermittent catheterisation over an indwelling catheter if it is feasible.
- *Catheters* for long-term use should always be silicone with a 10-mL balloon.
- *Catheter insertion* should be performed using a no-touch technique and clean, but not necessarily sterile, gloves.
- *Catheter changes* should only be done when there is malfunction or contamination or according to the manufacturers' recommendations.
- *Urine samples* should be taken from a sampling port, not by disconnecting the bag nor from the bag drainage outlet.
- *Debris* may be reduced by acidification of the urine with ascorbic acid. Encrustation ends up affecting half of all long-term catheters and is associated with infection by *Proteus* spp. When a patient starts to develop encrustation, plan a regular catheter change before the encrustation becomes troublesome.

Infection

- Inflammation around the urethral meatus may be related to encrustation of the catheter or infection.

Bypass

- This is caused by obstruction of the catheter or by detrusor instability, not by the catheter's being too small.
- Check that the bag is lower than the bladder; change the catheter and see if the old one was blocked; use a small bulb size (e.g., 5 mL); exclude and, if necessary, treat bladder stones and infection; and if there is no improvement, use anticholinergic drugs (e.g., oxybutynin).

Catheterising a Patient in Chronic Retention

- *Haematuria* is inevitable if the bladder has been distended for some time. Clamping to release the urine in stages does not prevent this.
- *Diuresis* may occur after the obstruction is relieved. Diuretic doses may need to be reduced. Admit patients whose diuresis is severe.

Difficulty Voiding

Bladder Outflow Problems in Males and Benign Prostatic Hypertrophy

GUIDELINES

National Institute for Health and Care Excellence. (2010; updated 2015). *Lower urinary tract symptoms in men: Management. NICE clinical guideline 97.* Retrieved from https://www.nice.org.uk/guidance/cg97.

National Institute for Health and Care Excellence. (2015; updated 2021). *Suspected cancer: Recognition and referral. NICE clinical guideline 12.* Retrieved from http://www.nice.org.uk.

- BPH is the most common cause of bladder outflow problems in males and occurs with increasing age and with variable symptoms.

History

- Take a history for relevant symptoms and score them (see Appendix 24). BPH is very common, with 41% of males older than 50 years old reporting moderate or severe symptoms.
- Consider differential diagnoses, including UTI, diabetes, prostatitis, medications, or lifestyle factors such as fluid and alcohol intake.
- Identify whether the patient has:
  - Voiding or obstructive symptoms (poor flow, hesitancy, terminal dribbling, and incomplete emptying)
  - Filling or overactive bladder symptoms (frequency, urgency, urge incontinence, small volume urinating, and nocturia)
- Is there nocturia out of proportion to other LUTS? Nocturia three or more times a night raises the possibility of nocturnal polyuria, which can be defined as a nocturnal urine volume greater than 35% of the total 24-hour urine volume (Marinkovic, Gillen, & Stanton, 2004). This suggests a disturbance of the normal diurnal excretory rhythm. It can occur in patients with chronic renal disease, diabetes mellitus, diabetes insipidus, and right-sided heart failure or can be an adverse effect of phenytoin, digoxin, lithium, diuretics, and excess vitamin D. All of these need treatment followed by reassessment of the LUTS. In the absence of a treatable cause, it may respond to restriction of fluid at night, diuretics in the morning, compression stockings for those with oedema, or desmopressin at night.
- Are there filling symptoms with no evidence of obstruction? Manage as for urge incontinence.

Examination

- Examine the abdomen for signs of chronic retention and pelvic or renal masses.
- Consider performing a digital rectal examination to examine for prostate size, to exclude sinister features, and as an aid to management decisions.

Investigations

a. Perform a dipstick urinalysis.

b. Test the blood for urea, creatinine, electrolytes, and fasting glucose or haemoglobin A1C (HbA1C) and consider (with informed consent) a prostate-specific antigen (PSA), though males with BPH are no more likely than others to have prostate cancer.

c. Consider ordering a USS (with postvoid residual volume) when there is a suspicion of chronic retention or an obstructive uropathy (e.g., palpable bladder, raised creatinine, overflow incontinence); uroflowmetry may also be available locally. Refer if the postvoiding residual volume is greater than 100 mL.

Immediate Management

- Admit those with acute urinary retention or acute kidney failure.
- Refer to be seen urgently (in the United Kingdom within 2 weeks) those with macroscopic haematuria (in the absence of infection or persisting after treatment of infection), a nodular or firm or irregular prostate, an increased PSA for the patient's age, or abnormal urinary cytology where done.
- Refer to be seen urgently (in the United Kingdom within 2 weeks) those older than 45 years of age with persistent microscopic haematuria.
- Consider a nonurgent referral for males older than 60 years of age with recurrent or persistent UTIs.
- Refer, at a timescale appropriate to the individual, those with chronic kidney disease (CKD) or with refractory symptoms affecting the quality of life.

The Management of Those Not Needing or Wanting Referral After Viewing Investigation Results

- Offer the patient a choice from the following options according to how bothered he is by his symptoms and whether he is at increased risk of progression (see later) of the obstruction. Explain that surgery is by no means inevitable.

  a. *Lifestyle advice and consider watchful waiting.* This is a key first-line approach to management. Advice includes advising a fluid intake reduced to 2 L/day and avoiding caffeine. Recommend bladder training to those with filling symptoms. Briefly, this means gradually lengthening the time between passing urine. Explain that avoiding excess fluid or alcohol intake and avoiding constipation help to reduce the risk of acute retention. Review medications that might predispose to retention (especially anticholinergics).

  b. *Drugs:*
     - *Use an alpha-blocker* in those with mild symptoms without risk factors for progression and when a quick symptomatic response is required. They are generally the first-line drugs for BPH. If there is benefit, it is felt within 4 to 6 weeks and lasts for at least 3 years. A trial in the individual patient is therefore feasible using the IPS score to follow a

trend (see Appendix 24). All alpha-blockers share this effect; a considerable saving can be made by choosing the least expensive. A reduction in blood pressure from the less selective alpha-blockers such as doxazosin might be beneficial in patients with hypertension.

- *Use a 5-α reductase inhibitor* (finasteride, dutasteride) in those at higher risk of progression such as those with a very large prostate or increased PSA. No symptomatic benefit may be seen for 3 to 6 months. If there is benefit, it is sustained while the drug is continued. Libido and erection problems occur in fewer than 10% of males, and there are risks of gynaecomastia, reduced ejaculate volume, and presence of the drug in semen (such that condoms are advised). PSA rates are, on average, halved, to be remembered when performing future PSAs. National Institute for Health and Care Excellence (NICE) recommends that a new PSA baseline is established after 6 months of treatment with 5-α reductase inhibitor and should be monitored regularly thereafter.

- *Antimuscarinics:* When BPH has caused a predominantly overactive bladder presentation, consider these drugs in addition to bladder training. There is little evidence to suggest that they can precipitate acute urinary retention even in the presence of severe BPH.

- *Saw palmetto:* has only weak and conflicting evidence for efficacy in treating BPH symptoms.

  c. *Surgery* (usually transurethral resection of prostate (TURP)) is much more effective than drugs in improving symptoms and flow rates but only in two-thirds of those who undergo it. It is most likely to be successful in those most bothered by their symptoms. It does, however, carry not only the short-term risks of any operation but also, in the case of TURP (Brookes et al, 2002), the risk of incontinence in one-third, although only 6% are bothered by it. After TURP, 9% need reoperation within 5 years. The rates for sexual dysfunction vary according to the type of surgery, but the main techniques all worsen ejaculatory dysfunction.

- Review patients at 6 to 12 weeks if they are taking an alpha-blocker; otherwise review at 3 to 6 months.
- Consider whether medications are working and tolerated, whether further medications need to be used in combination, whether lifestyle advice should be repeated, and whether a referral to a urologist is now indicated.
- Check creatinine and PSA annually.

Risk Factors for Progression of Bladder Outflow Problems in Males

- Large prostate (>30 cc)
- PSA greater than 1.4 ng/mL regardless of age

- Age older than 70 years
- IPS score greater than 7 (at least *moderate* severity)
- A low flow rate (<12 mL/sec)
- A postvoiding residual volume greater than 100 mL on USS

Carcinoma of the Prostate

> **GUIDELINE**
>
> National Institute for Health and Care Excellence. (2015; updated 2023). *Suspected cancer: Recognition and referral. NICE clinical guideline 12.* Retrieved from https://www.nice.org.uk/guidance/ng12.

- Prostate cancer raises difficult issues relating to screening and the question of the value of treatment in asymptomatic males in whom carcinoma is discovered incidentally. Symptomatic patients benefit from referral.
- Nearly 10,000 males die annually in the United Kingdom from prostate cancer.

Prostate-Specific Antigen Counselling and Interpretation (Public Health England, 2016)

- Population screening for cancer of the prostate is not recommended in the United Kingdom but should be available for male patients who request it and are able to give informed consent.
- A number of high-profile campaigns have raised public awareness of prostate cancer and PSA testing, and GPs should be prepared to discuss the risks and benefits of testing.

Risk Factors for Cancer of the Prostate

- *Age.* Half of males aged older than 80 years have prostate cancer, but most are asymptomatic and will die of other causes. Guidance suggests that PSA screening should not be offered to an asymptomatic male older than 75 years with less than 10 years' life expectancy.
- *Family history.* A family history of cancers of the prostate, breast, ovary, bladder, and kidney increase the risk.
- *Race.* Males of Black ethnic origin have a rate that is double that of White males. Asian males have the lowest rates.

Counselling for Patients Who Request Prostate-Specific Antigen Screening

- Explain the following points:
  - A rectal examination is considered as well as the blood test.
  - If screening results are positive, a biopsy may be needed. The biopsy itself is uncomfortable, risks infection, and is followed by haematuria or haematospermia for up to 3 weeks in one-third of patients. The mortality rate is 1 in 10,000.
  - Only about 25% of males who have positive PSA results turn out to have cancer. About 15% of males

with normal PSA results may have cancer. Even biopsy misses up to 20% of cancers.
- It is not clear that early treatment saves lives or improves other outcomes, and the treatments that may be offered can have potentially severe adverse effects, including effects on sexual functioning and continence. Studies are conflicting on the benefits of screening, and the chief medical officer of England has advised to continue to screen asymptomatic males if they ask for it and are appropriately informed.
- When the patient has symptoms or signs suggestive of prostate cancer (see NICE guidance on referring suspected cancer, earlier), PSA testing is more likely to be useful. Consider performing a digital rectal examination (DRE) and a PSA when there is unexplained haematuria, LUTS, erectile dysfunction, bone pain, low back pain, or weight loss. Refer urgently patients with abnormal DRE results or when the PSA is increasing or above the age-specific thresholds (see upcoming discussion). Repeat the PSA after 1 to 3 months if results are borderline and refer urgently they are increasing.
- The stress and anxiety of knowing that you have or might have cancer is considerable and affects life insurance applications.

Prostate-Specific Antigen Interpretation

1. The upper limit of normal increases with age. In the United Kingdom, NICE advises the following reference ranges:
   - Age younger than 40 years: use clinical judgement
   - Ages 40 to 49 years: 2.5 ng/mL
   - Ages 50 to 59 years: 3.5 ng/mL
   - Ages 60 to 69 years: 4.5 ng/mL
   - Ages 70 to 79 years: 6.5 ng/mL
   - Age older than 70 years: use clinical judgement
2. Probability of cancer at different levels of PSA:
   - PSA 4 to 10 ng/mL: 25%
   - PSA 11 ng/mL or greater: 66%
   - PSA greater than 60 ng/mL: usually indicates metastatic prostate cancer
3. Repeat a borderline level in 2 weeks (or according to local guidance); the result can alter by up to 30%.
4. Double the result if the patient has been taking finasteride or dutasteride for 6 months or more. Conversely, an enlarged prostate caused by BPH can double the PSA level without indicating cancer.
5. Rectal examination does not increase the PSA, but more invasive manoeuvres (including catheterisation) can, as can UTI, prostatitis, and BPH.

Treatment Options

This remains controversial. NICE guidance has been issued (see earlier, NICE clinical guideline 175), and there are various options:
- *Active surveillance.* This is especially appropriate for males whose life expectancy is less than 10 years and those reluctant to face radical treatment.

- *Radical (potentially curative) therapy.* Surgery carries a risk of incontinence that is mild in 4% to 21% and total in up to 7%. Erectile dysfunction varies between 20% and 80%.
- *Hormone therapy or orchidectomy* (androgen deprivation) is indicated for incurable disease that is not organ confined. Early treatment in the form of androgen deprivation prolongs survival in advanced local and in metastatic disease.
- Hormone escape disease refers to a rising PSA despite hormonal measures. The life expectancy is about 6 months. Drug options are:
  - Luteinising hormone–releasing hormone analogues (e.g., goserelin and leuprorelin), which can improve quality of life but not life expectancy. They may also cause hot flushes, reduced libido, erectile dysfunction, gynaecomastia, and an initial tumour flare.
  - Nonsteroidal antiandrogens (e.g., flutamide and bicalutamide), which can be used as adjunctive therapy for total androgen blockade.

Urinary Stones

> **GUIDELINE**
>
> National Institute for Health and Care Excellence. (2020). *Renal or ureteric colic—acute. NICE CKS.* Retrieved from https://cks.nice.org.uk/topics/renal-or-ureteric-colic-acute.

- *Consider:* a family history of urinary stones, dehydration, urinary infection (especially by *Proteus* spp.), hypercalcaemia, hyperuricaemia, and chronic obstructive uropathy.
- *Analgesia.* Use an NSAID given by any route. Opioids such as tramadol may be necessary. NICE advises against the use of antispasmodics.
- Check for microscopic haematuria with a dipstick. The presence of haematuria supports the diagnosis, but its absence does to exclude it (NICE, 2020). The presence of nitrites suggests possible infection. Check MSU and serum urea, electrolytes, and creatinine.
- Arrange, ideally within 24 hours, urgent CT of the kidneys, urethra, and bladder:
  - To establish the diagnosis
  - To assess the size, position, and number of stones
  - To look for obstruction
  - To identify medical or anatomic conditions that may predispose to stones
- Admit for:
  - Uncontrolled pain
  - Inability to drink adequate liquids
  - Infection
  - Complete unilateral or bilateral obstruction on imaging
  - Known renal insufficiency
  - Known to have a single kidney
- *Refer to outpatients* all those not requiring admission.

- Instruct the patient to save any stone passed by passing urine through a filter (e.g., a stocking). Send it for analysis.

After the Patient Has Been Discharged from Follow-up

- If conservative management has been chosen, support the patient with the information that 90% of small stones (<5 mm) pass spontaneously and that 50% of stones that are 5 to 10 mm in diameter also pass.
- Give lifestyle advice, including
  - Maintain adequate hydration.
  - Reduce salt intake.
  - Avoid carbonated drinks.
  - Maintain normal calcium intake.
  - Maintain a balanced diet and healthy weight.
- Check that an attempt has been made to find a cause (i.e., serum calcium and uric acid and a 24-hour urinary calcium). If there is a family history or the patient has recurrent stones, the following should also be checked:
  - 24-hour urine for pH, oxalate, phosphate, and uric acid
  - Random urine for cystine
- If an abnormality is found:
  - Treat *hypercalciuria* and calcium phosphate calculi with a low-calcium diet and consider the use of bendroflumethiazide or potassium citrate.
  - Treat *hyperuricaemia* and urate calculi with allopurinol.
  - Give dietary advice for oxalate stones (avoid chocolate, tea, rhubarb, spinach).

Asymptomatic Proteinuria in Males and Nonpregnant Females

> **GUIDELINE**
>
> National Institute for Health and Care Excellence. (2021). *Chronic kidney disease: Assessment and management. NICE clinical guideline 203.* Retrieved from https://www.nice.org.uk/guidance/ng203.

Identification of Proteinuria

- NICE advises against using reagent strips (dipsticks) for identifying proteinuria in children and young people and in adults unless the dipstick can identify low concentrations of albumin and express this as the albumin:creatinine ratio (ACR).
- Identify proteinuria by checking urine ACR. This should be tested for in:
  - People with diabetes (type 1 or 2)
  - People with an estimated glomerular filtration rate (eGFR) below 60 mL/min/1.73 m^2
  - Adults with an eGFR greater than 60 mL/min/1.73 m^2 in whom there is a strong suspicion of CKD
  - Children and young people with a creatinine above their age-specific range

- Those with a history of acute kidney injury (AKI) in the previous 3 years
- People with cardiovascular disease (CVD) (including hypertension)
- People with a family history of kidney disease
- Those known to have structural kidney disease
- People with multisystem disease that may involve the kidneys
  - People with gout
- Urine ACR greater than 3 mg/mmol should be considered clinically significant.
- If urine ACR is greater than 3 mg/mmol but less than 70 mg/mmol, repeat with an early-morning sample.
- If urine ACR is greater than 70 mg/mmol, a repeat sample is not needed.
- For management of CKD, see later.

Investigative Strategy if a Dipstick Shows Proteinuria + or ++

- History, including urinary tract symptoms, family history of renal disease, and medications
- Examination, including abdomen and loins, blood pressure, weight, and oedema
- Investigations:
  - MSU and check the dipstick for haematuria (1+ is significant)
  - Urine for ACR to quantify the degree of proteinuria
  - Serum urea, creatinine and electrolytes, and eGFR
  - Fasting blood sugar or HbA1c
  - Serum protein electrophoresis and urinary Bence Jones protein if other features (e.g., anaemia, bone pain) suggest myeloma or the patient is older than 50 years old
- *Note: For protein +++ or more, consider prompt referral* (by telephone discussion with the nephrologists). The protein loss is likely to be heavy enough to lead to nephrotic syndrome (proteinuria >3.5 g/day or urinary ACR >300 mg/mmol).

Haematuria

- Screening haematuria is not routinely recommended (poor specificity).
- Aspirin, warfarin, and so on are not an *excuse* for haematuria.
- The patient should collect an early-morning urine sample in a plain white bottle for dipstick analysis. False-positive results occur after exercise, during menstruation, and with UTIs.
- An MSU is usually not necessary in primary care to confirm the nonvisible haematuria.
- A finding of 1+ or more is significant when persistent in two of three early-morning urine samples over 4 to 6 weeks.
- Common causes are:
  - *Urologic:* BPH, prostatitis, urologic cancers (especially older than 45 years old) or calculi

- *Renal:* glomerular disease is relatively more common in those younger than 40 years old, especially immunoglobulin A nephropathy and polycystic kidney disease

Nonvisible Haematuria

- NICE advises that persistent invisible haematuria should prompt investigation for urinary tract malignancy (along the 2-week wait pathway in the United Kingdom) for those older than 45 years of age. More routine referral can be considered for those younger than 45 years.
- Particularly in those younger than 40 years, consider glomerular disease (see later).

Visible Haematuria

- Check that it is not caused by menstruation or other bleeding.
- Check the urine with a dipstick and send MSU for culture and blood for urea, creatinine, and electrolytes.
- When the MSU is negative for red blood cells, consider beeturia, obstructive jaundice, and (rarely) porphyria. However, if these are not present and repeat dipstick results are still positive, believe the dipstick. Red cells may have lysed on the journey to the laboratory.
- Refer any patient with painless macroscopic haematuria urgently (via the 2-week pathway in the United Kingdom) to a urologist. The exception is haematuria during a proven UTI, which resolves fully after treatment.

GUIDELINE

National Institute of Health and Care Excellence. (2015). *Suspected cancer: Recognition and referral. NICE guideline 12.* Retrieved from https://www.nice.org.uk/guidance/ng12.

Investigative Strategy for Persistent Unexplained Microscopic Haematuria

- Always consider the history and examination. Is the patient ill, or does the patient have red flags for urologic cancer? Urologic symptoms plus haematuria makes a urology referral to exclude underlying pathology appropriate.
- Consider age, blood pressure, and the presence of significant proteinuria. A renal cause is more likely if the patient is younger than 40 years old; is unwell; or there is proteinuria, a raised BP, or ankle oedema. Quantify the proteinuria. An ACR over 30 mg/mmol or a protein:creatinine ratio (PCR) over 50 mg/mmol is significant.
- Assess renal function by measuring serum urea, electrolytes, creatinine, and an eGFR.
- Referral:
  - *Refer to exclude cancer* as described earlier.
  - If cancer is excluded, consider nephrology referral if the eGFR is persistently below 60 mL/min/1.73 m^2,

the ACR is 30 mg/mmol or more, or the BP is 140/90 mm Hg or more.
- If the patient is younger than 40 years old, first consider nephrology referral, with appropriate urgency if necessary if any of the factors listed are present.
- When no cause is found after referral, monitor annually with blood pressure, creatinine, eGFR, and an ACR urine test. Consider urology re-referral if haematuria becomes symptomatic or macroscopic. Consider nephrology re-referral if the ACR deteriorates as above or if the eGFR decreases persistently to under 30 mL/min/1.73 m^2 or decreases by more than 5 per year or more than 10 per 5 years (NICE CKD clinical guideline; see Guidelines box).

Chronic Kidney Disease

GUIDELINE

National Institute for Health and Care Excellence. (2021). *Chronic kidney disease: Assessment and management. NICE clinical guideline 203.* Retrieved from https://www.nice.org.uk/guidance/ng203.

- The incidence of CKD is rising because of an ageing population and increases in the incidence of the main causes (e.g., diabetes). There is an accompanying growing incidence of the need for renal replacement therapy (RRT) for patients with end-stage CKD.
- Most patients with CKD are asymptomatic. Nearly half of all patients with CKD are the stage 3A or 3B, with much smaller numbers for stages 4 and 5.
- The principal causes of CKD in the United Kingdom are (from common to uncommon): diabetes mellitus, hypertension (diabetes and hypertension cause three-quarters of all CKD), vasculitis and glomerulonephritis, pyelonephritis, renovascular disease, and obstructive uropathies. Adult polycystic kidney disease (APKD), medications, and amyloidosis are less common. CKD, diabetes, and proteinuria are interlinked and are strong, independent risk factors for CVD and increased mortality rates.
- Management should be based on an eGFR. The serum creatinine alone is an insensitive measurement of renal function, only becoming abnormal after considerable renal function decline. NICE guidance aims to increase the detection of CKD in at-risk groups and thus assist in reducing the rates of associated CVD and death and in identifying and referring those at risk of progression to end-stage CKD requiring RRT.
- Calculating eGFRs:
  - Use the Modification of Diet in Renal Disease formula based on values for creatinine, urea, and albumin and the patient's age, race, and gender.
  - Age is never an excuse for a low eGFR. Consider the whole picture, trend, and comorbidity when considering further assessment and management.

Assessment and Management of Chronic Kidney Disease

Patients at Risk of Developing Chronic Kidney Disease
- Screen those with predisposing factors for CKD (e.g., hypertension, diabetes, CVD, persistent haematuria or proteinuria, nephrotoxic drugs, structural renal problems or calculi, BPH, a family history of stage 5 CKD, or multisystem disease (e.g., systemic lupus erythematosus)).
- Perform annual serum creatinine, eGFR, and ACR.

Action to Be Taken on Finding an eGFR Under 60 mL/min/1.73 m^2 or a Normal eGFR With Other Signs of Kidney Damage
- Consider if the patient is ill, raising the suspicion of glomerulonephritis. If so, act according to the clinical picture, not just the laboratory results.
- Consider a repeat creatinine and eGFR with the patient fasted and well hydrated, off oral NSAIDs. Consider past creatinine levels to assess the stability of the result. Note that the eGFR may fall by 25% as a result of taking an angiotensin-converting enzyme (ACE) inhibitor. If giving an ACE inhibitor, monitor closely and stop if there is more than a 25% deterioration in eGFR or more than a 30% increase in creatinine. Such deterioration raises the possibility of renal artery stenosis.
- Beware of misinterpreting the eGFR because serum creatinine is dependent on muscle mass. In those with high muscle mass, the eGFR will be underestimated, and in those with low muscle mass (including people with amputations or paraplegia), it will be overestimated. Equally, significant oedema and pregnancy cause problems with using the eGFR.
- Beware of overinterpreting eGFR changes when values are greater than 60 mL/min/1.73 m^2. Look instead for a greater than 20% increase in creatinine.
- Repeat a new finding of eGFR less than 60 mL/min/1.73 m^2 in 2 weeks and ensure three eGFRs are assessed over 3 months. At least two below 60 mL/min/1.73 m^2 suggest a true reduced eGFR and CKD. Consider the rate of progression and whether it is likely to be a problem based on the patient's age and comorbidity. Significant progression is more likely if there is also significant proteinuria.
- Previous iterations of NICE CKD guidance recommended the use of cystatin C–based estimation of eGFR on those who have an eGFR persistently between 45 and 59 mL/min/1.73 m^2 who have no other markers of renal disease. This is no longer recommended.
- Consider renal USS if there is a family history of APKD or there are obstructive urinary symptoms, persistent haematuria, significant progression of eGFR decline, or possibly in CKD stages 4 or 5.
- Monitor blood and urine tests according to the CKD stage identified and in discussion with the patient. Plan future monitoring to identify progression early. Most complications

occur at eGFRs less than 60 mL/min/1.73 m². Check urea, creatinine, electrolytes, eGFR, blood pressure, and ACR at least annually. Check the calcium and phosphate in CKD stages 4 and 5; check the haemoglobin in CKD stages 3B, 4, and 5. Consider checking eGFR every 6 months for people with CKD 3 and every 3 months for those with CKD 4.

- Be aware that for many people, CKD will not progress.

Further Management

- *Consider referral:* CKD stages 4 or 5 (for consideration of RRT), ACR greater than 70 mg/mmol or PCR greater than 100 mg/mmol (heavy proteinuria suggests progression and/or underlying disease), ACR greater than 30 mg/mmol or PCR greater than 50 mg/mmol with persistent haematuria (1+ on dipstick), significant eGFR deterioration (>5/year, >10/5 years), suspected renal artery stenosis or genetic kidney disease, or uncontrolled hypertension despite four antihypertensives.
- *Medications review:* Consider drugs that may be causing a reduced eGFR and those whose dosage is affected by reduced renal function.
- Consider the need for smoking cessation and healthy lifestyle advice.
- Control hypertension to 120 to 139/less than 90 mm Hg (120–129/<80 mm Hg with diabetes or ACR >70 mg/mmol). Use an ACE inhibitor for first-line treatment.
- Give an ACE inhibitor (or angiotensin-2 receptor antagonist) to the maximal dosage if the patient has diabetes and significant microalbuminuria an ACR greater than 70 mg/mmol, or CKD and hypertension and ACR greater than 30 mg/mmol.
- Optimise the management of risk factors for CKD progression: CVD, significant proteinuria, hypertension, diabetes, smoking, chronic use of oral NSAIDs, and urinary outflow obstruction. Asian and Black ethnicity are also risk factors for progression.
- Anaemia (haemoglobin <11 g/dL), acidosis, and metabolic bone disease are all complications increasingly prevalent from CKD stage 3B downward and may require referral or primary care-initiated assessment, dependent upon local guidance. In CKD stages 3/4/5 iron deficiency anaemia is likely at ferritin levels below 100 µg/L. NICE has published guidance on anaemia in CKD: after excluding other causes, iron can be given to get the ferritin to greater than 200 µg/L. If this fails, refer for consideration of erythropoietin therapy aiming in adults for a haemoglobin of 10.5 to 12.5 g/dL.
- If monitoring shows an ACR greater than 70 mg/mmol, no repeat is needed; this is heavy proteinuria requiring referral. However, an ACR of 30 to 70 mg/mmol needs to be repeated on the first-morning sample to confirm the proteinuria. Haematuria is also grounds for referral when persistent. In diabetes, an ACR greater than 2.5 mg/

mmol in males or greater than 3.5 mg/mmol in females is significant and needs repeat confirmation on an early-morning ACR.

Note: The above plan assumes that the patient does not have another condition that makes an active approach inappropriate.

Acute Kidney Injury

- AKI is the rapid deterioration of kidney function. It can be divided into three stages, with stage 3 AKI representing the most serious injury to the kidneys.
- Treatment of patients with AKI is primarily targeted at the causes of the injury, which are numerous but include infection, medication, heart failure, and blood loss (traumatic or intraoperative). However, various treatment and assessment steps should be undertaken regardless of the cause.
- AKI is common and predisposes to the development of CKD (see earlier) in the months and years following.
- *AKI stage 1* is defined by either an increase of creatinine more than >1.5 to 2 times above baseline or an increase of 26 µmol/L in the previous 48 hours. Management of AKI stage 1 should include:
  a. Assessment of fluid status
  b. Urine dip for infection, haematuria, and protein
  c. Assessment for other sources of infection
  d. Cessation of nephrotoxic drugs (e.g., NSAIDs, diuretics) until creatine is back to baseline
  e. Encourage fluid intake (unless fluid overloaded)
  f. Consider withholding antihypertensives if systolic blood pressure is below 100 mm Hg
  g. Repeat blood test for renal function and electrolytes in 5 to 7 days
- *AKI stage 2* is defined as an increase in creatinine of two to three times above baseline. Management of AKI 2 should include:
  a. Measures as for AKI 1.
  b. Stop ACE inhibitors, angiotensin 2 receptor blockers, and metformin.
  c. Consider suspending or reducing dose of opiates, gabapentinoids, sulfonylureas, insulin, benzodiazepines, allopurinol, and anticoagulants.
  d. Consider seeking specialist advice.
  e. Repeat renal function and electrolytes in 48 hours; if deteriorating or potassium is below 6 mmol/L, consider admission.
- *AKI stage 3* is defined an increase in creatine more than three baseline or more than 1.5 times above baseline with creatinine greater than 354 µmol/L. These patients should be admitted unless there is a compelling reason not to (e.g., the patient already is known to be in the last days of life and wishes to die at home).

References

Anonymous, Drug Therapy Bulletin (1998) Managing Urinary tract infections in women. *Drug and Therapeutics Bulletin*, 36, 30-32.

Brookes, S. T., Donovan, J. L., Peters, T. J., Abrams, P., & Neal, D. E. (2002). Sexual dysfunction in men after treatment for lower urinary tract symptoms: Evidence from randomised controlled trial. *BMJ (Clinical research ed.)*, 324, 1059–1061.

Brumfitt, W., & Hamilton-Miller, J. M. T. (1994). Consensus viewpoint on management of urinary infections. *Journal of Antimicrobial Chemotherapy*, 33, S147–S153.

Cody, J. D., Jacobs, M. L., Richardson, K., Moehrer, B., & Hextall, A. (2012). Oestrogen therapy for urinary incontinence in post-menopausal women. *Cochrane Database of Systematic Reviews*, 10(10), CD001405. doi:10.1002/14651858.CD001405.pub3

Marinkovic, S. P., Gillen, L. M., & Stanton, S. L. (2004). Managing nocturia. *BMJ (Clinical research ed.)*, 328, 1063–1066.

MeReC (1995) Urinary Tract infection. *MeReC Bulletin*, 6(8) 29-32

National Institute for Health and Care Excellence. (2020). *Renal or ureteric colic—acute. NICE CKS*. Retrieved from https://cks.nice.org.uk.

Public Health England. (2016). *PSA testing and prostate cancer: Advice for well men aged 50 and over.* https://www.baus.org.uk/_userfiles/pages/files/Patients/Leaflets/PSA%20advice.pdf

18

Ear, Nose, and Throat

Shivun Khosla & Robert Hone

CHAPTER CONTENTS

The Ear

Otologic History

- Pain: site, onset, character, radiation, associated symptoms, timing, exacerbating and relieving factors, severity
- Discharge
  - Constant versus intermittent
  - Colour
  - Odour
  - Painful versus painless
- Hearing
  - Loss sudden (<3 days) or more gradual (>3 days)
  - Quality of life impact
- Tinnitus
  - Unilateral or bilateral
  - Pitch
  - Pulsatility
  - Constant or intermittent
- Vertigo
  - Imbalance (disequilibrium) versus true rotational versus lightheaded
  - Length of episodes
  - Associated with head movements
  - Associated otology symptoms
- Other symptoms
  - Aural fullness
  - Headache
  - Any neurology or visual disturbance
  - Recent upper respiratory tract infection (URTI)

Otologic Examination

- Inspection
  - Cartilage swelling
  - Pinna position
  - Mastoid swelling
  - Facial nerve function
  - Skin changes
  - Scars
- Palpation
  - Tragal tenderness
  - Mastoid tenderness
  - Otoscopy

a. Canal health, erythema, and swelling
b. Tympanic membrane integrity and the middle ear
c. Discharge colour, blood staining, and pulsatility
- Tuning fork examination (256/512 Hz)
  - Weber test
  - Rinne test
- Whispered hearing test (if heard suggests hearing >30 dB HL)
- Cranial nerve examination
- Dix–Hallpike examination

Common Symptom Differentials

Otalgia

- *Otologic:* infection or inflammation of the ear canal, tympanic membrane, or middle ear
- *Referred*
  - Dental disease
  - TMJ dysfunction syndrome
  - Cervicogenic pain
  - Aerodigestive tract acute infection or inflammation
  - Occult aerodigestive tract malignancy

Otorrhoea

- Otitis externa
- Acute suppurative otitis media with tympanic perforation
- Myringitis (inflammation of the ear drum)
- Organic aural foreign body
- Chronic suppurative otitis media (squamous or mucosal)

Hearing Loss

- Wax impaction
- Middle ear effusion
- Sudden onset of sensorineural hearing loss
- Age-related presbyacusis
- Consider recent intravenous (IV) medications, chemotherapy, loud sound, trauma, and meningitis

Vertigo

- Benign paroxysmal positional vertigo (lasts seconds to minutes and usually occurs on head movement)
- Vestibular migraine (hours to days, migraine symptoms or history or triggers)
- Ménière disease (minutes to hours, recurrent attacks, tinnitus, and fluctuating hearing)
- Acute ischaemic stroke

External Ear Disease

Furunculosis

- Infection in a hair follicle in the auditory canal typically by *Staphylococcal* organisms.
- It is intensely painful with isolated and localised swelling.
- It can coalesce to form a carbuncle.
- *Treatment* is by opening with sterile needle or scalpel antibiotics with or without oral antibiotics, and warm compresses.

Auricular Cellulitis

- Diffuse inflammation of the pinna and lobule
- May spread to surrounding periauricular soft tissue as a facial cellulitis
- Typically caused by gram-positive cocci organisms
- Management with water avoidance, marking the region and high-dose antibiotics suitable for skin and soft tissue infection
- Low threshold for referral for appropriate IV therapy

Perichondritis

- Infection or inflammation of the underlying auricular cartilage
- Presents with swollen cartilage but sparing of the ear lobule
- Typically, spread of the infection from the ear canal
- Organisms: *Pseudomonas aeruginosa, Staphylococcus aureus, and Streptococcus* spp.
- Treatment requires aggressive antibiotic use: high-dose oral or IV
- Recurrent episodes are suspicious for underlying immunosuppression or autoimmune disease

Otitis Externa

- Inflammatory disorder of the external ear canal
- Typically starts with itching followed by pain, discharge, and tragal tenderness
- Can lead to facial cellulitis or suppuration or abscess formation in the canal
- Risk factors include water infiltration, dermatologic conditions of the canal (eczema, psoriasis), use of cotton buds, auditory aid use, and immunosuppression (diabetes mellitus)
- Organisms: *P. aeruginosa, S. aureus, Aspergillus niger, Candida* spp.
- Principles of management
  a. Avoid precipitating causes (e.g., swimming).
  b. Provide gentle mopping of the ear canal using cotton wool as a wick left in situ to soak up discharge.
  c. Identify organisms using ear swab for microscopy, culture, and sensitivity.
  d. Acidification of the canal using acetic acid solutions is toxic to most organisms if the tympanic membranes are intact and should be tried as first-line treatment for 1 week.
  e. In refractory cases, topical treatment using combination antibiotic and steroid based on local sensitivities is second-line treatment (e.g., gentamicin/hydrocortisone, neomycin/polymyxin B/hydrocortisone).
  f. In patients with tympanic perforation or ventilation tubes, fluoroquinolone antibiotics are recommended as first-line treatment because they are nonototoxic.
  g. If there is significant discharge, no improvement, or canal stenosis, refer to local microsuction services.
- Otomycosis: fungal infection that can be precipitated by topical antibiotic use
  - Typically has a constant brown-cream discharge or black spores consistent with *Aspergillus* spp.

- Requires frequent microsuction and specialist evaluation with long duration of topical antifungal agents (e.g., clotrimazole 1% solution, flumethasone pivalate 0.02%/clioquinol 1% drops) until at least 2 weeks after macroscopic resolution and absence of symptoms.
- Malignant otitis externa (OE)
  - Life-threatening complication of OE causing skull base osteomyelitis
  - Occurs almost exclusively in immunocompromised or diabetic patients
  - The main symptom is pain significantly out of proportion to examination finding possibly with recent OE
  - May have concomitant lower cranial nerve neuropathy (cranial nerves VI–XII)
  - *P. aeruginosa* is the main causative agent
  - Management is with ear, nose, and throat (ENT) specialists for prolonged IV antibiotic therapy and regular aural toilet. Surgery or hyperbaric oxygen is occasionally considered

Disorders of the Tympanic Membrane

Bullous Myringitis

- Inflammatory disorder of the tympanic membrane of unknown aetiology, possibly *Mycoplasma* infection
- Presents with painful ear and serosanguinous discharge
- May be confused with shingles or Ramsay Hunt syndrome
- Clinical examination shows a blistered eardrum
- Treatment with analgesia and topical antibiotic and steroid drops
- Typically self-limiting

Granular Myringitis

- Confluent or separate granulation tissue on the tympanic membrane
- More common after aural surgery such as cartilage tympanoplasty
- Present with aural irritation, discharge, and hearing loss
- Treatment is with topical steroid drops; if ongoing problems, refer for specialist opinion

Perforation

- Most commonly caused by:
  - Trauma, including iatrogenic, penetrating, and barotrauma
  - Sequelae of acute middle ear infection
  - Chronic ear disease
- Presenting complaints typically of hearing loss, tinnitus, chronic aural discharge, or recurrent ear infections
- Can be classified on their position (central vs marginal), size (pinhole, subtotal, or total), maturity (new vs mature) and activity (wet vs dry)

- 97% of acute perforations heal within 4 weeks with observation alone
- Myringoplasty or tympanoplasty can be performed to repair the defect to create a dry, safe ear; effect on hearing loss is more variable.

Acute Otitis Media

- Typically affects children aged 3 to 7 years
- Typically presents with otalgia, fevers, change in behaviour, and pulling or tugging at the ear
- Clinical examination reveals an erythematous, bulging drum
- Discharge, sometimes pulsatile, caused by transmitted pulse from the middle ear; may be mucopurulent with blood staining and indicates eardrum perforation; perforation relieves pain
- Organisms: rhinovirus, respiratory syncytial virus, entero rhinovirus, adenovirus, and coronavirus are most common
- Complicated bacterial overlay: *Streptococcus pneumoniae, Moraxella catarrhalis, Haemophilus influenzae*
- Management
  - Most children recover within 3 days of onset of symptoms.
  - Antibiotics reduce pain and fever in children younger than the age of 2 years between days 3 and 7 and in bilateral cases of acute otitis media (AOM). They have no impact on pain within the first 48 hours or incidence of hearing impairment at 1 month.
  - Appropriate analgesia and antipyretic use is recommended as first-line therapy.
  - Topical drops using local anaesthetic and analgesic can help with symptoms (phenazone with lidocaine) if there is no tympanic membrane perforation.
  - Antibiotics should be considered in those with significant systemic upset and no improvement after 4 days, children younger than 2 years of age with bilateral AOM, children of any age with aural discharge, and those with higher risk of complications (e.g., chronic ear disease, immunosuppression, trisomy 21, cleft palate).
  - The first-line antibiotic is typically amoxicillin with a course duration of initially 5 days. Amoxicillin–clavulanic acid can be considered for refractory cases. Clarithromycin or erythromycin is recommended for those with true penicillin allergy.
  - Use of delayed prescribing with good explanation of rationale can reduce antibiotic use and appears to be safe.
  - In children with ventilation tubes, use of topical antibiotics (fluoroquinolone) in addition to oral antibiotics can expedite recovery and reduce the risk of biofilm formation on the ventilation tube.

Complications

- Complications of AOM can be intracranial or extracranial.

- Early antibiotic use does not reduce the risk of progression to AOM complications.
- Mastoiditis
  - Is a subperiosteal abscess that forms over the mastoid bone
  - Presents with systemic upset, postauricular swelling with or without palpable abscess and displacement of the pinna forwards, and effacement of the skin crease
  - Necessitates urgent ENT opinion for consideration of IV therapy as a minimum and may need surgical drainage.
- Meningitis
  - Meningoencephalitis can occur secondary to AOM or mastoiditis and presents with typical signs of meningism after an URTI.

Recurrent Acute Otitis Media

- Defined as four confirmed episodes of AOM within a 6-month period
- Prevention may be facilitated by avoiding cigarette exposure
- Referral to an ENT specialist to investigate causes and consider surgical intervention depending on cause

Otitis Media With Effusion

- Fluid within the middle ear without signs of inflammation and can be serous or mucoid
- *Children*
  - Glue ear is a common sequalae of URTI.
  - Half of affected children resolve spontaneously with 3 months, but 2% to 3% of those younger than 7 years of age have prolonged hearing impairment requiring specialist review.
  - A period of watchful waiting of 3 months with appropriate hearing assessments is appropriate.
  - Referral to paediatric audiology services facilitates confirmation of the diagnosis, gradation of the severity and assessment of overall disability, and facilitate auditory aiding if required.
  - There is no role for antibiotics, antihistamines or oral or intranasal corticosteroids.
  - Use of autoinflation devices (e.g., Otovent) is a beneficial, low-cost intervention that can improve symptoms.
  - There is a low translation from children having specialist assessment to having surgery.
- In children having surgery:
  - Ventilation tube insertion may have a short-term impact on hearing but very little sustained improvement after 12 months.
  - Concomitant adenoidectomy can halve the number of children requiring repeat ventilation tube insertion.
- Refer directly to an ENT specialist if:
  - Persistent hearing loss confirmed as otitis media with effusion (OME) for more than 3 months

- Significant impact on speech, learning, or social functioning
- Associated with persistent pain
- Other disabilities that may further impact the above and where hearing optimisation is vital.
- Adults
  - OME typically follows URTIs and barotrauma.
  - It is more common with a second bimodal peak after age 70 years and in patients with known eustachian tube problems.
  - Persistent effusion of more than 6 weeks' duration needs specialist investigation to rule out nasopharyngeal lesions, especially if it is unilateral.
  - Management includes use of autoinflation devices, hearing aids, and ventilation tubes.
  - Eustachian tube surgery has significantly lower success in patients with eustachian tube dysfunction with OME than eustachian tube dysfunction alone.
  - Intranasal treatments should only be instigated in the presence of nasal symptoms and evidence of rhinitis.

Chronic Suppurative Otitis Media

- Can be active or inactive
  - Active: inflammation causing pain and mucopurulent discharge
  - Inactive: tympanic membrane perforation or retraction without symptoms.
- Classically divided into squamous and mucosal subtypes
- Mucosal chronic suppurative otitis media (CSOM)
  - An actively discharging middle ear with a "wet" and perforated tympanic membrane
  - CSOM is caused by inflammation of the middle ear respiratory mucosa.
  - Chronic discharge can be managed with microsuction or cotton wool wick mopping by patients at home.
  - Microscopy, culture, and sensitivity are recommended because these cases can need prolonged, or longer term treatments and identifying causative agents is useful in directing management.
  - Topical quinolone antibiotics are typically more effective than oral antibiotics, but sometimes both need to be used in combination based on symptoms and sensitivities from microscopy, culture, and sensitivity.
  - ENT referral should be given for consideration of tympanoplasty for patients with frequent episodes or episodes refractory to medical treatments.
- Squamous CSOM
  - This is an inactive disease related to tympanic membrane retraction into the middle ear caused by negative middle ear pressure.
  - It can result in erosion of ossicles and other structures.
  - Active disease relates to cholesteatoma (ear canal skin growing in the wrong place) with foul-smelling, usually painless discharge.

- Complications include facial nerve palsy, vestibulopathy, skull base erosion, and meningitis.
- ENT referral should be given for suspected cases because treatment is almost always surgical.

Hearing Loss

- Hearing loss is typically divided into conductive and sensorineural.
- One-third of patients aged 70 years and half of those aged 80 years have hearing impairment that warrants aiding for main speech frequencies.
- There is significant emerging evidence that hearing impairment correlates to earlier onset of memory loss, social isolation, and progression to cognitive impairment and dementia.
- Patients with hearing loss should be managed in primary care in line with current recommendations.

Sensorineural Hearing Loss

- The main differentiator is an onset of hearing loss of less than 72 hours or longer than 3 days.
- Otoscopic examination results are frequently normal.
- The tuning fork testing should be performed to confirm suspicion of sensorineural hearing loss.
- Refer patients with:
  - *Unilateral hearing loss less than 72 hours in onset:* requires emergency referral to an ENT specialist. Patients should be counselled on the risks of medication with view to starting oral prednisolone 1 mg/kg up to 60 mg with or without proton pump inhibitor cover once daily for 7 days and then tapered up to day 14.
  - *Unilateral hearing loss with a longer history* should be evaluated as per recommendations for hearing loss in primary care and be referred to audiology or an ENT specialist as per local pathway for further investigation of the cause (e.g., vestibular schwannoma).
- Be active in detecting hearing loss in older adults and encourage patients to consider hearing aids to reduce their rate of cognitive decline.
- Encourage patients to persevere with auditory aids after they are supplied because it takes some time to get the full benefit from hearing aids whilst discrimination of sounds is relearnt.

Conductive Hearing Loss

- Assume all conductive hearing loss is treatable.
- Examine the ear canal and drum to decide the most likely cause of hearing loss. Tuning fork tests with 256- and 512-Hz tuning forks facilitate confirmation of a conductive hearing loss.
- *If wax is present and occluding the ear canal* (>80% or adjacent to ear drum):
  1. Treat with regular olive oil for 2 weeks or sodium bicarbonate drops for 5 days.

2. If there is no improvement, consider removal using syringing or referral via local pathway for microsuction.
3. If hearing is not improved after removal, refer to an ENT specialist.

- All patients with conductive hearing loss not caused by wax should be referred to an ENT specialist.

Dizziness

- The diagnosis for patients with dizziness comes mainly from the history. Examination is used to support the diagnosis, and investigations are usually not necessary.
- It is important to distinguish between true rotational vertigo, disequilibrium (unsteadiness), and lightheadedness (usually cardiovascular in origin and unlikely related to ENT)

True Vertigo

- Is the illusion of movement of the subject or of their surroundings, most commonly rotatory
- Can be associated with nausea and vomiting
- Causes can be peripheral (after VIII nerve leaves brainstem) or central
- *Episodic*
  - *Vertigo lasting seconds or minutes* indicates a short-lived stimulation or depression in the labyrinth or central connections.
  - *Vertigo lasting minutes to hours* usually is a result in altered physiology or metabolism in the labyrinth.
- *Prolonged*
  - *Vertigo lasting more than 24 hours* can be from a peripheral deficit (e.g., vestibular neuronitis, labyrinthitis, or vestibular hypofunction) or a central lesion (e.g., brain stem lesion, acute ischaemic episode, multiple sclerosis), although the latter group has other suggestive signs or symptoms.
- Examination
  a. General inspection and assessment of gait on entry to the consulting room
  b. Otoscopy and cranial nerve examination and HINTS (head impulse, nystagmus, and test of skew)
  c. Head impulse testing in which fixation is on the tester's nasal bridge and the head is turned from the side to the midline in short, sharp movements with the neck relaxed (a positive test result shows movement of the eyes with head movement with corrective saccade back to the point of fixation and indicates peripheral vestibular hypofunction on the ipsilateral side; use with caution in patients with cervical neck problems)
  d. Detailed assessment of nystagmus (patients with peripheral lesions have fast phase nystagmus towards healthy side, and this is increased in amplitude when looking towards the affected side; in central lesions, nystagmus can be horizontal, vertical, or rotary)

e. The test of skew is performed by fixation on the tester's nasal bridge again and covering one of the patient's eyes with quick switching to cover the contralateral eye. (A positive test is with vertical or diagonal corrective eye movements and is suggestive of a central cause for symptoms.)

- Treatment
  - Vestibular sedatives such as prochlorperazine 12.5 mg intramuscularly can be useful acutely if significant nausea and vomiting with a short course of 5 mg three times a day orally for up to 1 week to control symptoms. Avoid long-term courses as compensation while on vestibular sedatives means patients will be reluctant to stop in the future.
  - Longer term treatment should centre on compensation, which occurs naturally, especially in younger, more active patients, and can be augmented by vestibular physiotherapy if the aetiology is peripheral.
- Vestibular rehabilitation exercises
  - *In bed:*
    a. Eye movements: up and down, side to side, finger focus as it moves from arm's length to 30 cm away and back
    b. Head movements: moving the head forward and backward and side to side
  - *Sitting:* head movements: rotating the head from side to side, bending down, and standing up straight with the eyes open and then closed
  - *Standing:* turning through 360 degrees, throwing a small ball from hand to hand
  - *Moving:* walking across a room, up and down a slope, and up and down stairs with the eyes open and closed

Vestibular Migraine

- Common cause of vertigo
- Symptoms include:
  - Spontaneous or positional vertigo (variable duration, 5 minutes–72 hours)
  - Nausea and imbalance
  - May have concomitant migraine but not with every episode
  - Other symptoms of aura: phonophobia, photophobia
- Patients tend to have a history of migraine and family history of migraine.
- Diagnostic criteria suggest at least five episodes of vestibular symptoms with half of the episodes associated with unilateral, pulsating migrainous headache or other form of aura.
- Treatment
  - Acute attacks can be managed as migraine with use of triptan medications.
  - Prophylaxis can be with a dietary modification to avoid triggers and a variety of medications including tricyclics, beta-blockers, calcium channel antagonists, and antiepileptic medications as with other migraine variants.

Benign Paroxysmal Positional Vertigo

- Benign paroxysmal positional vertigo (BPPV) is a disorder of the peripheral vestibular system caused by short excess stimulation of the saccule and utricle of the labyrinth from debris in the semicircular canals.
- The posterior semicircular canal is the most commonly affected (95%).
- True rotational vertigo lasts seconds, typically on head movement: bending forward, looking up, and turning over in bed are common triggers.
- It can occur in combination with other disorders of balance or in isolation.
- The history is suggestive, and the Hallpike test is diagnostic for posterior canal BPPV.
- The Hallpike test
  1. Sit the patient on the couch and check that the patient does not have any neck or back problems. Hold the patient's head in both hands, turn it 45 degrees towards the test ear, and ask the patient to fixate on a constant point while keeping their eyes open. Maintain the head position as you swiftly move the patient to a position of extension up to 30 degrees beyond the horizontal.
  2. Maintain this position observing for torsional, geotropic nystagmus (eye rotation toward the ground) that lasts seconds and fades with repetition.
  3. Return to the upright and test the contralateral ear.
  4. Patients with a positive test result can proceed to Epley manoeuvre (canalith repositioning).
- *Management of BPPV*
  a. Patient education is an important part of management with slow standing and head movement to minimise symptoms.
  b. The Epley manoeuvre is a safe and effective treatment for patients with posterior canal BPPV (Hilton & Pinder, 2014).
  c. The Epley manoeuvre can be completed in less than 5 minutes and does not require specialist training with instructional videos available from British Society of Otology and ENT UK.

Ménière Disease

- This is an uncommon disorder characterised by a triad of symptoms that happen as clusters over several weeks.
  - Aural pressure or fullness
  - Low-frequency hearing loss that fluctuates
  - Episodic vertigo lasting 20 minutes to 24 hours
- More common in middle-aged females.
- Referral to an ENT specialist should be made to confirm diagnosis and rule out alternative disorders.
- Medical treatment
  - Patients with a diagnosis should inform the DVLA (Driving and Vehicle Licencing Agency) of the condition.
  - No randomised controlled trials exist for acute management with betahistine, benzodiazepines, or anticholinergics.

- Betahistine and diuretics are commonly used medications, but the most recent Cochrane review concluded there was no evidence that they are effective or ineffective because the evidence quality was low or very low quality (Webster et al, 2023a).
- Dietary modification is commonly recommended; however, a recent Cochrane analysis found the role of dietary or lifestyle modification to be uncertain (Webster et al, 2023b).
- *Acute attacks:* These are treated with a short course of vestibular sedative such as prochlorperazine 5 mg or cinnarizine 30 mg, both administered three times a day.
- *Recurrent attacks:* Betahistine 16 mg three times a day can be prescribed, but recent evidence shows that it is no better than placebo (Adrion et al, 2016).
- Referral to an ENT specialist is recommended for attacks that are refractory to management.
- Intratympanic steroids or aminoglycosides can be used, but the latter has a risk to hearing.
- There is no evidence for systemic pharmacological prophylaxis in the management of Ménière disease or syndrome.

Unsteadiness

- Unsteadiness lasting several seconds indicates a temporary overload of vestibular or central balance systems. It occurs most frequently on rapid movement and associated with minor inadequacy of the proprioceptive or labyrinthine systems.
- Unsteadiness that is prolonged, especially in older adults, is usually multifactorial and is caused by inadequacy in most components of the balance system, including the peripheral vestibular system, eyesight, proprioception, and central integration.

Lightheadedness

- Patients with lightheadedness often report a momentary sensation of spinning; this does not mean that the vestibular system is the cause of their symptoms.

Tinnitus

- Thirteen percent of UK adults experience prolonged tinnitus with 90% having associated hearing loss.
- For most people, this improves with time with 1% to 2% of the population having tinnitus severely impacting on their quality of life.
- Exclude drug-induced causes (nonsteroidal antiinflammatory drug (NSAIDS), loop diuretics, tricyclics, aminoglycoside).

- Refer patients with:
  - Tinnitus with hearing loss: auditory aiding can often help
  - Unilateral, persistent tinnitus lasting longer than 3 months for exclusion of cerebellopontine angle tumours
  - Neck or skull bruits suggestive of carotid artery stenosis or arteriovenous fistula
  - Tinnitus severe enough that it impacts the quality of life
  - Tinnitus associated with systemic or neurologic disease
- *Treatments*
  - Nonspecific support and counselling are very helpful.
  - Consider completion of a tinnitus handicap inventory score to grade the severity of tinnitus.
  - Refer patients to the British Tinnitus association website (https://tinnitus.org.uk) for information and masking strategies.
  - Screen for concomitant depressive disorder and manage as appropriate. Suicide is a known consequence of depression and tinnitus. There is no evidence that antidepressive medication is helpful in the treatment of tinnitus.
  - *Amplification*: A hearing aid can be useful to amplify ordinary background noise.
  - *Tinnitus retraining therapy*: This combines counselling with sound therapy to reduce the attention that the patient pays to the tinnitus. There is evidence that this is more effective than tinnitus masker.
  - *Cognitive-behavioural therapy*: This does not change the subjective loudness of tinnitus but has a significant improvement in depression scores and quality of life.

Lower Motor Neurone Facial Nerve Palsy

- Lower motor neurone facial nerve palsy can be caused by:
  - Middle ear pathology (e.g., acute infection, cholesteatoma, necrotising OE)
  - Tumours (cerebellopontine angle, parotid)
  - Trauma (temporal bone fracture, penetrating trauma to the skull base or parotid)
  - Infection or inflammation within the nerve (Ramsay Hunt syndrome, Lyme disease, mononeuritis multiplex)
  - Idiopathic (Bell palsy)

Bell Palsy

- This is a diagnosis of exclusion after complete neurotologic examination to rule out the above listed causes.

- It is characterised by unilateral facial nerve weakness, which may or may not have associated deep ear pain.
- It is more common in pregnant females and patients with diabetes after URTI.
- Referral
  - All cases of lower motor neurone facial nerve weakness should be referred urgently to an ENT surgeon to:
    a. Confirm diagnosis of Bell's palsy.
    b. Arrange appropriate follow-up and investigation if there are ongoing symptoms after 6 weeks.
    c. Consider cosmetic and functional surgery if weakness impacting the patient's quality of life at 9 months.
- Assessment of eye closure is invaluable, and failure to completely close the eye warrants referral to ophthalmology specialist input.
- Management in primary care
  - *Protect the eye.* Taping the eye closed at night, not using a patch, reduces the risk of corneal ulceration alongside regular use of Hypromellose or carbomer eye drops during the day and thick gel or ointment at night such as Lacrilube.
  - *Oral prednisolone.* Early use of prednisolone significantly improves the chance of complete recovery at 3 and 9 months (Sullivan et al, 2007). The recommended dosage is 1 mg/kg (maximum, 60 mg) for 5 days, **then** taper 10 mg/day to stop.
  - *Oral antivirals.* Low-quality evidence suggests that the addition of antiviral agents to steroids might reduce rate of late sequelae over steroids alone. It is recommended in North America for patients with severe palsy.
  - *Physiotherapy.* There is no evidence that it has any significant benefit (Teixeira et al, 2011).

PATIENT INFORMATION

Bell's Palsy Association. Available at https://bellspalsy.org.uk.

The Nose

Rhinitis

- Rhinitis is defined as a general inflammation of the lining of the nose and broadly divided into two categories:
  - Nonallergic rhinitis
    - Acute viral with or without bacterial overlay
    - Nonallergic rhinitis with eosinophilia
    - Hormonal rhinitis: typically seen in pregnancy
    - Occupational rhinitis: wood dusts, solvents, sulphur dioxide, and nitrogen dioxide gas
    - Drug induced: NSAIDS, antihypertensives
    - Rhinitis medicamentosa: overuse of decongestants
    - Vasomotor rhinitis: older adulty patients, more commonly males presenting with dripping clear rhinorrhoea
  - Allergic rhinitis
  - Seasonal
  - Perennial

Viral Rhinitis

- Most commonly presents as the common cold.
- Organisms tend to be rhinovirus, coronavirus, parainfluenza, and influenza virus.
- Typically has three stages:
  1. Prodromal stage of systemic upset and fatigue
  2. Catarrhal stage: rhinorrhoea, sneezing
  3. Mucoid stage: thick mucoid discharge
- Management
  - There is no evidence that antibiotics improve purulent nasal discharge.
  - There is some evidence that over-the-counter medications containing antihistamines, decongestants, analgesics, or combination help with recovery in all but young children.
  - Regular use of oral vitamin C appears to reduce the duration and severity of symptoms.

Allergic Rhinitis

- Affects 10% to 15% of children and 25% of adults in the United Kingdom
- Strong association with asthma (80% of people with asthma have allergic rhinitis)
- Classified as seasonal or perennial with severity based on impact on impact on daily function
- Common aeroallergens include tree, grass, and ragweed pollen; cat and dog dander; house dust mite faeces; and moulds such as *Aspergillus* and *Alternaria* spp.
- Management
  - Allergen avoidance where practicable such as regular dusting, mattress protection, and acaricides for carpets and furniture.
  - Low-quality evidence suggests that saline nasal rinsing can help with symptoms of allergic rhinitis.
  - Adults should be started on oral antihistamine or intranasal corticosteroid monotherapy as first-line treatment based on their predominant symptom; children should be initiated on a selective H_1-antagonist.
  - Second- and third-generation oral H_1-antagonists (e.g., fexofenadine, loratadine, cetirizine) are a good first-line treatment for mild to moderate symptoms such as reducing nasal itching, sneezing, and watery rhinorrhoea but less for nasal obstruction.
  - Intranasal corticosteroids are superior to oral or topical H_1-antagonists at relieving symptoms of nasal obstruction, and ones with low systemic bioavailability are recommended first-line treatment (mometasone, fluticasone propionate for prophylaxis). The patient should use it once or twice per day based on manufacturers' instructions. Teach proper technique for administration to reduce side effects. In seasonal rhinitis, they should be started 2 weeks before anticipated onset of symptoms and continued until rhinitis is likely to have subsided.
  - Ipratropium bromide spray can be used as an alternative if rhinorrhoea is the predominant symptom.

- Sodium cromoglicate eye drops can be used as an adjunct in allergic rhinoconjunctivitis.
- Patients with ongoing symptoms despite good concordance with treatment should be referred to an allergy specialist.

Rhinosinusitis

GUIDELINE

Fokkens, W., Lund, V., Hellings, P., Kern, R., Reitsma, S., Toppila-Salmi, S., Bernal-Sprekelsen, M., Mullol, J., Alobid, I, Anselmo-Lima, W. T., Bachert, C., Baroody, F., von Buchwald, C., Cervin, A., Cohen, N., Constantinidis, J., De Gabory, L, Desrosiers, M., Diamant, Z., ... Zwetsloot C. P. (2020). European position paper on rhinosinusitis and nasal polyps. *Rhinology*, 20;58(Suppl. 29),1–464. Retrieved from https://epos2020.com/Documents/supplement_29.pdf.

- Rhinosinusitis is an inflammatory disorder affecting the nose and paranasal sinuses.
- Symptoms include nasal obstruction or nasal discharge with or without facial pressure or reduced smell
- *Acute*
  - Most typically viral in origin
  - Management
    a. Simple analgesia
    b. Steam inhalation
    c. Short use (<7 days) of intranasal decongestants may help symptoms but will not expedite recovery.
- Acute bacterial rhinosinusitis may complicate and is suggested by:
  - Persistent pyrexia (temperature >38°C)
  - Unilateral symptoms
  - Worsening facial pain
  - Double sickening (improvement followed by deterioration)
- If acute bacterial rhinosinusitis is suspected, then antibiotics may play a role in management.
- Refer urgently:
  - Any facial cellulitis or periorbital swelling
  - Systemic signs of sepsis or meningitis
- Refer routinely if the patient has more than four episodes of defined acute bacterial rhinosinusitis in 1 year.

Chronic Rhinosinusitis

- Duration longer than 12 weeks.
- Defined by same symptoms as acute rhinosinusitis with endoscopic findings suggestive of disease.
- Now subdivided by dominant pathophysiological mechanism—eosinophil driven versus neutrophil driven
- May or may not be associated with nasal polyposis.
- Nasal polyps can be associated with adult-onset asthma and NSAID intolerance.
- Initial treatment is medical.
  - Intranasal corticosteroid with saline nasal irrigation is the first-line treatment and should be reviewed at 12 weeks.

- Short-course, tapered oral prednisolone can be added as an adjunct in those with eosinophil-driven disease and those with sinonasal polyposis.
- High-dose steroid nasal drops (Flixonase Nasule 400 μg/ampoule) with half applied to each nostril, twice a day used in the headupside-down position for upto 6 weeks can be used for refractory cases before transitioning back to an intranasal corticosteroid spray.
- A 2-week oral antibiotic course can be used with thick nasal discharge as the predominant symptom.
- Refer patients with persistent symptoms that are refractory to medical therapy.

Sinonasal Masses

- Tumours of the nasal cavity are rare and can be benign or malignant.
- Suspicious features are unilateral epistaxis or blood-stained serous discharge, unilateral nasal obstruction, referred otalgia, visual symptoms, and facial numbness.
- These patients should be referred to an ENT specialist under locally agreed suspected cancer pathways.

Epistaxis

- Sixty percent of people have experienced epistaxis at some point in their lifetime.
- Epistaxis has a bimodal distribution peaking at age 10 years and again after age 45 years.
- About 80% to 95% is anterior epistaxis from Little's area of vessels on the anterior nasal septum.
- Most episodes of epistaxis are self-limiting and do not require medical intervention.

Management

- *Acute epistaxis*
  a. First aid measures should be used, including sitting forwards and pinching the cartilaginous portion of the nasal tip firmly for 15 minutes.
  b. If bleeding stops, topical use of Naseptin cream (or if peanut allergic, mupirocin ointment) twice a day for 2 weeks can reduce inflammation in the nasal vestibule and subsequent nose bleeds.
  c. In ongoing bleeding, if a vessel is visible, unilateral targeted silver nitrate nasal cautery can be used to stop the bleeding.
  d. Silver nitrate cautery with antiseptic cream offers a small but statistically significant benefit over antiseptic cream alone in treating epistaxis in paediatric patients.
  e. If cautery is ineffective or a vessel is not visible, patients may require transfer to hospital for assessment and nasal packing.
  f. If bleeding is managed in primary care, patients should be advised not to blow their nose, avoid strenuous exercise, and avoid hot drinks for 24 hours.
  g. Oral tranexamic acid may reduce episodes of rebleeding within the following 10 days.

- *Recurrent epistaxis*
  a. Management of acute episodes is as above.
  b. Consider referral to an ENT specialist if there are ongoing disabling episodes or signs and symptoms of potential underlying cause (angiofibroma, sinonasal tumour, bleeding disorders).

Obstructive Sleep Apnoea Syndrome

- Obstructive sleep apnoea syndrome (OSAS) a sleep-related breathing disorder characterised by complete or partial episodic obstruction of the upper airway during sleep causing apnoea or hypopnoea.
- In adults, it is a diagnosis made after sleep study.
- Affects about 1.8% of children (Brunetti et al, 2001) and up to 49% of middle aged males and 24% of middle-aged females.

Children

- Ask the parents for the child's sleep quality and pattern with defined and witnessed pauses lasting seconds.
- Ask about restlessness, easy arousal, and sweating during sleep and work of breathing during sleep.
- Evaluate daytime symptoms of reduced concentration, excessive tiredness, or hyperactivity.
- Document weight; faltering growth is rare and is a sign of severe sleep-disordered breathing and warrants urgent investigation.
- Assess the child's nasal patency and palatine tonsillar tissue.
- Refer to an ENT specialist if symptoms of sleep-disordered breathing (not just snoring) with adenotonsillar hypertrophy.

Adults

- Screen for OSAS using the STOPBANG questionnaire (Box 18.1).
- Ask about excessive tiredness, snoring, and fatigue using Epworth Sleepiness scale (Box 18.2).
- Ask about collateral history of pauses, gasping, or choking.
- Assess for risk factors for OSAS and medical conditions that may impacted by it such (e.g., hypertension, diabetes).

• BOX 18.1 **STOPBANG Questionnaire to Assess for Obstructive Sleep Apnoea Syndrome**

S: Do you snore loudly?
T: Do you often feel tired, fatigued, or sleepy during the daytime?
O: Has anyone observed you stop breathing during sleep?
P: Do you have, or are you being treated for, high blood pressure
B: Body mass index >35 kg/m^2
A: Age older than 50 years
N: Neck circumference >40 cm
G: Gender male
Interpretation: One point for each positive answer. A score of 2 or less is low risk. A score of 3 or 4 suggests a need for further evaluation. A score of 5 or more is high risk.

• BOX 18.2 **Epworth Sleepiness Scale**

For each of the below situations, ask the patient how likely they are to fall asleep.
   No chance of dozing = 0 points
   Slight chance of dozing = 1 point
   Moderate chance of dozing = 2 points
   High chance of dozing = 3 points
1. Sitting and reading
2. Watching TV
3. Sitting inactive in a public place (e.g., theatre or meeting)
4. As a passenger for >1 hour without a break
5. Lying down to rest in the afternoon when circumstances permit
6. Sitting and talking to someone
7. Sitting quietly after lunch without alcohol
8. In a car, whilst stopped in traffic for a few minutes
Interpretation: 0–7, unlikely to be abnormally sleepy. 8–9, an average amount of daytime sleepiness. 10–15, excessive sleepiness in certain situations; consider further investigations. >15, excessively sleepy.

- Refer patients to a local sleep clinic:
  - High risk of OSAS on screening
  - Concomitant respiratory condition. Chronic obstructive pulmonary disease, evidence of cardiac or ventilatory failure, or need to operate machinery warrants urgent referral.
- Refer patients to an ENT specialist:
  - Suspicion of treatable sinonasal pathology exacerbating sleep disorder (e.g., nasal septal deviation, sinonasal polyposis)
- Driving
  - Patients with suspected sleep apnoea must be advised not to drive when they are excessively tired.
  - Patients with confirmed sleep apnoea are required to inform the DVLA and insurance company and not drive until OSAS is controlled.

Throat and Mouth

Sore Throat

- Approximately 20% of sore throats are bacterial, namely beta-haemolytic *Streptococci* group A (GABHS), C, and G.
- The sensitivity and specificity of throat swabs are 30% and 80%, respectively, with 40% of individuals carriers of GABHS; therefore, swab positivity does not prove infection and is not recommended as routine.

Bacterial Tonsilitis

- Streptococcal tonsillitis cannot be reliably diagnosed clinically, although it is more likely in children younger than age 11 years with:
  - Myalgia
  - Tender swollen cervical lymphadenopathy
  - Tonsillar exudates

- The CENTOR or FEVERPAIN criteria are not accurate in screening children or adults for streptococcal tonsillitis but are widely used to guide decision making around antibiotic prescribing.
- CENTOR = Cough absent, Exudate on tonsils, lymph Nodes that are tender, Temperature over 38 degree. One point is awarded for the presence of each. The maximum score is 4 and a score of 3 or 4 increases the chance of streptococcus infection to 34 to 56%.
- FEVERPAIN = FEVER during the previous 24 hours, Purulence (on tonsils or pharynx), Attend within three days of onset, Inflamed tonsils, No cough/coryza. One point is awarded for each up to a maximum of 5 points. A score of 4 or 5 is associated with a 62–65% chance of streptococcal infection.
- Use of antibiotics improves sore throat and headache by day 3 but not significantly by day 7 with no significant impact on fever.
- Antibiotics do not seem to protect against nonsuppurative complications of streptococcal tonsillitis, or if they do, the incidence in developed countries is so rare that it should not influence management.
- The antibiotic of choice is typically phenoxymethylpenicillin four times a day for 7 to 10 days or if the patient has a true allergy to penicillin, clarithromycin twice a day, but this should be tailored to local microbiology recommendations.
- Antibiotics have no effect on the incidence of bacterial or viral URTI in the subsequent 6 months.
- Patients given a single dose of steroids (e.g., 30 mg of prednisolone or 8 mg of dexamethasone) are twice as likely to experience pain relief at 24 hours.
- If a penicillin is used, a 10-day course is more successful than a 5-day course in eradicating streptococci from the throat.

Management

- The aim is to balance:
  1. Unnecessarily widespread use of antibiotics with the disadvantages of antibiotic resistance, overreliance on general practitioner consultation, and drug side effects
  2. Facilitate access to antibiotics required for unwell patients or those at higher risk of complication
- Antibiotics should not be used for symptomatic relief of sore throat.
- Recommend regular use of analgesics and antipyretics with appropriate age-based doses. Ibuprofen three times a day with food is the drug of choice, augmented when required with paracetamol four times a day.
- If giving a prescription for antibiotics, delaying a prescription for 3 days can reduce use by two-thirds with no significant difference in clinical outcomes.
- The antibiotic of choice is typically phenoxymethylpenicillin 250 mg four times a day for 10 days or if the patient has a true allergy to penicillin, 500 mg of clarithromycin twice a day, but this should be tailored to local microbiology recommendations.

- In patients who are members of a closed community with an outbreak of suspected or confirmed streptococcal pharyngitis (e.g., schools), have a lower threshold for antibiotic prescribing.
- Patients with sore throat associated with trismus, dysphonia, dysphagia, breathing difficulty, or stridor should be referred for immediate ENT assessment.
- In patients with prolonged tonsillitis:
  a. Arrange blood tests for a full blood count (FBC), C-reactive protein, liver function tests, infectious mononucleosis serology and ASOT (Antistreptolysin O Titre) titre.
  b. Consider escalating antibiotics to a cephalosporin or co-amoxiclav because beta-lactamase–producing organisms may be destroying the penicillin.
- Have a low threshold for face-to-face assessment and antibiotic prescribing in patients who are immunosuppressed.
- Treat patients who have a history of complicated tonsillitis (e.g., previous quinsy) more readily with antibiotics.

Peritonsillar Abscess

- This is a complication of acute bacterial tonsillitis in which an abscess forms between the tonsil capsule and superior constrictor muscle.
- Clinically, it presents with peritonsillar swelling over the soft palate and medialisation of the tonsil and uvular displacement to the contralateral side.
- Quinsy is usually polymicrobial, including oral cavity anaerobes.
- In observational studies, patients with one quinsy have up to a 14% chance of further quinsy.

Management

- Suspected quinsy should be referred to an ENT specialist for further assessment.
- Steroids give good symptomatic relief (prednisolone 30 mg) and reduce hospitalisation.
- Penicillin and metronidazole in combination is effective in almost 99% of cases.
- There is no significant evidence to suggest incision and drainage is superior to aspiration in managing peritonsillar abscess.

Infectious Mononucleosis

- This is a systemic disorder most commonly caused by *Herpesviridae* infection (typically Epstein-Barr virus (EBV) or cytomegalovirus).
- It is typically spread via the oral route or, in immunosuppressed patients, reactivation when a carrier.
- The most commonly affected age group is 15 to 24 years of age.
- Patients typically present with a sore throat, neck swelling, and constitutional symptoms with the clinical

examination in keeping with cervical lymphadenopathy and hypertrophic tonsils with greyish exudates.

- Patients suspected of having glandular fever should have blood tests to check:
  a. FBC: Atypical lymphocytes with lymphocytosis may be seen; thrombocytopaenia and autoimmune haemolytic anaemia can also occur
  b. A serologic diagnostic test (e.g., for antiheterophile antibodies or EBV immunoglobulin M)
  c. Liver function testing: About 90% of patients have raised alanine aminotransferase and aspartate aminotransferase levels.
- A 72-hour course of oral prednisolone (30 mg/day) can give short-term relief of sore throat, but the benefit is not sustained if given for a longer duration than this.
- Patients should be advised to avoid heavy lifting and contact sports for 4 weeks from the diagnosis to reduce risk of splenic rupture.
- Patients with associated liver dysfunction should have it repeated in primary care within 6 weeks of diagnosis and avoid alcohol.
- Postviral fatigue occurs in up to 10% of patients.

Tonsillectomy

- In adults, tonsillectomy for recurrent acute tonsillitis is both clinically and cost effective with few days of sore throat in the treated group over 24 months.
- In children, surgery offers chance of avoiding two moderate to severe throat infections over 2 years.
- *Indications for referral*
  - Recurrent acute tonsillitis: seven episodes in 1 year, five in 2 years, or three in 3 years
  - Suspicion of obstructive sleep apnoea in children younger than 16 years of age
  - Recurrent peritonsillar abscess
  - Unilateral tonsillar enlargement: suspicion for malignancy
  - Bacterial carriers who have not responded to antibiotics in certain contexts (e.g., PFAPA (Periodic Fever, Aphthous Stomatitis, Pharyngitis, Adenitis), GABHS (Group A beta haemolytic streptococcus) with rheumatic fever)
  - Guttate psoriasis with exacerbations from sore throats

Oral Thrush

- This is a clinical diagnosis of nonpainful, easily removable plaque on the oral mucosa and tongue with a nonpainful erythematous surface underneath.
- It is more commonly seen in neonates, older adults, steroid inhaler users, and those with systemic immunosuppression.
- Acute erythematous oral candidiasis presents with soreness and burning mainly affecting the palate and tongue with atrophy of the underlying tissue.
- It is most common in patients after a course of oral antibiotics.

Management

- Rule out and treat any predisposing cause (e.g., new diagnosis of diabetes, human immunodeficiency virus (HIV)).
- Lifestyle modification: Smoking cessation, inhaler techniques, and denture cleaning advice can reduce infections.
- A 14-day course of miconazole oral gel is the first-line treatment for children older than the age 4 months and adults.
- Consider Nystatin suspension in those who can gargle as second-line treatment or oral fluconazole if there is persistent infection.

Supraglottitis

- Supraglottis is an inflammatory disorder of the pharynx and larynx.
- It typically presents with an acute onset sore of throat, dysphonia, and dysphagia; increased respiratory effort and stridor are late signs of advanced swelling and airway obstruction.
- In children, epiglottitis is the most common manifestation.
- In adults, it is more common in smokers.
- Patients need immediate referral to an ENT specialist and rapid ambulance transfer to a place of safety.

Dysphagia

- Persistent dysphagia can be a presenting complaint of upper digestive tract malignancy, and patients should be referred directly for upper gastrointestinal endoscopy first-line treatment.
- The upper aerodigestive tract (benign and malignant conditions) and neurologic conditions can also cause dysphagia.
- Dysphagia alongside other concerning symptoms such as a referred neck lump, otalgia, or dysphonia should warrant urgent referral to an ENT specialist.
- Acute pharyngeal dysphagia (over days) with the inability to swallow saliva, with or without sore throat, warrants immediate ENT assessment.

Dysphonia

- Persistent hoarse voice for greater than 6 weeks in patients 45 years of age and older warrants urgent referral to ENT for endoscopic evaluation of the larynx.
- Consider rereferral, even when normal prior nasendoscopy, especially in smokers and those with excessive alcohol intake if their hoarse voice does not improve after 3 months.
- Consider the patient's voice use in the context of their hoarse voice; overuse can be seen in children and occupational voice users.
- Encourage good vocal hygiene.
- Speech and language therapy referral should be considered in those with ongoing voice problems.
- Professional voice users should seek the advice of a voice coach.

Globus Sensation

- This is a nonpainful sensation of a lump in the throat.
- The likelihood of malignancy is extremely low in the absence of other red flag symptoms of head and neck cancer and a normal ENT examination.

Sore Mouth

Red or White Patches

- In patients with oral cavity lesions, an assessment from their dentist is recommended.
- Refer all red patches as suspected erythroplakia to an oral surgeon urgently.
- Persisting white patches that do not respond to treatment for oral thrush or are in unusual sites for them (e.g., buccal mucosa) should be referred as suspected leukoplakia (1% per annum risk of malignant transformation).

Vincent Angina

- This is an ulcerated gingivostomatitis which can spread to the tonsils; caused by infection by fusiform bacteria and spirochetes.
- Treatment is with 400 mg of metronidazole twice a day for 3 days.

Aphthous Ulceration

- This is the most common ulcerative disease of the mouth, affecting up to 25% of people during their lifetime.
- It is associated with stress, menstruation, smoking, higher socioeconomic status, misfitting dental appliances, and age younger than 40 years.
- Check FBC, iron levels, vitamin B_{12}, and folate and zinc levels because these can all be associated with recurrent aphthous ulcers. Tissue transglutaminase, HIV, and erythrocyte sedimentation rate can be added if suspicion of systemic disorders.
- *Minor ulcers* are smaller under 1 cm in size; the majority heal within 14 days.
- *Major ulcers* are 1 to 3 cm in size and can take 6 weeks to heal.
- Treatment for infrequent minor ulcers may not be required.
- Topical treatments include:
  - Lidocaine in gels or benzydamine mouth wash for analgesic effect
  - Chlorhexidine gluconate oral solution or doxycycline mouthwash for antimicrobial effect
  - Hydrocortisone oromucosal tablets or betamethasone soluble tablets can be used with duration titrated to response.
- Severe, recurrent ,or nonresolving ulcers require evaluation by an oral medicine specialist.

References

Adrion, C., Fischer, C. S., Wagner, J., Gürkov, R., Mansmann, U., Strupp, M., & BEMED Study Group (2016). Efficacy and Safety of betahistine treatment in patients with Ménière's disease: Primary results of a long term, multicentre, double blind, randomised, placebo controlled, dose defining trial (BEMED trial). *BMJ (Clinical research ed.), 352*, h6816.

Brunetti, L., Rana, S., Lospalluti, M. L., M. L., Pietrafesa, A., Francavilla, R., Fanelli, M., & Armenio, L. (2001). Prevalence of obstructive sleep apnea syndrome in a cohort of 1,207 children of southern Italy. *Chest, 120*(6), 1930–1935.

Hilton, M., & Pinder, D. (2014). The Epley (canalith repositioning) manoeuvre for benign paroxysmal positional vertigo. *Cochrane Database of Systematic Reviews*, (2), CD003162.

Sullivan, F. M., Swan, I. R., Donnan, P. T., Morrison, J. M., Smith, B. H., McKinstry, B., Davenport, R. J., Vale, L. D., Clarkson, J. E., Hammersley, V., Hayavi, S., McAteer, A., Stewart, K., & Daly, F. (2007). Early treatment with prednisolone or acyclovir in Bell's palsy. *New England Journal of Medicine, 357*, 1598–1607.

Teixeira, L. J., Valbuza, J. S., & Prado, G. F. (2011). Physical therapy for Bell's palsy (idiopathic facial paralysis). *Cochrane Database of Systematic Reviews*, (12), CD006283.

Webster, K. E., Galbraith, K., Harrington-Benton, N. A., Judd, O., Kaski, D., Maarsingh, O. R., MacKeith, S., Ray, J., Van Vugt, V. A., & Burton, M. J. (2023a). Systemic pharmacological interventions for Ménière's disease. *Cochrane Database of Systematic Reviews*, (2), CD015171.

Webster, K. E., George, B., Lee, A., Galbraith, K., Harrington-Benton, N. A., Judd, O., Kaski, D., Maarsingh, O. R., MacKeith, S., Murdin, L., Ray, J., Van Vugt, V. A., & Burton, M. J. (2023b). Lifestyle and dietary interventions for Ménière's disease. *Cochrane Database of Systematic Reviews*, (2), CD015244.

19

Eye Problems

Sana Rasool

CHAPTER CONTENTS

General Points

> **PATIENT INFORMATION**
>
> Patient information leaflets for a number of eye conditions are available at http://www.moorfields.nhs.uk/listing/conditions.

Visual Acuity Testing

- Tests of visual acuity have a reliability of 98% and is essential referral information but only if the following steps are taken:
  a. The Snellen chart should be the recommended distance from the patient for the size of chart used. The distance should be marked, and the patient should stand behind the mark.
  b. The chart should be illuminated with 480 lux (e.g., a spotlight).
  c. Visual acuity should be tested with and without glasses.
- Smartphone-based visual acuity testing may be of particular benefit in remote testing or when a Snellen chart is not available. Many apps are available depending on the device used, and this gives a reasonable idea as to what the visual acuity may be, which would assist in deciding on the urgency of a potential referral (Tiraset et al, 2021).

Instilling Drops Into the Eye

- *Instilling drops.* Pull the lower eyelid down with the patient looking up. Squeeze one drop onto the lower fornix.
- *Instilling ointments or gels.* As above but squeeze 1 cm onto the inner surface of the eyelid. Warn the patient it will blur the vision for a short while.

The Gritty, Irritable Red Eye

Acute Infective Conjunctivitis

In adults and children:
- Viral conjunctivitis is the most common overall cause of infectious conjunctivitis, with up to 90% of cases being caused by adenoviruses.

- The most severe ocular manifestation of adenoviral conjunctivitis is epidemic keratoconjunctivitis, which is when both the conjunctiva and cornea are involved, leaving long lasting corneal changes and therefore decreased visual acuity.
- Adenoviral conjunctivitis is highly contagious; the infected individual can transmit the disease for up to 14 days after they are infected. Use of artificial tears and cold compresses may help alleviate symptoms.
- Antibiotic eye drops do not play a role in treating viral conjunctivitis and may in fact spread the disease to the contralateral eye by cross contamination from an infected bottle. The use of antibiotic eye drops unnecessarily will also increase the risk of bacterial resistance (Azari & Arabi, 2020).
- The history and examination traditionally give grounds for distinguishing between bacterial and viral infection but there is no evidence to support this (Rietveld et al, 2003).
- The combination of bilateral mattering of the eyelids upon waking up in the morning, lack of itching, and no previous history of conjunctivitis are strong predictors of bacterial conjunctivitis.
- However, even in proven bacterial conjunctivitis, antibiotics only modestly improve the rate of resolution. More than half resolve without treatment in 2 to 5 days (Sheikh & Hurwitz, 2005).
- Individual data meta-analysis showed that acute conjunctivitis in primary care can be thought of as a self-limiting condition. Patients with a purulent discharge or a mild severity of red eye may have a small benefit from antibiotics (Au Jefferies, Perera, & Evert, 2011).

If the visual acuity is normal and the cornea is clear, advise the patient to:
- Wipe away discharge.
- Wash hands after touching the eyes.
- Use separate towels.
- Inform the patient that they are highly infectious.
- It seems logical to recommend that children should stay away from school even though this is not the recommendation of the Public Health Agency (2017).
- Treat only if there is purulent discharge with a mild red eye. It may be appropriate to advise the patient to return in 3 days to collect a prescription for antibiotic drops if symptoms are not resolving (Everitt, Little, & Smith, 2006). Prescribe chloramphenicol eye drops every 2 hours for 2 days and then four times a day for a further 5 days. Gentamicin is only indicated if there is gram-negative infection.
- If symptoms are still present at 1 week but there are no complications, stop all treatment and review weekly. Adenoviral infection typically takes 2 to 3 weeks to resolve.
- Refer to eye casualty at any stage if the visual acuity is reduced or the cornea is involved.
- *Orbital cellulitis:* Admit immediately.

In neonates:
- The likelihood and the dangers of sexually transmissible disease are greater than in older children and adults.
- If the eye is mildly sticky, take a swab and review.
- If the discharge is purulent, take swabs for viral, bacterial, and chlamydial infection and a smear for gonococci. Then start chloramphenicol eye drops hourly and refer for an ophthalmic opinion the same day.
- Admit for intensive antibiotic therapy if:
  a. Herpes simplex, chlamydia, or gonococcus has grown
  b. The clinical situation worsens, with a red eye, cloudy cornea, blepharitis, marked preauricular lymphadenopathy or an unwell child
- Notify as ophthalmia neonatorum.

Allergic Conjunctivitis

Findings include itching, mucoid discharge, chemosis, and eyelid oedema.

Acute

- Reassure the patient that the eye will not be harmed and that the problem will settle soon.
- Advise patients not to rub their eyes.
- Discontinue contact lens use whilst symptomatic.
- Apply cool compresses with or without refrigerated artificial tears.
- If patients require further short-term treatment, use antihistamines with or without vasoconstrictors (e.g., olopatadine or antazoline with xylometazoline). Vasoconstrictors cause rebound hyperaemia if taken for more than 2 weeks.

Chronic or Recurrent Allergic Eye Disease

- Establish, if possible, what the allergen is and reduce or avoid contact.
- Preferred use is for an antihistamine with mast cell stabilising properties (e.g., olopatadine). Instruct the patient they must use this for at least 2 weeks because mast cell stabilizers require a loading period of several weeks and are better to be given before the antigen exposure. If there is concurrent rhinitis, consider using a steroid nasal spray (e.g., Nasonex spray twice a day (BD)) rather than an oral antihistamine.
- *Prophylaxis.* Give sodium cromoglicate, nedocromil sodium, or lodoxamide drops four times a day (QDS). Benefit may not be seen for 2 weeks. Where symptoms are seasonal, start treatment before the season starts.
- Consider giving an oral nonsedating antihistamine if symptoms are still not controlled. (not in patients with dry eye because this can exacerbate symptoms).

- *Severe cases not responding to the above.* Refer to ophthalmology for consideration of weak topical steroid (e.g., prednisolone).
- If a patient's condition worsens dramatically after starting to use drops, consider contact sensitivity. The usual cause is the preservative in the drops.

Blepharitis

- The mainstays of treatment are patient education and counselling.
- Emphasise that this is a chronic disease with intermittent exacerbations and that cure is generally not possible.
- Reassure the patient that the condition will not threaten sight. Explain that it results from either colonisation of eyelashes or Meibomian gland dysfunction. Treatment is long term.
- Avoid eye makeup (especially mascara and eyeliner).
- *Eyelid hygiene comprises three stages:*
  1. *Compresses.* Heat the area with a hot washcloth (not scalding) for 5 to 10 minutes
  2. *Massage.* Directly after compresses, massage the eyelids down and towards the eyelid margin to empty the ducts.
  3. *Wash.* Using a dedicated eyelid cleanser and a cotton bud, gently scrub the eyelid margins, initially bd then twice weekly thereafter. Previously, the use of baby shampoo was recommended, but there could be a loss of goblet cell function with this, so this is no longer recommended (Sung et al, 2018).
- Treat patients as if they have dry eyes because the tears evaporate more rapidly. See later discussion for treatment regimen but do not continue if there is no benefit.
- If there is no improvement, give chloramphenicol ointment to be applied to the eyelid margins bd for 1 month.
- Treat those not still responding and those with acne rosacea with long courses of oral antibiotics, such as doxycycline 100 mg bd for 1 month and then once a day (OD) for 3 months or tetracycline (contraindicated in pregnancy, breastfeeding, and children younger than 12 years). Consider topical azithromycin 1% solution twice a day for 3 days a week for 6/52 (Luchs, 2008).
- Consider referral to an ophthalmologist for those:
  a. With remaining symptomatic despite treatment for a few months, particularly if unilateral (masquerade syndrome of sebaceous cell carcinoma).
  b. Who have associated skin disease.
  c. When there is suspicion of corneal involvement. The inflammation is secondary to hypersensitivity to the cell wall protein of staphylococcus and may require topical steroid and antibiotic drops for a

short period. Encourage the patient to continue eyelid hygiene.
  d. Orbital or preseptal cellulitis is suspected.
  e. An eye becomes painful or red.
  f. Rapid onset of visual loss.

Dry Eye

- Early detection and treatment may help prevent corneal ulcers and scarring.
- Treat any blepharitis (see earlier).
- Check that the patient is not taking any drugs that might exacerbate the condition (e.g., antihistamines).
- Encourage the patient to alter their environment by minimising air conditioning and heating and to try to increase the humidity, if appropriate.
- Advise the intake of omega 3/6 fatty acids.
- Lubrication is the mainstay of treatment.
- *Artificial tears.* Encourage the patient to use these as often as necessary. Start with hypromellose 0.3%. Start at qds and increase up to every 30 minutes. Higher strengths may give relief for longer. If using more than six times daily, drops should be preservative free, although these are often expensive single-use formulations.
- Substitute products that last longer (e.g., sodium hyaluronate).
- *Gels.* These increase duration by clinging to the surface (e.g., carbomers use up to qds).
- *Ointments.* Prescribe paraffin-containing ointments for use at night only because they create a greasy tear film that is difficult to see through.
- Refer:
  a. Urgently if there is a sudden increase in discomfort, redness, or deterioration in vision. These patients are at increased risk of microbial keratitis.
  b. Routinely patients who are having to instil drops very frequently. Many other treatments may be appropriate: topical glucocorticoids or cyclosporine, autologous serum, vitamin A or oral antioxidants, punctual plugs, or eyelid surgery.

Trauma

- Check the visual acuity. Refer if this is diminished or has decreased when the patient is seen next.

Foreign Body

- Suspect a foreign body in any unilateral red eye with or without a history of 'something going into the eye'.
- Always fully evert the upper eyelid when looking for a foreign body. If a foreign body is seen, it can usually be removed from the conjunctiva without difficulty.
- If there is a history of pain while hammering metal or of exposure to glass splinters, refer to exclude an intraocular foreign body.

Corneal Foreign Body

1. Insert local anaesthetic. Start with proxymetacaine, and when the stinging has stopped, deepen the anaesthesia with amethocaine 1% drops. Continue until the drops feel cold but do not sting.
2. Remove the foreign body with a cotton wool bud or the tip of a sterile needle. Do not dig into the cornea; at its centre, it is only 1 mm thick.
3. After removal, prescribe antibiotic eye ointment bd for 2 days as prophylaxis.
4. Give a cycloplegic (e.g., Cyclopentolate 1% TDS) if pain continues.
5. Do not apply an eye pad.
6. Examine after 24 hours:
   a. With fluorescein to be sure the epithelium has healed
   b. To exclude a rust ring if the foreign body was metallic. If present, refer to an ophthalmologist urgently for it to be removed.

Chemical Burns

- These are acid or alkali burns (usually in the form of cement, lime, caustic soda, or ammonia). Whereas acid burns cause coagulation necrosis, alkali burns are the more serious, causing saponification of phospholipid membranes, leading to rapid epithelial cell death and caustic penetration. Ammonia can cause severe injury in 2 minutes.
- Irrigate with tap water or normal saline for 20 minutes or with alkali burns until the pH is normal (pH, 6.5–7.5).
- Examine the cornea with fluorescein and send to eye casualty if it is not clear.
- *Cement.* Look for cement adhering to the eye, under the eyelids, or in the conjunctival fornices. If found, give local anaesthetic drops (e.g., benoxinate) and remove it, however distressing this is to the patient. Refer immediately after this.
- *Detergent.* If the conjunctiva shows punctate epithelial loss, treat with chloramphenicol and review in 3 days.

Ultraviolet Light Burns

- *Arc eye* is usually caused by exposure to ultraviolet C through welding or using a sunbed without eye protection. Patients are usually unaware until 6 to 12 hours after exposure.
- Treatment is supportive with anticipation that damaged epithelium will regenerate within 24 to 72 hours.
- Give local anaesthetic drops (e.g., benoxinate) *once* but do not repeat them; they slow corneal healing.
- Treat with chloramphenicol ointment for lubrication and prevention of super infection qds for 2 to 3 days.
- The worst of the two eyes can be padded if it offers some relief.
- Give sufficient sedatives and analgesics to ensure a night's sleep. Opioids are likely to be needed. Cessation of blinking during sleep enables the corneal epithelium to heal.
- Review the patient in 2 to 3 days.

Corneal Abrasion

- Use topical anaesthetic once for examination purposes only.
- Confirm the abrasion with fluorescein dye after examining the eye and excluding other injuries (e.g., hyphaema and open globe).
- In contact lens wearers, use a pen light to look for an infiltrate.
- Treat with chloramphenicol ointment qds for 24 hours and then bd for 1 further week.
- For a large abrasion, give a cycloplegic (e.g., cyclopentolate 1% drops bd) if pain continues. Warn the patient about driving and difficulty reading. Consider oral nonsteroidal antiinflammatory drugs (NSAIDS; e.g., ibuprofen) or topical ophthalmic NSAID drops (e.g., diclofenac sodium) (Weaver & Terrell, 2003).
- Do not apply an eye pad.
- Give oral analgesia if the pain is severe.
- Refer if:
  a. There is a decrease in acuity of greater than 2 lines of the Snellen chart.
  b. There is a large defect (>50% of the epithelium).
  c. There is a purulent discharge or white infiltrate.
  d. The epithelium has not healed after 3 days.
- *Recurrent abrasions (erosions).* Recurrences tend to occur in the early morning during opening of that eye, when tear secretion is less. Give long-term (At least 3 months) artificial tears during the day and ointment at night (see the discussion of dry eyes). Explain that recurrences can continue for months or years. Refer to an ophthalmologist if not improving. Laser ablation may be needed.

Blunt Injuries

Refer all patients who receive blunt injuries (e.g., from a squash ball) because they may give rise to bleeding into the anterior chamber of the eye (hyphaema), and the pressure may increase.

Problems With Contact Lenses

Conjunctivitis

- Advise the patient to remove the lens and leave it out until recovered. (Keep the lens and its container in case it is needed for culture.)
- Check that the patient is cleaning and disinfecting the lenses every night (or using disposable single-use lenses).
- Prescribe antibiotic eye drops.
- Arrange for slit-lamp examination to exclude keratitis, either by the lens provider or the local ophthalmology emergency department.
- *Corneal abrasion.* See earlier.
- *Microbial keratitis.* A white infiltrate viewed with a pen light needs to be referred to the ophthalmology emergency department immediately. There is a risk of perforation and endophthalmitis.
- *Other problems* need slit-lamp examination to distinguish them. Advise the patient to leave the lenses out and contact the lens prescriber or refer the patient to an ophthalmologist.

NHS facilities are available to lens wearers if pathological problems have arisen.

Painful Red Eye That Is Not 'Gritty'

- Most need referral to eye casualty:
  a. Keratitis, ocular herpes simplex, corneal ulcer, scleritis and uveitis the same day
  b. Acute glaucoma immediately
- General practitioners may treat:
  a. *Episcleritis* with an oral NSAID if there is discomfort (e.g., diclofenac or flurbiprofen for 2 weeks). Topical NSAIDS (e.g., diclofenac qds) are also appropriate. Refer if not improved within 1 month.
  b. *Recurrent uveitis.* Treatment with topical steroids can be started, provided:
     - Their use has been previously sanctioned by a consultant.
     - The visual acuity is normal.
     - A dendritic ulcer is excluded with fluorescein and magnified examination of the cornea but arrange for specialist assessment. Ophthalmic supervision is always necessary because intensive topical steroids may be needed. Treat with topical antivirals if the history is suggestive of herpes while awaiting assessment.

Ophthalmic Herpes Zoster

- Give a high-dose antiviral drug at the first sign of zoster in the ophthalmic division of the trigeminal nerve (i.e., when the rash appears on the forehead, usually before any involvement of the eye) (e.g., acyclovir 800 mg five times a day). Untreated, about half would develop eye involvement.
- Refer to an ophthalmologist if there is:
  - Hutchinson sign (involvement of the nasociliary nerve which supplies the side of the nose and the skin of the inner corner of the eye)
  - A red eye
  - Visual complaints (Opstelten & Zaal, 2005)
  This referral is for an early but not immediate appointment. The complications for which ophthalmic expertise is needed (e.g., keratitis or uveitis) tend to occur 1 week or more after the onset of the rash.
- Be alert to the long-term complications of eye involvement:
  - Loss of corneal sensation may make the eye vulnerable to neuropathic ulceration or exposure keratopathy.
  - Scarring of the eyelid by an extensive periorbital vesicular rash may lead to incomplete closure, putting the cornea at risk.
  Patients with either of these problems need to use lubricating eye ointments for the long term with or without surgery.

Eyelash, Eyelid, and Lacrimal Problems

Acute Dacryocystitis

- Treat aggressively for presumed staphylococcal or streptococcal infection (e.g., with flucloxacillin and amoxicillin) for 1 week.

- Review after 24 hours. If the symptoms are worse, refer for an ophthalmologic opinion that day.
- Refer after the patient has recovered for an ophthalmological opinion and possible surgery.

Chalazion

- Advise the patient to use a warm compress (e.g., a face flannel) over the lump and massage towards the eyelid margin. Antibiotic ointments or drops are traditionally given (on to the eye in the hope that they will penetrate the chalazion through the conjunctival surface) despite the lack of evidence of benefit.
- Treat secondary infection with oral antibiotics (see dacryocystitis).
- Review the patient after they have recovered and treat any blepharitis present (see earlier discussion).
- Refer if a hard lump has failed to resolve after 3 months, is affecting vision, or is particularly troublesome for incision and curettage.
- *Prevention of recurrence.* Encourage eyelid hygiene (see earlier).

Styes

- Treat the infected eyelash follicle with topical antibiotics.
- If there is marked swelling of the eyelid, consider oral antibiotics.

Twitching

- *Myokymia.* Reassure the patient that twitching of a small area of the orbicularis muscle is common and is not sinister. It is often exacerbated by tiredness.
- *Facial twitching.* Refer to a neurologist or paediatrician.
- *Blepharospasm.* Forcible contractions of the entire orbicularis muscle should be referred to an ophthalmologist. Further investigation may be necessary (e.g., magnetic resonance imaging (MRI)), and botulinum toxin injections can give short-term relief.

Watery Eye

- This may result from inflammation or stenosis of the nasolacrimal duct or malposition of the eyelid.
- Treat any infection with topical antibiotics.
- Consider a trial of artificial tears (e.g., carbomer). The patient's natural basal secretion of tears may be deficient, causing reflexive overwatering as compensation.
- Refer patients who are bothered by it to an ophthalmologist. They may benefit from exploration of the nasolacrimal duct or eyelid surgery. Massage of the lacrimal sac does not help unless there is a mucocoele.

Acute Disturbance of Vision

- Establish that the loss is acute and not just sudden awareness of a preexisting field loss or cataract.
- Distinguish transient from continuing visual losses and treat as appropriate. For migraine and transient ischaemic attack, see Chapter 11.

Acute Painless Loss of Vision

Central Retinal Artery Occlusion

If seen within 24 hours:

- Arrange for the patient to be seen immediately in eye casualty. Restoration of blood flow within 90 to 100 minutes leads to no retinal injury.
  If any delay is anticipated:
  a. *Temporal arteritis.* If the history and examination suggest temporal arteritis, give 1000 mg of methylprednisolone by slow intravenous (IV) injection.
  b. Give aspirin 300 mg (unless contraindicated).
  If seen after 24 hours:
- There is no treatment for the eye, and the object is to try to prevent retinal artery occlusion of the other eye.
- Refer to an ophthalmologist but less urgently.
- Give aspirin 75 mg/day.
- Take blood for an erythrocyte sedimentation rate (ESR). If the clinical picture suggests temporal arteritis, give steroids while awaiting the result.
- Look for evidence of more widespread cardiovascular disease, especially a carotid bruit. Check blood pressure, fasting blood sugar, and lipids.
- Consider the possibility that the occlusion was embolic. If so, refer to a vascular surgeon or cardiologist according to where you suspect the embolus originated.

Central or Branch Retinal Vein Occlusion

- Workup:
  a. Blood pressure
  b. Blood sugar
  c. Full blood count and ESR for polycythaemia and leukaemia
- Refer to eye casualty. The patient may need photocoagulation for chronic macular oedema and ischaemia following a vein occlusion. Various treatment options now exist in the form of intravitreal anti–vascular endothelial growth factor (VEGF) injections for branch or central vein occlusion with macula oedema. Monitoring by an ophthalmologist is required after occlusion to assess for retinal ischaemia and the risk of glaucoma. Complications can develop early; 50% develop neovascular glaucoma within 3 months (Royal College of Ophthalmologists, 2022).

Decreased Vision With Pain

Acute Closed-Angle Glaucoma

- Suspect it when:
  - The patient is unwell, with vomiting and eye or head pain; the eye is red and tender, the cornea is hazy, and the pupil is semidilated.
  - There may be a past history of episodes of blurred vision, associated with haloes round lights, that have been aborted by exposure to a bright light or by going to sleep. In these situations, the pupil constricts, pulling the pupillary iris out of the angle.

- Refer suspected cases urgently to eye casualty or admit. If treatment is delayed, irreversible damage to the optic nerve may occur in addition to adhesions between the iris and cornea, requiring surgical drainage.
- If it is not possible to get the patient to hospital immediately, give acetazolamide 500 mg IV or two 250-mg tablets orally and instil pilocarpine 2%, 0.5% Timolol 0.5%, and 1% apraclonidine 1% into the eye, 1 minute apart.
- Treat nausea and vomiting with prochlorperazine 12.5 mg intramuscularly.
- Do not attempt to dilate the pupil of anyone with suspected acute-angle glaucoma.

Optic Neuritis

- Progressive reduction in vision over a few days with the nadir at 1 to 2 weeks, with pain on eye movements. Colours appear washed out. Symptoms may be worse after a hot shower or bath.
- One-third of the patients have papillitis; the remainder have retrobulbar inflammation.
  - Improvement occurs within 2 weeks, and full recovery is usual within 3 months.
  - About 50% to 70% of individuals aged 20 to 40 years with retrobulbar neuritis in the United Kingdom will develop multiple sclerosis (MS), almost all of them within 5 years. A second episode increases that risk fourfold (Kanski, 1989).
- Refer urgently patients having their first attack to ophthalmology. Gadolinium-enhanced MRI provides confirmation of optic neuritis and aids prognosis and treatment decisions. Arrange for the patient to be seen again if symptoms are not improving after 2 weeks.
- Refer patients with a second attack to a neurologist (if not already done) because of the chance that this is MS.
- In younger patients, consider infectious or postinfectious causes of optic neuritis. In older patients (older than 50 years), consider ischaemic optic neuropathy.
- Ophthalmology or neurology may advocate IV steroids in severe or bilateral visual loss because they speed recovery (and decrease short-term risk of MS development) but they give no benefit to long-term visual outcome or MS development. Oral steroids are contraindicated because they cause an increased rate of recurrence of optic neuritis.

Acute Distortion of Vision

- Refer urgently. Older patients may have acute wet age-related macular degeneration (AMD), especially if the diagnosis has already been made in the other eye. Typically, they report that straight lines appear crooked.
- If vision is still better than 6/96, they may benefit from intraocular injections of an anti-VEGF approved by National Institute for Health and Care Excellence (NICE) provided they fit the criteria (Royal College of Ophthalmologists, 2024).

Floaters and Flashes

- Refer urgently patients who report:
  a. Multiple floaters, especially if associated with flashing lights. They may have a posterior vitreous detachment, which carries a 5% chance of causing a retinal tear.
  b. The appearance of a single large blob, which then fragments. They may have a vitreous haemorrhage.
- Be readier to refer if:
  a. There is a family history of retinal tear or detachment.
  b. The other eye has already had a detachment. Almost 25% of patients develop a detachment in the second eye.
  c. The patient has high myopia.
  d. There is a history of cataract surgery, which increases the risk of retinal detachment ninefold.
- Refer immediately if there is a field loss or decrease in acuity. These imply that retinal detachment has occurred. It may be visible ophthalmoscopically. Instruct the patient to lie with the face on the side of the detachment (i.e., the side opposite the field defect) on the pillow while waiting for the ambulance.

Note: Retinal tears are unlikely to be detected by conventional ophthalmoscopy. A normal fundus is therefore no grounds for inaction.

INFORMATION FOR PATIENTS WITH RETINAL DETACHMENT

Royal College of Ophthalmologists. (n.d.). *Understanding retinal detachment.* Retrieved from http://www.rcophth.ac.uk (search on 'information booklets').

Gradual Loss of Vision

- Refer to the optometrist who can ascertain whether there is refractive error (normally acuity will improve with a pinhole) and provide spectacles or perform a more thorough examination as to any other causes and refer appropriately.
- Suggest the following to all patients with visual difficulty:
  a. Use adequate lighting (e.g., an angle-poise lamp), especially for reading and close work.
  b. Rearrange the room to sit with the main window behind the patient and the television away from the window.
  c. If visual acuity is 6/18 or worse, refer routinely because they may be eligible for partial sight registration.
  d. Recommend the patient information leaflets available from the Royal National Institute of Blind People (RNIB) at http://www.rnib.org.uk and search for 'leaflets'.

Cataracts

- *In a child.* Refer as a matter of urgency. Any opacity of the ocular media can have a catastrophic effect on the development of vision and should be diagnosed and treated promptly.

- *In a young adult.* Refer but also investigate for diabetes or any other systemic disease that a clinical history might lead you to suspect.
- *In an older adult*
  - Exclude diabetes.
  - *Refer to an optometrist all patients* who have not had a recent refraction because a myopic shift often accompanies the onset of cataract, and a change in spectacle lenses can often postpone the need for cataract surgery.
  - They should be able to *refer directly to an ophthalmologist* if no improvement in vision is possible with refraction and the following are present:
    a. The patient is having significant visual problems affecting quality of vision or activities such as driving or reading.
    b. The patient is willing to undergo surgery. There is little point in referring those who are happy with their current level of vision and would not accept an invitation for surgery.
- There is no absolute Snellen acuity below which surgery is indicated. It depends on the patient's individual needs and circumstances. Many patients are content with vision that is 6/18 or better unless they drive or do fine work.
- Some patients find their cataract is more disabling than would be predicted from the level of Snellen acuity. This happens particularly in posterior subcapsular cataract when localised opacities scatter light, causing difficulty with reading and with glare when driving. After surgery, 85% to 90% will achieve vision that is adequate for driving (Allen & Vasavada, 2006).

Problems After Cataract Surgery

- *A red eye after surgery* may be caused by an allergy to the antibiotic and steroid drops given postoperatively. Rarely, in 0.1% to 0.5% of patients, it is caused by postoperative endophthalmitis. It would therefore be prudent to refer promptly any postoperative patient with a red eye, especially if there is reduced vision and pain.
- *More long-term deterioration of vision after surgery.* Refer the patient back; 20% develop opacification of the posterior capsule within 2 years of operation. They need laser treatment.

Age-Related Macular Degeneration

- AMD occurs in older adult patients who present with progressive loss of central vision and, frequently, distortion effects. When looking at straight lines, they appear wavy. The vision is best in dim light. The eye appears normal except for the choroidoretinal changes.
- Refer all patients for optometric assessment unless there is a sudden deterioration suggestive of wet AMD to confirm the diagnosis and to refer to an ophthalmologist if appropriate.
- Reassure patients that although they have lost some of their central reading vision, they will never be completely

blind and that further deterioration will be slow. The average time it takes for vision to deteriorate to less than 3/60 (eligible for blind registration) is 5 to 10 years.

- Encourage the patient to stop smoking. Smokers carry a three- to fourfold increased risk of AMD. There is evidence that stopping smoking reduces the incidence and progression of the disease (Kelly et al, 2004).
- *Prevention.* There is now evidence to show that nutritional supplements, including antioxidant vitamins and lutein and zeaxanthin, are beneficial in slowing the progression of AMD. (AREDS2 Research Group, 2013).

PATIENT INFORMATION

Macular Disease Society. Crown Chambers, South St, Andover, Hampshire, SP10 2BN. Tel: 0300 3030 111. Available at http://www.macularsociety.org.
    Royal College of Ophthalmologists. (n.d.). *Understanding age-related macular degeneration.* Retrieved from http://www.rcophth.ac.uk (search on 'information booklets').

Chronic Simple Glaucoma

- Treatment to lower intraocular pressure (IOP) has been shown to slow the progression of the disease (Wormald, 2003).
- Loss of visual acuity is a late sign of chronic glaucoma. By this stage, disc cupping and field loss are likely to be advanced and irreversible.
- The incidence increases with age. In the United Kingdom, it is 1 in 5000 at age 40 to 49 years and only really increases after age 60 years. After 85 years of age, it is 1 in 10.
- The risk increases:
  a. With a family history (×10)
  b. In paitents with high myopia (×3)
  c. In patients with diabetes (×3)
  d. In African Caribbeans
  e. In users of topical steroid drops for over 5 days

Screening and Referral

- Eye tests are advised every 2 years or more frequently if the patient is in a high-risk group.
- Screening for glaucoma should be completed by the optometrist who will perform tonometry (pressure measurement), visual field analysis, and fundoscopy as well as possibly gonioscopy and pachymetry (angle and corneal thickness analysis).
- Testing is free in Scotland and elsewhere for children and adults older than 60 years of age. Many of those in the high-risk groups are also eligible for free testing, such as those:
  - Older than 40 years of age with a family history of glaucoma
  - With glaucoma or diabetes
- *Driving.* Advise the patient to notify the Driver and Vehicle Licensing Agency, (DVLA) if there is significant bilateral visual field loss.

PATIENT INFORMATION

International Glaucoma Association. Woodcote House, 15 Highpoint Business Village, Henwood, Ashford, Kent, TN24 8DH. Tel: 01233 64 81 70. Available at http://www.glaucoma-association.com.
    Royal College of Ophthalmologists. (n.d.). *Understanding glaucoma.* Retrieved from http://www.rcophth.ac.uk (search on 'information booklets').

- Treatment is managed by the hospital eye department. Each patient will have a different target IOP, depending on various factors such as the patient's central corneal thickness, if they have progressive glaucomatous disc changes, or if they only have vision in one eye. Drops that can be used are:
  a. *Prostaglandin analogues* (latanoprost, travoprost, and bimatoprost), which increase aqueous outflow through the uveoscleral pathway and can reduce IOP by 30% to 35%. Systemic side effects are minimal; eyelashes may lengthen and darken, and light irises may permanently darken.
  b. *Beta-blockers* (timolol, carteolol, betaxolol, levobunolol, and metipranolol), which reduce the secretion of aqueous. They can cause systemic symptoms and may unmask latent and previously undiagnosed heart failure and airway obstruction (Kirwan et al, 2002). Systemic effects can be reduced by finger pressure on the caruncle or by shutting the eyes for several minutes after instilling the drops. This approach may also increase ocular absorption of the drug.
  c. *Carbonic anhydrase inhibitors* (dorzolamide, brinzolamide, or oral acetazolamide), which reduce the secretion of aqueous. Oral acetazolamide is the most effective but has significant side effects. Topical forms have few side effects. Neither should be used in patients with sulphonamide allergy.
  d. *Parasympathomimetic drugs* (e.g., pilocarpine) are now used only infrequently. They constrict the pupils and pull on the trabecular meshwork, increasing the flow. Pilocarpine eye drops frequently cause headaches, but they tend to disappear after the first few weeks of use. Pilocarpine constricts the pupil and may cause blurred vision if central lens opacities are present.

Allergy to Drops

This may present with intense itching and irritation of the eyes and eyelids, which is exacerbated by instillation of the drops. The allergy may be to the active drug or preservative (usually benzalkonium chloride). Stopping treatment (with monitoring of the pressure) should result in rapid improvement. Some topical agents are available in a preservative-free form.

Laser Treatment

Laser treatment in the form of trabeculoplasty or even ciliary body ablation may be appropriate in certain circumstances. In some patients, this may be first-line treatment:

a. *Trabeculoplasty.* Argon or diode 'burns' are applied to the trabecular meshwork. It is used only where the drainage angle is open.

b. *Ciliary body ablation.* This is usually done with a diode laser to burn the ciliary body and reduce production of Aqueous humour. The process may need to be repeated to keep the pressure low, and patients normally need to continue drug treatment.

Other laser methods (iridotomy and iridoplasty) are used in angle-closure glaucoma.

Surgical Treatment

Trabeculectomy or glaucoma drainage devices can be used when medical or laser treatment has failed. A channel is created to allow flow from the anterior chamber. After it has been performed, bacterial conjunctivitis can develop more readily into endophthalmitis.

Visual Handicap

- More than two-thirds of people who are eligible are not registered as blind or partially sighted. The majority of these people receive no social care services whatsoever.
- Two-thirds of all people with visual impairments have an additional disability or serious health problem.
- More than 50% of visually impaired people live alone, yet few have been offered any training in daily living skills. Almost half of all visually impaired people cannot cook for themselves because of hazards in the kitchen (RNIB, 2002).

Certification and Registration

- Certification is by a consultant ophthalmologist on form CV1.
- *Blind certification* is for those with visual acuity below 3/60 or with a VA of up to and including 6/60 but with gross visual field restriction.
- *Certification as partially sighted* is not defined by statute. It is appropriate for patients with visual acuity of 6/60 or worse with full visual fields or those with visual acuity better than that but with restriction of visual fields. A patient with a homonymous hemianopia, for instance, is likely to be eligible.
- *Registration* is voluntary and would normally be offered at the time of certification. Registration entitles a person to a range of benefits and concessions and help from some local voluntary groups. The receipt of a CVI by the social services department entitles that person to have their name added to the register. This also acts as a trigger for social services to arrange an assessment of the person's social care needs.
- Patients with low vision but not certified as blind or partially sighted should be encouraged to self-refer to social services using the Low Vision Leaflet available from high street opticians. They are also likely to benefit from a low visual aid referral, which is normally through the ophthalmology department.

Benefits

- Registration means that a social worker will contact the patient and provide:
  a. Access to a mobility officer, a teacher of Braille, and daily living courses
  b. Free audio aids
  c. Details of the RNIB talking-book service.
- In addition, the registered blind (but not necessarily the partially sighted) are eligible for:
  a. A slightly higher rate of income support
  b. Extra housing benefit, income support, and council tax benefit
  c. Increased income tax allowance
  d. Reduced fares and a Blue Parking Badge
  e. Ffree sight tests
  f. A reduction in the TV licence fee

The Royal National Institute for the Blind (provides information, support, and advice for anyone with a serious sight problem. helpline@rnib.org.uk. Helpline: 0303 123 9999 (interpreters are available). helpline@rnib.org.uk. Available at http://www.rnib.org.uk.

Prescribing for Patients With Contact Lenses

PATIENT INFORMATION

The British Contact Lens Association. Available at http://www.bcla.org.uk (search on 'do's and don'ts').

Topical Applications
Avoid:
a. Eye ointments
b. Eye drops containing preservatives (in soft lenses)
c. Topical steroids
d. Coloured drops: fluorescein and rose bengal
e. Sympathomimetics

Systemic Drugs
Avoid:
a. Drugs that reduce or alter tear secretion: oral contraceptives, hormone replacement therapy, drugs with anticholinergic activity (e.g., tricyclic antidepressants), beta-blockers, diuretics, and isotretinoin
b. Drugs that reduce blinking: benzodiazepines
c. Drugs that stain the lens: nitrofurantoin, rifampicin, and sulfasalazine
d. Drugs that are concentrated in the lens and can irritate the eye: aspirin

Myopia Management

- This remains a service provided by the private sector that is not regulated.

- Although legally in the United Kingdom, any registered medical practitioner may perform refractive surgery, the Royal College of Ophthalmologists recommends that it should only be performed by a fully trained ophthalmologist who has undergone additional specialist training in refractive surgery. They may or may not also be an NHS consultant.
- Advise patients to download the leaflet 'Refractive Surgery' available online from the Royal College of Ophthalmologists at http://www.rcophth.ac.uk (search on 'refractive surgery').
- Additionally, many nonsurgical options are available for myopia which are currently undergoing trials. Atropine eye drops are available to slow down the rate of progression of myopia; however, this is still only available privately. There are also spectacles and contact lenses to specifically reduce the rate of progression of myopia, which some opticians may be able to prescribe (Yam et al, 2022).

Further Reading

Chong, E. W., Wong, T. Y., Kreis, A. J., Simpson, J. A., & Guymer, R. H. (2007). Dietary antioxidants and primary prevention of age-related macular degeneration: Systematic review and meta-analysis. *BMJ (Clinical research ed.), 335*, 755–799.

Crick, R. P., & Tuck, M. W. (1995). How can we improve the detection of glaucoma? *BMJ (Clinical research ed.), 310*, 546–547.

Curi, A., Matos, K., & Pavesio, C. (2004). *Acute anterior uveitis. Clinical Evidence, 14*: 739-43 . Retrieved from www.clinicalevidence.com.

Doona, M., & Walsh, J. B. (1995). Use of chloramphenicol as topical eye medication: Time to cry halt? *BMJ (Clinical research ed.), 310*, 1217–1218.

Evans, J. R. (2004). Antioxidant vitamin and mineral supplements for age-related macular degeneration (Cochrane Review). In: The Cochrane Library, Issue 2.

Isenberg, S. J., Apt, L., Valenton, M., Del Signore, M., Cubillan, L., Labrador, M. A., Chan, P., & Berman, N. G. (2002). A controlled trial of povidone-iodine to treat infectious conjunctivitis in children. *American Journal of Ophthalmology, 134*(5), 681–688.

Lancaster, T., Swart, A. M., & Jick, H. (1998). Risk of serious haematological toxicity with use of chloramphenicol eye drops in a British general practice database. *BMJ (Clinical research ed.), 316*, 667.

Miller, E. R., 3rd, Pastor-Barriuso, R., Dalal, D., Riemersma, R. A., Appel, L. J., & Guallar, E. (2005). Meta-analysis: High-dosage vitamin E supplementation may increase all-cause mortality. *Annals of Internal Medicine, 42*, 37–46.

Mitchell, R., & Edwards, R. (1997). Prescribing for patients who wear contact lenses. *PRESCRIBER-LONDON-, 8*, 107-112.

Pippin MM, Le JK. Bacterial Conjunctivitis. [Updated 2023 Aug 17]. In: StatPearls [Internet]. Treasure Island (FL): StatPearls Publishing; 2024 Jan-. Available from: https://www.ncbi.nlm.nih.gov/books/NBK546683/

Solebo, A. L., Angunawela, R. I., Dasgupta, S., & Marshall, J. (2008). Recent advances in the treatment of age-related macular degeneration. *British Journal of General Practice, 58*, 309–310.

Wormald, R., Evans, J., Smeeth, L., Henshaw K. (2004). *Photodynamic therapy for neovascular age-related macular degeneration (Cochrane review)*. In: The Cochrane Library, Issue 2.

References

Allen, D., & Vasavada, A. (2006). Cataract and surgery for cataract. *BMJ (Clinical research ed.), 333*, 128–132.

AREDS2 Research Group. Lutein/zeaxanthin and omega-3 fatty acids for age-related macular degeneration. The Age-Related Eye Disease Study 2 (AREDS2) Controlled Randomized Clinical Trial. *JAMA*, published online May 5, 2013

Au Jefferies, J., Perera, R., & Evert, H. (2011). Acute Infective conjunctivitis in primary care: Who needs antibiotics? Individual patient data meta-analysis. *British Journal of General Practice, 61*(590), 542–548.

Azari, A. A., & Arabi, A. (2020). *Conjunctivitis: A systematic review. Journal of Ophthalmic & Vision Research, 15*(3), 372–395.

Everitt, H. A., Little, P. S., & Smith, P. W. (2006). A randomised controlled trial of management strategies for acute infective conjunctivitis in general practice. *BMJ (Clinical research ed.), 333*, 321–324.

Kanski, J. J. (1989). *Clinical ophthalmology* (2nd ed.). London: Butterworths.

Kelly, S. P., Thornton, J., Lyratzopoulos, G., Edwards, R., & Mitchell, P. (2004). Smoking and blindness. *BMJ (Clinical research ed.), 328*, 537–538.

Kirwan, J. F., Nightingale, J. A., Bunce, C., & Wormald, R. (2002). β Blockers for glaucoma and excess risk of airways obstruction: Population based cohort study. *BMJ (Clinical research ed.), 325*, 1396–1397.

Luchs, J. (2008). Efficacy of topical azithromycin ophthalmic solution 1% in the treatment of posterior blepharitis. *Advances in Therapy, 25*(9), 858.

Opstelten, W., & Zaal, M. J. (2005). Managing ophthalmic herpes zoster in primary care. *BMJ (Clinical research ed.), 331*, 147–151.

Public Health Agency. (2017). *Guidelines on the infection control in schools and other childcare settings*. Retrieved from https://www.gov.uk/government/publications/health-protection-in-schools-and-other-childcare-facilities.

Rietveld, R. P., van Weert, H. C., ter Riet, G., & Bindels, P. J. (2003). Diagnostic impact of signs and symptoms in acute infectious conjunctivitis: Systematic literature search. *BMJ (Clinical research ed.), 327*, 789.

Royal College of Ophthalmologists (2024). *Age Related Macular Degeneration Services: Recommendations*. Retrieved from https://www.rcophth.ac.uk/wp-content/uploads/2021/08/Commissioning-Guidance-AMD-Services-Recommendations.pdf

Royal College of Ophthalmologists. (2022). *Guidelines on retinal vein occlusion*. Retrieved from https://www.rcophth.ac.uk/resources-listing/retinal-vein-occlusion-rvo-guidelines/.

Royal National Institute for the Blind. (2002). *Progress in sight: National standards of social care for visually impaired adults*. Retrieved from www.rnib.org.uk. Search for 'Social services'.

Sheikh, A., & Hurwitz, B. (2005). Topical antibiotics for bacterial conjunctivitis: Cochrane systematic review and meta-analysis update. *British Journal of General Practice, 55*, 962–964.

Sung, J., Wang, M. T. M., Lee, S. H., Cheung, I. M. Y., Ismail, S., Sherwin, T., & Craig, J. P. (2018). Randomized double-masked trial of eyelid cleansing treatments for blepharitis. *The Ocular Surface, 16*(1), 77–83.

Tiraset, N., Poonyathalang, A., Padungkiatsagul, T., Deeyai, M., Vichitkunakorn, P., & Vanikieti, K. (2021). Comparison of visual acuity measurement using three methods: Standard ETDRS chart, near chart and a smartphone-Based eye chart application. *Clinical Ophthalmology (Auckland, N.Z.), 15*, 859–869.

Weaver, C. S., & Terrell, K. M. (2003). Do ophthalmic nonsteroidal anti-inflammatory drugs reduce the pain associated with simple corneal abrasion without delaying healing? *Annals of Emergency Medicine, 41*, 134–140.

Wormald, R. (2003). Treatment of raised intraocular pressure and prevention of glaucoma. *BMJ (Clinical research ed.), 326*, 723–724.

Yam, J. C., Zhang, X. J., Zhang, Y., Wang, Y. M., Tang, S. M., Li, F. F., Kam, K. W., Ko, S. T., Yip, B. H. K., Young, A. L., Tham, C. C., Chen, L. J., & Pang, C. P. (2022). Three-year clinical trial of Low-Concentration Atropine for Myopia Progression (LAMP) Study: Continued versus washout: Phase 3 report. *Ophthalmology, 129*, 308–321.

20

Skin Problems

Anchal Agarwal Goyal, Helen Dilworth, Kieran Dinwoodie & Rakhee Choukhany Gupta

CHAPTER CONTENTS

Atopic Eczema

GUIDELINES

NICE (National Institute for Health and Care Excellence). (2018). Retrieved from https://cks.nice.org.uk/topics/dermatitis-contact. PCDS (Primary Care Dermatology Society). (n.d.). Retrieved from https://www.pcds.org.uk/clinical-guidance/eczema-contact-allergic-dermatitis-including-latex-and-rubber-allergy.

Background

- Atopic eczema is a chronic, relapsing, itchy skin condition. *If it's not itchy, it's not eczema.*
- There is a strong overlap with atopic family history; conditions such as asthma, rhinitis, and hay fever.
- It occurs in genetically susceptible individuals when they are exposed to environmental irritants or allergens.
- It may be exacerbated but not caused by trigger factors such as stress or hormonal changes.
- Environmental factors have an important role, particularly exposure to pets, house dust mites, and pollen.
- It usually has episodic flares and remissions.
- It usually improves in adult life.
- About 80% of cases occur before the age of 5 years.
- The age affects the distribution:
  - *Infancy.* It primarily involves the face, the scalp, and the extensor surfaces of the limbs.
  - *Children.* Localisation to the flexures of the limbs is more likely.
  - *Adults:* flexural involvement. Eczema on the hands can be the primary manifestation.

Complications

Infection

- Superficial fungal infections are also more common.
- Bacterial infection with *Staphylococcus aureus* may present as typical impetigo or worsening of eczema, including increased redness, oozing, and crusting.
- Herpes simplex infection: This presents with grouped vesicles and punched-out erosions. **Eczema herpeticum is a dermatologic emergency.**

Psychological

- Causes considerable distress. Consider the Dermatology Quality of Life (DLQI) score.
- Preschool children: increased fearfulness and dependence on parents
- School children: time off school, impaired performance, teasing and bullying
- Sleep disturbance

Erythroderma

- Usually occurs in people with worsening or unstable eczema

General Advice

- It is not possible to fully counsel a patient on eczema management in a 10-minute consultation. Also, patients only remember a small amount of what we tell them. Instead give the basics and print off a patient information leaflet or signpost to resources such as the National Eczema Society, which also has a helpline at 0800 448 0818.
- Emollients are the cornerstone of management.
- Reassure patients that topical steroids are safe and effective during flares with ointments being preferable to creams.
- Avoid irritants such as soaps and fragrances and instead use emollients for washing.
- In children, reassure the parents that eczema often improves with time, and dietary modification is usually not required unless the child has a known allergy and is on an exclusion diet.
- In adults, explain that eczema is a chronic illness characterised by flares that can usually be controlled with appropriate treatment.
- Avoid scratching (keep nails short; use baby scratch mitts).
- Avoid trigger factors e.g., synthetic clothing, soap, detergents, animals, and heat.
- Bathe or shower daily for no longer than 10 minutes; then pat dry and apply emollient.
- Bath emollients are ineffective and not recommended.

General Advice for Bottle-Fed and Breastfed Infants

- The mothers of breastfed infants in whom allergy is suspected to be the cause of moderate or severe eczema may require referral for dietary advice.
- A 6- to 8-week trial of hydrolysed protein formula milk or amino acid formula milk may be tried in bottle-fed infants younger than 6 months of age in whom eczema is not controlled by emollients or mild topical steroids.
- If the infant responds well to a change in formula milk, they will require referral to a dietician.
- If there is no response, then the infant should have cow's milk–based formula restarted with monitoring of eczema.

Emollients

- The best emollient is often the one the patient likes and uses regularly.
- Avoid soap and use soap substitutes such as emollients instead.
- Emollients are the mainstay of treatment for patients with eczema.
- Most emollients are plain, but some contain active ingredients. These are generally best avoided. Active ingredients include urea (Balneum plus and Eucerin intensive) and lanolin (E45 and Oilatum bath additive).

- Do not prescribe aqueous cream because it can cause skin reactions.
- Ointments are usually poorly tolerated compared with creams, which affects patient compliance with ointments.
- Application of an emollient every 2 to 3 hours should be considered normal. Patients often underestimate the amount they should use.
- Prescribe emollients in large quantities such as 500 g/week for an adult or 250 g/week for a child.
- It may be more convenient to use better tolerated products (creams and lotions) during the day and use ointments at night.
- It is particularly important to use emollients after bathing (within 3 minutes).
- Apply by smoothing them into the skin along the line of hair growth.

Topical Steroids

- Steroids are safe and effective when used correctly.
- They are available in different strengths.
- If used incorrectly, side effects include skin thinning, telangiectasia, stretch marks, easy bruising, and hypertrichosis.
- They should be used cautiously on eyelid skin because excessive use can cause glaucoma.
- Fingertip units guide the amount of steroid to be applied to a body site:
  - One hand: 1 fingertip unit
  - One arm: 3 fingertip units
  - One foot: 3 fingertip units
  - One leg: 6 fingertip units
  - Face and neck: 2.5 fingertip units
  - Trunk (front and back): 14 fingertip units
  - Entire body: about 40 fingertip units
- Table 20.1 includes a list of commonly prescribed topical steroids.

Treatment of Mild and Moderate Flares

- Prescribe a generous amount of emollient and advise frequent and liberal use. Make sure enough is prescribed (i.e., 500 g/week) and advise the patient to keep using it regularly when the flare is cleared.
- Prescribe a moderately potent topical steroid for inflamed areas (e.g., betamethasone valerate 0.025%, clobetasone butyrate). Continue treatment for 48 hours after the flare has settled. Steroids should be applied once a day but can be increased to twice a day.
- For delicate areas such as the face and flexures, start with a mild-potency topical steroid and increase to a moderately potent corticosteroid if needed.
- If there are areas of infected skin, treat them with a topical antibiotic. These should not be used for a longer than 1 week because of the risk of antibiotic resistance.
- Consider maintenance topical steroids to control areas of skin prone to frequent flares. Consider one of the following maintenance regimens:
  - *A step-down approach:* prescribing the lowest potency and amount of topical steroid to control the condition

TABLE 20.1 Basal Cell Carcinoma Subtypes

Subtype	Presentation	Differential Diagnosis	Management
Superficial	Thin plaques with a fine border, telangiectasia; often bleeds on minimal excoriation	Fungal infection: usually very itchy and does not bleed Bowen disease: scaly patch Eczema: especially if multiple; usually there is a history of eczema and good response to topical steroids	Cryotherapy Topical imiquimod or Aldara Refer to dermatology
Nodular	Pearly appearance; nodule or papule with telangiectasia	Dermatofibroma(firm, pinch sign positive)	Usually surgical Refer to dermatology If surgery is not an option, then radiotherapy or hedgehog inhibitors are considered
Ulcerated	Crust-covered ulcer with a rolled border; telangiectasia	Squamous cell carcinoma; primary chancre of syphilis (history would help)	Usually surgical Refer to dermatology If surgery is not an option, then radiotherapy or hedgehog inhibitors are considered
Pigmented	Pigmented, well-defined nodules; can be ulcerated	Seborrhoeic keratosis: typical stuck-on warty appearance Malignant melanoma: usually history of preexisting mole	Surgical; refer to dermatology
Morphoeic	Appears as sclerosed yellowish ill-defined plaques; more aggressive	Scar tissue Scleroderma: difficult to differentiate, and sometimes diagnostic biopsy is the only option	Surgical; most require Mohs surgery, which is highly specialised

- *Intermittent treatment:* weekend therapy on Saturdays and Sundays only (This is probably the preferred option based on the evidence of risks vs benefits.)
- Topical calcineurin inhibitors (tacrolimus and pimecrolimus) are a second-line option. However, they should only be prescribed by a specialist (including general practitioners with a specialist interest in dermatology). They do have evidence similar to that of moderately potent steroids. They do not cause skin atrophy. However, long-term side effects are unknown, and there is a theoretical long-term risk of malignancy.
- If there is severe itch, consider prescribing a 1-month trial of a nonsedating antihistamine.

Treatment of Severe Flares

- Prescribe a generous amount of emollient and advise frequent and liberal use.
- Prescribe a potent topical steroid (e.g., betamethasone valerate 0.1%). Aim for a maximum of 5 days of use. Again, steroids should be prescribed once a day and only increased to twice daily if skin does not improve.
- For delicate areas such as the face and flexures, use a moderately potent topical steroid (e.g., betamethasone valerate 0.025%, clobetasone butyrate 0.05%). Aim for a maximum of 5 days of use.
- If itching is severe and affecting sleep, prescribe a sedating antihistamine (e.g. chlorphenamine) for adults and children aged 6 months and older.
- If there is severe, extensive eczema causing psychological distress, consider a short course of oral corticosteroids (30 mg of prednisolone for 5-7 days then wean down over next 6 weeks by 5 mg per week), but the patient needs to use regular emollients with this to avoid a flare on cessation of steroids.
- If there are signs of infection, consider an oral antibiotic.
- Consider maintenance steroid therapy as per treatment of moderate flares.
- *Refer:*
  - Admit to hospital if the patient has eczema herpeticum or erythrodermic eczema.
  - Refer for routine dermatology appointment if:
    The diagnosis has become uncertain.
    Current management has not controlled eczema satisfactorily (person having one or two flares a month) or the person is reacting adversely to many emollients.
    Facial eczema has not responded to appropriate treatment.
    Contact allergic dermatitis is suspected.
    There is recurrent secondary infection.
    Eczema is associated with significant social or psychological problems; DLQI is helpful to assess.
  - Refer people in whom food allergy is suspected to either immunology or paediatrics (children younger than 6 months who have widespread eczema that has not responded to emollients or mild topical steroids).

RESOURCE

National Eczema Society. Helpline: 0800 448 0818. Available at http://www.eczema.org.

Contact Dermatitis

GUIDELINES

NICE (National Institute for Health and Care Excellence). (2018). Retrieved from https://cks.nice.org.uk/topics/dermatitis-contact.
    PCDS (Primary Care Dermatology Society). (n.d.). *Eczema: Contact allergic dermatitis (including latex and rubber allergy).* Retrieved from https://www.pcds.org.uk/clinical-guidance/eczema-contact-allergic-dermatitis-including-latex-and-rubber-allergy.

Background

- Contact dermatitis is an inflammatory skin reaction that occurs in response to an external agent acting as an irritant or allergen.
- Irritant contact dermatitis accounts for 80% of all contact dermatitis cases with allergic contact dermatitis accounting for the remaining 20%.
- Atopic eczema is strongly associated with irritant contact dermatitis.
- The hands and face being affected in preference to other body parts helps to distinguish contact dermatitis from other forms of dermatitis.
- Irritant contact dermatitis often includes burning, itching, painful, dry, fissured skin with less pronounced borders.
- Irritant contact dermatitis is an inflammatory response that occurs after damage to the skin, usually by chemicals.
- Allergic contact dermatitis is a type IV delayed hypersensitivity reaction. The most common substances are poison ivy, nickel, and fragrances.
- Allergic contact dermatitis often includes itching, vesicles, and distinct borders.
- In practice, irritant contact dermatitis and allergic contact dermatitis often coexist.
- Pompholyx eczema is a specific type of hand and foot eczema characterised by vesicles. It is thought to be multifactorial and related to sweating because flares occur in hot weather or humid conditions. However, there is a strong association with irritant and allergic contact dermatitis.
- Physical conditions such as heat, cold, repeated frictional exposure, and low humidity can also increase the likelihood and severity of contact dermatitis.
- Common irritants include:
  - Water
  - Detergents and soaps

- Solvents and abrasives
- Machining oils
- Acids and alkalis including cements
- Powders, dusts, and soils
- Common allergens include:
  - Cosmetics, particularly fragrances, and nail varnish
  - Metals such as nickel and cobalt in jewellery
  - Topical medications (including rare allergy to topical corticosteroids)
  - Rubber additives
  - Textiles, particularly from dyes and formaldehyde resins
  - Plants: composite group (chrysanthemum and sunflowers), daffodils, tulips, and primula are the most common
- Some occupations are particularly associated with contact dermatitis; these include workers who do 'wet work' with their hands. Common occupations include healthcare workers, beauticians, hairdressers, cooks, and cleaners plus those who work with chemicals.

Diagnostic Investigations

- A subgroup of people with contact dermatitis will need further investigations to identify the causative stimuli and to obtain treatments not available in primary care.
- The gold standard investigation is patch testing. This needs expert knowledge because interpretation is complex.

Differential Diagnosis

- Atopic dermatitis
- Dyshidrotic eczema
- Inverse psoriasis
- Latex allergy
- Palmoplantar psoriasis
- Scabies
- Tinea

Management

- Avoidance of the trigger is the most important thing, so try to identify the stimulus with a full occupational and recreational history.
- There should be frequent and liberal use of emollient.
- A soap substitute should be used instead of normal soap.
- Gloves should be used for all house and occupational work. Patients can use cotton, vinyl, or rubber gloves. Vinyl or rubber gloves should be used for wet work.
- Treat patients with localised acute dermatitis with a topical steroid appropriate to the severity and location of the dermatitis. (More information is available in the atopic eczema section.) It is worth remembering that affected skin on the hands and feet may need a potent or very potent topical steroid (e.g., Betnovate or Dermovate).

- Consider short-term use of a systemic corticosteroid if there is:
  - Significant impairment of function (e.g., eczema in the hands)
  - Extensive acute dermatitis (>20% of the body affected)
- Evidence suggests that antihistamines are not helpful in this condition. However, in practice, they are commonly prescribed.
- *Refer:*
  - Chronic, recurring dermatitis despite appropriate avoidance measures and appropriate strength corticosteroid treatment
  - Suspicion of contact dermatitis but no clear history of exposure
  - Suspicion of occupational contact dermatitis that does not respond to corticosteroid therapy

Do not request skin prick tests for allergic contact dermatitis because this is for type 1 hypersensitivity. Allergic contact dermatitis is type 4, so it requires patch testing.

Seborrhoeic Dermatitis

GUIDELINES

National Institute for Health and Care Excellence. (2022). Retrieved from https://cks.nice.org.uk/topics/seborrhoeic-dermatitis.
   Primary Care Dermatology Society. (n.d.). Retrieved from https://www.pcds.org.uk/clinical-guidance/seborrhoeic-eczema.

Background

- Seborrhoeic dermatitis is a common inflammation of the skin occurring in areas rich in sebaceous glands (scalp, nasolabial folds, ears, eyebrows, and chest).
- It commonly occurs in infants younger than 3 months of age as cradle cap and in adults.
- In infants, it usually gets better over a few weeks with only some cases persisting past 8 to 9 months. In adults, it is more likely to be a chronic condition which is likely to recur after treatment.
- It can vary from mild dandruff to dense adherent scale.
- The cause of seborrhoeic dermatitis is unknown, but it is thought to be associated with the presence of *Malassezia* yeasts.
- It may be more common and in chronic cases more severe in the winter months.
- It has a greater prevalence in immunocompromised people than in health adults. It has been established as a possible marker for early human immunodeficiency virus (HIV) infection, and this should be considered, particularly when there is severe disease.

Management

Infants

- Parents should be reassured that this is not a serious condition, does not bother the baby, and spontaneously resolves over 6 to 12 months.
- Advise parents to regularly wash the scalp with a baby shampoo and then use a gentle brush to loosen scales.
- Softening the scales with baby oil first can help remove the scales, and if they are particularly thick, soaking them overnight and in olive oil and then washing off in the morning can help.
- If these simple measures are not effective, prescribe a topical imidazole cream (clotrimazole or miconazole). Treat until symptoms resolve but ideally not for more than 4 weeks.

Seborrhoeic Dermatitis in the Scalp and Beard

- Reassure the person that seborrhoeic dermatitis is not caused by a lack of cleanliness or excessive dryness of the skin and is not transferable.
- Explain that treatment cannot cure seborrhoeic dermatitis but can control it. Symptoms often recur after treatment is stopped.
- Remove thick crusts or scales on the scalp before using an antifungal shampoo. This can be done by applying warm olive oil to the scalp for several hours and then washing with a coal tar shampoo.
- Prescribe ketoconazole 2% shampoo for adolescents and adults. (Selenium sulphide shampoo is an alternative.) Leave the shampoo on the affected area for 5 to 10 minutes before washing off. Shampoos should be used twice a week for at least 1 month. When symptoms are under control, their use can then be reduced to once a week. Shampoos can also be applied to the beard area.
- Treat flexural areas as intertrigo with use of combination topical therapy such as Trimovate.
- If the patient has severe itching of the scalp, consider co prescribing 4 weeks of treatment with a potent topical steroid scalp application (e.g., Betamousse or Elocon Scalp). These are not appropriate for the beard area because they may cause thinning of skin on the face.
- Topical steroids are not appropriate for long-term use.
- Alternatives for resistant symptoms include metronidazole gel and benzoyl peroxide (BPO).

Seborrhoeic Dermatitis of the Face and Body

- Prescribe ketoconazole 2% cream twice daily for 4 weeks. (Clotrimazole or miconazole can also be used.)
- Consider adding a mildly potent topical corticosteroid (e.g., hydrocortisone 1%) to help settle inflammation. They should only be used short term (1–2 weeks).
- Ketoconazole shampoo can also be used as a body wash.

Severe or Recalcitrant Symptoms

- Systemic itraconazole 100 mg/day for 3 weeks can be considered along with dermatology referral.
- Again, HIV testing should be considered.

Management of Ocular Symptoms

- Eyelid hygiene with cotton wool soaked in cool boiled water may be enough.
- Artificial tears should be applied liberally if eyes are dry or sore.
- Treatment with a tetracycline can be used for 6 to 8 weeks if symptoms are particularly troublesome. Erythromycin is an alternative if the patient is unable to take tetracycline.
- *Refer:* Patients responding inadequately to treatment should be referred to secondary care. In such cases, a prolonged course of low-dose isotretinoin (off-label use) may be considered.

Acne Vulgaris

Background

- Acne vulgaris is one of the commonest skin disorders affecting the adolescent population.
- It usually starts at puberty, peaks at around 16 to 20 years of age, and tends to resolve in most people by mid 20s. In about 7% of patients, it persists into their 40s and 50s or may resolve and recur in later life.
- Acne scarring is more likely if treatment is delayed.
- There are four aetiologic factors.
  - Excessive sebum production leading to seborrhoea. It is androgen mediated.
  - Comedone (blackheads or whiteheads) formation caused by excessive proliferation of keratinocytes in intrafollicular ducts.
  - Ductal colonisation with *Propionibacterium acnes.*
  - Inflammation leading to papule, pustule, and nodule formation.
- Acne can be graded in various ways. The simplest way to grade it is as follows:
  1. Noninflammatory or comedonal acne
  2. Inflammatory acne, which is subdivided into mild, moderate, and severe acne

Presentation

- Thes are polymorphic lesions mainly on the face (99%), back (60%), and chest (15%).
- Seborrhoea along with scarring and postinflammatory erythema or pigment changes are common features.
- These may all contribute to significant physical and psychosocial impact.
- It has usually been present for months. It tends to be worse in autumn and winter because of a lack of sunlight.
- Mild inflammatory acne usually presents with inflamed comedones (open or closed), papules, and pustules.
- Moderate inflammatory acne usually presents with inflamed papules and pustules.

- Severe inflammatory acne usually presents with nodules and cysts. These can be painful. Acne scarring can cause psychological distress.
  Some special subtypes of acne are:
- *Acne conglobata.* This is rare and characterised by multiple and extensive inflammatory papules, tender nodules, and abscesses, which commonly coalesce to form malodorous draining sinus tracts, usually presents in the second to third decade of life.
- *Acne fulminans.* Typically seen in teenage boys. It has an acute presentation with cystic ulcerating acne. It is commonly associated with systemic illness such as myalgia or arthralgia.
- *Drug- or chemical-induced acne.* This usually presents in atypical sites and in the wrong age group. Common triggers are systemic steroids, anticonvulsants, isoniazid and adrenocorticotropic hormone, chlorinated hydrocarbons (in insecticides, fungicides, and so on), and cosmetics.
- *Prepubertal acne.* Descriptive terms used for acne in pre-adolescent children are generally based on age and include *neonatal, infantile, midchildhood,* and *prepubertal* or pre-adolescent acne.

Diagnosis

- The diagnosis is clinical and does not usually require any investigations.
- The differential diagnosis includes:
  - *Perioral dermatitis:* perioral noncomedonal erythematous papules; tends to worsen with topical steroids but responds to oral tetracycline.
  - *Seborrhoeic eczema:* dry, scaly, erythematous, itchy skin on the scalp and upper trunk.
  - *Rosacea:* noncomedonal erythema or telangiectasia with flushing. It is seen in older people, and truncal involvement is rare. It may be associated with rhinophyma.

Management

- Irrespective of treatment, the following should be discussed with all patients:
  a. Acne can be chronic and take a long time to respond to treatment.
  b. No response to treatment may be seen in the first 6 to 8 weeks.
  c. Continuing treatment for at least 6 to 8 months if responding to treatment is important.
  d. Stress-induced and premenstrual flares may be seen, and sunlight usually causes a temporary improvement.
- Treatment should be based on the severity of acne and the aetiology or pathogenesis.

Topical Treatment

- Topical treatment is indicated on it is own in mild inflammatory acne, in conjunction with oral treatment in moderate acne, or as maintenance treatment after completion of oral treatment.
- The choice of treatment depends on the type of acne as follows:
  a. Comedolytic and antiinflammatory therapies:
     Benzoyl peroxide 2.5% and 5%
     Azelaic acid 20% cream (Gollnick & Layton, 2008)
     Topical retinoids (e.g., adapalene, all-trans retinoic acid, isotretinoin)
  b. Topical antibiotics: clindamycin, erythromycin
  c. Combinations therapies: Duac or Treclin gel, which include a comedolytic therapy and antibiotic
  d. Epiduo gel contains adapalene and BPO
  e. Topical dapsone is also available for treatment of acne

Systemic therapy

- Oral antibiotics should be considered in acne not responding to topical treatment or where acne is difficult to reach (e.g., on the back). Common regimens include:
  a. Oxytetracycline 500 mg twice daily. Not used in children younger than 12 years of age. Warn patients regarding photosensitivity.
  b. Lymecycline 408 mg once daily. Side effects are the same as those of tetracycline.
  c. Doxycycline 100 mg/day or, if not tolerated, 50 mg od. Side effects include photosensitivity.
  d. Erythromycin 500 mg bd. Common side effects are gastrointestinal.
  e. Trimethoprim 200 mg three times a day has been recommended as a third-line management as an off-licence indication
  Treatment should be reviewed for efficacy and tolerability after 8 to 12 weeks.
- Combined oral contraceptive pills can be considered in females. Co-cyprindiol (Dianette) can also be considered. It is not licensed as a contraceptive in the United Kingdom but is used in moderate to severe acne in adult females. Patients should be informed about side effects such as an increased risk of venous thromboembolism.
- Spironolactone at a dose from 50 to 200 mg can be used in adult acne as antiandrogen treatment.
- Oral retinoids should not be prescribed or managed in primary care.
- *Refer:*
- Refer to a dermatologist:
  a. Severe inflammatory acne
  b. Patients with any grade of acne with scarring
  c. Patients who have failed to respond to treatment
  d. Diagnostic uncertainty
- All patients who had treatment for acne can be referred to plastic surgery for scar revision. However, they need to wait for 12 to 18 months after treatment to see if the skin remodels itself.

Acne Rosacea

GUIDELINE

Primary Care Dermatology Society. (2018). *Rosacea. Clinical guidance.* Retrieved from http://www.pcds.org.uk (search on 'rosacea').

- This is a chronic condition with a clinical appearance similar to that of acne vulgaris. However, there are marked erythema and telangiectasia. There is associated papules and pustules but no comedones (helps differentiate from acne vulgaris).
- It usually presents on face, particularly on cheeks, nose, chin, forehead, and tip of the nose and most commonly presents in those aged older than 40 years.
- It is aggravated by sunlight, hot and spicy foods, alcohol, and hormonal therapy.
- The differential diagnosis includes:
  - Acne vulgaris: usually has comedones and an earlier age of presentation
  - Seborrhoeic eczema: usually scaly, around the nasolabial areas and scalp; can be itchy; no pustules
  - Perioral dermatitis: usually in younger people and restricted to around the mouth
  - Systemic lupus erythematosus: usually differentiated by lack of papules and pustules, and patients are usually systemically unwell

Complications

- Blepharitis
- Conjunctivitis
- Keratitis
- Lymphoedema of the face
- Rhinophyma

Management

- Provide information leaflets and discuss aggravating factors.
- Encourage using sunscreen regularly.
- Treatment depends on the clinical presentation of rosacea.
- Oral antibiotics are the mainstay of treatment for papulopustular rosacea, usually oxytetracycline 250 mg bd for 2 to 3 months. If there is no response, then a further course should be prescribed, or sometimes long-term treatment may be required. Alternative regimens include doxycycline 100 mg/day, erythromycin 250 mg bd, lymecycline 408 mg od, or minocycline 100 mg/day.
- Topical treatment for erythema with 0.75% metronidazole gel or cream (Rozex or Metrogel) bd.
- Azelaic acid 20% for erythema (Gollnick and Layton, 2008).
- Topical ivermectin 1% cream for 12 weeks is indicated for papulopustular rosacea.
- Treatment of telangiectasia includes brimonidine gel (Mirvaso). Warn patients regarding hypopigmentation and the possible bleaching effect, which is temporary and settles after treatment is stopped.
- Encapsulated 5% BPO (EPSOLAY) has been approved by the US Food and Drug Administration (FDA) for the treatment of patients with inflammatory rosacea (not available in the United Kingdom).
- Laser treatment is recommended for persistent facial erythema with telangiectasia.
- Low-dose isotretinoin is recommended for resistant rosacea.
- Low-dose propranolol has been recommended for transient erythema (flushing).
- Oxymetazoline cream 1% (RHOFADE) as an alpha receptor agonist is helpful in reducing persistent facial rosacea (not available in the United Kingdom).

Psoriasis

GUIDELINE

NICE (National Institute of Health and Care Excellence). (2022). *CKS psoriasis.* https://cks.nice.org.uk/topics/psoriasis/

- Psoriasis is a chronic inflammatory multisystem disease with predominantly skin and joint manifestations. It is characterised by scaly skin lesions, which can be in the form of patches, papules, or plaques. Although it is usually chronic, the guttate form typically resolves within 3 to 4 months of onset (Ashton & Leppard, 2009).
- It affects 2% of the world's population.
- The inheritance is likely controlled by several genes, which is why the familial occurrences are variable. When one parent has psoriasis, 8% of offspring develop psoriasis, and when both parents are affected, 41% of offspring get psoriasis. Human leukocyte antigen (HLA) types commonly linked with psoriasis are HLA- B13, B17, Bw57, and Cw6. Also, CD8+T cells are also known to be involved (Wolff & Johnson, 2009).
- It can be precipitated by hormonal changes, infections (e.g., streptococcal sore throat causing guttate psoriasis), trauma, drugs (lithium, glucocorticoids, antimalarial drugs, interferon, beta-blockers), alcohol, and emotional stress (Wolff & Johnson, 2009).
- It commonly starts between the ages of 15 and 25 years but can occur at any age. The diagnosis is usually clinical.
- Males and females are equally affected.
- Clinical presentations: although there can be variations in distribution, the lesions generally appear red in colour, have clearly defined borders, and have an easily shedable silvery scale. Scratching and removing scales reveal minute blood droplets (Auspitz sign).

Different types of psoriasis:
- Chronic plaque psoriasis
- Guttate psoriasis
- Scalp psoriasis
- Nail psoriasis
- Erythrodermic psoriasis
- Pustular psoriasis and palmoplantar psoriasis
- Inverse psoriasis and psoriasis vulgaris
- Generalised acute pustular psoriasis (von Zumbusch)

Psoriasis is associated with several other conditions:
- Psoriatic arthritis
- Traditional cardiovascular risk factors (hypertension, hyperlipidaemia, diabetes)
- Inflammatory bowel disease
- Obesity
- Metabolic syndrome

Management

General points to consider are:
- Be aware of the possibility of joint involvement and refer to a rheumatologist if psoriatic arthropathy is affected.
- Psoriasis can be associated with mood disturbance; therefore, this should be enquired about at review.
- Emollients are the main stay of treatment.
- Psoriasis is often thought of as a nonitchy skin condition. However, patients often do find itch a problem, and antihistamines can help.
- All patients with psoriasis should have yearly follow-up to address cardiovascular risk factors. Despite being associated with an increased risk of cardiovascular disease, it is not included in most cardiovascular risk assessment tools.
- Compliance with treatment is improved by good patient understanding of the condition. Signposting to online web resources and patient information leaflets should be considered.
- Carrying out a PASI (Psoriasis Area and Severity Index) score and DLQI (Dermatology Life Quality index) at the start of treatment and on follow-up helps with more objective evidence of improvement and aids in the decision to refer to secondary care if no improvement is seen.

Chronic Plaque and Scalp Psoriasis (Wolff & Johnson, 2009)

- *Emollients.* Bland emollients with no active ingredients are usually recommended to avoid further skin irritation. Usually a more cream- or lotion-based preparation for daytime use and an ointment-based preparation for nighttime use are more practical and allow more compliance. Examples include Epaderm cream and ointment, Cetraben lotion, and 50:50 ointment.
- *Salicylic acid.* Useful for scalp plaques. Examples include Sebco or Cocois scalp ointment (apply at night) and Capasal shampoo (wash the scalp in the morning).
- *Vitamin D$_3$ analogues.* Calcipotriol (Dovonex), calcitriol (Silkis), tacalcitol (Curatoderm), or Capitrol + betamethasone (Dovobet, Enstillar foam) may achieve better

compliance and now have licence for use as maintenance treatment twice weekly for resistant cases. *Contraindications* include calcium metabolism disorders, severe renal or liver impairment, and patient allergic to ingredients in the preparation. Use with caution in erythrodermic or pustular patients.
- *Dithronol or anthralin cream.* Used in large plaques only. Start with lowest strength (0.1%) and gradually over 4 to 6 weeks up to the highest tolerated strength (up to 2%). Cream preparation is preferred. Leave it on for 30 to 60 minutes and then wash it off. Stop using it when the lesions are flat. It is applied 30 minutes after applying emollient. *Contraindications:* It can cause severe irritant reaction on the skin and temporary staining of skin, hair, fabrics, and bathroom tiles and fittings. Avoid smoking and contact with fire.
- *Coal tar.* Newer preparations are less messy and more practical to use than old preparations. It is available as ointments and scalp preparations in the United Kingdom. Shampoos include Capasal, Alphosyl, Polytar, and T gel, and skin preparations include Exorex and Psoriderm for trunk plaque psoriasis. Avoid using in severe cases and pustular or erythrodermic patients. *Contraindicated* in the first trimester of pregnancy, patients with skin infections or genital or rectal psoriasis, and over broken skin.

Guttate Psoriasis (Wolff & Johnson, 2009)

- Usually triggered after a streptococcal throat infection. It is worth checking antistreptolysin O titres; treat with oral antibiotics if titres are high.
- The mainstay of treatment is reassurance because this condition tends to self-resolve in 3 to 4 months. Symptomatic treatment in the form of Dovobet and emollients may help. Ultraviolet (UV) B light helps for widespread disease.

Flexural Psoriasis

- Encourage smoking and alcohol cessation, and weight loss.
- Topical treatments include cream- or lotion-based emollients and topical steroids.
- Calcitriol can be used for maintenance in frequently relapsing cases.
- Treat secondary fungal or bacterial infections.

Erythrodermic and Pustular Psoriasis

- Patients need dermatology input and treatment as inpatients. Treat with bland emollients such as 50:50 and refer to a dermatologist for same-day assessment.
- *Refer:* Most cases of psoriasis can be managed in primary care. Referral to secondary care or dermatology should be made if:
  - Unsure regarding diagnosis
  - Extensive disease

- Moderate to severe disease severity
- Not responding to topical treatments or topical treatments not tolerated
- Generalised pustular psoriasis and erythrodermic presentations (same-day referral)
- Severe impact on psychological, physical, and social well-being
- Patients may benefit from education on treatment from skin care nurses

Lichen Planus

- Lichen planus is a chronic autoimmune condition usually distributed in the flexural aspects of the wrists, ankles, and lumbar region of the back. Mouth, hair, nails, and genital areas can also be affected.
- It is characterised by the '6Ps'; purple, polygonal, planar (flat topped), pruritic papules and plaques.
- Wickham striae (white lines over lesions) are also present.
- It can be associated with hepatitis C.
- Certain drugs can cause a lichen planus–like condition, including thiazide diuretics, spironolactone, beta-blockers, and nonsteroidal antiinflammatory drugs.

Variants

- Cutaneous lichen planus (classical presentation)
- Oral lichen planus: persistent erosion and ulceration of the oral mucosa; diffuse peeling and redness of the gums
- Vulval lichen planus
- Lichen planopilaris can cause scarring alopecia
- Lichenoid drug eruption
- Bullous lichen planus

Investigations

- Diagnosis is usually clinical, but when uncertain, biopsy should be arranged to confirm
- Patch testing for oral lichen planus affecting the gums in those with amalgam fillings

Management

- Give the patient an information leaflet and inform them that 85% will improve by 18 months, but it can be a relapsing condition.
- Antipruritic management such as antihistamines or menthol cream can be used.
- Potent or superpotent topical steroids can be used until lesions improve. Lesions heal with postinflammatory hyperpigmentation, which may take months to clear up.
- For facial lesions, tacrolimus ointment or pimecrolimus cream may be an alternative to a steroid.
- For scalp lesions, offer a topical steroid scalp preparation. Start the treatment early to prevent scarring.
- Mucosal areas are difficult to manage. Inform the patient to see a dentist every 6 months to monitor for oral cancer.

- Systemic treatment in the form of oral steroids is recommended for widespread disease or severe local disease.
- Other options are Acetretin, hydroxychloroquine, and phototherapy.
- Other immunosuppressive agents such as methotrexate, azathioprine, and mycophenolate mofetil are also used under specialist supervision.
- *Refer* if:
  - There is clinical uncertainty.
  - It is refractory to treatment.
  - There is scalp, mucosal, or nail involvement.
  - There is aggressive disease or any suspicion of squamous cell carcinoma (SCC).

> **PATIENT SUPPORT ORGANISATION**
>
> UK Lichen Planus. Available at http://www.uklp.org.uk.

Infection and Infestation

Infection manifests itself in most medical specialities but is of particular importance in dermatology. This chapter is by no means a comprehensive listing; instead, it is designed to refresh knowledge and an attempt to look systematically at skin infection groupings and to remind busy general practitioners of the most common skin infections and infestations.

Viral Infections

Viral Warts and Verruca Vulgaris

- Warts are benign epithelial proliferation associated human papillomavirus (HPV). They are common and infection is transmitted by direct contact. Most clear by 2 years but they can last up to 10 years in adults.
- Diagnosis is usually clinical and can be aided by paring down the wart, which will often reveal small black dots representing coagulated capillaries.
- Malignant change is rare except in immunocompromised individuals.
  Types:
- Common wart: firm and raised, resembles cauliflower, on hands and feet
- Plane wart: round, flat topped, found on back of hands
- Filiform wart: long and slender, found on face and neck
- Palmar and plantar (verrucae): central dark dots in the middle and may be painful
- Mosaic: when warts coalesce
- The differential diagnosis includes:
  - Actinic keratosis
  - Seborrhoeic keratosis
  - Lichen planus
  - Knuckle pads
  - SCC (rare but increased on sun-exposed sites and in immunocompromised patients)
  - Palmoplantar keratoderma

Management

- Advise the patient that warts are not harmful, and most resolve spontaneously. To reduce the risk of transmission, wear a waterproof plaster when swimming and flip flops in the shower and avoid sharing shoes, socks, and towels. To avoid autoinoculation, do not scratch, bite, or suck warts.
- No medical therapy is often necessary or recommended. Only consider treatment if a wart is unsightly or painful or if the patient requests treatment for a persisting wart.
- *Salicylic acid* topical preparations of 10% to 26% applied daily after paring with occlusion if possible. Apply for 3 months. The main side effect is irritation, and they are contraindicated in areas of poor healing and the face.
- *Cryotherapy.* Keep the wart frozen for 5 to 30 seconds, repeating every 2 to 4 weeks for at least 3 months (six treatments). Advise about risks of pain, blistering, and hypopigmentation.
- A combination of salicylic acid and cryotherapy can be used.
- Children with verruca do not need to be banned from swimming but can instead wear verruca socks.
- Treatment failure is frequent, and recurrences are common.

Specific Wart Treatment Options

- *Plantar.* Paring of the skin; then salicylic acid up to 50% or cryotherapy every 2 weeks for up to 4 months. Another option for painful plantar warts is to treat with corn plasters.
- *Palmar.* Await self-resolution or use 2% to 10% salicylic acid cream or mild cryotherapy. Apply topical retinoic acid if the warts are persistent.
- *Facial wart.* Do not use salicylic acid. Gentle cryotherapy (5–10 seconds to the wart but avoid surrounding skin) is an option; repeat every 2 to 3 weeks. Make sure patients are consented for the risks associated with cryotherapy.
- *Warts in children.* Await self-resolution because children have much faster spontaneous clearing than in adults. Salicylic acid is an option. Cryotherapy is often poorly tolerated.
- *Recalcitrant warts* can be treated with oral acitretin therapy.
- Consider *referral* if:
  a. Symptomatic warts present for at least 2 years which are unresponsive to topical treatment and cryotherapy
  b. Uncertain diagnosis
  c. Immunocompromised patient
  d. Extensive mosaic warts
  e. Anogenital warts should be referred to a genitourinary medicine (GUM) clinic

Herpes Simplex

- Caused by herpes simplex virus (HSV) 1 and 2
- Acquired by direct contact
- The primary episode is prolonged and more severe. Vesicular eruption may be preceded by itching, burning, and tingling. When blisters appear, they can be very painful.
- Clinical symptoms are precipitated by local trauma, sun exposure, and general ill health.
- Diagnosis is largely clinical, but a viral swab should be obtained for confirmation during an acute episode.
- Provide patients with written information.
- Consider the option of no treatment for HSV infections that are mild and uncomplicated because episodes will self-resolve.
- See specific treatments in the sections covering HSV subtypes later.
- Advise patients to reduce the chances of transmission to others by not kissing, participating in oral sex, or sharing cups whilst they are symptomatic.
- Advise caution to contact lens wearers during an episode to reduce the chance of herpes keratoconjunctivitis.
- Admission may be required for those who:
  - Are immunocompromised
  - Are systemically unwell
  - Are unable to swallow and are at risk of dehydration
  - Who have suspected herpes keratoconjunctivitis
  - Who have suspected eczema herpeticum (see later)
- *Refer:*
  - If frequent, persistent, or severe HSV
  - If in third trimester of pregnancy with genital herpes
  - If lesions are refractory to oral treatment
  - If the diagnosis is uncertain

Herpetic Gingivostomatitis

- Presents with white vesicles on the tongue, buccal mucosa, palate, and lips
- Usually resolves by 2 weeks
- Treatment is acyclovir, 200 mg five times a day for 5 days

Herpes Labialis

- Presents as grouped vesicles on the lips and perioral skin.
- Usually resolves by 10 days.
- Advise on appropriate UV protection because sunlight is a trigger.
- Local abrasive and cosmetic treatments can precipitate the attack.
- Use topical acyclovir (available over the counter) five times a day for 5 to 10 days starting at the first sign of attack.
- If recurrent (more than five episodes per year), consider long-term acyclovir 400 mg bd at least for 1 year; then reassess.

Genital Herpes

- It may cause dysuria, mimicking features of urinary tract infection.
- Treatment is with acyclovir 200 mg five times a day for 5 days.
- Both the patient and their partner or partners need a full sexually transmitted infection (STI) screening, which may best be undertaken by the GUM clinic

Eczema Herpeticum
- This occurs in those with atopic eczema. The lesions occur on the eczematous skin and are punched-out erosions or vesicles that are often widespread. There may be systemic upset, including fever and lethargy, and there may be enlarged inguinal or axillary lymph nodes.
- Treat with systemic acyclovir; this usually requires admission for treatment with intravenous acyclovir, particularly if there is systemic upset.
- Consider giving antibiotics for superadded bacterial infection, which may occur.

Neonatal Herpes Simplex Virus
- High risk if mother has genital herpes at the time of delivery, particularly if it is a primary episode. It can range from localised to disseminated.
- Have a low threshold for seeking advice from a paediatrician.
- Disseminated HSV can be life threatening: early recognition and urgent referral are required.

Herpes Zoster or Shingles
- The infection occurs because of reactivation of the varicella zoster virus that lies dormant in the nerves after an infection with chicken pox infection or varicella vaccination.
- It often affects people with weak immunity.
- Patients older than 70 years of age (who are not immunocompromised) in the United Kingdom are now entitled to a shingles vaccine, which is expected to reduce the burden of shingles in this vulnerable group.
- The first manifestation of an attack is usually burning pain, which may be severe and can be accompanied by fever, headache, and malaise. The rash which follows the pain after 1 to 3 days is a blistering grouped vesicular eruption with a typical dermatomal distribution. If the rash crosses the midline, then consider alternative diagnoses.
- Patients are infectious until all lesions are crusted over (day 10–15 from rash onset) and should avoid contact with those who have never had chickenpox or who are immunocompromised.
- School or work need only be avoided if the rash is weeping or cannot be covered.
- Treatment is with acyclovir 800 mg five times a day for 7 days (alternatively, valaciclovir or famciclovir can be used). Ideally, this should be initiated within 72 hours of the onset of rash but consider starting it up to 1 week after onset of rash, particularly in those at high risk of complications.
- The role of oral steroids in the treatment of herpes zoster is controversial.
When to consider referral or admission:
- *Under ophthalmology* if there is ophthalmic involvement with a red eye or visual complaints. If there is ophthalmic shingles with no eye involvement, then start treatment and review in 1 week.
- *Under ear, nose, and throat* if Ramsay Hunt syndrome is present. This may present with deep ear pain or rash in the ear canal or on the auricle, and there may be associated facial droop, tinnitus, ipsilateral hearing loss, and vertigo.
- *Under medics* if the patient is immunocompromised and the rash is widespread.

Postherpetic Neuralgia
- Postherpetic neuralgia is persistent neuropathic pain or recurrence of pain more than 1 month after the onset of the rash but better considered after 3 months.
- The pain of postherpetic neuralgia can be severe and debilitating, although it is usually self-limiting, lasting around 3 to 5 weeks. It can last for months or years. It occurs in around one in five people after shingles and is more common in older adults, females, immunocompromised people, and those who have had a severe attack of shingles.
- Offer the patient an information leaflet.
- Step 1 management is paracetamol or codeine.
- Step 2 management are neuropathic analgesics, usually amitriptyline or gabapentin.
- Topical treatments, including capsaicin or lidocaine plasters, may be effective if oral medications have failed.
- Consider referral for pain management in those with refractory symptoms.

PATIENT SUPPORT ORGANISATION
Herpes Viruses Association, 41 North Road, London, N7 9DP. Helpline: 0845 123 2305. info@herpes.org.uk. Available at http://www.herpes.org.uk.

Bacterial Infection
It is worth remembering that skin infection can be either a primary disease process or a consequence of an underlying skin disease.

Staphylococci and Streptococci
Both these organisms account for some of the most common encounters, often causing significant morbidity and, potentially, death.

Impetigo
- Superficial infection of the upper layers of the skin most commonly encountered in children
- Usually highly contagious; the child is systemically well, with classic honey-coloured crusting lesions on the face or digits and readily spreadable locally; it rarely presents as bullous lesions
- Usually caused by *S. aureus* but occasionally *Streptococcus pyogenes*
- Treatment for localised lesions can be with topical mupirocin/fusidic acid. Give oral antibiotics (e.g., flucloxacillin or erythromycin) for more widespread or severe cases.

- Provide education to patients about how it is transmitted and how to prevent transmission.

Ecthyma

- The presentation is similar to impetigo, but deeper layers of skin are involved, leading to ulceration on the lower legs, buttocks, thighs, ankles, and feet. Patients tend to give a history of previous trauma such as insect bites. It is caused by *S. pyogenes*.
- Lesions are painful and tend to start with vesicles or pustules on inflamed skin, which deepens to form ulcers (≤3 cm in size) with an overlying greyish thick crust. Removal of the crust reveals a punched-out ulcer. It tends to heal slowly with scarring. Regional lymphadenopathy can be seen.
- It is more common in patients with diabetes and older adults with neglected skin. It is also more common in tropical climates.
- Complications include cellulitis, gangrene, bacteraemia, staphylococcal scalded skin syndrome, and toxic shock syndrome.
- The differential diagnosis includes:
  - *Ecthyma gangrenosum*. The appearance similar but is caused by *Pseudomonas* spp. It is associated with significant mortality.
  - *Orf or ecthyma contagiosum*. Consider this diagnosis if there is relevant history of exposure to sheep or goats.
  - *Pyoderma gangrenosum*. This tends to have a similar appearance but usually has a typical purplish appearance on the edges of the ulcer.
  - *Arterial ulcers* especially if the patient has a history of arterial disease.
  - Investigations should include blood tests to rule out neutropenia and diabetes, as well as wound swabs.

Treatment

- Treatment depends on the extent of the lesions. If they are localised, antibacterial washes such as Hibiscrub and topical mupirocin/fusidic acid can be used.
- More extensive infections require oral flucloxacillin or phenoxymethylpenicillin if group A streptococcus has been isolated.
- Treatment may be required for several weeks. If there are clinical concerns or doubt about diagnosis or management, then refer to secondary care because surgical debridement may be necessary for extensive infection.

Folliculitis

- Folliculitis presents with multiple small papules or pustules on an erythematous base with or without a hair follicle visible in the centre. Sometimes it can present with deeper lesions as painful nodules that may result in scarring and permanent hair loss. It is usually caused by *S. aureus* (and very occasionally caused by gram-negative organisms).
  Common subtypes based on distribution are:
- Beard: folliculitis barbae

- Lower legs: pseudofolliculitis (secondary to hair removal or shaving)
- Trunk or buttocks: *Malassezia* or *Pseudomonas* folliculitis
- Scalp: folliculitis decalvans
- Eosinophilic folliculitis
  Treatment
- Avoid or treat the causative factor.
- Antibacterial washes such as chlorhexidine or Hibiscrub can be used.
- A topical or oral antistaphylococcal antibiotic can be used depending on disease extent. It may require 4 to 6 weeks of treatment.
- If *Malassezia* infestation is present, then consider ketoconazole cream or shampoo regularly until clear and then once or twice weekly for maintenance.
  Refer if:
- If there is diagnostic doubt.
- There is poor response to treatment because these patients can be considered for isotretinoin or phototherapy.

Furuncles, Carbuncles, and Abscesses

- A furuncle or a boil is a deeper infection of the hair follicle with subcutaneous tissue involvement leading to abscess formation. A carbuncle forms when multiple inflamed hair follicles coalesce to form a single lump which discharges pus.
- Treatment is with an oral antistaphylococcal antibiotic (e.g., flucloxacillin) if infection is caught early, but it may require surgical incision and drainage.

Erysipelas

- Erysipelas is the name given to a more superficial form of cellulitis, and it is usually seen after a breach in the skin. Common sites are the face and legs, and it can present bilaterally.
- It is caused by *Streptococcus* group A (pyogenes) and occasionally by *Staphylococcus* spp. Other pathogens may be causative in immunocompromised patients.
- Patients present with well-demarcated erythema and oedema which is hot and tender to touch.
- The patient is usually systemically well unless septic.
- Treatment is with oral flucloxacillin 500 mg to 1g qds (Four times a day) or clarithromycin 500 mg bd (Twice daily). If there is facial involvement, consider co-amoxiclav. Treatment may need to be prolonged for 10 to 14 days.
- Refer if the patient is systemically unwell or not responding to oral treatment.

Cellulitis

- Cellulitis is commonly encountered in primary care. It is usually caused by *S. aureus* but can also be caused by *S. pyogenes* and, uncommonly, *Haemophilus influenzae*.
- Cellulitis involves the deep dermis, and the patient is systemically unwell. The area will be red, hot, painful, and generally swollen with an ill-defined border and may have an obvious point of entry for infection.
- Risk factors include:

- Gravitational eczema
- Leg ulcers
- Tinea infection
- Trauma
- Lymphoedema
- High body mass index
- Diabetes
- Immunocompromised
- It is highly unusual to encounter bilateral lower leg cellulitis, often chronic venous stasis with red legs will be wrongly labelled as bilateral cellulitis, leading to incorrect treatment.
- The differential diagnosis includes:
  - *Chronic venous insufficiency.* Usually bilateral. No associated tenderness or heat. The patient is systemically well. This follows a more chronic history.
  - *Allergic contact dermatitis.* Usually there is a history of contact with an allergen. It presents acutely with associated blisters and itching.

Treatment

- If infection is limited, treatment is with oral flucloxacillin. Otherwise, the patient will require intravenous flucloxacillin or penicillin with the addition of clindamycin if severe.
- Always treat underlying causes such as tinea or ulcers.
- Weight management is important.
- Advise rest, elevation, and analgesia.
- Mark the area and observe for tracking.
- *Refer* if the patient is systemically unwell or not responding to oral treatment.

Recurrent Cellulitis
- Cellulitis is recurrent if the patient has two or more episodes of cellulitis per year.
- Treatment is with prophylactic antibiotics such as penicillin V 250 mg bd for 1 year and then 250 mg od (once daily). For penicillin-allergic patients, the treatment is with clarithromycin 250 mg od or erythromycin 250 mg bd.
- Stop treatment after 2 years. If symptoms recur after 2 years, restart prophylaxis and continue long term.

Necrotising Fasciitis

- This is a rare but an important surgical emergency and must be referred for immediate management. It is often a polymicrobial infection involving the deep planes of the skin, including fascia. Although often numerous bacteria may be involved, including anaerobes, *S. pyogenes* is the most rapid, often being termed 'flesh eating', and the patient is moribund within a couple of hours.
- Presentation
  - Level of pain is out of proportion to the clinical presentation
  - Greyish violaceous area with erythema
  - Crepitus
  - Blisters that become necrotic
  - Systemically unwell

- Treatment involves pattern recognition in a septic, deteriorating patient with emergency onward referral for debridement, intensive support, and antibiotics. It requires multidisciplinary input.

Erythrasma

- Erythrasma presents with macerated areas that are often patchy and involve either the interdigital or intertriginous areas, or they may also appear as reddish-brown plaques in the axillary areas. It is caused by *Corynebacterium minutissimum.*
- Treatment is either topical clindamycin or topical erythromycin.

Gram-Negative Bacilli

- Most commonly *Pseudomonas* spp., usually *P. aeruginosa.* Infection generally develops on skin which is already damaged, for example, in severe tinea infection. The skin becomes macerated and develops a foul smell and may appear with a greenish tinge because of pigment production from the bacteria.
- Treatment is aimed at treating the underlying skin condition.

Lyme Disease

- Lyme disease is caused by the spirochaete organism *Borrelia*, transmitted by the *Ixodes* tick. The type of *Borrelia* depends on which continent the tick is encountered.
- Ticks removed before 24 hours of attachment are unlikely to be problematic; however, cutaneous lesions developing within 1 month of tick removal should be considered for evaluation of early Lyme disease.
- A history of being in woodland areas and of tick bites is useful. It is usually seen in the spring and summer.
- The most common presentation is that of erythema chronicum migrans, a distinctive rash which starts as an erythematous papule, expanding to an annular erythema with central clearing. It can be seen between 1 to 33 days after exposure and fades over 3 to 4 weeks, but only 70% to 80% of patients develop the typical rash.
- There may be a mild flulike illness, and about two-thirds of untreated patients develop symptoms, including arthritis, neuroborreliosis, Bell's palsy or other cranial nerve involvement and, cardiac borreliosis, and peri- or myocarditis leading to conduction defects.
- Long-term sequelae include chronic arthritis and neurologic problems.
- Advise patients travelling to at risk areas to:
  a. Wear white (for easy spotting of ticks) long-sleeved clothes, long trousers tucked into socks, and long boots.
  b. Use pesticides or repellents.
  c. Check the whole body for ticks closely when home and repeat this the following day.
  d. If a tick is seen, use tweezers and firmly remove it in whole.
  e. Disinfect the skin.

- The presence of the typical rash merits immediate treatment.
- Serology for antibodies to *B. burgdorferi*. However, these may be negative in the first few weeks after infection.
- Treatment is with doxycycline (100 mg bd or tds) three times a day, amoxicillin, or erythromycin (less effective) for 2 to 3 weeks.

Fungal Infections

Tinea

- Tinea is characterised by an erythematous, scaling, itchy rash.
- Consider it if there is an asymmetrical rash with scale and a leading edge.
- Take skin scrapings from the advancing edge of the rash.
- False-negative results are not uncommon, and samples should be repeated with treatment given if there is strong clinical suspicion of tinea.
- For mild tinea, use topical agents, but if widespread or severe, then oral therapies are indicated.
- Terbinafine is first-line oral agent, but alternatives are imidazole preparations. If using terbinafine, then get baseline liver function tests (LFTs) before initiation and repeat them after 6 weeks of treatment.
- Advise patients not to share towels or hats and to disinfect combs, scissors, pillows, and bed covers.

Scalp Infection

- This is common in children.
- Features are hair loss and scaling.
- Take skin scrapings and hair follicles for mycology.
- Offer the patient an information leaflet.
- Topical management with terbinafine or imidazoles for 2 to 4 weeks can be considered for limited infection.
- Systemic treatment with terbinafine or imidazoles for 2 to 4 weeks should be given if infection is extensive or the rash is very inflamed.
- If a kerion is present, refer to dermatology:
  - Because of the risk of scarring, oral therapy is offered, and this is usually terbinafine, although itraconazole can also be used.
  - For children, griseofulvin is first-line treatment.
  - Also use antifungal shampoo for the first 2 weeks of therapy.
  - Treat family members with antifungal shampoo for 2 weeks.

Hands

- A white discolouration in the skin folds is often present.
- Always examine the feet, hands, and nails because spread is common.

Feet

- Interdigital skin gets broken down and is a common cause of secondary cellulitis.
- Give topical treatment unless there is coexistent nail involvement in which case systemic therapy is indicated.

- Advise the patient to wear breathable footwear to reduce the chance of recurrence.

Nails

- This presents with subungual hyperkeratosis and yellow or white discolouration of the nails.
- Offer the patient an information leaflet. Self-care is often appropriate if the patient is not bothered by the nail or is concerned about the side effects of treatment.
- For nail clippings, first cut the nail back; then remove the friable debris to be sent for mycology. This will reduce false-negative results.
- Explain that cure rates are often 60% to 80%.
- Topical treatment is only for isolated superficial infections. Preparations such as tioconazole or Loceryl can be used.
- Systemic treatment is with terbinafine 250 mg od and should be for 6 weeks for fingernails and 3 months for toenails. Alternatively, pulsed therapy of itraconazole can be used, giving 400 mg od or 200 mg BD for 1 week every month for 1 week every month. Two cycles are needed for fingernails, and four cycles are required for toenails. Get baseline LFTs before starting oral treatment.
- Inform the patient that even with successful treatment, it can take months for the toenail to grow out and look healthy again.
- In children, weight-adjusted terbinafine or griseofulvin can be used.
- If the patient has recurrent infection, then long-term twice-weekly topical antifungal (terbinafine or imidazoles) can be used.

Tinea Incognito

- This is a fungal skin infection that occurs when the condition has been misdiagnosed and inappropriately treated with steroid creams. These creams can improve the clinical appearance and itch, but the infection continues to spread.

Candidiasis

Oral

- In healthy adults, candidiasis may be the symptoms of underlying immunodeficiency, so think about risk factors for diabetes, malnutrition, cancer, and HIV.
- Review known triggers if present such as poor denture hygiene, inhaler technique, and diabetic control.
- First-line treatment is miconazole gel or nystatin, but if extensive, then offer oral fluconazole.

Skin

- Advise the patient to avoid tight-fitting clothes and keep the area as dry as possible to avoid reinfection.
- If the patient is obese, give lifestyle counselling on weight loss.
- For localised infection, use topical imidazole creams or terbinafine. If the rash is very inflamed or itchy, consider adding a topical steroid to the antifungal cream.

- Creams should be used for 7 days, and if there is no improvement, then review the diagnosis and treatment.

Pityriasis Versicolour

- This most commonly presents in children and teenagers as round or oval macules and papules that have a fine scale and may coalesce. Usually, it is asymptomatic but is occasionally mildly itchy. It typically occurs on the chest, back, and upper arms. It is caused by yeasts of the genus *Malassezia*.
- It is a self-limiting, noncontagious condition that is usually easily treated, although skin change back to normal can take months.
- Ketoconazole shampoo or selenium sulphide (contraindicated in pregnancy) shampoos can be used if extensive.
- Topical imidazoles can be applied if localised. Use for 2 weeks.
- If treatment fails, then take skin scrapings to confirm the diagnosis and consider using systemic therapy such as itraconazole or fluconazole.
  Consider referral:
a. If the diagnosis is uncertain and scrapings are negative
b. If there is extensive disease
c. If the patient is immunocompromised, pregnant, or younger than 12 years old requiring systemic therapy

Parasitic Infections

Scabies

- Scabies typically presents with widespread itching and a rash that may exhibit papules, vesicles, or nodules and linear burrows that classically affect the interdigital web spaces and flexor aspects of the wrists, elbows, groin, and axillae.
- It affects many family members in the household.
- Treat the patient and all household and sexual contacts with permethrin 5% (or malathion as alternative) immediately and after 1 week.
- Advise patients to machine wash clothes and bed linens at 50°C.
- Treat itch and concurrent bacterial infection if present.
- If crusted scabies is present, then consider an underlying immunodeficiency.
- Inform patients that itch may last up to 4 weeks after treatment.
- Consider urea or crotamiton emollients to treat ongoing itch.
- Oral ivermectin is an off-licence indication in the use of scabies that have not responded to the FDA-approved treatments.
- Contact the Health Protection Agency if there is an outbreak in an institution such as school or nursing home.
  When to consider referral:
- If the patient has crusted scabies or if the diagnosis is in doubt
- If there is ongoing active infection despite two courses of treatment

Head Lice

- Head lice are parasites that can be found on the head, eyebrows, and eyelashes.
- The infection is characterised by the presence of the louse, which is 2 to 3 mm in size, and eggs (nits) at the base of hair.
- The infection causes itch, which can lead to secondary infection on the scalp.
- It can spread easily by direct contact in less than 30 seconds.
- Affected children can still attend school.
- Treat all affected family members on the same day. Options include dimethicone, Malathion, or wet combing.
- Insecticide preparations should be used twice (repeated again at 7 days), and detection combing should be undertaken 3 days after treatment to make sure lice are eradicated.
- Permethrin cream 1% has been approved by the FDA and can be safely used in children 2 months of age and older.

Pubic Lice

- If transmitted via sexual contact, then refer to a GUM clinic for further STI screening and contact tracing. Alternatively, screen for chlamydia and other STIs, inform the patient to avoid sexual contacts until all have been treated, and undertake contact tracing for sexual contacts over the past 3 months.
- Treat with topical malathion 0.5% or permethrin 5% to be used twice 7 days apart.
- If present in a child, then, although nonsexual contact is most common, consider the possibility of sexual abuse.

Lesions and Malignancies

- There are many different types of skin lesions and malignancies. Discussing them all would be beyond the scope of this book. Some of the common skin lesions and malignancies that are seen in general practice are described here.
- Common terminologies used when describing skin lesions (Ashton & Leppard, 2009):
  - *Macule*: pigmented or nonpigmented flat lesion which is not palpable.
  - *Papule*: raised pigmented or nonpigmented lesion which is palpable and smaller than 0.5 cm in diameter.
  - *Nodule*: raised pigmented or nonpigmented lesion which is palpable and larger than 0.5 cm in diameter.
  - *Plaque*: a plateau-like elevation above the skin surface where the diameter is greater than the thickness of the lesion.

Benign Skin Lesions

Seborrhoeic Keratosis (Ashton & Leppard, 2009)

- This is the most common of the benign epithelial lesions. It is commonly seen after the age of 30 years. It can range from a few scattered lesions to hundreds in some older adult patients. They are usually asymptomatic, but they can be itchy or become inflamed.

- Lesions range from small, barely elevated papules to plaques with a warty surface and a typical 'stuck-on' appearance. They can be nonpigmented or pigmented.
- Patients usually present worried because they think they have a melanoma. They give a history of a long-standing pigmented 'mole' that has grown in size or become itchy or inflamed. A thorough examination in which multiple similar lesions are found mostly on the torso is reassuring.
- The differential diagnosis includes:
  - *Solar lentigo*: generally macular and lacks the warty appearance
  - *Actinic keratosis*: scaly, rough appearance; seen on sun-exposed areas
  - *Pigmented basal cell carcinoma (BCC)*: appears more pearlescent and nodule like
  - *Melanoma*: uneven pigmentation; irregular border
- *Management* is with reassurance. If inflamed, curettage or cryotherapy can be offered.
- *Refer* if there is diagnostic uncertainty.

Dermatofibroma or Histiocytoma (Ashton & Leppard, 2009)

- This is a common, probably reactive, benign skin tumour more commonly seen on the extremities. Commonly seen in adults, it can be asymptomatic but unsightly. Occasionally, they are tender. They range from 3 to 10 mm in size.
- They often (but not always) present after trauma such as insect bite.
- They present as a papule or nodule with a smooth surface. They are firm in consistency, and the characteristic feature is the 'dimple' or pinch sign (the tumour indents on lateral pressure with the fingers because it is adherent to overlying skin but free from underlying structures). They can be shiny or scaly.
- Reassure the patient.
- Refer if there is diagnostic uncertainty or if it is causing troublesome symptoms.

Sebaceous Hyperplasia (Wolff & Johnson, 2009)

- These are common benign lesions that are often mistaken for BCC. They are usually secondary to enlarged sebaceous glands around a single hair follicle, usually on the face. They are common in older people and patients who have had solid organ transplant and are taking ciclosporin.
- They present as small (2–5 mm in diameter), flesh- or yellow-coloured papules with telangiectasia and central punctum. Usually there are multiple lesions in one area.
- The differential diagnosis is a small BCC, which is usually solitary.
- *Management*, if there is diagnostic uncertainty, is with excision or removal by light electrocautery under local anaesthetic.

Keratoacanthoma (Du Vivier, 2013)

- These are rapidly growing benign tumours which tend to simulate SCC but usually self-resolve in 4 to 6 months. They tend to rapidly grow for 3 months and reach up to 3 cm in diameter before regressing spontaneously over the next 3 months. They are most commonly seen in older age groups, patients who have had chronic sun exposure, and in transplant recipients taking immunosuppressants.
- They present as a small spot that rapidly grows in size, causing alarm. They are erythematous or flesh coloured well-defined nodules, with a central keratin-filled crater. Its appearance mimics an erupting volcano. It is commonly seen in sun-exposed areas such as the face, nose, ears and cheeks, and dorsum of the hands and forearms. They are usually solitary but very occasionally can be multiple.
- The differential diagnosis includes SCC (difficult to clinically differentiate) and hypertrophic solar keratosis.
- *Refer* for surgical excision or curettage and cautery depending on site because they cannot be clinically distinguished from SCCs. Multiple lesions may require systemic retinoids or methotrexate.

Precancerous Skin Lesions

Actinic (Solar) Keratosis (Ashton & Leppard, 2009)

- These occur predominantly on chronically sun-exposed skin. They are rough, occasionally sore or itchy spots. They may be single or multiple, dry, rough, adherent, scaly, yellowish-brown lesions. They are more easily felt than seen because of their roughness. The surrounding skin can be normal or erythematous.
- They are commonly seen on face, bald scalp, and dorsum of the hands and forearms of patients older than 50 years of age.
- The differential diagnosis includes:
  - *Bowen disease*: flat, scaly lesions commonly seen on the shins
  - *Seborrhoeic keratosis*: warty stuck-on appearance
  - *Superficial BCC*: pearlescent appearance and telangiectasia
- If left untreated, some can progress to SCC.
- *Advise prevention* or further worsening by recommending a high-factor UVB or UVA sunscreen (usually SPF 30+).
- *Treatment* options include:
  a. *Cryotherapy.* Usually freeze for 5 to 10 seconds after the white halo has appeared.
  b. *5% 5-fluorouracil (5-FU) or Efudix.* Usually apply twice daily for 4 weeks on and then 4 weeks off. If a vast area is involved, then it is best to divide into quarters or sections and apply treatment in cycles. Warn the patient regarding erythema and erosions. If the reaction is too intense, it can be applied once daily or on 5 of 7 days per week.
  c. *5% imiquimod or Aldara.* Highly effective but can cause an intense reaction, which can put patients off.

The treatment regimen is 3 of 7 days per week for 4 weeks.

d. *Zyclara (3.75% imiquimod).* Can be used for facial lesions. The treatment regimen is to use once daily at night for 2 weeks and rest for 2 weeks.

e. *3% Diclofenac of Solaraze gel.* Used twice daily for 3 months. Better tolerated but not as effective as Aldara and Efudex.

f. *Picato gel.* This gets good compliance as 3-day treatment only.

g. Other treatments not commonly used are laser treatment, photodynamic therapy, and facial peels.

- If the patient finds the reactions secondary to topical treatment too intense, then advise to use for 5 of 7 days per week and use topical steroids on the rest days to help the skin recover.
- *Refer* if not responding to treatment or the patient is not tolerating treatment.

Bowen Disease (Squamous Cell Carcinoma in Situ) (Du Vivier, 2013)

- This is described as an intraepidermal carcinoma of the skin that can occasionally progress to SCC. Usually asymptomatic, patients usually present with a persistent solitary rough patch.
- It is a well-defined, solitary, plaque which may be slightly raised, scaly, and erythematous. Similar but nonscaly lesions on the glans or vulva are called *erythroplasia.* HPV-induced Bowenoid changes in the vulval or penile area are called *Bowenoid papulosis.* It carries premalignant potential and hence should be treated. Common sites are sun-exposed areas such as face, dorsum of the hands and forearms, and shins.
- *Management* options include:
  a. Cryotherapy
  b. Efudix or 5- FU: Use once or twice daily for 4 weeks.
  c. Aldara or imiquimod: Use three times per week for 12 weeks.
  d. Referral for surgical treatment such as curettage and cautery and excision.
- Treat lesions on the shins with care because they can lead to leg ulceration caused by poor healing.

Cutaneous Horn

- These are horny outgrowths from the skin. These are of importance because at the base of these lesions, there could be an underlying actinic keratosis, Bowen disease, or SCC.
- *Refer* to secondary care.

Atypical or Dysplastic Naevus (Wolff & Johnson, 2009)

- Although not malignant, it is considered a potential precursor to melanoma. It occurs because of dysfunctional proliferation of atypical melanocytes. They can arise from preexisting moles or de novo.
- Sometimes patients present with a mole that looks different from their other moles or has been gradually evolving.

However, sometimes these are picked up coincidentally when the patient presents for other pathology (e.g., whilst examining the chest for a cough).

- They are usually differentiated from benign naevi by their large and variegate appearance with irregular borders, and the tend to stand out amongst other moles.
- The differential diagnosis is malignant melanoma (MM). They are difficult to distinguish.
- *Refer* for excision because of their malignant potential.

Malignant Skin Lesions

GUIDELINE

National Institute for Health and Care Excellence. (2015). *Suspected cancer: Recognition and referral. NICE guideline 12.* https://cks.nice.org.uk/topics/skin-cancers-recognition-referral/.

Basal Cell Carcinoma (Rodent Ulcer)

- This is the commonest type of skin cancers. It is usually secondary to chronic sun exposure, although genetic mutations are known to cause these, too. It is locally invasive and erodes gradually through the skin but hardly ever metastasises, hence the name 'rodent ulcer' (Du Vivier, 2013).
- *Key features*
  - Pearly margins
  - Telangiectasia
  - Usually firm but can be cystic
  - Tends to bleed when excoriated
  - Commonly seen in middle-aged or older adult fair-skinned individuals with a history of chronic sun exposure (e.g., gardeners, sailors, people who worked abroad in tropical areas)
  - Commonly seen on the face but can be present anywhere on the body
- There are various subtypes (see Table 20.2) (Wolff & Johnson, 2009)
  a. *Superficial BCC.* This is the commonest subtype. They appear as thin plaques with fine borders and

TABLE 20.2	Commonly Prescribed Topical Steroids for Eczema	
Potency	**Examples**
Mild	Hydrocortisone (0.5%, 1%, 2.5%)
Moderate	Clobetasone butyrate (Eumovate) Betamethasone valerate 0.025% (Betnovate RD)
Potent	Betamethasone valerate 0.1% (Betnovate) Mometasone furoate (Elocon) Fluocinolone acetonide (Synalar)
Very potent	Clobetasone propionate (Dermovate)

telangiectasia. They are best seen with use of a hand lens.

b. *Nodular BCC.* These can present as well-defined nodules or papules, classically described as 'pearly' (i.e., skin-coloured smooth surface with telangiectasia).

c. *Ulcerated BCC.* Some nodular BCCs can progress to form an ulcer in the middle covered with crust and rolled-out borders and telangiectasia.

d. *Pigmented BCC.* Some BCCs can be pigmented and mimic a nodular or superficial spreading melanoma.

e. *Morphoeic or sclerosing BCC.* This is a difficult one to diagnose but fortunately is not very common. It presents as a macular scarlike area. It often has an ill-defined, hypopigmented, and sclerosed appearance. It can progress to ulcerated or nodular BCC. It is more aggressive in nature.

- *Refer* for excision on a routine basis (Ashton & Leppard, 2009).

Squamous Cell Carcinoma (Wolff & Johnson, 2009)

- SCC is a malignant metastasising tumour that arises from the keratinocytes within the epidermis. It can arise de novo or evolve from preexisting precancerous skin conditions such as Bowen disease or an actinic keratosis. It can also be an underlying pathology in chronic non-healing ulcers.

- The main risk factor is chronic sun exposure; therefore, it is most commonly seen in outdoor workers and people who live or travel to tropical countries. It is also more common in immunosuppressed people. Other risks are phototherapy and sunbed users, exposure to polycyclic hydrocarbons (tar, mineral oils), arsenic ingestion, and HPV.

- Patients usually present with a solitary keratotic papule or nodule that has either persisted for months or has been gradually growing in size. Usually there are no associated symptoms such as pain or bleeding or itching. The appearance can be of a scaly to indurated plaque or nodule. It can have an ulcerated or crusted surface. It is commonly seen in sun-exposed areas such as the face, forearms, bald scalp, ears, and lower legs.

- A history of a nodule developing on the background of a scaly or plaquelike area should also raise suspicions of SCC.

- The differential diagnosis includes:
  - *Bowen disease:* usually scaly plaque with no induration.
  - *Keratoacanthoma:* short history, rapid growth, and tends to self-resolve in 4 to 6 months. However, it is clinically difficult to differentiate from SCC, so it is best to treat as SCC until proven otherwise.
  - *BCC:* especially the early stages and the well-differentiated ones. However, BCCs are pearlier in appearance with telangiectasia and tend to be less indurated.
  - *Chondrodermatitis nodularis helicalis:* on the free border of helix or ear. Usually develops spontaneously, has rapid growth, tends to be smaller than 1 cm in size, and is tender, unlike SCCs.

- *Refer* for excision, which has to be complete (both peripheral and deep margins). This should be along a 2-week suspected cancer pathway.

- Patients with recurrent SCCs are offered systemic treatment such as Acitretin to reduce the incidence of further lesions developing.

Malignant Melanoma

- MM is the one of the most malignant neoplasms of the skin. These are tumours that arise from the pigmented cells within the dermoepidermal junction called melanocytes. Two-thirds of these arise de novo, and only one-third arise from preexisting moles (Wolff & Johnson, 2009).

- High-risk features are:
  - Fair-skinned people with red hair (i.e., skin type 1)
  - History of severe sun burns in younger years
  - People with multiple moles (>50)
  - People with dysplastic naevi
  - Family history or personal history of melanoma

- There are five main subtypes (Wolff & Johnson, 2009):
  1. *Lentigo maligna melanoma.* Malignant cells are limited to the epidermis. The growth of this tumour is usually in horizontal plane rather than vertical. Presentation is usually as a 1- to 3-cm macular pigmented lesion on the sun-exposed areas, usually in an older adult patient. These can evolve into superficial spreading melanoma or nodular melanoma.
  2. *Melanoma in situ.* Not diagnosed clinically and mainly a histopathologic diagnosis. It is a term used when the melanoma cells are confined to the epidermis, above the basement membrane. These lesions are usually flat or macular with irregular borders and marked variegation of pigmentation.
  3. *Superficial spreading melanoma.* Malignant cells usually lie along the dermoepidermal junction. The growth is more in the horizontal plane. The presentation is usually of an enlarging macular irregularly pigmented lesion with irregular borders. The surrounding skin may show inflammation.
  4. *Nodular melanoma.* The growth is mostly in the vertical plane rather than the horizontal plane. The presentation is usually of a darkly pigmented, dome-shaped nodule. The surface tends to break down and bleed or ooze and crust over. Sometimes lesions are not darkly pigmented and can be flesh coloured or erythematous; they are then called *amelanotic melanoma.*
  5. *Acral melanoma.* These tend to occur on the palms, soles, and nail beds. Any nontraumatic de novo pigmentation or change in a mole in these areas should be referred for further assessment to rule out malignant potential.

- Any patient who presents with a change (shape, size, colour, or itchiness or bleeding) in a longstanding mole or history of developing new moles after the age of 30 years should be referred to rule out an MM (Box 20.1).

This is a good and simple way of assessing a mole when assessing for superficial spreading melanoma.
A: Asymmetry in shape; one half is different from the other
B: Borders: irregular borders
C: Colour: more than one shade of pigment to the lesion
D: Diameter >6 mm or 'ugly duckling' appearance: stands out as an odd-looking mole amongst others
E: Enlargement: history of an increase in size

- Referral should be urgent under the suspicion of cancer pathway for assessment and excision. The primary excision is usually carried out with a 2-mm margin, and after histologically confirmed, wide local excision is carried out ranging from 5 mm to 2 cm with option for superficial lymph node biopsy and targeted chemotherapy based on the type and stage of melanoma.
- All melanomas except in situ melanomas are followed up by specialist from 1 to 10 years depending on staging.

PATIENT INFORMATION

Most patient information leaflets can be accessed on the British Association of Dermatologists' website. Available at http://www.bad.org.uk.

Venous or Varicose Eczema

GUIDELINE

National Institute for Health and Care Excellence. (2022). *Venous eczema and lipodermatosclerosis. Clinical knowledge summaries.* https://cks.nice.org.uk/topics/venous-eczema-lipodermatosclerosis/.

- Features range from haemosiderin deposits to active eczema with chronic changes of atrophie blanche, lipodermatosclerosis, and an increasing risk of active ulceration.
- Give patients general advice, including:
  - Avoid prolonged standing or sitting with the legs down.
  - Elevate the legs when sitting when possible.
  - Stay physically active.
  - Avoid skin injury.
  - Use regular emollients.
- *Topical steroids* can be used for a flare of eczema, moderately potent (e.g., Eumovate) to potent (e.g., Betnovate), for 7 to 10 days. Topical steroids can be continued twice weekly as a maintenance regimen if recurrent flares. In lipodermatosclerosis, very potent topical steroids may be required. For persistent venous eczema, consider a trial of potent topical steroid ointment under medicated bandages such as ZIPZOC.
- *Treat infections* with antibiotics according to swab sensitivities.

- Consider *compression stockings* for resistant cases. Check ankle-brachial pressure index (ABPI) and use below-knee compression stockings if there is no evidence of arterial insufficiency (class 2 is suitable for most people or class 1 if these are not tolerated).
  - ABPI less than 0.3 or greater than 1.3: Avoid compression stockings.
  - ABPI greater than 0.3 but less than 0.8: Only class 1 (mild) stockings can be used.
  - ABPI greater than 0.8 but less than 1.3: Up to class 3 stockings can be used.
- Consider the differential of allergic contact dermatitis in spreading eczema.
- Consider referral:
  a. For patch testing if allergic contact dermatitis is suspected
  b. Inability to control condition despite full primary care intervention
  c. If there is evidence of fibrosis or evidence of ulceration
  d. If ABPI is less than 0.8, refer to a vascular specialist.

PATIENT SUPPORT ORGANISATION

National Eczema Society. 11 Murray Street, London, NW1 9RE. Helpline: 0800 089 1122. Available at http://www.eczema.org.

Leg Ulcers

GUIDELINE

National Institute for Health and Care Excellence. (2021). *Leg ulcer—venous. Clinical knowledge summaries.* Retrieved from https://cks.nice.org.uk/topics/leg-ulcer-venous/.

- Of leg ulcers, 70% are venous and 10% are arterial, with the rest including neuropathic, pressure ulcers, autoimmune conditions, or skin malignancy.
- Involve nursing colleagues with experience in wound management early in the presentation.
- Remember to treat associated conditions such as pain, eczema, and oedema and to inform patients with regards to signs of infection.
- Take a history to determine if the cause is arterial, neuropathic, or cellulitic.
- Give healthy lifestyle advice, especially diet and exercise, smoking cessation, and alcohol advice, because it promotes healing and reduces the risk of recurrence.
- Ensure the ulcer is cleaned and dressed at least weekly.

General Advice

- Mobility keeps the calf muscle pumps active and helps reduce oedema.

- Avoid tight-fitting footwear and avoid trauma to the legs.
- Elevate the legs when immobile. Ideally, elevation should be to the level of the heart if possible (i.e., lying in bed rather than using footstools).

Management

- Use an emollient frequently.
- A moderately potent topical steroid can be used for surrounding venous dermatitis.
- Antibiotics are only indicated if there is clinical suspicion of infection and should not be initiated on swab results without clinical suspicion.
- Compression stockings are effective in reducing recurrent ulcers and chronic lower leg swelling, but check ABPI via Doppler. Only use compression therapy if ABPI less than 0.8; it is not a diabetic or neuropathic ulcer; and there is no phlebitis, deep vein thrombosis, or cellulitis. Discontinue compression therapy if features of arterial insufficiency or infection occur.
- Compression bandaging should be applied as follows:
  - For people who are immobile, three- or four-layer bandaging is most suitable.
  - For people who are mobile, two-layer bandaging is more practical.
  - For most patients, below-knee compression stockings are most suitable. Remember to prescribe two at a time and for patients to get a new prescription every 4 months because the stockings lose elasticity.
- If an ulcer is failing to heal, then screen for iron deficiency and diabetes. Also consider the differential diagnosis, which can include skin malignancy.
- It is common for ulcers to recur, so support stockings are needed long term.
- *Refer:*
  - *Refer routinely* to a vascular surgeon if the ABPI is less than 0.8 or if there are significant varicosities.
  - *Refer urgently* to a vascular surgeon if the ABPI is less than 0.5 or if ischaemic changes occur because of compression stockings.
  - *Refer to a dermatologist* if there is no improvement despite primary care therapy or if there is deterioration; malignancy is suspected; or there is an atypical pattern of ulceration, which may signify an underlying disease process (e.g., pyoderma gangrenosum, vasculitis, contact dermatitis).
  - Consider referral if there is no improvement after 3 months.

PATIENT SUPPORT ORGANISATION

The Lindsay Leg Club Foundation. Ipswich, PO Box 689, IP1 9BN. Tel: 01473 749565. Available at http://www.legclub.org.

Hidradenitis Suppurativa or Acne Inversa

GUIDELINES

Primary Care Dermatology Society. (2014; updated 2017). *Hidradenitis suppurativa. Clinical guidance.* Retrieved from http://www.pcds.org.uk (search on 'hidradenitis suppurativa). British Association of Dermatologists. Retrieved from http://www.bad.org.uk.

- Hidradenitis suppurativa is a chronic suppurative, often cicatricial disease of the apocrine gland–bearing skin. It usually affects the axilla, anogenital region, and occasionally scalp (called *cicatricial perifolliculitis*) (Wolff et al., 2009).
- The clinical course can range from relatively mild cases with recurrent appearances of papules, pustules, and some inflammatory nodules to severe cases presenting with deep fluctuant abscesses, sinus formation, and scarring.
- It affects about 1% of the population. The female:male ratio is 3:1. It usually occurs between the ages of 20 and 40 years (Ashton & Leppard, 2009).
- The exact aetiology remains unclear; however, contributing factors include hormones, obesity, coexisting polycystic ovarian syndrome or inflammatory bowel disease (more common with Crohn disease), acne, infection (unsure if commensal or not), genetics, and smoking (Wolff & Johnson, 2009).
- All patients with hidradenitis suppurativa should have a baseline Hurley staging (Table 20.3) recorded at diagnosis, which helps with monitoring disease progression and treatment.
- The diagnosis is mainly clinical. Swabs can be done if resistance suspected, and biopsies are rarely done if there is diagnostic uncertainty.
- Rule out other metabolic syndromes such as diabetes or thyroid dysfunction. If there are persistent bowel symptoms, rule out associated inflammatory bowel disease.

TABLE 20.3	**Hurley Staging for Hidradenitis Suppurativa**
Hurley Stage	**Presentation**
1	Solitary or multiple isolated abscess formation without scarring or sinus tract formation
2	Recurrent abscesses; single or multiple widely separated lesions with sinus tract formation
3	Diffuse involvement with multiple interconnected sinus tracts and abscesses and scarring

Treatment (British Association of Dermatologists, Ashton & Leppard, 2009)

- Start treatment early to reduce the chance of future scarring.
- Advice regarding weight loss and lifestyle measures should be given early.
- Smoking cessation should be advised.
- Using antibacterial wash in the shower such chlorhexidine or Dermol can help reduce frequency of acute flare-ups. Clindamycin 1% solution can be used in mild solitary nodules.
- Avoid shaving too often. Wear loose-fitting clothes and maintain good personal hygiene.
- Usually treated with prolonged courses of antibiotics such as lymecycline or doxycycline (initially 100 mg once daily and can be increased to 200 mg/day for 6–8 months if tolerating well). The photosensitive effect should be discussed and sunscreen advised.
- Metformin (normal or slow release if not tolerating normal) 500 mg to 1 g can be added to help with weight loss.
- If the above is not effective, the patient can have a 12-week trial of rifampicin (300 mg bd) and clindamycin (300 mg bd) with blood (LFT) monitoring.
- Using Hidrawear garments if stage 3 disease may help with keeping wounds clean.
- Refer for surgical removal of abscesses or scars when causing contractures.
- Intralesional corticosteroid injections in selected lesions only.
- Provide enough dressings to help keep acute lesions clean.
- *Refer* to dermatology if medical therapies are ineffective or if widespread scarring disease is present. Treatment options in secondary care include cyclosporine, isotretinoin, acitretin, Dapsone, tumour necrosis factor-α inhibitors such as infliximab and adalimumab (Du Vivier, 2013). More recently Secukinumab has been approved by NICE as a treatment option.

PATIENT SUPPORT ORGANISATIONS

The Hidradenitis Suppurativa Trust. Cliffe House, Anthonys Way, Rochester, ME2 4DY. enquiries@hstrust.org. Available at http://www.hstrust.org
Hidradenitis Suppurativa foundation. Available at http://www.hs-foundation.org.
My HS Team. Available at http://www.myhsteam.com.

PATIENT INFORMATION

British Association of Dermatologists. Available at http://www.bad.org.uk.
Dermnet NZ. Available at http://www.dermnetnz.org.

Hyperhidrosis

GUIDELINES

National Institute for Health and Care Excellence. (2018). *Hyperhidrosis. Clinical knowledge summaries*. https://cks.nice.org.uk/topics/hyperhidrosis/.
Primary Care Dermatology Society. (2014). *Hyperhidrosis*. Retrieved from http://www.pcds.org.uk/clinical-guidance/hyperhidrosis.

- Excessive sweating can be classified by location (focal or generalised) and the presence of an underlying cause (primary or secondary).
- Primary focal hyperhidrosis has no underlying cause and affects the scalp, face, axillae, palms, or soles.
- Secondary hyperhidrosis focal affects a specific site and is caused by an underlying condition.
- Generalised hyperhidrosis affects the entire skin surface area and is usually secondary to other medical conditions or induced by drugs.
  - Common drugs include antidepressants, alcohol, and substance abuse.
  - Medical conditions include, but are not limited to, anxiety, pregnancy, infections, malignancy, menopause, hyperthyroidism, and hyperpituitarism.

Investigations

- In obvious primary hyperhidrosis, these are not indicated.
- If generalised hyperhidrosis is a differential, then further investigation is required and often includes a full blood count (FBC), urea and electrolytes, LFT, erythrocyte sedimentation rate or C-reactive protein, fasting blood glucose, and thyroid function tests (TFT). If clinically indicated, then chest radiography (neoplasm) and HIV serology should be obtained.

Management

- Provide the patient with an information leaflet.
- Advise the patient to avoid caffeine and spicy foods and avoid tight-fitting clothes.
- Use a 20% aluminium chloride hexahydrate roll-on at night. Apply at night on dry skin and wash it off in the morning until symptoms are controlled. Do not apply within 12 hours of shaving. When control achieved, then use weekly.
- If the feet are most affected, then use aluminium dusting powder.
- For skin irritation caused by aluminium, 1% hydrocortisone ointment can be used for up to 2 weeks.
- Pro-Banthine or oxybutynin can be used as a second-line medication.
- If anxiety is an issue, then offer cognitive-behavioural therapy as an alternative to propranolol or antidepressants, which can worsen sweating.

- Review in 1 to 2 months to reassess.
- If not controlled, then consider referral to a dermatologist.
- Management of generalised hyperhidrosis is targeted at finding the cause and treating it. If the aetiology remains unclear and ongoing sweating occurs, then consider referral to a dermatologist.

PATIENT SUPPORT ORGANISATIONS

Hyperhidrosis UK. Available at http://www.hyperhidrosisuk. org.
    International Hyperhidrosis Society (United States). Available at http://www.sweathelp.org.

Urticaria and Angioedema

- This is commonly called hives. Urticaria is composed of wheals (transient erythematous papules or plaques). They are usually pruritic and well-defined superficial in nature (Wolff & Johnson, 2009).
- Angioedema, on the other hand, is a larger oedematous area that involves the dermis and subcutaneous tissue. It is deep and ill defined (Wolff & Johnson, 2009).
- They can both be acute recurrent or chronic recurrent.
- *Acute urticaria.* Acute onset and recurring over less than 30 days. It consists of large wheals, often associated with angioedema. It is immunoglobulin E (IgE) dependent and complement related (Wolff & Johnson, 2009).
- *Chronic urticaria.* Recurring over more than 30 days. It can present as small and large wheals. It is non IgE mediated and mostly idiopathic. Females are affected twice as commonly as males. Most chronic urticarias that last more than 6 months tend to persist over prolonged periods (Wolff & Johnson, 2009).
- Urticaria can also be classified into the following subtypes (Wolff & Johnson, 2009):
  1. Idiopathic: most common
  2. Immunologic: IgE related (food allergy, infections, reactions to external agents on body), complement mediated (C1 esterase inhibitor deficiency), autoimmune or immune contact urticaria, and vasculitic.
  3. Nonimmunologic or physical: heat, cold, cholinergic, pressure, solar, dermographism or medication related
  4. Hereditary angioedema
  5. Angioedema–urticaria–eosinophilia syndrome
- Symptoms (Ashton & Leppard., 2009):
  - *Urticaria:* mainly itch or pruritis
  - *Angioedema:* can present with swelling of the face, lips, and tongue. This can affect speech, food intake, and breathing.
- Signs
  - *Urticaria:* well-defined, raised, erythematous plaques ranging from 1 to more than 8 cm. They tend to resolve over a 24-hour period and appear in different part of the body.

- *Dermographism* is usually positive to varying degrees.
- *Angioedema:* skin-coloured, transient enlargement of the area, mainly the face (eyelids, lips, tongue) caused by subcutaneous oedema. Dermographism not always positive.
- *Investigations.* The diagnosis is usually clinical based on presentation and examination findings. Most patients do not have active rash when seen in clinic, but photographs from flareups and positive dermographism in clinic are helpful.
- For acute idiopathic urticaria (lasting <6 weeks), no investigations are usually indicated. In chronic or recurrent cases in which a secondary cause is suspected, the following can be considered:
  - FBC to look for eosinophilia (not always present)
  - TFTs, antithyroglobulin antibody
  - Antimicrosomal antibody
  - Skin biopsies can be done for an atypical presentation or diagnostic uncertainty

Management (Ashton & Leppard, 2009)

- Prevention: if stimulus is known, then avoid acute attacks by avoiding stimulus.
- Give lifestyle advice, including avoidance of overheating such as taking hot baths, alcohol, eating spicy foods, and caffeine.
- Treatment
  a. *Topical antipruritic* creams such as Eurax or Dermacool 2-5% can be used to help with symptoms.
  b. *Oral antihistamines.* These patients usually require a cocktail of various antihistamines over a 24-hour period to provide a round-the-clock antihistamine effect. Options include nonsedating antihistamines during the day, including cetirizine, fexofenadine, and loratadine. Sedating antihistamines such as chlorphenamine, hydroxyzine, or promethazine can be used at night.
  c. In severe acute urticaria associated with angioedema, a short course (5 days) of oral prednisolone may be needed.

  When to refer:
- Consider referral to secondary care if above not effective or of minimal benefit. Options include using off-licence doses of antihistamines and Omalizumab in secondary care with regular monitoring (Wolff & Johnson, 2009).
- Refer urgently to a dermatologist if the patient has suspected urticarial vasculitis. (This is tender urticaria with associated joint pains, bruising, or static wheals that are present for more than 24 hours or contact urticaria.) (Ashton & Leppard, 2009).
- Rarely, the patient should be referred to an immunologist for radioallergosorbent testing or skin prick testing if the condition is thought to be caused by food, drug, or latex allergies.

Urticaria Pigmentosa (Ashton & Leppard, 2009)

- This is a rare condition related to excessive mast cells in the skin.
- *Presentation* is with orange-brown pigmented macules that can coalesce to form larger patches. It is seen in children and young adults. It is nonscaly, but Darrier sign positive (on rubbing, wheals appear because of histamine release from mast cells). Most patients are asymptomatic and present with an unsightly rash. Systemic symptoms such as headache, flushing, wheeze, shortness of breath, syncope, and diarrhoea are very uncommon.
- *Treatment.* Avoid mast cell degranulating agents such as aspirin, alcohol, morphine, and codeine.
- If itchy, the patient can try antihistamines or psoralen and UVA to help mask the rash.

PATIENT INFORMATION

British Association of Dermatologist. *Patient information leaflets.* Available https://www.bad.org.uk/pils/urticaria-pigmentosa/.
Dermnet NZ. Available at https://dermnetnz.org/topics/maculopapular-cutaneous-mastocytosis.

Alopecia

GUIDELINES

National Institute for Health and Care Excellence. (2018). *Alopecia areata.* https://cks.nice.org.uk/topics/alopecia-areata/
British Association of Dermatologists. (2012). *Guidelines for the management of alopecia areata.* https://onlinelibrary.wiley.com/doi/full/10.1111/j.1365-2133.2012.10955.x.

- Alopecia may be either:
  - Nonscarring (no inflammation, follicular openings present, atrophy absent)
  - Scarring (inflammation usually present, no follicular openings, atrophy present)
- Causes of nonscarring alopecia include:
  - *Alopecia areata*: scalp looks normal, exclamation hairs at edges, 'pull test positive'
  - *Tinea Capitis*: subtle scale may be seen
  - *Trichotillosis* (compulsive hair pulling): different length hairs
  - *Traction alopecia*: from hair styling
- Causes of scarring alopecia include:
  - Infection (bacterial or fungal)
  - Lichen planopilaris

- Frontal fibrosing alopecia
- Folliculitis decalvans
- Lupus
- Investigations:
  - FBC, ferritin, and TFT (consider syphilis if diffuse alopecia)
  - Enquire about childbirth, recent surgery, and causative medications
  - Fungal culture
  - Consider ANA (Antinuclear antibody)

Management

- Provide a patient information leaflet and consider counselling and psychological support.
- Advise sunblock on bald patches.
- Nonextensive (<50% hair affected): No treatment is often indicated because spontaneous remission occurs in up to 80% of patients.
- Extensive alopecia (>50% hair affected) areata: wigs.
- Trial of potent or very potent steroids for 3 months (in nonpregnant patients who do not want referral). If referring, consider trialling this treatment whilst awaiting review.
- Protopic 0.1% can be used as a steroid-sparing alternative.
- Intralesional steroid injection such as triamcinolone may be tried, but warn the patient about the possibility of atrophy.
- *Refer:*
  a) If there is more than 50% hair loss or no regrowth
  b) Patient preference

PATIENT SUPPORT ORGANISATIONS

Alopecia UK. Available at http://www.alopecia.org.uk.
National Alopecia Areata Foundation. Available at http://www.naaf.org.

References

Ashton, R., & Leppard, B. (2009). *Differential diagnosis in dermatology.* Radcliffe. (3rd ed., pp. 186, 231, 242–244, 267, 271–275, 285–286, 288–290).

Du Vivier, A. (2013). *Atlas of clinical dermatology.* Elsevier. (4th ed., pp. 150–152, 170–171, 192–194, 196–214, 233–250).

Gollnick, H., & Layton, A. (2008). Azelaic acid 15% gel in the treatment of rosacea. *Expert Opinion on Pharmacotherapy, 9*(15), 2699–2706. doi:10.1517/14656566.9.15.2699.

Wolff, K., & Johnson, R. A. (2009). *Fitzpatrick's color atlas and synopsis of clinical dermatology.* McGraw Hill. (6th ed., pp. 53–71, 215–216, 222, 224–226, 274–296, 300, 308–333).

21

Allergic Problems

Adam Staten

CHAPTER CONTENTS

Food Allergies

GUIDELINES AND SYSTEMATIC REVIEWS

National Institute for Health and Care Excellence. (2011). *Food allergy in children and young people. Diagnosis and assessment of food allergy in children and young people in primary care and community settings. NICE clinical guideline 116.* Retrieved from https://www.nice.org.uk/guidance/cg116.

Boyce, J. A., Assa'ad, A., Burks, A. W., et al. (2010). Guidelines for the Diagnosis and Management of Food Allergy in the United States: Summary of the NIAID-Sponsored Expert Panel Report. Journal of Allergy and Clinical Immunology, *126*(6), 1105–1118.

de Silva, D., Geromi, M., Panesar, S. S., Muraro, A., Werfel, T., Hoffmann-Sommergruber, K., Roberts, G., Cardona, V., Dubois, A. E., Halken, S., Host, A., Poulsen, L. K., Van Ree, R., Vlieg-Boerstra, B. J., Agache, I., Sheikh, A., & EAACI Food Allergy and Anaphylaxis Guidelines Group (2014a). Acute and long-term management of food allergy: Systematic review. Allergy, *69*(2), 159–167.

de Silva, D., Geromi, M., Halken, S., Host, A., Panesar, S. S., Muraro, A., Werfel, T., Hoffmann-Sommergruber, K., Roberts, G., Cardona, V., Dubois, A. E., Poulsen, L. K., Van Ree, R., Vlieg-Boerstra, B., Agache, I., Grimshaw, K., O'Mahony, L., Venter, C., Arshad, S. H., Sheikh, A., ... EAACI Food Allergy and Anaphylaxis Guidelines Group (2014b). Primary prevention of food allergy in children and adults: Systematic review. Allergy, *69*(5), 581–589.

- The UK incidence of severe food allergic reactions leading to hospitalisation has increased in recent years (Baseggio Conrado et al, 2021).
- Adverse reactions to food may result from allergy (hypersensitivity), which may be immunoglobulin E (IgE) or non-IgE mediated, or intolerance (reactions that are not clearly immunologically mediated.

- The severity of allergic reactions is highly variable, with symptoms ranging from mild cutaneous symptoms (e.g., exacerbation of atopic eczema or dermatitis and urticaria) predominantly experienced in those with non–IgE-mediated food allergy to systemic life-threatening anaphylaxis, which may be seen in those with IgE-mediated food allergy.
- Patients often use the term 'allergy' to refer to any of a number of food-related adverse reactions; double-blind, placebo-controlled studies, however, show that only a minority of these reactions have an allergic basis (Rona et al, 2007; Sampson 2005).
- In addition to the immediate effects of allergic reactions, food allergies can have a significant impact on patients' everyday lives. Activities such as food shopping, eating outside the home, and travelling abroad can become challenging. An accurate diagnosis and good long-term management are therefore crucial in maintaining quality of life and minimising anxiety (Munoz-Furlong, 2003).

Diagnosis

- Differentiating food allergy from intolerance is important because the former typically requires meticulous avoidance of the food(s) in question; continued exposure to the triggering food(s) in those with IgE-mediated food allergy increases the risks of major systemic allergic reactions such as anaphylaxis (Sheikh & Walker, 2002; Wood, 1999).
- Attempt to differentiate food allergy from intolerance by the following features of the history and examination:
  a. *Family history.* Food allergy usually occurs in those with a personal or family history of allergic disorders (e.g., atopic eczema, hay fever, asthma).
  b. *Type of food.* Although almost any protein-based food may provoke allergic symptoms in sensitised

individuals, most reactions occur in relation to exposure to a small group of foods (Table 21.1) (Teuber et al, 2006).

  c. *Speed of onset.* Symptoms that occur soon after food intake (usually <1 hour and often within minutes) are suggestive of IgE-mediated allergy.

  d. *Effect of reexposure.* Reexposure to the same food(s) tends to produce similar reactions in those with food allergy; the picture is often much more variable in those with intolerance.

  e. *Pollen–food allergy syndrome* (known until recently as oral allergy syndrome) is an IgE-mediated hypersensitivity to raw fruits, root vegetables, and some nuts. It is most likely to occur in patients with tree pollen allergy (i.e., those with spring hay fever). Contact urticaria or angioedema of the lips and oropharynx occurs through a cross-reactivity between specific epitopes in pollens and fresh fruits or vegetables, manifesting as an itchy oropharynx and swelling of the lips and tongue. More severe reactions may occur but are unusual.

  f. *The clinical picture.* Food allergy typically triggers symptoms indicative of inflammation in one or more organ systems. These include features of angioedema (particularly of the lips and tongue), urticaria, conjunctivitis, rhinitis, bronchospasm, gastrointestinal oedema (cramps, vomiting and diarrhoea), and anaphylaxis. Food-related symptoms of tiredness, joint and muscle pains, sleep disturbance, and emotional upset are all more suggestive of a diagnosis of food intolerance.

Management

Symptomatic Treatment

- Treat symptomatically with H_1-antihistamines; if life-threatening features are present (respiratory difficulty or symptoms suggestive of hypotension), then treat as for anaphylaxis (see later discussion).

Further Management

- Attempt to unequivocally identify the food(s) responsible for triggering reactions. Take a detailed history of reactions from the patient and carer and, if necessary, refer to the list of the most common trigger foods to deduce likely culprits (see Table 21.1). Confirm clinical suspicion with objective allergy test if IgE-mediated disease is suspected (skin-prick test or serum-specific IgE) or a trial of dietary exclusion if non–IgE-mediated food allergy is suspected.

- Refer to an allergist if provision for suitable testing is unavailable, in the event of diagnostic uncertainty, or if the patient has experienced a life-threatening reaction.

- Recommend the avoidance of food(s) found to trigger symptoms. Advise careful checking of food ingredients (e.g., by reading food labels, asking waiting staff and caterers when eating outside the home).

- Encourage patients to be proactive in seeking relevant information. For example, organisations such as Allergy UK and the Anaphylaxis Campaign (see the Useful Contacts box), as well as many larger food manufacturers and catering chains now publish allergen information online.

- Recommend that patients with pollen–food allergy syndrome avoid the offending fruits or vegetables in their raw forms. In most cases, the allergen is removed by peeling or destroyed by heating, and the peeled or cooked fruits or vegetables can then be safely consumed.

- Enlist the help of a dietician to ensure that patients fully understand about the foods that they need to avoid, help them manage avoidance when eating in and outside the home, and ensure their diet is nutritionally adequate.

- Issue self-injectable adrenaline to those with a history of anaphylaxis and recommend a medical identity bracelet or necklace.

- Refer patients with severe food intolerance(s) to a gastroenterologist. Any long-term exclusion diet should be supervised by a dietician (Grimshaw, 2006).

- Review patient periodically to ensure long-term management is effective.

Reintroducing Foods After a Period of Avoidance

- Children with allergy to milk and eggs commonly develop tolerance to these foods as they grow older. In those with a history of reactions that are not considered to be life threatening, the careful reintroduction of these foods at a later date may be appropriate.

- Consider reintroducing:
  a. *Milk* at the age of 3 years (by which time 85% of children with a history of milk allergy will be tolerant)
  b. *Eggs* at the age of 6 to 10 years (by which time 55%–80% of children with a history of egg allergy will be tolerant) (Teuber et al, 2006).

- *Persistent symptoms.* Refer to specialist services.

Note: Peanut, fish, and seafood allergies are, in the majority of individuals, lifelong (Teuber et al, 2006), and attempts at reintroduction are not normally recommended, though some specialist clinics do supervise oral immunotherapy, a process in which very small amounts of the allergen are introduced to the diet, and the degree of exposure is increased gradually (Stiefel et al, 2017). This should never be done without specialist supervision.

TABLE 21.1	Foods Commonly Responsible for Triggering Allergic Reactions	
Children	**Adults**
Milk	Fish and seafood
Egg whites	Tree nuts
Peanuts	Peanuts
Wheat	Additives
Soya beans	Fruits

Prevention

- Pregnant and breastfeeding females do not need to change their diets or take supplements in an attempt to prevent allergies in infants.
- Previously, those with a family history of allergic disorders were advised to avoid peanuts during pregnancy, lactation, and weaning until the age of at least 3 years, but evidence now suggests that this may actually increase the risk of peanut allergy through preventing the development of immunologic tolerance (Du Toit et al, 2008; McLean & Sheikh, 2010).
- Recent research suggests that early introduction of peanut products to infants as young as 4 months of age is likely to reduce allergy, and some researchers suggest that population-level introduction of peanut products in infancy would be an effective public health strategy (Roberts et al, 2023). Guidelines for this do not currently exist.
- Encourage lactating mothers of infants with a parent or sibling with an atopic disease to exclusively breastfeed for 4–6 months as there is some evidence of a protective function in children with atopic heredity although the role in breastfeeding and atopy in general is controversial (Lin et al, 2020).

USEFUL CONTACTS

For Patients

The Anaphylaxis Campaign. 1 Alexandra Road, Farnborough, Hampshire GU14 6SX. Tel: 01252 546100; Helpline: 01252 542029. info@anaphylaxis.org.uk. Available at http://www.anaphylaxis.org.uk.

Allergy UK. Planwell House, LEFA Business Park, Edgington Way, Sidcup, Kent, DA14 5BH. Helpline: 01322 619898. info@allergyuk.org. Available at http://www.allergyuk.org.

MedicAlert Foundation. The MedicAlert Foundation, 327 Upper Fourth Street, Milton Keynes, MK9 1EH. Tel: 01908 951045. info@medicalert.org.uk. Available at http://www.medicalert.org.uk.

Supermarkets can provide information on products that are 'free from' certain ingredients.

For Professionals

British Society for Allergy and Clinical Immunology. Studio 16. Cloisters House 8 Battersea Park Road London SW8 4BG. Tel: 0207 501 3910. Available at http:// www.bsaci.org.

Anaphylaxis

GUIDELINES

Resuscitation Council UK. (2008; updated 2021). *Emergency treatment of anaphylactic reactions: Guidelines for healthcare providers.* Retrieved from https://www.resus.org.uk/library/additional-guidance/guidance-anaphylaxis/emergency-treatment.

- Anaphylaxis is a severe, life-threatening generalised or systemic hypersensitivity reaction. It is rapid in onset and may cause death.
- Anaphylaxis is commonly triggered by foods, drugs, and the venom of stinging insects. It may also be induced by exercise, latex, and a number of other factors. Some cases are idiopathic.
- The UK rate of hospitalisation because of anaphylaxis has steadily increased in the past 2 decades (Baseggio et al, 2021).
- Government figures estimate that there are between 20 and 30 deaths from anaphylaxis in the United Kingdom each year, and many of them are potentially preventable.
- The classification of reactions into anaphylactic (IgE-mediated hypersensitivity reactions) and anaphylactoid (non–IgE-mediated mast cell degranulation) is of little practical relevance to the management of anaphylaxis and is now largely avoided.
- Anaphylaxis can have a significant long-term impact on a patient's everyday life beyond the immediate ill effects of a reaction. Managing an unfamiliar set of risks may be challenging for patients, particularly immediately after diagnosis. The possibility of further reactions can lead to increased anxiety. Allergen avoidance requires careful vigilance and may adversely affect the patient's family and social life. Good long-term management is therefore essential in maintaining quality of life.

Diagnosis

- Anaphylaxis presents a range of signs and symptoms, which can sometimes result in diagnostic difficulties. A diagnosis is likely when all three of the following criteria are met:
  - Sudden onset and rapid progression of symptoms
  - Life-threatening airway, breathing, or circulation problems
  - Skin or mucosal changes (flushing, urticaria, angioedema)
- There may also be gastrointestinal symptoms such as vomiting.
- Exposure to a known allergen for the patient supports the diagnosis.
- Isolated skin or mucosal changes do not indicate anaphylaxis.
- The diagnosis of anaphylaxis should always be followed up by specialist-led investigation into the underlying cause.

Management

- Management is best considered in two stages: treatment of the acute attack and follow-up care.

Acute Management

The key steps for the treatment of an anaphylactic reaction are shown in the algorithm (Table 21.2; see Appendix 26).
1. Commence life support (basic and advanced) if indicated.
2. Give oxygen.

TABLE 21.2	Routes of Administration and Drug Dosages for Agents Used in the Emergency Treatment of Patients With Anaphylaxis	
Drug (Route of Administration)	**Age-Related Dosage**	
Adrenaline 1:1000 (IM)	Younger than 6 years: 150 μg (0.15 mL)	
	6–12 years: 300 μg (0.3 mL)	
	Older than 12 years (small or prepubertal children): 300 μg (0.3 mL)	
	Older than 12 years: 500 μg (0.5 mL)	
Crystalloid fluid (IV)	Children: 10 mL/kg Adults: 500–1000 mL	

IM, Intramuscular; *IV,* intravenous.

3. Give adrenaline (epinephrine) 1:1000 solution (injected intramuscularly into the anterolateral aspect of the middle third of the thigh) if not already administered. (Many patients with a history of anaphylaxis will have been issued with adrenaline for self-injection.) The Resuscitation Council cautions against the use of the intravenous (IV) route except by experienced practitioners treating patients with profound shock (Working Group of the Resuscitation Council, 2008).
4. Give nebulised salbutamol and ipratropium if there is severe bronchospasm.
5. Repeat adrenaline 5 to 10 minutes after the first dose if there is no clinical improvement.
6. Give IV crystalloid fluid infusion if symptoms of hypotension persist (a repeat dose may be necessary) (Working Group of the Resuscitation Council, 2008).
7. After treatment, the patient should be observed for a minimum of 6 hours in a clinical area suitable for resuscitation if necessary (Working Group of the Resuscitation Council, 2008).

- *Trigger.* Refer to an allergist to identify the trigger objectively and for consideration of desensitisation therapy in those with venom-triggered reactions (Working Group of the Resuscitation Council, 2008). This should involve a detailed history and subsequent investigations, which may include skin-prick testing, serum-specific IgE tests, and allergen challenge.
- *Allergen avoidance.* Reinforce all allergen advice issued to patients and families, tailored to individual age and circumstances; dietetic referral may be indicated in cases of food allergy. Encourage the patient or parent to be proactive in seeking relevant information (e.g., checking product labels on foods, pharmaceuticals, and cosmetic products). Advise avoidance, when possible, of products carrying 'may contain' allergen labels.
- *Adrenaline.* Issue an adrenaline autoinjector for self-administration (and educate the patient on when and

how to use it). Delayed use of adrenaline can lead to fatality, so advise patients not to hesitate in self-administering it. In addition to verbal explanation, use a trainer autoinjector and ask the patient to demonstrate its correct use. Ensure the autoinjector dosage is correct. Advise patients to take note of their autoinjector expiry dates and make arrangements for repeat prescription. Note that adrenaline autoinjector users can subscribe to an expiry alert service by letter, email, or SMS text message (see the Useful Contacts box later). Multiple autoinjectors may need to be prescribed to cover different sites, such as one for home and one for school or the workplace.
- *Alert bracelet.* Recommend purchase of a medical identity bracelet, necklace, or smart card documenting the history of anaphylaxis and that adrenaline is carried.
- *Asthma control.* Optimise asthma management in those with a history of asthma because the risk of fatality is increased in this group.
- Liaise with the patient's nursery, school, school nurse, or /work as appropriate.
- Review the patient 6 months after diagnosis and thereafter every year and after any subsequent reactions. Reviews should be used to support patients' self-management as appropriate (e.g., reinforcing allergen avoidance advice, encouraging carrying an adrenaline autoinjector, retraining in autoinjector use, or referring to a specialist for retesting). A management plan incorporating training in adrenaline use, support, and follow-up may prove useful (Choo & Sheikh, 2007; Hourihane, 2001; Nurmatov et al, 2008).

USEFUL CONTACTS

For Patients

The Anaphylaxis Campaign. 1 Alexandra Road, Farnborough, Hampshire GU14 6SX. Tel: 01252 546100; Helpline: 01252 542029. info@anaphylaxis.org.uk. Available at http://www.anaphylaxis.org.uk.

Allergy UK. Planwell House, LEFA Business Park, Edgington Way, Sidcup, Kent, DA14 5BH. Helpline: 01322 619898. info@allergyuk.org. Available at http://www.allergyuk.org.

MedicAlert Foundation. The MedicAlert Foundation, 327 Upper Fourth Street, Milton Keynes, MK9 1EH. Tel: 01908 951045. info@medicalert.org.uk. Available at http://www.medicalert.org.uk.

Supermarkets can provide information on products that are 'free from' certain ingredients.

For Professionals

British Society for Allergy and Clinical Immunology. Studio 16. Cloisters House 8 Battersea Park Road London SW8 4BG. Tel: 0207 501 3910. Available at http:// www.bsaci.org.

Education for Health. The Athenaeum, 10 Church Street, Warwick CV34 4AB. Tel: 01926 493313. info@education-forhealth.org. Available at http://www.educationforhealth.org.

Adrenaline prescribing information. Includes autoinjector demonstration and details of the expiry alert system. Available at http://www.epipen.com; www.jext.co.uk.

References

Baseggio Conrado, A., Ierodiakonou, D., Gowland, M. H., Boyle, R. J., & Turner, P. J. (2021). Food anaphylaxis in the United Kingdom: Analysis of national data, 1998-2018. *BMJ (Clinical research ed.)*, *372*, n251 doi:10.1136/bmj.n251.

Choo, K., & Sheikh, A. (2007). Action plans for the long-term management of anaphylaxis: A systematic review of effectiveness. *Clinical and Experimental Allergy*, *37*, 1090–1094.

Du Toit, G., Katz, Y., Sasieni, P., Mesher, D., Maleki, S. J., Fisher, H. R., Fox, A. T., Turcanu, V., Amir, T., Zadik-Mnuhin, G., Cohen, A., Livne, I., & Lack, G. (2008). Early consumption of peanuts in infancy is associated with a low prevalence of peanut allergy. *Journal of Allergy and Clinical Immunology*, *122*, 984–991.

Grimshaw, K. E. C. (2006). Dietary management of food allergy in children. *Proceedings of the Nutrition Society*, *65*, 412–417.

Hourihane, J. (2001). Community management of severe allergies must be integrated and comprehensive, and must consist of more than just epinephrine. *Allergy*, *56*, 1023–1025.

Lin, B., Dai, R., Lu, L., Fan, X., & Yu, Y. (2020). Breastfeeding and atopic dermatitis risk: A systematic review and meta-analysis of prospective cohort studies. *Dermatology*, *236*(4), 345–360. doi:10.1159/000503781.

McLean, S., & Sheikh, A. (2010). Does avoidance of peanuts in early life reduce the risk of peanut allergy? *BMJ (Clinical research ed.)*, *340*, c424. doi:10.1136/bmj.c424.

Munoz-Furlong, A. (2003). Daily coping strategies for patients and their families. *Pediatrics*, *111*, 1654–1661.

Nurmatov, U., Worth, A., & Sheikh, A. (2008). Anaphylaxis management plans for the acute and long-term management of anaphylaxis: A systematic review. *Journal of Allergy and Clinical Immunology*, *122*, 353–361.

Roberts, G., Bahnson, H. T., Du Toit, G., O'Rourke, C., Sever, M. L., Brittain, E., Plaut, M., & Lack, G. (2023). Defining the window of opportunity and target populations to prevent peanut allergy. *Journal of Allergy and Clinical Immunology*, *151*(5), 1329–1336. doi:10.1016/j.jaci.2022.09.042.

Rona, R. J., Keil, T., Summers, C., Gislason, D., Zuidmeer, L., Sodergren, E., Sigurdardottir, S. T., Lindner, T., Goldhahn, K., Dahlstrom, J., McBride, D., & Madsen, C. (2007). The prevalence of food allergy: A meta-analysis. *Journal of Allergy and Clinical Immunology*, *120*, 638–646.

Sampson, H. A. (2005). Food allergy: Accurately identifying clinical reactivity. *Allergy*, *60*(Suppl. 79), 19–24.

Sheikh, A., & Walker, S. (2002). Ten-minute consultation: Food allergy. *BMJ (Clinical research ed.)*, *325*, 1337.

Stiefel, G., Anagnostou, K., Boyle, R. J., Brathwaite, N., Ewan, P., Fox, A. T., Huber, P., Luyt, D., Till, S. J., Venter, C., & Clark, A. T. (2017). BSACI guideline for the diagnosis and management of peanut and tree nut allergy. *Clinical and Experimental Allergy*, *47*(6), 719–739. doi:10.1111/cea.12957.

Teuber, S. S., Beyer, K., Comstock, S., & Wallowitz, M. (2006). The big eight foods: Clinical and epidemiological overview. In S. J. Malecki, A. W. Burks, & R.M. Helm (Eds.), *Food Allergy* (pp. 49–79). Washington, DC: ASM Press.

Working Group of the Resuscitation Council (UK). (2008). *Emergency treatment of anaphylactic reactions. Guidelines for healthcare providers*. London: Resuscitation Council (UK). Retrieved from www.resus.org.uk/pages/reaction.pdf.

22
Diabetes and Endocrinology

Mohit Kumar

CHAPTER CONTENTS

Diabetes Mellitus

GUIDELINES

National Institute for Health and Care Excellence. (2016). *Type 2 diabetes: Prevention in people at high risk. NICE public health guideline 38.* Retrieved from https://www.nice.org.uk/guidance/ph38.

National Institute for Health and Care Excellence. (2019). *Diabetic foot problems: Prevention & management. NICE clinical guideline 19.* Retrieved from https://www.nice.org.uk/guidance/ng19.

National Institute for Health and Care Excellence. (2020). *Diabetes in pregnancy: Management from preconception to the postnatal period. NICE clinical guideline 3.* Retrieved from https://www.nice.org.uk/guidance/ng3.

National Institute for Health and Care Excellence. (2022a). *Type 1 diabetes in adults: Diagnosis and management. NICE clinical guideline 17.* Retrieved from https://www.nice.org.uk/guidance/ng17.

National Institute for Health and Care Excellence. (2022b). *Type 2 diabetes in adults: Management. NICE clinical guideline 28.* Retrieved from https://www.nice.org.uk/guidance/ng28.

- Diabetes mellitus has become a global epidemic with a rapidly expanding prevalence exceeding predictions. Recent UK data suggest:
  - Almost 4.3 million people are diagnosed with diabetes in the United Kingdom.
  - An estimated 850,000 are undiagnosed.
  - More than 6% of the total population are affected.
  - Current NHS expenditure for diabetes care is in the region of 10% of the total budget.
- Approximately 88% have type 2, 10% have type 1, and 2% are subgroups with secondary or other diabetes.
- There is an alarming increase in the number of children with type 2 diabetes.
- The key roles in primary care management of diabetes are:
  - Prompt recognition and diagnosis
  - Identification of at-risk individuals and intervention to prevent type 2 diabetes
  - Identification of all patients with diabetes in practice within a registry and a means for recall that enables annual review

- Prevention of microvascular and macrovascular complications through management of glycaemia and cardiovascular risk factors; with appropriate management or referral for established complications
- Encourage patient self-management
- Optimise pregnancy outcomes for patients with diabetes
- Appropriate liaison or referral to secondary care

Diagnosis

- The World Health Organization (WHO) criteria are the internationally accepted diagnostic criteria for diabetes. They are defined as:
  a. The presence of symptoms of hyperglycaemia (polyuria, polydipsia, and weight loss) with:
     - Random plasma glucose of 11.1 mmol/L or greater
     or
     - Fasting plasma glucose (FPG) of 7 mmol/L or greater
     or
     - Two-hour plasma glucose of 11.1 mmol/L or greater after a 75-g oral glucose tolerance test (OGTT)
     or
     - Glycated haemoglobin A1c (HbA1c) of 48 mmol/mol or greater (6.5%)
  b. In the absence of hyperglycaemic symptoms, a further glucose test on a separate day should be performed.
- *Impaired fasting glucose:* FPG of 6.1 to 6.9 mmol/L
- *Impaired glucose tolerance:* 2-hour OGTT of 7.8 to 11 mmol/L

Glycated Haemoglobin A1c

- The role of haemoglobin A1c (HbA1c) in diagnosis of diabetes has been recognised. However, it is less sensitive than an FPG measurement, and an HbA1c less than 48 mmol/mol (6.5%) does not exclude diabetes.
- It should *not* be used in:
  - Exclusion of suspected type 1 diabetes
  - Children
  - Short duration of osmotic symptoms (i.e., <3 months)
  - Pregnancy
  - Suspected medication-induced secondary diabetes (e.g., steroids, antipsychotics)
  - Suspected pancreatic diabetes
  - Those with haemoglobinopathies or known factors that affect red cell turnover

What Type of Diabetes?

- This question can sometimes be challenging, but some clues can make a diagnosis more likely (Table 22.1).

TABLE 22.1	Typical Features of Type 1 and 2 Diabetes	
Type 1 Diabetes	**Type 2 Diabetes**
Young age (younger than 40 years)	Generally older
Often presents in childhood	More indolent presentation
Presence of ketones	Metabolic syndrome
Acute osmotic symptoms	Obesity
Normal or low BMI	South Asian predisposition (at lower BMI)
~1 in 25 chance of developing the condition if a first-degree relative is affected	Stronger genetic predisposition
Autoantibodies present	Absence of autoantibodies
C-peptide low and eventually undetectable	C-peptide increased unless significantly advanced disease with beta-cell destruction

BMI, Body mass index.

- Other subtypes of diabetes may have features of either type 1 or type 2:
  1. Pancreatic diabetes (type 3c)
     - Known pancreatic pathology
     - Features of pancreatic exocrine dysfunction (e.g., steatorrhoea, malabsorption)
  2. Secondary diabetes
     - Associated causative agent (e.g., steroids, antipsychotics)
     - Features of endocrinopathy (e.g., acromegalic or cushingoid appearances)
  3. Latent autoimmune diabetes in adults
     - Slow and delayed presentation of type 1 diabetes
     - Autoantibodies present
     - Low and declining levels of C-peptide
     - Often misdiagnosed as type 2, particularly in patients not phenotypically type 2 diabetes
     - Quicker progression to insulin therapy than type 2
  4. Genetic diabetes (e.g., maturity onset diabetes of the young):
     - Strong family history
     - Age younger than 40 years and not requiring insulin

Primary Care Investigations

- Make the diagnosis using WHO criteria.
- Assess the need for emergency treatment:
  a. Hyperglycaemia with ketones
  b. Children with glycosuria
     - Do a point-of-care glucose test and discuss with paediatrics if the patient has hyperglycaemia.

- *Do not* wait on laboratory test results to come back and *do not* arrange for the child to come back for a second laboratory test to confirm the diagnosis regardless of symptoms.
    c. Suspicion of type 1 diabetes
    d. Blood glucose greater than 30 mmol/L
    e. Acutely unwell and hyperglycaemic
- Other tests are usually limited to secondary care
    a. C-peptide
    b. Autoantibodies (Anti-GAD/IA-2/Zn transporter 8)
    c. Genetics

Referral

- Those with type 1 diabetes are generally managed in secondary care.
- Those with type 2 diabetes are generally managed in primary care unless:
    - Significant micro- or macrovascular complications
    - Failure to reach glycaemic and blood pressure targets despite maximal therapy
    - Unclear diagnosis
    - Younger than 40 years of age
- Females with gestational diabetes or preexisting diabetes in pregnancy should be referred immediately to a combined diabetes and obstetrics team.

Type 2 Diabetes Mellitus

Screening for Type 2 Diabetes and Those at Risk

- Around 850,000 people in the United Kingdom are thought to have undiagnosed type 2 diabetes. Many patients have the disease for 7 to 10 years preceding diagnosis and present with established complications. Despite this, there is a lack of evidence to suggest population screening for type 2 diabetes is cost effective or that it would improve population health. However, high-risk individuals should be screened, including:
    - All adults aged 40 years or above, unless pregnant
    - People aged 25 to 39 years of South Asian, Chinese, Black African, African-Caribbean, or other high-risk ethnicity
    - Those with a condition known to increase risk of type 2 diabetes (e.g., polycystic ovarian syndrome (PCOS), obesity)
- National Institute of Health and Care Excellence (NICE) has published guidance on preventing type 2 diabetes in those at high risk.
- The first priority is to identify high-risk patients using a validated risk assessment tool (e.g., the Diabetes Risk Score Assessment tool, available at the Diabetes UK's website at http://www.diabetes.org.uk):
    1. Low or intermediate risk
        a. Advice on lifestyle intervention
        b. Reassurance whilst stressing that the result does not mean no risk
        c. Reassess in 5 years
    2. High risk score
        a. Perform FPG or HbA1c.
        b. Fasting blood glucose (FBG) below 5.5 mmol/L or HbA1c below 42 mmol/mol is moderate risk.
            - Inform the patient of their increased risk of developing type 2 diabetes.
            - Discuss risk factor modification.
            - Direct the patient to appropriate local weight loss or fitness programmes.
            - Reassess in 3 years.
        c. FBG of 5.5 to 6.9 mmol/L or HbA1c of 43 to 47 mmol/mol is high risk.
            - Inform the patient that they are at high risk for developing type 2 diabetes, but it is still preventable.
            - Offer referral to intensive lifestyle-change programme with emphasis on increasing physical activity to at least 150 minutes moderate activity per week, weight loss, and dietary advice to increase wholegrain foods and vegetables with a reduction in fatty foods and simple carbohydrates. Refer to a diabetes prevention programme if available.
            - Review the patient's progress and biochemistry on a minimum annual basis.
        d. FBG at or above 7 mmol/L or HbA1c at or above 48 mmol/mol:
            - If asymptomatic, retest on another day as per WHO guidelines for overt diabetes.
            - If not diagnostic of diabetes, then intervention as per high risk.

Pharmacologic Therapies in Preventing Type 2 Diabetes

- NICE suggests metformin can be used to prevent progression to type 2 diabetes in patients whose FBG and HbA1c are deteriorating despite best efforts in lifestyle intervention and in those in whom such intervention is inappropriate (especially if body mass index >35 kg/m^2).
- Orlistat can also be considered in patients progressing biochemically to type 2 diabetes with obesity in whom intensive lifestyle intervention has failed. It needs to be used alongside a low-fat (<30%) diet, and weight loss goals should be reviewed regularly to monitor effectiveness.

Management of Type 2 Diabetes

- The focus of type 2 diabetes management is ultimately to prevent development of the microvascular (retinopathy, neuropathy, nephropathy) and macrovascular (coronary artery, cerebrovascular, and peripheral vascular disease) complications associated with it. This is achieved by targeting glycaemia and controlling cardiovascular risk factors.

- At diagnosis and annual review, patients should have the following:
  a. Explanation of type 2 diabetes, complications, and means of reducing risk
  b. Weight and height
  c. Blood pressure
  d. Cardiovascular examination, including peripheral pulses
  e. Examination of the feet for neuropathy and ulcers
  f. Visual acuity
  g. Referral to national retinal screening programme
  h. Smoking status documented and advice given
  i. Discussion of oral healthcare
  j. Ask males about erectile dysfunction
  k. Mood assessed
  l. Driving status and advice with regard to Driver and Vehicle Licensing Agency (DVLA) regulations
  m. Consideration of referral to dietician and diabetes specialist nurse for education on lifestyle intervention
  n. Referral to a locally available type 2 diabetes education programme
  o. Discussion about contraception and preconception care for females of childbearing age
  p. Assessment of cardiovascular risk
- Laboratory tests should be sent for:
  a. Urea and electrolytes
  b. Glucose and HbA1c; Table 22.2 defines HbA1c units and corresponding average blood glucose levels
  c. Liver function tests (LFTs)
  d. Lipids
  e. Urinary albumin-to-creatinine ratio (ACR)
- Patients taking medication for treatment of diabetes qualify for a medical exemption certificate in the United Kingdom allowing them free prescriptions; therefore, form FP92A should be completed.

TABLE 22.2	Haemoglobin A1c in Relation to Mean Blood Glucose Levels	
Haemoglobin A1c (mmol/mol)	Haemoglobin A1c (%)	Mean Blood Glucose (mmol/L)
31	5	5.4
42	6	7.0
53	7	8.6
64	8	10.1
75	9	11.7
86	10	13.3
97	11	14.9
108	12	16.5
119	13	18.1
130	14	19.6

Glycaemic Control

- The United Kingdom Prospective Diabetes Study (UK-PDS) was a randomised control study from 1977 to 1997 that showed a 25% reduction in microvascular complications with intensive glycaemic control versus conventional targets (HbA1c 7% vs 7.9%). These risk reductions were largely seen in retinopathy and nephropathy. There was no impact on macrovascular disease outcomes from improvements in glycaemic control.
- Current guidelines advise that glycaemic targets are discussed and individualised to each patient.
- The Scottish Intercollegiate Guidelines Network (SIGN) suggests aiming for an HbA1c below 53 mmol/mol (<48 mmol/mol early in the diagnosis), and NICE suggests below 48 mmol/mol if there is no risk of hypoglycaemia.
- Relaxed targets are appropriate in some circumstances (e.g., severe hypoglycaemia risk, end-of-life care, frailty).

Treatments

- Lifestyle intervention with education on diet and physical activity should be trialled for 3 to 6 months. Discuss the aim of 5% to 10% weight loss if the patient is overweight.
- If HbA1c remains above target, then consider pharmacotherapy.
- Treatment of type 2 diabetes is becoming more complex and less algorithm based with increasing evidence emerging on the newer hypoglycaemic agents and potential cardiovascular benefits they confer.
- Optimisation of therapy takes time, and the urge to intensify therapy needs to be balanced with time to achieve desired effect. This can lead to treatment inertia, meaning patients remain suboptimally controlled for months, and in some cases years, despite further options for treatment intensification. To minimise this, review of therapy at least every 3 months is suggested until HbA1c is within target.

Metformin and First Intensification of Treatment

- This remains the first-line oral agent for glycaemic control in type 2 diabetes.
- It is cost effective and has data showing cardiovascular benefits (UKPDS).
- Biguanide: The mechanism of action not entirely understood, but it decreases hepatic gluconeogenesis and improves insulin sensitivity.
- Start with 500 mg/day and titrate to a maximum tolerated dose of 2 g/day (standard release).
- Patients may experience gastrointestinal (GI) side effects and should be reassured that these are often mild and should settle. A modified-release preparation may be helpful.
- Risk of lactic acidosis may require a break from therapy during acute illness.

- Contraindications are severe liver failure and renal failure with estimated glomerular filtration rate (eGFR) less than 30 mL/min (with dose reduction at higher eGFR).
- After metformin tolerability has been established, irrespective of HbA1c reduction, a sodium–glucose cotransporter-2 (SGLT2) inhibitor should be added for all patients with:
  - Chronic heart failure
  - Atherosclerotic cardiovascular disease (CVD)
  - High cardiovascular risk (QRISK 2 >10% if age 40 years or older or presence of one or more cardiovascular risk factor if age older than 40 years)
- If metformin is not tolerated, an SGLT2 inhibitor (see later) should be commenced as the first-line treatment.
- Further treatment intensification may be with sulphonylurea, pioglitazone, a (dipeptidyl peptidase-4 DPP-4) inhibitor, or a glucagon-like peptide-1 (GLP-1) agonist.
- Insulin therapy may be considered at any point when the HbA1c is below the agreed target.

Sodium–Glucose Cotransporter 2 Inhibitors

- These include empagliflozin, dapagliflozin, and canagliflozin.
- They act by blocking the SGLT2 receptor in the proximal tubule of the kidneys, preventing reabsorption of glucose and water, resulting in glycosuria.
- *Benefits:* weight loss, reduction in blood pressure, and absence of hypoglycaemia unless used with other hypoglycaemic agents. Additional benefits from clinical trials include reduction in cardiovascular mortality, improvement in heart failure, and renoprotection. This cardiorenal protection has led to the promotion of SGLT2 inhibitors in NICE (and multiple other) guidelines.
- *Side effects:* volume depletion, hypotension, electrolyte disturbance, genitourinary infections, ketoacidosis.
- Ketoacidosis has been reported in patients with type 2 diabetes taking an SGLT2 inhibitor, even at near-normal glucose levels (euglycaemic diabetic ketoacidosis). Patients need to be counselled on symptoms of ketoacidosis (nausea, vomiting, abdominal pain, anorexia) and advised to seek medical attention if they develop these. Sick day rules of drug breaks whilst unwell should be discussed.
- *Contraindications:* renal impairment depending on level and agent, history of ketoacidosis, and recurrent genitourinary sepsis.
- Use with caution in patients at increased risk of volume depletion.

Sulphonylurea

- The most commonly used is gliclazide. It works by stimulating pancreatic insulin secretion. Side effects include hypoglycaemia and weight gain. Contraindications include eGFR below 30 mL/min because of the risk of severe hypoglycaemia.

- The typical starting dosage is 80 mg once daily, titrated to a maximum of 160 mg twice daily. A lower dosage of 40 mg/day should be given if there is concern for hypoglycaemia.
- Patients should be made aware of the symptoms of hypoglycaemia and be trained to check their own blood sugars at relevant times.
- DVLA restrictions should be discussed.

Dipeptidyl Peptidase-4 Inhibitors

- Options include saxagliptin, sitagliptin, linagliptin, alogliptin, and vildagliptin. The choice between these should be based on local policy.
- Incretin-based therapy blocks DPP-4, preventing inactivation of GLP-1 and subsequent inhibition of glucagon release, increased insulin secretion from the pancreas, and decreased gastric emptying. These events lead to reduced blood glucose levels.
- Expected to reduce HbA1c by approximately 0.5%.
- *Benefits:* weight neutral, low risk of hypoglycaemia unless used with insulin or sulphonylurea.
- *Side effects:* GI side effects, nasopharyngitis, pancreatitis. Dose adjustment is needed for renal impairment with exception of linagliptin. Although there are no data to suggest increase in cardiovascular death associated with DPP-4 use, given current conflicting data, they should be used with caution in those at high risk of heart failure.

Pioglitazone

- Thiazolidinedione is a peroxisome proliferator-activated receptor-γ agonist that decreases peripheral insulin resistance.
- It decreases triglycerides but increases high-density lipoprotein and low-density lipoprotein cholesterol.
- The dosage is 15 to 45 mg once daily.
- *Side effects:* fluid retention, weight gain, increased risk of heart failure, small increased risk of bladder cancer, increased risk of bone fractures, and liver dysfunction.
- *Contraindications:* preexisting heart failure or high risk of heart failure, previous or active bladder cancer or significant family history of bladder cancer, hepatic impairment, haematuria of unknown aetiology.
- Use with caution in those at risk of falls or at increased risk of bone fracture (e.g., osteoporosis).
- Monitor liver function before treatment, after 2 months, and periodically thereafter.

Glucagon-Like Peptide 1 Agonists

- These include liraglutide, dulaglutide, and semaglutide, all of which are injectable. Oral semaglutide is available. They work by enhancing pancreatic insulin secretion in a glucose-dependent manner, inhibiting glucagon release, and delaying gastric emptying, thus promoting satiety.
- There are various regimens from twice-daily injection to once weekly.

- *Benefits:* promotes weight loss whilst reducing hyperglycaemia, low risk of hypoglycaemia if not used alongside insulin or sulphonylureas.
- *Side effects:* GI side effects that may be intolerable, skin reactions at injection sites, pancreatitis, theoretical risk of increased pancreatic and medullary thyroid cancer but not proven.
- *Contraindications:* gastroparesis, pancreatic pathology, previous or preexisting thyroid cancer, hepatic impairment.
- They are expensive.
    - Most health boards have specific criteria to monitor effectiveness of treatment before funding for more than 6 months.
    - NICE suggests a minimum HbA1c reduction of 1% AND weight loss of 3% or more be achieved within 6 months of starting treatment, or therapy should be discontinued.
    - Cardiovascular outcome trials have also shown significant cardiovascular benefit of GLP-1 agonist therapy in the LEADER (Liraglutide and Cardiovascular Outcomes in Type 2 Diabetes), SUSTAIN-6 (Semaglutide and Cardiovascular Outcomes in Patients with Type 2 Diabetes) and REWIND (Dulaglutide and cardiovascular outcomes in type 2 diabetes) trials.

Dual GLP-1/GIP Receptor Agonist
- Tirzepatide is a novel drug in this class.
- Once weekly injection, starting at 2.5 mg and titrated up monthly.
- *Benefits:* weight loss and hyperglycaemia reduction (both in excess of GLP-1 receptor agonists) without risk of hypoglycaemia if not used alongside insulin or sulphonylurea.
- Side effects as per GLP1 agonists – GI symptoms, pancreatitis, gall stone disease, hypersensitivity reactions, theoretical risk of pancreatitis and medullary thyroid cancer.
- *Contraindications:* gastroparesis, pancreatic pathology. There is limited data in patients with severe hepatic and renal impairment. Caution should be exercised if used in patients with non-proliferative retinopathy requiring therapy, proliferative retinopathy and macular oedema.
- Cardiovascular outcome trial data is awaited.
- NICE recommended if
    - Triple oral therapy is not tolerated, ineffective or contraindicated, and
    - BMI of 35 kg/m^2 or more with comorbidities associated with obesity, or
    - BMI less than 35 where insulin therapy would affect occupation or tirzepatide therapy would improve other weight associated comorbidities.

Insulin
- Once-daily neutral protamine Hagedorn (NPH) insulin is usually sufficient for initiation of insulin in patients with type 2 diabetes.

- A total daily dose of 0.3 to 0.5 units/kg is a reasonable starting dose (maximum first dose, 10 units).
- Metformin should continue.
- Other hypoglycaemic agents should be reviewed for continuation, stopping, or dose adjustment.
- Insulin analogues such as detemir and glargine may be preferred for those at risk of overnight or severe hypoglycaemia.
- If NPH insulin is insufficient, twice-daily mixed preparations can be tried.
- Before starting insulin, the patient must:
    a. Have education on insulin administration and blood glucose monitoring from a diabetes educator.
    b. Have open access to a clinician capable of advising on dose adjustments during initiation.
    c. Know how to recognise and treat hypoglycaemia.
    d. Discuss driving regulations and occupational hazards.

Other Therapies
- *Meglitinides* can be used for patients intolerant to sulphonylurea.
    - Similar to sulphonylureas
    - More expensive
- Acarbose
    - Blocks intestinal alpha glucosidase, preventing starchy compounds being broken down to simple sugars.
    - Not as effective, and intolerable GI side effects can occur.

Home Glucose Monitoring

- Required for *all* patients taking insulin and for patients taking sulphonylurea who drive or are at risk of hypoglycaemia.
- It is not generally required for patients with type 2 diabetes on other regimens unless they are planning pregnancy. It may be considered if starting corticosteroid treatment or to confirm suspected hypoglycaemia.
- Intermittently scanned continuous glucose monitoring (isCGM or 'Flash') (e.g., Freestyle Libre) has been approved for patients with:
    - Recurrent or severe hypoglycaemia
    - Impaired hypoglycaemia awareness
    - A condition or disability meaning they cannot undertake capillary blood glucose monitoring but could use isCGM
    - They would otherwise need to undertake capillary monitoring eight times per day or more

Hypoglycaemia
- All patients taking insulin or sulphonylurea should be educated on the symptoms of hypoglycaemia and how to treat it.
- They should be advised to check their blood glucose to confirm hypoglycaemia (<4 mmol/L) if they have symptoms.
- If conscious and swallow safe, then they should take 15 to 20 g of oral glucose e.g.:
    - 200 mL fresh fruit juice

- Four jelly babies
- Four or five dextrose tablets
- Blood glucose should be rechecked 15 minutes later and treatment repeated if needed.
- When resolved, the patient should eat some complex carbohydrate (e.g., sandwich).
- If unconscious or swallow not safe, the caregiver should give intramuscular (IM) glucagon 1 mg and call an ambulance.
- Medically trained staff will be able to administer intravenous (IV) glucose (150 mL 10% glucose or 75 mL 20% glucose).
- Identify and correct the cause of hypoglycaemia.

Sick Day Rules for Patients on Insulin Therapy

- If possible, patients should keep up their dietary intake.
- If unable, oral fluids are important to prevent dehydration.
- A trial of easily digested foods (soup, jelly) may be effective.
- Check blood glucose at least every 4 hours.
- *Do not* omit insulin therapy.
- If hypoglycaemia occurs, treat with sugary drinks.
- If the patient has refractory hypoglycaemia, seek medical advice.
- If blood glucose above 15 mmol/L, check for ketones.
- If ketones are positive, administer 10% of total daily insulin dose in short-acting insulin and repeat blood glucose and ketones after 2 hours. If not resolving, repeat the step, but if worsening, seek medical help.
- If the patient has hyperglycaemia but no ketones, they can give a correction dose of short-acting insulin. A correction dose can be calculated as 100/total daily insulin dose. For example, a patient taking 50 units of insulin per day would have a correction dose of 2 units, assuming that 1 unit of insulin will correct blood glucose by 2 mmol/L.
- This can be repeated after 2 hours also, but if worsening, seek medical advice.

Blood Pressure Management

- *Targets*
  - SIGN suggests targeted blood pressure below 130/80 mm Hg for all patients with diabetes.
  - NICE suggests targets of below 135/85 mm Hg (or <130/80 mm Hg if the patient has nephropathy with albuminuria). A target of 145/85mm Hg may be acceptable in patients older than 80 years of age.
  - The UKPDS study showed every 10–mm Hg reduction in systolic blood pressure reduced 10-year risk of cardiovascular death by 15%.
  - Intensive blood pressure control to these targets reduces the development of microvascular complications.
  - Further intensification to below these values is not recommended (ACCORD Action to Control Cardio-

vascular Risk in Diabetes Study Group. Effects of intensive blood pressure control in type 2 diabetes).
- Treatments
  - An angiotensin-converting enzyme (ACE) inhibitor is first-line therapy, in addition to intensive lifestyle intervention. If intolerant, an angiotensin receptor blocker (ARB) should be used instead.
  - Calcium channel blockers or thiazide-like diuretics should be added as second-line treatment.
  - Blood pressure should be monitored once or twice monthly until consistently within target.

Other Cardiovascular Risk Factors

Lipids

- Statin therapy should be offered to all patients with diabetes whose 10-year cardiovascular risk is 10% or more, regardless of cholesterol level. This generally includes all patients with diabetes aged older than 40 years and younger patients with microvascular complications.
- Primary prevention doses are:
  - Atorvastatin 20 mg (NICE)
  - Simvastatin 40 mg or atorvastatin 10 mg (SIGN)
- Secondary prevention doses are higher, with atorvastatin 80 mg recommended.

Antiplatelet Therapy

- This is not recommended for primary prevention.

Smoking

- All patients should be advised to stop and be referred to smoking cessation services.

Diabetic Nephropathy

- Microalbuminuria is the first sign of diabetic kidney disease and is associated with increased cardiovascular morbidity and mortality.
- It is defined as:
  - 24-hour urinary albumin of 30 to 300 mg
  - Urinary ACR greater than 2.5 mg/mmol in males (>3.5 mg/mmol in females)
- Overt diabetic nephropathy is defined by an ACR above 30 mg/mmol and is a strong indicator of cardiovascular risk and progression to end-stage renal failure.
- Urinary ACR and eGFR should be monitored at least annually in patients aged 12 years and older with diabetes.
- If microalbuminuria present, an ACE inhibitor should be started irrespective of blood pressure because it will slow progression to overt nephropathy and can reverse microalbuminuria.
- An SGLT2 inhibitor should be considered if not already administered and there are no contraindications.
- The addition of finerenone after the use of ACE inhibitor or ARB plus SGLT2 inhibitor is recommended

if the patient has chronic kidney disease stage 3 or 4 with albuminuria (if eGFR $\geq$25 mL/min/m^2) to reduce the risk of progression of renal disease and reduce the risk of cardiovascular disease.
- Intensive glycaemic and blood pressure control is vital to preventing progression.

Diabetic Retinopathy and Maculopathy

- Up to 40% of patients with type 2 diabetes have retinopathy at diagnosis.
- All patients with type 2 diabetes should undergo retinal screening at diagnosis and at least annually thereafter.
- Retinal screening is best performed as part of the national screening programme using digital photography.
- Fundoscopy is not reliable.
- Retinopathy is defined as:
  - Background retinopathy
  - Preproliferative retinopathy
  - Proliferative retinopathy
- Proliferative or referable preproliferative retinopathy should be referred to an ophthalmologist.
- Urgent referral should be given if neovascularisation is near the macula or there is associated vitreous haemorrhage.
- Those with macular oedema should also be referred urgently.
- Intensive blood pressure and glycaemic control should be targeted to prevent progression, and patients must stop smoking.

Diabetic Foot Disease and Neuropathy

- The principal risk factors for the development of foot ulceration in patients with diabetes are neuropathy and peripheral vascular disease.
- All patients with diabetes should have their feet screened at diagnosis and then at least annually and if any foot problems occur. Assessment must include the peripheral circulation (pulses), sensation (with a 10-g monofilament), the presence of structural abnormalities, and any history of previous ulceration. The feet should be risk stratified (low, moderate, high, or active foot disease) and a management plan discussed.
- Foot care education should be given to all patients with diabetes. It is important to discuss the person's current risk of developing foot problems and who to contact if a foot emergency should arise. Moderate- and high-risk feet should have input from the foot protection service.
- All patients with active ulceration and signs of sepsis, ulceration with critical limb ischaemia, gangrene, or deep-seated soft tissue or bone infection should be referred urgently to the acute hospital and the multidisciplinary foot care service informed.

- For all other active foot problems and suspected Charcot foot (swelling, redness, and warmth of a foot with or without pain, especially if the skin is intact), refer urgently to the multidisciplinary foot care service.
- For the management of neuropathic pain, NICE recommends offering a choice of amitriptyline, duloxetine, gabapentin, or pregabalin initially. If one is not effective or tolerated, then one of the remaining three agents should be offered.

Erectile Dysfunction

- Erectile dysfunction is common and a marker of underlying CVD.
- Ask about symptoms at annual review and offer a phosphodiesterase type 5 inhibitor if the patient has no contraindications.
- If pharmacologic therapy is unhelpful, refer to a local erectile dysfunction service.
- Testosterone therapy is controversial and should not be commenced without consulting an endocrinologist. If a testosterone deficiency is suspected, the fasting morning testosterone level should be checked on two occasions to confirm.

Driving Regulations

- In the United Kingdom, patients treated with insulin may hold a group 1 (car or motorcycle) or a group 2 (lorry or bus) licence; however, the DVLA must be informed. Group 1 licences are reviewed every 3 years or sooner in the context of any of these events:
  - More than one severe hypoglycaemic attack (requiring third-party assistance) in the preceding 12 months whilst awake for group 1 licence holders
  - Impaired hypoglycaemic awareness
  - Vision below the minimum eyesight standards (because of any condition)
  - Neuropathy or peripheral vascular disease that impacts on their ability to drive a standard manual car
- Requirements for patients holding a group 2 licence are tighter, and assessment is annual. In addition, the DVLA needs to be informed if:
  - The patient is taking any medication for diabetes regardless of its perceived hypoglycaemic risk.
  - Even only one severe hypoglycaemic attack has occurred in a 12-month period, which must be reported immediately.
  - Proof of blood glucose monitoring to demonstrate acceptable control and at times appropriate to driving must be available. Three months of such monitoring (on a downloadable glucometer with date and time function) is reviewed by the patient's doctor before renewal of the patient's licence).

General Advice for Driving With Diabetes

- Check blood glucose immediately before driving.
- Aim to be above 5 mmol/L before commencing driving.
- Check blood glucose every 2 hours as a minimum on long journeys but sooner if there are symptoms of hypoglycaemia.
- Keep quick-acting carbohydrate in the car at all times to enable prompt treatment.
- Provide follow-up treatment of hypoglycaemia with complex carbohydrate (e.g., sandwich).
- If blood glucose is below 4 mmol/L at any point, turn off the engine, remove the keys, leave the driver's seat, treat the hypoglycaemia, and do not resume driving until at least 45 minutes after a blood glucose above 5 mmol/L has been achieved and the patient feels well enough to continue safely.

Gestational Diabetes

GUIDELINE

National Institute for Health and Care Excellence. (2020). *Diabetes in pregnancy: Management from pre-conception to the postnatal period. NICE clinical guideline 3.* Retrieved from https://www.nice.org.uk/guidance/ng3.

- Gestational diabetes mellitus (GDM) is defined as glucose intolerance with onset or first recognition during pregnancy. Maternal risk factors for GDM are shown in Table 22.3; females should be assessed for these factors in early pregnancy and if present should be offered screening with a 75-g OGTT at 24 to 28 weeks of gestation or earlier if they have a history of GDM in a previous pregnancy.

Screening and Diagnosis

- Current treatment of GDM is influenced by a number of large clinical trials showing that treatment of GDM with insulin improves pregnancy outcomes, including birthweight and macrosomia, and demonstrating a continuum of risk for maternal glucose levels and adverse pregnancy outcomes.

TABLE 22.3 Risk Factors for Gestational Diabetes

Body mass index (BMI) >30 kg/m²

Previous macrosomic baby weighing ≥4.5 kg

Previous gestational diabetes mellitus

Family history of diabetes (first-degree relative with diabetes)

Minority ethnic family origin with a high prevalence of diabetes

TABLE 22.4 Diagnostic Criteria for Gestational Diabetes Mellitus

	IADPSG	NICE
Fasting plasma glucose (mmol/L)	≥5.1	≥5.6
1-hour glucose (mmol/L)	≥10	
2-hour glucose (mmol/L)	≥8.5	≥7.8

IADPSG, International Association of the Diabetes and Pregnancy Study Groups; *NICE*, National Institute of Health and Care Excellence.

- The optimal way to diagnose GDM, however, remains controversial. The most widely adopted diagnostic criteria were developed by the International Association of the Diabetes and Pregnancy Study Groups, and these criteria have been endorsed by various other bodies, including the American Diabetes Association. In 2015, NICE updated its guidelines with diagnostic criteria as outlined in Table 22.4.
- The majority of centres in the United Kingdom use these criteria; other centres, particularly in the United States, use alternative criteria, including two-step approaches using a 50-g and then 100-g OGTT.

Treatment

- After being diagnosed with GDM, patients should be taught to undertake blood sugar monitoring to assess fasting and postprandial glycaemia and to guide treatment. Dietary modification is the mainstay of treatment, and all patients should be seen by a dietician as soon as possible after diagnosis. Other lifestyle advice, including exercise, should be offered.
- Metformin is used in the majority of females who fail to reach their glycaemic targets with diet alone. Although it crosses the placenta, it is thought to be safe for use in pregnancy, with no significant effect on perinatal development. Approximately 50% of females treated with metformin will require additional therapy with insulin.
- Insulin therapy is used in females who fail to reach glycaemic targets with dietary measures or with metformin and in those for whom metformin is not tolerated. Undiagnosed type 2 diabetes should be considered in females with a fasting glucose of 7 mmol/L or greater or 2-hour glucose of 11mmol/L or greater; these patients should be treated initially with insulin, with or without metformin.
- Glibenclamide, a sulphonylurea, does not cross the placenta in significant amounts and has been used in a number of studies in pregnancy, although there has been limited data on long-term pregnancy outcomes.

Issues After Pregnancy

- After pregnancy, the majority of patients with GDM no longer require any treatment.
- Patients should be advised of the risk of GDM in all subsequent pregnancies and to seek medical advice if further pregnancy is desired.
- Patients should be offered testing at 6 weeks postpartum and annual testing thereafter to assess for underlying type 2 diabetes.

Type 1 and Type 2 Diabetes in Pregnancy

- Type 1 and type 2 diabetes are associated with a number of adverse foetal and maternal outcomes, including congenital malformations, preeclampsia, miscarriage, and macrosomia.
- Females with preexisting diabetes should be referred for prepregnancy counselling and have regular checks of HbA1c, aiming for HbA1c below 48 mmol/mol (6.5%) before conception. Females with HbA1c greater than 86 mmol/mol (10%) should be advised against pregnancy. High-dose folic acid should be commenced, and medications such as statins and ACE inhibitors should be stopped before considering pregnancy. In females with type 2 diabetes, the safety of modern medications such as DPP-4 inhibitors, SGLT-2 inhibitors, and GLP-1 analogues has not been studied extensively in pregnancy, and these medications should be stopped before pregnancy. Insulin is usually required in this case.
- To help reduce the risk of preeclampsia, females should be treated with aspirin 150mg/day from 12 weeks of gestation.

Thyroid Disease

GUIDELINES

National Institute for Health and Care Excellence. (2020).*Thyroid disease: Assessment and management. NICE clinical guideline 145.* Retrieved from https://www.nice.org.uk/guidance/ng145.
National Institute for Health and Care Excellence. (2022). *Thyroid cancer: Assessment and management. NICE clinical guideline 230.* Retrieved from https://www.nice.org.uk/guidance/ng230.

- Thyroid disease is common. Thyroid function tests (TFTs) are among the most frequently requested tests in primary care, and an understanding of how to interpret them and what to do next is essential for daily working as a general practitioner.
- Most laboratories report thyroid-stimulating hormone (TSH) and free thyroxine (T_4) as standard, but some include total T_4 and triiodothyronine (T_3). T_4 and to a lesser extent T_3 are bound in plasma by thyroid-binding globulin, and the unbound component is physiologically active. T_3 is more active than T_4.

Hypothyroidism

- Symptoms include lethargy, weight gain, cold intolerance, muscle cramps, slowed cognition, constipation, dry hair and skin, hoarse voice, and fluid retention.
- Severely hypothyroid patients may present with:
  - Myxoedematous appearance—periorbital puffiness, macroglossia, thin hair
  - Cardiac failure
  - Hypothermia
  - Peripheral neuropathy
  - Encephalopathy
  - Coma

Primary Hypothyroidism

- Primary hypothyroidism is most common and results from the failure of the thyroid to produce adequate thyroid hormone. Biochemically, it is high TSH and low T_4.
- Causes include:
  - Autoimmune (Hashimoto): thyroid peroxidase (TPO) antibody positive, usually with goitre
  - After radioiodine therapy or thyroid surgery
  - Iodine deficiency (endemic goitre)
  - Postradiotherapy to the head or neck
  - Congenital
  - Drugs: lithium, amiodarone, chemotherapy agents

Secondary Hypothyroidism

- Secondary hypothyroidism is caused by failure of the pituitary gland to produce TSH. Results in low (or inappropriately normal) TSH with low T_4. It is usually associated with other pituitary hormone deficiencies.
- Causes
  - Pituitary tumours
  - After pituitary surgery or radiotherapy
  - Postcranial irradiation
  - Empty sella
  - Rarer pituitary disorders (e.g., infiltrative, infarction or haemorrhage)
- In secondary hypothyroidism, exclude cortisol deficiency as a matter of urgency. Do not initiate thyroid replacement until glucocorticoid deficiency is excluded.

Investigations in Primary Care

a. TFTs
b. TPO antibodies for primary hypothyroid (once only)
c. Urgent 9 am cortisol level if secondary hypothyroid or refer for *urgent* short Synacthen test if high suspicion of glucocorticoid deficiency
d. Full blood count for associated anaemia and macrocytosis
e. Urea and electrolytes for hyponatraemia

Treatment

- Give levothyroxine. In younger patients without cardiac disease, give 1.6 µg/kg rounded to the nearest 25 µg. For older, comorbid patients and those with

heart disease, 25 to 50 µg should be started with gradual titration.
- Repeat TFTs 6 weeks after initiation and titrate the dose in 25- to 50-µg increments. Repeat testing and dose escalation should not occur before this. Aim for normal TSH and T_4. In females planning pregnancy, the target TSH for the first trimester should be aimed for.
- In secondary hypothyroidism, the TSH should not be used to guide treatment. T_4 should be aimed to be in the upper half of the reference range.
- T_3 therapy is controversial, and there is little evidence to suggest greater benefit than T_4, A small number of patients report improved symptoms.
- Despite normalisation of TFTs, patients may complain of symptoms. Levothyroxine should not be increased.
- Review medications because some drugs can affect absorption of thyroxine (antacids, proton pump inhibitors, iron).

Referral
- Most primary hypothyroidism is managed in primary care.
- Refer:
  a. All secondary hypothyroidism
  b. Primary hypothyroidism
     - Paediatric patients
     - High doses (i.e., >200 µg/day) when compliance is good
     - Large goitre causing obstructive symptoms
     - Pregnancy or within 6 months postpartum

Subclinical Hypothyroidism
- High TSH but normal T_4
- Treatment still debated but generally accepted if:
  - TSH is above 10 mU/L or the patient has symptoms
  - Repeated testing trending towards overt hypothyroidism
  - Consider if significant cardiac disease
- A 6-month trial may be considered if the patient is younger than 65 years of age.
- It is more likely to adopt a wait-and-see approach in older adult patients because TSH increases with age.

Hyperthyroidism
- Symptoms: flushes, anxiety, tremor, palpitations, heat intolerance, loose stools, oligomenorrhoea, hair loss, eye symptoms in Graves disease

Primary Hyperthyroidism
- Suppressed TSH, high T_4, and/or high T_3
- Causes
  - Graves disease: positive TSH-receptor antibodies (TRAB) usually; TRAB-negative variant also with typical features on thyroid imaging
  - Toxic multinodular goitre
  - Toxic nodule

- Thyroiditis: subacute de Quervain, postpartum
- Drug induced: amiodarone
- Factitious: thyroxine abuse
- Very rarely thyroid cancer

Secondary Hyperthyroidism
- Secondary is very rare
- Causes:
  - TSH-oma
  - Thyroid hormone resistance
- Results in normal or high TSH with high T_4/T_3 ratio

Graves Disease
- Autoimmune thyrotoxicosis with diffuse goitre
- Associated with TRAB antibodies
- Associated eye symptoms:
  - Gritty, dry eyes
  - Pain
  - Proptosis and eyelid lag
  - Periorbital oedema
  - Diplopia or ophthalmoplegia
  - Altered colour vision
  - Visual loss

Investigations in Primary Care
a. TFTs
b. TRAB and TPO antibodies
c. Ultrasound only if concern about thyroid cancer

Treatment
- Nonselective beta-blockers can be used for symptom management.
- Consider starting antithyroid treatment. Pregnancy needs to be discussed in females of childbearing age (risk of treatment vs uncontrolled thyrotoxicosis); pregnancy should ideally be avoided.
- Patients with thyroiditis do not usually require antithyroid treatment, and prescribing it may precipitate profound hypothyroidism.

Antithyroid Drugs
- These are usually first-line treatment in autoimmune disease. Patients typically receive 12 to 18 months of antithyroid therapy before a trial off it.
- Carbimazole
  - Varying doses from 10 to 40 mg/day depending on the severity of thyrotoxicosis and response to treatment
  - Counsel patients about the risk of agranulocytosis:
    a. Stop therapy and seek urgent medical attention if you have a severe sore throat, mouth ulcers, or fever.
    b. An urgent full blood count should be taken to ensure that the white blood cell count is normal; and if so, the patient can recommence treatment.
- Propylthiouracil (PTU)
  - Used in the first trimester of pregnancy or if intolerant to carbimazole.

- The dosage is 200 to 400 mg/day in divided doses initially.
- Lower risk of agranulocytosis than carbimazole.
- Hepatitis more common.
- Check LFTs 4 to 6 weeks after initiating treatment and periodically thereafter. Discontinue and seek advice if results are abnormal.
- Monitor TFTs every 6 to 8 weeks until the patient is euthyroid and every 3 months thereafter while the patient is on maintenance therapy.

Radioactive Iodine
- Given to those who relapse or show resistance to antithyroid medication
- Likely required in toxic nodular disease
- High risk of hypothyroidism after treatment
- Not suitable for carers of young children or in pregnancy because of radiation risks

Thyroid Surgery
- This is frequently used if planning pregnancy or if the patient has thyroid eye disease or large goitre.
- The patient will need levothyroxine after surgery.
- Other risks include recurrent laryngeal nerve damage, hypoparathyroidism, haemorrhage, and infection.

Referral
- All patients with hyperthyroidism should be referred.
- Patients with Graves disease who become pregnant should be referred to endocrinology and obstetrics as early as possible.
- Patients with sight-threatening thyroid eye disease should be referred as an emergency to an ophthalmologist:
  - Globe subluxation
  - Symptoms of corneal ulceration
  - Visual loss
  - Impaired colour vision

Thyroid Nodules
- Thyroid cancer is rare (<1% of all cancers).
- TFTs are usually (but not always) normal in thyroid cancer.
- Increasing concern if:
  - Rapid growth
  - Larger than 1 cm
  - Lymphadenopathy
- All patients with thyroid nodules should be referred.
- Followed up at least annually by endocrinology or oncology:
  - The target TSH is based on Dynamic Risk Stratification done after surgery with or without radioiodine therapy.

Sick Euthyroid Syndrome
- Ideally, TFTs should not be checked in those with acute or subacute illness.

- Typically, there is inappropriately normal or suppressed TSH with low T_4/T_3 ratio, but various patterns are seen.
- Any decision to commence treatment in such cases needs monitoring closely.

Thyroid Disease in Pregnancy
- Females with hypo- or hyperthyroidism should be referred to endocrinology as soon as pregnancy is confirmed.
- Females with hypothyroidism should increase their levothyroxine dose by 25% to 30% as soon as pregnancy confirmed:
  - Target TSH is less than 2.5 mU/L in the first trimester.
  - TSH levels are normally lower in the first trimester because of biochemical similarities to human chorionic gonadotropin (hCG).
  - Diagnosis and treatment of patients with subclinical hypothyroidism in pregnancy are controversial.
- Females with hyperthyroidism usually require smaller doses of antithyroid medication and may be able to stop it in pregnancy:
  - PTU is preferred in the first trimester because of the higher risk of teratogenicity associated with carbimazole.
  - TRAB antibodies should be checked in pregnancy in females with a history of Graves disease; if the results are positive, there is a risk of neonatal Graves disease.
  - Females with Graves disease are at risk of recurrence in the postnatal period; TFTs should be checked 4 to 6 weeks after delivery.

Hypoadrenalism

REVIEWS AND GUIDANCE

Bornstein, S. R., Allolio, B., Arlt, W., Barthel, A., Don-Wauchope, A., Hammer, G. D., Husebye, E. S., Merke, D. P., Murad, M. H., Stratakis, C. A., & Torpy, D. J. (2016). Diagnosis and Treatment of Primary Adrenal Insufficiency: An Endocrine Society Clinical Practice Guideline. *Journal of Clinical Endocrinology & Metabolism, 101*(2), 364–389. https://doi.org/10.1210/jc.2015-1710.
Charmandari, E., Nicolaides, N. C., & Chrousos, G. P. (2014). Adrenal insufficiency. *Lancet, 383*, 2152–2167.

- Hypoadrenalism can be primary (most commonly autoimmune or Addisons disease), secondary (most commonly hypopituitarism caused by pituitary adenoma), or tertiary (most commonly exogenous glucocorticoid administration).
- Fatigue is a presenting feature common to all causes. Patients with primary hypoadrenalism may demonstrate skin pigmentation (increased adrenocorticotropic hormone (ACTH) levels) and symptoms of mineralocorticoid deficiency. In secondary and tertiary hypoadrenalism,

mineralocorticoid secretion is normal; therefore, plasma potassium levels are normal.

- All causes can present with a hypoadrenal crisis; symptoms consist of abdominal pain, vomiting, dehydration, and hypotension. This is a medical emergency.
- *Primary hypoadrenalism*
  - Prevalence has increased in recent years, likely because of an increase in autoimmune hypoadrenalism cases.
  - It is more common in females than males.
  - The incidence peaks between 30 and 50 years of age.
- *Secondary hypoadrenalism*
  - More common than primary hypoadrenalism
  - Tends to present at a later age, around 60 years
- *Tertiary hypoadrenalism*
  - Patients receiving oral glucocorticoid treatment for more than 2 weeks are at risk; therapy should not be stopped abruptly.
  - Inhaled, topical, intramuscular, and intraarticular steroids may also cause tertiary hypoadrenalism.

Diagnosis

- Measure serum cortisol levels before and after stimulation with synthetic ACTH (Synacthen). Patients should not be taking any form of exogenous steroids. False-negative results can occur in acute secondary or tertiary hypoadrenalism. (The adrenal glands take time to atrophy, and response to ACTH is preserved in the short term.) The cutoff for diagnosis varies according to the assay used and should be confirmed locally.
- Differentiating between primary, secondary, and tertiary hypoadrenalism is based on history (drug history, presence of other autoimmune conditions, family history), and further investigations may include plasma ACTH levels, aldosterone and renin measurements, adrenal androgens, adrenal autoantibodies, and depending on clinical suspicion, pituitary function tests or adrenal or pituitary imaging. These are undertaken by the endocrine team.

Treatment

- Glucocorticoid replacement is given, most commonly with hydrocortisone (complete form FP92A to exempt prescription charges in the United Kingdom) in divided doses mimicking a diurnal rhythm (e.g., 10 mg, 5 mg, 5 mg). Prednisolone at 3 to 5 mg/day is sometimes used.
- Mineralocorticoid replacement is only required in those with primary adrenal insufficiency and is not needed if the daily dose of hydrocortisone is greater than 50 mg.
- Adrenal androgen replacement is not currently recommended in the United Kingdom because of a lack of evidence regarding efficacy.
- In the United Kingdom, all patients should be given the NHS steroid emergency card.

- All patients should be educated in sick day rules:
  a. Take a double or triple hydrocortisone dose during intercurrent illnesses. This needs to be reduced slowly if illness persists for more than a few days.
  b. Seek medical assistance if vomiting or unable to tolerate oral hydrocortisone treatment and wear a medic alert bracelet or carry a steroid card.
  c. Have IM hydrocortisone (100 mg) for self-administration in case of emergencies; patients should be familiar in how and when to use it.
  d. Inform medical staff promptly of steroid dependence if they are unwell or undergoing invasive procedures so timely replacement treatment can be initiated.
- Abrupt cessation of steroids can precipitate adrenal crisis; patients should always be prescribed and dispensed adequate amounts of hydrocortisone to cover holiday periods and sick days.
- Monitoring of treatment is usually undertaken by specialist endocrine team and involves assessing adequacy of replacement while minimising the risks of overreplacement (hypertension, diabetes, reduced bone mineral density).
- Adrenal crisis is a life-threatening emergency that requires prompt treatment. Give 100 mg of hydrocortisone IM or IV and urgent referral to hospital.

Hypercalcaemia

> **GUIDELINE**
>
> National Institute for Health and Care Excellence. (2019). *Primary hyperparathyroidism: Diagnosis, assessment and initial management.* NICE clinical guideline 132. Retrieved from https://www.nice.org.uk/guidance/ng132.

- Calcium is the most abundant mineral and has vital roles in cellular function, cardiovascular stability, and bone health. It is under homeostatic control of parathyroid hormone (PTH), with lesser roles for vitamin D and magnesium. Approximately half is bound to albumin in blood, and it is the unbound component that is physiologically active. Levels need to be corrected to albumin concentration as a result.
- Normal levels of corrected calcium are 2.2 to 2.6 mmol/L.
- Severe hypercalcaemia is generally considered at 3 mmol/L and above, but symptoms or end-organ damage at lower levels can occur.

Symptoms

- Thirst
- Frequent urination
- Bony pain
- Nausea and vomiting
- Constipation
- Renal colic

- Lethargy
- Confusion
- Altered mood

Causes

Parathyroid Hormone Dependent (High or Inappropriately Normal Parathyroid Hormone)

- Primary hyperparathyroidism (PHPT; common)
- Tertiary hyperparathyroidism:
  - Occurs after a prolonged period of hypocalcaemia
  - Seen in end-stage renal disease and malabsorptive conditions
- Chronic vitamin D deficiency
- Familial hypocalciuric hypercalcaemia (FHH)
  - Rare defect of the calcium sensing receptor gene
  - Autosomal dominant
  - Mild hypercalcaemia usually of no important sequelae
- Lithium

Parathyroid Hormone Independent (Low Parathyroid Hormone)

- Drugs: calcium supplements, thiazide diuretics, high-dose vitamins A and D
- Humoral hypercalcaemia of malignancy caused by PTH-related peptide secretion by tumours, particularly breast and squamous cell lung cancers
- Bony metastases
- Multiple myeloma
- Renal failure

Initial Tests

a. Serum corrected calcium above 2.6 mmol/L
b. Urea and electrolytes
c. PTH
d. Vitamin D
e. Urinary calcium to creatinine ratio (<0.01 suggestive of FHH)
f. Serum protein electrophoresis and urinary Bence Jones protein
g. Further tests guided by results

Primary Hyperparathyroidism

- Of PHPT cases, 85% are caused by single adenoma. The remainder are caused by parathyroid hyperplasia; less than 1% of cases are caused by parathyroid carcinoma.
- Common in postmenopausal females.
- Many patients have mild to moderate hypercalcaemia and are asymptomatic.
- Consider genetic cause e.g., multiple endocrine neoplasia (MEN) 1 if:
  - Younger than 40 years
  - Parathyroid hyperplasia
  - Strong family history of PHPT
  - Other endocrine tumours

Treatment

- *Rehydration.* Advise the patient to drink 3 L of water per day unless contraindicated.
- Loop diuretics are not indicated and may increase the risk of nephrocalcinosis.
- Stop offending drugs.
- Parathyroidectomy if
  - Younger than 50 years of age
  - Serum calcium greater than 2.85 mmol/L
  - Confirmed nephrolithiasis or nephrocalcinosis
  - Kidney injury as a result of hypercalcaemia
  - Osteoporosis
  - Symptoms of hypercalcaemia
- Some patients are too frail or do not meet criteria for surgery.
  - Observe symptoms and calcium levels.
  - Bone density scan should be done every 2 to 3 years. Advise weightbearing exercise, lifestyle changes, and antiresorptive therapy for osteoporosis when appropriate.
  - Cinacalcet 30 mg/day, titrated up, may be suggested.

If the patient later meets criteria for surgery (e.g., development of osteoporosis) and is fit enough for surgery, then referral should be made at that point.

Hirsutism

> ## GUIDELINES
>
> Escobar-Morreale, H. F., Carmina, E., Dewailly, D., Gambineri, A., Kelestimur, F., Moghetti, P., Pugeat, M., Qiao, J., Wijeyaratne, C. N., Witchel, S. F., & Norman, R. J. (2012). Epidemiology, diagnosis and management of hirsutism: A consensus statement by the Androgen Excess and Polycystic Ovary Syndrome Society. *Human Reproduction Update, 18,* 146–170.
>
> Martin, K. A., Chang, R. J., Ehrmann, D. A., Ibanez, L., Lobo, R. A., Rosenfield, R. L., Shapiro, J., Montori, V. M., & Swiglo, B. A. (2008). Evaluation and treatment of hirsutism in premenopausal women: An Endocrine Society clinical practice guideline. *The Journal of Clinical Endocrinology and Metabolism, 93,* 1105–1120.
>
> Teede, H. J., Tay, C. T., Laven, J. J. E., et al. (2023). Recommendations from the 2023 international evidence-based guideline for the assessment and management of polycystic ovary syndrome. *The Journal of Clinical Endocrinology and Metabolism, 108*(10). 2447–2469.

- Hirsutism (an excess of terminal hair growth) is common. Most females have either no physiological abnormality or benign pathology (most commonly polycystic ovary syndrome); however, there are a number of rare but important conditions to consider and exclude.
- Hirsutism is caused by elevated androgens, originating from an adrenal or ovarian source and peripheral conversion of testosterone to the more active compound dihydrotestosterone. This peripheral conversion may explain why many females are symptomatic despite having serum testosterone within the normal range.

TABLE 22.5 Causes of Hirsutism and Clinical Features

Cause of Hirsutism	Associated Clinical Features
Polycystic ovary syndrome	Menstrual disturbance Long duration of symptoms Obesity or features of insulin resistance
Congenital adrenal hyperplasia	Family history of congenital adrenal hyperplasia Ethnicity: Ashkenazi Jewish, Hispanic
Virilising tumour (ovarian or adrenal)	Rapid onset Other signs of virilisation (clitoromegaly, voice change) Abdominal mass Significantly elevated serum androgens
Ovarian hyperthecosis	Postmenopausal onset: often gradual but can have virilisation and significantly elevated androgens
Iatrogenic	Drug history (e.g., androgens, including DHEA, cyclosporine, minoxidil, dexamethasone, some anticonvulsants, antipsychotics, and antidepressants). Transfer of testosterone from gels
Endocrinopathy	Other relevant features of Cushing syndrome, acromegaly, thyroid dysfunction, or prolactinoma Uncommon for hirsutism to be a presenting feature
Idiopathic hyperandrogenism	Hirsutism with no other clinical features and elevated serum androgens
Idiopathic hirsutism	Hirsutism with no other clinical features and normal serum androgens

DHEA, Dehydroepiandrosterone.

- Investigation of mild hirsutism with no associated clinical features has a low probability of detecting underlying disease and a significant risk of false-positive results and is therefore not recommended.
- Serum testosterone is usually significantly elevated (more than twice upper limit of normal) in malignant disease.
- The laboratory measurement of testosterone is challenging, partly because of variation in sex hormone–binding globulin (SHBG) seen in a number of conditions, including obesity and diabetes. Measurement of the free androgen index (which takes account of SHBG) is useful, as is measurement of testosterone in specialist laboratories using tandem mass spectroscopy rather than immunoassays. Liaising with local services for the interpretation of difficult cases is advised.

Table 22.5 lists the common causes of hirsutism and associated clinical features.
- PCOS is the most common diagnosis. The diagnosis depends on finding two of the following three features:
  - Androgen excess
  - Ovulatory dysfunction
  - Polycystic ovaries
- Dehydroepiandrosterone sulfate and androstenedione may be measured if testosterone is normal. TFTs, prolactin, and 17-hydroxyprogesterone (17OHP) should be checked to screen for mimics. Synacthen-stimulated 17OHP is the diagnostic test for congenital adrenal hyperplasia.

Treatment

- *Lifestyle*
  - Weight loss and improved insulin sensitivity improve many features of PCOS, including unwanted hair growth.
  - Metformin can be used as an insulin-sensitising agent; however, the effect on hirsutism is minimal.
  - It is important to regularly consider cardiovascular risk, hyperglycaemia, sleep apnoea, and endometrial cancer risks in females diagnosed with PCOS.
- *Hair removal*
  - Plucking, waxing, and shaving are effective and cheap, but they must be performed frequently.
  - The illusion of thicker hair is caused by the shaved tip of hair having a blunt edge.
  - Laser and electrolysis treatments are more expensive but can be effective for up to 6 months, are most effective in light-skinned females with dark hair, and are not suitable for use on extensive areas of skin.
- Warn patients planning to seek either of the last two options to check that the practitioner is a member of the appropriate professional body
- *Pharmacologic treatment*
  - Pharmacologic treatment should not be evaluated for efficacy before 6 months.
  - The oral contraceptive pill (OCP) is the first-line treatment.
  - If no improvement is seen, an antiandrogen (spironolactone or cyproterone acetate) can be added, but OCPs must be prescribed concurrently (or alternative definitive contraception) because of the risk of female foetal virilisation.

- Spironolactone (50–200 mg) can be used; it may cause hyperkalaemia, diuresis, and hypotension.
- Cyproterone acetate is generally well tolerated, but there is a risk of hepatotoxicity; LFTs should be monitored. Combination treatment in the form of Dianette carries a higher risk of venous thromboembolism than other forms of low-dose OCP.
- Finasteride inhibits 5α-reductase activity. It is generally well tolerated.
- Topical treatment (i.e., eflornithine cream) is only effective in reducing hair regrowth and should only be used in combination with hair removal methods.

Referral

- Patients with rapid virilisation or significantly elevated testosterone levels should be referred to endocrinology.
- In addition, if the diagnosis is unclear or there is no response to treatment, endocrine referral is warranted.
- Patients with new-onset postmenopausal hirsutism with hyperandrogenism should be referred for urgent evaluation.

Gynaecomastia

- Gynaecomastia is benign proliferation (>0.5 cm) of glandular breast tissue as distinct from a discrete breast mass (when carcinoma must be excluded) or diffuse enlargement caused by adiposity and obesity.
- It is usually bilateral but can be unilateral.
- It is a normal physiological phenomenon in many boys during the neonatal period and adolescence. It is also a common finding in older, middle-aged males without underlying pathology.
- It can be associated with a number of endocrine and non-endocrine conditions as well as many drugs (Table 22.6).

TABLE 22.6 **Causes of Gynaecomastia**

Nondrug Causes	Drugs
Physiological (neonatal, adolescence, old age)	Digoxin
Hypogonadism	Spironolactone
hCG-producing tumours (testis, lung)	Cannabis
Liver disease	Acid suppression: ranitidine, cimetidine, omeprazole
Renal disease	Opiates
Hyperthyroidism	Oestrogens
	Androgen deprivation therapy (e.g., bicalutamide; prostate cancer)
	Anabolic steroids
	Antiretrovirals
	Metoclopramide, domperidone

hCG, Human chorionic gonadotropin.

Clinical Evaluation

- Assess for thyroid status, signs of chronic liver disease, and associated features of hypogonadism (loss of body hair, female pattern of fat distribution, loss of muscle mass).
- Perform testicular and abdominal examination for the presence of a palpable mass.
- Take a full drug history, including any herbal remedies and recreational drugs.

Biochemical Tests

- Testosterone (early-morning fasting sample, repeat at least once if low), luteinising hormone (LH), hCG, alpha-fetoprotein, oestradiol, and LFTs, particularly if there is a rapid onset with pain.
- Elevated hCG or oestradiol suggests possible neoplasm, and testicular ultrasound examination is indicated, proceeding to imaging of the adrenals and liver if negative.
- Most patients will have normal investigations, and the cause is idiopathic.

Management

- The majority of adolescent gynaecomastia cases resolve without intervention.
- In most adult cases, removal of any contributing medication, reassurance, and observation is sufficient.
- Tamoxifen can be used in some cases with recent onset but is rarely required.

Hypogonadism in Adult Males

GUIDELINES

Bhasin, S., Cunningham, G. R., Hayes, F. J., Matsumoto, A. M., Snyder, P. J., Swerdloff, R. S., Montori, V. M., & Task Force, Endocrine Society (2010). Testosterone therapy in men with androgen deficiency syndrome: An Endocrine Society clinical practice guideline. *Journal of Clinical Endocrinology and Metabolism, 95,* 2536–2559.

Jayasena, C. N., Anderson, R. A., Llahana, S., Barth, J. H., MacKenzie, F., Wilkes, S., Smith, N., Sooriakumaran, P., Minhas, S., Wu, F. C. W., Tomlinson, J., & Quinton, R. (2022). Society for Endocrinology guidelines for testosterone replacement therapy in male hypogonadism. *Clinical Endocrinology, 96,* 200–219.

- The term *hypogonadism* refers to a reduction in sperm or testosterone production. Table 22.7 lists its classifications.
- Symptoms suggestive of androgen deficiency in male adults are loss of libido, erectile dysfunction, hot flashes or sweats (if severe and of rapid onset), and breast discomfort. Less specific symptoms include reduced energy levels, low mood, poor concentration, sleep disturbance, reduced muscle bulk, and increased body fat.
- *Enquire* about illnesses (e.g., mumps) or trauma that could have affected the testicles and drugs that interfere with testicular function or testosterone metabolism (e.g., glucocorticoids, opioids, and alcohol).

TABLE 22.7 Classification of Hypogonadism

	LH/FSH	Testosterone	Prolactin	Aetiology
Primary hypogonadism	Elevated	Low	Normal	Testicular failure
Secondary hypogonadism	Inappropriately normal or low	Low	Normal or elevated	Hypothalamic or pituitary disease

FSH, Follicle-stimulating hormone; *LH*, luteinising hormone.

- *Examination* should include testicular size and the development of secondary sexual characteristics. Other physical findings include a reduction in facial or body hair, small or shrinking testes, incomplete or delayed sexual development, inability to conceive, and height loss or low-trauma fractures. Visual fields should be checked.
- *Biochemical assessment* consists of a fasting venous serum sample for total testosterone between 8 and 10 AM along with gonadotrophins (LH, follicle-stimulating hormone) in patients with symptoms. A repeat sample should be taken to confirm the diagnosis along with prolactin, 9 AM cortisol, and TFTs in secondary hypogonadism. Assessment should not be made during acute or subacute illness. Measurement of SHBG and albumin may aid the diagnosis if the calculated free testosterone level helps to differentiate borderline cases; it is usually done by an endocrinologist.
- *Refer* to an endocrinologist patients with symptoms, with osteopenia or osteoporosis, with evidence of pituitary disease, or with markedly low testosterone levels from primary testicular failure for further investigation and a decision about testosterone replacement therapy. Research suggests that increasing testosterone in hypogonadal symptomatic males older than 65 years of age may provide some benefit in sexual function and mood but not in respect to vitality or walking distance.
- Conditions in which testosterone administration is associated with a high risk of adverse outcome include prostate cancer, an unevaluated prostate nodule or raised prostate-specific antigen, breast cancer, a haematocrit greater than 50%, severe lower urinary tract symptoms, and poorly controlled congestive heart failure.

Appendix *Medical Management of Obesity*

Pharmacologic Management

- Consider pharmacologic management with if adequate weight loss has not been achieved with appropriate dietary and behavioural measures

Drug	Starting Criteria	Stopping Criteria
• Liraglutide (Saxenda): 3 mg SC daily)	BMI ≥35 kg/m^2 or ≥32.5 kg/m^2 in higher risk ethnic groups • *Plus* nondiabetic hyperglycaemia • *Plus* high risk of cardiovascular disease *Plus* prescribed by a specialist weight management service	Nil
• Orlistat (120 mg with meals)	BMI ≥30 kg/m^2 BMI ≥28 with an associated risk factor	Continue over 3 months only if at least 5% of body weight is lost
• Semaglutide (Wegovy): 2.4 mg SC weekly)	• BMI ≥35 kg/m^2 • BMI ≥30 kg/m^2 and meet criteria for specialist weight management service referral (lower threshold by 2.5 kg/m^2 in high-risk ethnic groups) • *Plus* at least one weight-related comorbidity *Plus* prescribed by a specialist weight management service	Consider stopping if there is <5% weight loss after 6 months Maximum, 2 years of use

Surgical Management

- Consider referral for bariatric surgery if
  - BMI ≥40 kg/m^2 or
  - BMI 35–40 kg/m^2 with at least one comorbidity that would improve with weight loss
  - Lower threshold by 2.5 kg/m^2 in high-risk ethnic groups
  - *Plus* commitment to long-term follow-up

BMI, Body mass index; SC, subcutaneous.

Further Reading

The Action to Control Cardiovascular Risk in Diabetes (ACCORD) Study Group. (2010). Effects of intensive blood pressure control in type 2 diabetes. *New England Journal of Medicine, 362,* 1575–1585.

Bhasin, S., Cunningham, G. R., Hayes, F. J., Matsumoto, A. M., Snyder, P. J., Swerdloff, R. S., Montori, V. M., & Task Force, Endocrine Society (2010). Testosterone therapy in men with androgen deficiency syndromes: An Endocrine Society clinical practice guideline. *Journal of Clinical Endocrinology and Metabolism, 95,* 2536–2559.

Bornstein S. R., Allolio B., Arlt W., Barthel A., Don-Wauchope A, Hammer G. D., Husebye E. S., Merke D. P., Murad H., Stratakis C. A., Torpy D. J. (2016). Diagnosis and management of primary adrenal insufficiency. Endocrine Society Clinical Practice Guideline.

Bilezikian, J. P., Khan, A. A., Silverberg, S. J., Fuleihan, G. E., Marcocci, C., Minisola, S., Perrier, N., Sitges-Serra, A., Thakker, R. V., Guyatt, G., Mannstadt, M., Potts, J. T., Clarke, B. L., Brandi, M. L., & International Workshop on Primary Hyperparathyroidism. (2022). Evaluation and management of primary hyperparathyroidism: Summary Statement and Guidelines from the Fifth International Workshop. *Journal of Bone and Mineral Research, 37,* 2293–2314.

Charmandari, E., Nicolaides, N. C., & Chrousos, G. P. (2014). Adrenal insufficiency. *Lancet (London, England), 383,* 2152–2167.

Diabetes Improvement Plan. (2014). *Scottish government publications.* Retrieved from https://www.gov.scot/publications/diabetes-improvement-plan-diabetes-care-scotland-commitments-2021-2026/

Diabetes UK. (2023). *Facts and stats.* Retrieved from www.diabetes.org.uk.

Diabetes UK. (n.d.). *Diabetes risk score assessment tool.* Retrieved from https://riskscore.diabetes.org.uk/start

Escobar-Morreale, H. F., Carmina, E., Dewailly, D., Gambineri, A., Kelestimur, F., Moghetti, P., Pugeat, M., Qiao, J., Wijeyaratne, C. N., Witchel, S. F., & Norman, R. J. (2012). Epidemiology, diagnosis and management of hirsutism: A consensus statement by the Androgen Excess and Polycystic Ovary Syndrome Society. *Human Reproduction Update, 18,* 146–170.

Husebye, E. S., Allolio, B., Arlt, W., Badenhoop, K., Bensing, S., Betterle, C., Falorni, A., Gan, E. H., Hulting, A. L., Kasperlik-Zaluska, A., Kämpe, O., Løvås, K., Meyer, G., & Pearce, S. H. (2014). Consensus statement on the diagnosis, treatment and follow-up of patients with primary adrenal insufficiency. *Journal of Internal Medicine, 275,* 104–115.

Jayasena, C. N., Anderson, R. A., Llahana, S., Barth, J. H., MacKenzie, F., Wilkes, S., Smith, N., Sooriakumaran, P., Minhas, S., Wu, F. C. W., Tomlinson, J., & Quinton, R. (2022). Society for Endocrinology guidelines for testosterone replacement therapy in male hypogonadism. *Clinical Endocrinology, 96,* 200–219.

Legro, R. S., Arslanian, S. A., Ehrmann, D. A., Hoeger, K. M., Murad, M. H., Pasquali, R., Welt, C. K., & Endocrine Society. (2013). Diagnosis and treatment of polycystic ovary syndrome: An Endocrine Society clinical practice guideline. *Journal of Clinical Endocrinology and Metabolism, 98,* 4565–4592.

Marso, S. P., Bain, S. C., Consoli, A., Eliaschewitz, F. G., Jódar, E., Leiter, L. A., Lingvay, I., Rosenstock, J., Seufert, J., Warren, M. L., Woo, V., Hansen, O., Holst, A. G., Pettersson, J., Vilsbøll, T., & SUSTAIN-6 Investigators. (2016). Semaglutide and cardiovascular outcomes in patients with type 2 diabetes. *New England Journal of Medicine, 375*(19), 1834–1844. doi:10.1056/NEJMoa1607141.

Marso, S. P., Daniels, G. H., Brown-Frandsen, K., Kristensen, P., Mann, J. F., Nauck, M. A., Nissen, S. E., Pocock, S., Poulter, N. R., Ravn, L. S., Steinberg, W. M., Stockner, M., Zinman, B., Bergenstal, R. M., Buse, J. B., LEADER Steering Committee, & LEADER Trial Investigators. (2016). Liraglutide and cardiovascular outcomes in type 2 diabetes. *New England Journal of Medicine, 375,* 311–322.

Martin, K. A., Chang, R. J., Ehrmann, D. A., Ibanez, L., Lobo, R. A., Rosenfield, R. L., Shapiro, J., Montori, V. M., & Swiglo, B. A. (2008). Evaluation and treatment of hirsutism in premenopausal women: An Endocrine Society clinical practice guideline. *Journal of Clinical Endocrinology and Metabolism, 93,* 1105–1120.

Metzger B. E., Lowe L. P., Dyer A. R., Trimble E. R., Chaovarindr U., Coustan D. R., Hadden D. R., Mccance D. R., Hod M., Mcintyre H. D., Oats J. J. N., Persson B., Rogers M. S., Sacks D. A., (HAPO Study Cooperative Research Group). (2008). Hyperglycaemia and adverse pregnancy outcome. *New England Journal of Medicine, 358,* 1991–2002.

National Institute for Health and Care Excellence. (Updated 2022). *Type 1 diabetes in adults: diagnosis and management. NICE clinical guideline 17.* Retrieved from https://www.nice.org.uk/

National Institute for Health and Care Excellence. (Updated 2016). *Type 2 diabetes: Prevention in people at high risk. NICE clinical guideline 38.* Retrieved from www.nice.org.uk.

National Institute for Health and Care Excellence. (Updated 2020). *Diabetes in pregnancy: Management from pre-conception to the postnatal period. NICE clinical guideline 3.* Retrieved from www.nice.org.uk.

National Institute for Health and Care Excellence. (Updated 2019). *Diabetic foot problems: Prevention and management. NICE clinical guideline 19.* Retrieved from www.nice.org.uk.

National Institute for Health and Care Excellence. (Updated 2022). *Type 2 diabetes in adults: Management. NICE clinical guideline 28.* Retrieved from www.nice.org.uk.

National Institute for Health and Care Excellence. (2020). *Thyroid disease: assessment and management. NICE clinical guideline 145.* Retrieved from www.nice.org.uk

National Institute for Health and Care Excellence. (2022). *Thyroid cancer: Assessment and management. NICE clinical guideline 230.* Retrieved from www.nice.org.uk

National Institute for Health and Care Excellence. (2019). *Primary hyperparathyroidism: diagnosis, assessment and initial management. NICE clinical guideline 132.* Retrieved from www.nice.org.uk

Scottish Intercollegiate Guidelines Network. (2013). *Management of diabetes. SIGN guideline 116.* Retrieved from www.sign.ac.uk.

The Nuffield Department of Population Health Renal Studies Group, & SGLT2 inhibitor Meta-Analysis Cardio-Renal Trialists' Consortium. (2022). Impact of diabetes on the effects of sodium glucose co-transporter-2 inhibitors on kidney outcomes: Collaborative meta-analysis of large placebo-controlled trials. *Lancet (London, England), 400,* 1788–1801.

Teede, H. J., Tay, C. T., Laven, J., Dokras, A., Moran, L. J., Piltonen, T. T., Costello, M. F., Boivin, J., Redman, L. M., Boyle, J. A., Norman, R. J., Mousa, A., Joham, A. E., & International PCOS Network. (2023). Recommendations from the 2023 International Evidence-based Guideline for the Assessment and Management of Polycystic Ovary Syndrome. *Human Reproduction (Oxford, England), 38*(9), 1655–1679. https://doi.org/10.1093/humrep/dead156.

UK Prospective Diabetes Study Group. (1990). UKPDS 6. Complications in newly diagnosed type 2 diabetic patients and their association with different clinical and biochemical risk factors. *Diabetes Research, 13,* 1–11.

UK Prospective Diabetes Study Group. (1998a). Effect of intensive blood-glucose control with metformin on complications in overweight patients with type 2 diabetes (UKPDS 34). *Lancet (London, England), 352*, 854–865.

UK Prospective Diabetes Study Group. (1998b). Intensive blood-glucose control with sulphonylureas or insulin compared with conventional treatment and risk of complications in patients with type 2 diabetes (UKPDS 33). *Lancet (London, England), 352*, 837–853.

UK Prospective Diabetes Study Group. (1998c). Tight blood pressure control and risk of macrovascular and microvascular complications in type 2 diabetes (UKPDS 38). *British Medical Journal (Clinical Research Ed.), 317*, 703–713.

23

Persistent Physical Symptoms

Christopher Burton

CHAPTER CONTENTS

- This chapter considers the common problem of persistent physical symptoms. These are symptoms (e.g., pain, fatigue, dizziness) which either arose as part of a clearly recognised disease but have persisted after its resolution or symptoms which arose without an apparent primary cause. This can include both single symptoms such as musculoskeletal pain or abdominal bloating and clusters of symptoms in syndromes such as fibromyalgia and irritable bowel syndrome (IBS).

- These physical symptoms are sometime termed 'functional somatic symptoms' (because they are characterised by changes in function rather than structure) or problems of 'central sensitisation.' The term *medically unexplained symptoms* is still in common usage but is discouraged: it implies that such symptoms cannot be understood or are in some way different from other symptoms. Neither of these is true (Burton et al, 2020). We use the term *persistent physical symptoms* because it is both accurate and is preferred by patients.

- Symptoms can be understood as having both peripheral and central components. Peripheral components include tissue damage or inflammation and altered function (e.g., smooth muscle spasm). Central components include changes in the way the brain processes sensory information and changes in the way the mind interprets symptoms. Although in recent years, attention has focused on the mind interpretation of symptoms (the cognitive approach), recent research suggests increasing evidence for altered (and preconscious) brain processing of body signals.

- Symptoms can be understood as having both peripheral and central components. Peripheral components include tissue damage or inflammation and altered function (e.g., smooth muscle spasm). Central components include changes in the way the brain processes sensory

information and changes in the way the mind interprets symptoms. Although in recent years, attention has focused on the mind's interpretation of symptoms (the cognitive psychological approach), recent research suggests increasing evidence for altered neurologic processing of body signals.

- This peripheral–central combination is most easily understood through the example of pain. An initial injury can trigger symptoms through peripheral mechanisms (nociceptive pain). However, in some patients, the pain persists or can spread to affect areas unrelated to the original injury. This changing pain is known as *nociplastic pain* (Fitzcharles et al, 2021) or *central sensitisation*. Many persistent physical symptoms have both peripheral and central processes.

- In some of the functional syndromes such as IBS, it is clear that for a substantial number of patients, there are clear peripheral factors such as dietary intake of FODMAPs (fermentable oligosaccharides, disaccharides, monosaccharides, and polyols) (Staudacher & Whelan, 2017), and it is likely that additional peripheral features will be identified over time in other syndromes. It may be helpful to think of them as disorders of brain–body communication. It is not appropriate to think of symptoms and syndromes as mental problems just because currently known physical disease has been ruled out.

- Persistent physical symptoms and emotional distress (low mood and anxiety) often co-occur (Henningsen, Zimmerman, & Sattel, 2003). However, it is clear that emotional distress is neither necessary nor sufficient to cause persistent physical symptoms.

- There are many reasons for the interaction between symptoms and emotional distress. Symptoms are inherently distressing, and physical symptoms predispose patients to anxiety and depression. In a reciprocal way, susceptibility to anxiety or depression also predisposes patients to develop persistent physical symptoms. Even though these interactions are common, many patients with symptoms do not have anxiety or depressive disorders.

- Persistent physical symptoms may occur as a single symptom (e.g., dizziness), as one or more defined syndromes (e.g., tension-type headache, fibromyalgia, or IBS), or in a less specific pattern of multiple symptoms in multiple body systems on multiple occasions.
- The syndromes are sometimes referred to as *functional somatic syndromes*. There are a number of classifications of multiple symptoms and systems, though none is widely used in general practice. These include *somatic symptom disorder* in the *Diagnostic and Statistical Manual of Mental Illnesses*, fifth edition (which emphasises the presence of psychological or social features in addition to physical symptoms) and *bodily distress disorder,* which emphasises the diversity of symptoms and body systems involved.

Table 23.1 lists a range of disorders currently considered broadly within the spectrum of functional somatic syndromes.

- There are two situations in which patients deliberately present themselves as having symptoms which are simulated. These are malingering (in which symptoms are simulated for personal gain) and factitious illness (in which symptoms are simulated for no apparent gain other than access to healthcare). Both of these are uncommon and should not be confused with persistent physical symptoms as described in this chapter.

Prevalence

- In patients seeing a general practitioner (GP), between 15% and 30% have at least one symptom without apparent disease. Most of these symptoms resolve spontaneously and do not become persistent.
- At least 2% of adults have persistent physical symptoms (McGorm et al, 2010). Patients generally seek care in an episodic rather than continuous fashion but often end up with a number of different investigations or specialist referrals as each symptom is taken seriously and appropriately worked up. Most patients with persistent physical symptoms are not immediately identified by general practice teams. As a prompt, it may be useful to think of patients presenting with multiple symptoms in multiple body systems on multiple occasions.
- A small number of patients (~2 per 1000) have severely disabling persistent physical symptoms. They are often high users of healthcare, and some will be known to every general practice. They may have had extensive specialist referrals with negative results and may be seen as facing, and presenting, multiple challenges.
- It is important to remember that some symptoms without apparent disease are actually early or subtle symptoms of a disease which becomes apparent over time. Occasionally, this includes serious conditions such as cancer. When a specialist has made an appropriate assessment of symptoms which have been present for several months, this is uncommon (occurring in 1%–5% of patients). However, with recent symptoms in primary care, it may be more common, so GPs should always consider the possibility of organic disease alongside managing a persistent symptoms as just that.

Principles of Management

- When symptoms are new or have changed, always consider or reconsider organ-system disease.
- Principles of assessment are broadly similar across the spectrum of severity across the range of persistent physical symptoms.

Clinical Assessment

History

- Take a careful history and actively listen:
  - Many persistent physical symptoms have characteristic patterns, such as the unchanging nature of tension-type headache and the bloating and relation to meals of IBS. The absence of typical features of these syndromes should raise concern.
  - Sometimes patients volunteer a symptom which is much more suggestive of pathology; check for 'red flags', but it is better to listen first.
  - Many patients with new or persistent physical symptoms have specific concerns about the cause; active listening encourages patients that disclosing concerns or distress is part of a normal consultation. In

TABLE 23.1	Common Symptom Disorders by Specialty
Specialty	Common Symptom Disorders
Cardiology	Chest pain with normal coronary arteries, palpitations
Ear, nose, and throat	Dizziness, globus pharyngis, functional dysphonia
Gastroenterology	Functional dyspepsia, irritable bowel syndrome, proctalgia fugax
Gynaecology	Chronic pelvic pain
Maxillofacial	Facial pain, temporomandibular joint dysfunction
Musculoskeletal	Chronic widespread pain, fibromyalgia
Neurology	Nonepileptic attacks, functional weakness, tension-type headache
Respiratory	Unexplained breathlessness, hyperventilation
Urology	Chronic genital or prostatic pain
Generalised	Chronic fatigue syndrome, multiple chemical sensitivity

contrast, asking, 'Do you think stress could be causing this?' is often seen as threatening (Peters et al, 2009) and is best avoided.

- By actively listening and responding to the story, for instance by saying, 'That must have felt terrible', you convey empathy and give the patient the legitimate opportunity to describe the emotional aspect of their symptoms.
- You earn yourself the opportunity to make a judgement or recommendations based on having collected sufficient information. You can demonstrate this by summarising the history back to the patient and ensuring that what they have described and you have heard matches up.

Examination

- A new symptom or a change in an old one usually warrants examination.
- Introduce the examination positively with 'I would like to properly examine your . . .', not '. . . take a quick look at . . .'; the patient has to believe you when you find nothing abnormal.
- Consider anticipating normal findings: 'I think this is *X*, in which case the examination will be normal, but I need to check that', so when you find nothing, it is no surprise.
- Use the break in the consultation between the history and examination to ask the patient if they have any ideas or concerns about what might be causing their symptoms. You will not have eye contact, so it is a less threatening point in the consultation, and you can specifically direct the examination to areas of concern.
- Talk the patient through key points of your examination, either in advance 'I'm going to check your abdomen for any lumps or swellings' or afterwards say, 'The back of your eyes look perfect. I was checking to see if the pressure in your brain is normal, and it appears to be'.
- Use tests that indicate functional signs as explanation rather than to prove there's nothing wrong. If you can identify pain on light touch (allodynia) or increased sensitivity to pain (hyperalgesia) by pinching the skin of the abdominal wall, then demonstrate them as part of the 'proof' of your explanation. Similarly, if you can demonstrate normal movement in one situation and not in another (and you do not think the patient is malingering), then use it to point out that the body can do this, but the brain is sometimes inhibiting it.

Investigation

- Investigations have an important role in patients with new or changing symptoms. Doctors find them reassuring, and if anxious patients lead to anxious doctors, it is understandable that we turn to them.
- In making the decision whether to investigate further, the following principles can be useful:
  - Persistent physical symptoms do not cause abnormal results on screening tests. If these occur and are

nontrivial, then follow them up with more tests or referral.

- Beware of looking for tests which are likely to have abnormal results even though only weakly (or not at all) associated with persistent physical symptoms such as vitamin D levels.
- Normal results of diagnostic tests produce an immediate sense of relief in patients, but this is only temporary. Repeated testing and relief may lead to an escalating cycle of reassurance seeking.
- Patient satisfaction and symptom resolution are not altered by whether investigations are conducted immediately or deferred.
- If a plausible (nonpathological) explanation for symptoms is given before the investigation, a negative result is likely to lead to greater reassurance than if it is withheld until afterwards (or not given at all).
- GPs request more investigations than patients actually want. Sometimes tests are ordered as the only thing one can offer; often patients do not want more tests so much as either a reasonable explanation of what is causing their symptoms (rather than what they do not have) or some understanding of and support for their attempts to cope.

Beware of Overassessing

- It usually does not make sense to repeat investigations when nothing much has changed.
- When test results have all been normal and a reasonable specialist opinion (sometimes more than one) has concluded there is no serious cause, is it unlikely that a new specialist will find the missing problem.
- It is essential to remember that incidental and clinically unimportant findings are common (e.g., unexpected and clinically irrelevant lesions re found on 5%–10% of cranial magnetic resonance imaging scans).

Referral

- Specialists are good at recognising organ-system disease, but most have no more skills in managing persistent physical symptom than their GP colleagues. Multidisciplinary pain services are of value for some patients.
- Specialist teams for managing functional symptoms are currently rare; liaison psychiatry and psychology services may be able to assess and offer cognitive-behavioural therapy or other psychological therapies.
- Outcomes for patients with complex persistent physical symptoms who engage in treatments can be good, though not all will benefit.

Treatment

- There are no specific medical treatments for persistent physical symptoms, so most management is generic and may include explanation, selective prescribing (e.g., a low-dose tricyclic for chronic pain), and the use of simple cognitive or behavioural techniques.

Example 1: Functional Dyspepsia

You keep describing these stomach cramps, but the results of the endoscopy were normal. This tells me there is nothing wrong with the structure of your stomach, no disease, and no ulcer or infection. We often find this, that from time to time, the stomach doesn't work properly; it churns around or cramps up, giving the sort of symptoms you describe. This is a problem with the way your stomach functions (called *functional dyspepsia*) rather than a sign of any disease. Treatment often helps to smooth out that function, but it's important for you to know that even if this functional dyspepsia happens, it can't cause you further harm.

Example 2: Dizziness

We have tested your balance, and it works fine (this might have included Dix–Hallpike test and a stepping test), but when we did the tests, even though your balance performed normally, your brain told you things weren't OK. This condition is called *functional dizziness* (or disequilibrium).

What it means is that although your brain is getting the right signals from your inner ears, these signals are then setting off false alarms. False alarms are quite common and normal; sometimes they occur after an episode of illness and sometimes for no good reason at all. Unfortunately, what happens is that the more they bother you, the more your brain looks out for them, and then the more they happen. What is important here is that you find a way to trust your own balance more (we have seen that it works) and rely on these unsteadiness alarms in your brain less (because they're false alarms).

There are some techniques called vestibular rehabilitation which help, and they are available from (a range of websites or in the United Kingdom from the Ménière Disease Foundation). I want you to look at these and start practising them, and I will see you again in 4 weeks to see how you are starting to recover.

Explanation

- Brief interventions in primary care to reattribute physical symptoms to emotional states are unlikely to be effective and are actively resisted by patients (Rosendal et al, 2013).
- A recent large trial found that extended interventions by GPs with extended role led to significant and long lasting improvement (Burton, Mooney et al 2024)
- Many doctors tell patients what they do not have but then fail to provide an explanation for what is (or could be) causing their symptoms.
- Studies indicate that effective explanations should make sense to both the patient and doctor, should not convey blame, and should lead to therapeutic action (Dowrick et al, 2004).
- Explanations may be brief but also need to be flexible: an explanation for a relatively new symptom can be straightforward, but a simplistic explanation for a symptom that has been going on for a long time may be counterproductive.
- Box 23.1 contains two examples of explanation. Both include a plausible explanation, are blame free, and outline therapeutic action and partnership.
- Neither of these explanations included questions about stress, anxiety, or depression. However, if the patient raised them, they could certainly be fitted in. If issues of concerns have been handled gently during the consultation, sometimes a plausible positive explanation gives the patient the opportunity to volunteer their own concern (e.g., with the dizziness explanation, 'That's a relief, and there was me worrying I had a brain tumour') in a lightly self-deprecating fashion.
- Care for patients with persistent physical symptoms includes management of depressive and anxiety disorders when these are identified but should be as part of a wider formulation.

References

Burton C, Mooney C, Sutton L, et al. (2024) Effectiveness of a symptom-clinic intervention delivered by general practitioners with an extended role for people with multiple and persistent physical symptoms in England: the Multiple Symptoms Study 3 pragmatic, multicentre, parallel-group, individually randomised controlled trial. *The Lancet* 403, 2619-2629.

Burton, C., Fink, P., Henningsen, P., Lowe, B., & Rief, W. (2020). Functional somatic disorders: Discussion paper for a new common classification for research and clinical use. *BMC Medicine, 18*, 34.

Dowrick, C. F., Ring, A., Humphris, G. M., & Salmon, P. (2004). Normalisation of unexplained symptoms by general practitioners: A functional typology. *British Journal of General Practice, 54*(500), 165–170.

Fitzcharles, M. A., Cohen, S. P., Clauw, D. J., Littlejohn, G., Usui, C., & Häuser, W. (2021). Nociplastic pain: Towards an understanding of prevalent pain conditions. *The Lancet, 397*, 2098–2110.

Henningsen, P., Zimmermann, T., & Sattel, H. (2003). Medically unexplained physical symptoms, anxiety, and depression: a meta-analytic review. *Psychosomatic Medicine, 65*(4), 528–533.

McGorm, K., Burton, C., Weller, D., Murray, G., & Sharpe, M. (2010). Patients repeatedly referred to secondary care with symptoms unexplained by organic disease: Prevalence, characteristics and referral pattern. *Family Practice, 27*, 479–486.

Peters, S., Rogers, A., Salmon, P., Gask, L., Dowrick, C., Towey, M., Clifford, R., & Morriss, R. (2009). What do patients choose to tell their doctors? Qualitative analysis of potential barriers to reattributing medically unexplained symptoms. *Journal of General Internal Medicine, 24*(4), 443–449.

Rosendal, M., Blankenstein, A., Morriss, R., Fink, P., Sharpe, M., & Burton, C. (2013). Enhanced care by generalists for functional somatic symptoms and disorders in primary care. *Cochrane Database of Systematic Reviews, 10*, CD008142.

Staudacher, H. M., & Whelan, K. (2017). The low FODMAP diet: Recent advances in understanding its mechanisms and efficacy in IBS. *Gut, 66*, 1517–1527.

24

Palliative Care and Care of the Dying Patient

Ben Dietsch

CHAPTER CONTENTS

Basic Principles

GUIDELINES

Scottish Palliative Care Guidelines. Available at https://rightdecisions.scot.nhs.uk/scottish-palliative-care-guidelines.
Twycross, R., Wilcock, A., & Howard, P. (2017). *Palliative care formulary* (6th ed.). Available at http://www.palliativedrugs.com.
Watson, M., Lucas, C., Hoy, A., & Back, I. (2009). *Oxford handbook of palliative care*. Cambridge: Oxford University Press.

- Palliative care seeks to optimise the quality of living for patients with advanced, incurable life-limiting illness (LLI). As such, the approach addresses physical, psychological, social, and spiritual needs as identified by the patient.
- The National Institute for Health and Care Excellence (NICE) defined *end-of-life care* as care provided in the last year of life; however, palliative care can encompass a much longer period spent living with LLI.
- When referring to care of the dying patient, the author has in mind those with a likely prognosis of days to 1 week.
- Good management and decision making in palliative and end-of-life care require careful assessment of the presenting problem or symptom, an appreciation of the context of the person's underlying LLI, an understanding of the person's wishes, and considered communication to draw together these strands.
- Anticipatory planning for symptom control and end-of-life care needs is crucial to patients with LLI.
- The outcome of any discussions and decisions should be recorded clearly and in ways which make it readily accessible to other professionals involved in the person's care (e.g., on the patient's Summary Care Record or electronic Advance Care Plan (ACP)).
- Patients with capacity should be fully involved in decisions about treatment and encouraged to consider and document ACPs, including:
  - Advance Decisions to Refuse Treatment (ADRT), Do Not Attempt Cardiopulmonary Resuscitation (DNACPR) orders, and Treatment Escalation Plans
  - Advance statements describing what they would ideally like to happen at the end of life (e.g., Preferred Place of Care or Death, wishes around hospital admission or care at home)
  - What should happen if they develop an intercurrent illness
  - Who they would want included in any communication or decisions involving their treatment and care, including Lasting Power of Attorney
- If or when capacity to make specific decisions is lost, the information recorded in advance will assist in making best interests decisions.

- Recognising the context of the presenting problem(s) helps to determine appropriate management options (i.e., what is likely to be successful or not). For instance, some problems may be the natural mode of death, such as respiratory failure (in the context of advanced motor neurone disease (MND)), neutropenic sepsis (in advanced myelosuppression or neutropenia caused by extensive bone metastases or refractory haematologic malignancy), lower respiratory tract infection (in the context of advanced respiratory disease), or anorexia or cachexia (in the context of advanced dementia).

Emergencies

Metastatic Spinal Cord Compression and Cauda Equina Syndrome

GUIDELINE

National Institute for Health and Care Excellence. (2023). *Spinal metastases and metastatic spinal cord compression*. NICE clinical guideline 234. Available at https://www.nice.org.uk/guidance/NG234.

Presenting Features
- Consider spinal metastases or metastatic spinal cord compression (MSCC) in all patients with a past, current, or suspected diagnosis of cancer and the following signs and symptoms:
  - Pain suggestive of spinal metastases (severe and unremitting or progressive back pain, aggravated by straining, local spinal tenderness, nocturnal spinal pain preventing sleep, claudication) *and* neurologic signs and symptoms including radicular pain, weakness in any limb, difficulty in walking, sensory loss, numbness, or bladder or bowel dysfunction
- Consider cauda equina compression as a form of MSCC. Neurologic signs in cauda equina compression typically include symptoms suggestive of spinal metastases in the lower spine *and* low back pain, saddle anaesthesia or paraesthesia, bowel or bladder dysfunction, and weakness in one or both legs.

Management
- *Patients unlikely to benefit from further investigation or treatment.* Circumstances in which further imaging or treatment may not be appropriate include the following:
  - Patients whose spinal metastases have previously been deemed untreatable.
  - Those who are in the last days to week(s) of life (i.e., whose overall clinical condition means they are unsuitable for surgical intervention and not likely to live long enough to benefit from radiotherapy).
  - Those who have capacity to refuse investigation.
  - Patients in these circumstances should not be admitted to hospital for further investigation.

- Management of these patients may include a trial of dexamethasone 16 mg by mouth (PO) (daily dose; usually administered as 8 mg twice daily), provision of adequate analgesia, and provision for care needs and equipment.
- *Patients with the potential to benefit from investigation and treatment.* This is anyone not fulfilling the listed criteria, including those with established MSCC for whom intervention may be appropriate for pain relief if not to improve function.
  - Contact the local MSCC coordinator to arrange assessment and further management (surgery or radiotherapy):
    a. Immediately (often via acute oncology hospital service) if the patient has neurologic signs and symptoms suggestive of MSCC
    b. Urgently (within 24 hours) to discuss the care of patients with cancer and any symptoms suggestive of spinal metastases
  - In practice, when MSCC is suspected and further imaging is desired or appropriate, then:
    1. Urgent hospital admission for whole spine magnetic resonance imaging will be required.
    2. Dexamethasone 16 mg/day PO should be commenced (with proton pump inhibitor (PPI) cover).
    3. Patients should be kept immobile.

Superior Vena Cava Obstruction

GUIDELINE

Scottish Palliative Care Guidelines. (n.d.). *SVCO*. Available at http://www.palliativecareguidelines.scot.nhs.uk/guidelines/palliative-emergencies/Superior-Vena-Cava-Obstruction.aspx.

Presenting Features

- Patients with known diagnosis of malignancy and lymphadenopathy.
- Superior vena cava obstruction (SVCO) is most frequently caused by extrinsic compression by carcinoma of the lung, lymphoma, or other cancers or thrombosis formation.
- Signs and symptoms:
  - Breathlessness, headache, dizziness, feeling of fullness in head are common symptoms.
  - Signs include oedema of the conjunctivae, face, hands, or arm(s); dilated veins in the neck; dilated collateral veins in the arms and chest wall; stridor; and cyanosis.
- The onset may be acute (often when caused by thrombosis) or chronic.

Management

- Dexamethasone 16 mg/day PO to reduce peritumour oedema

- Oxygen if available.
- Urgent hospital admission for radiologic investigation; definitive management is often anticancer therapy (including radiotherapy or chemotherapy), thrombolysis, or endovascular stent.
- In patients with advanced malignancy, supportive symptomatic management with opioids and benzodiazepines should also be given (see 'Symptom Management Guidelines: Respiratory: Breathlessness').
- When hospital admission for further investigation or management is not appropriate or desired, dexamethasone and oxygen can be tried for symptom benefit (as earlier), and the focus should be on pharmacologic management of associated symptoms and distress.

Hypercalcaemia of Malignancy

GUIDELINES

National Institute for Health and Care Excellence Clinical Knowledge Summaries. (n.d.). *Hypercalcaemia—known malignancy.* Available at https://cks.nice.org.uk/topics/hypercalcaemia/management/known-malignancy/
Scottish Palliative Care Guidelines. (n.d.). *Hypercalcaemia.* Available at http://www.palliativecareguidelines.scot.nhs.uk/guidelines/palliative-emergencies/Hypercalcaemia.aspx.

Presenting Features

- The malignancies most often associated with malignant hypercalcaemia are myeloma, lung, breast, renal, and thyroid.
- Patients may have known (lytic) bone metastases but not always.
- Signs and symptoms (often worsen over days):
  - Common: malaise, weakness, nausea, constipation, polyuria
  - Severe: delirium, vomiting, seizure, coma
  - Corrected calcium (adjusted for albumin) often needs to be greater than 3 mmol/L to be symptomatic, but some patients can be symptomatic with an increase of anything above normal.

Management

- Confirm corrected calcium and renal function.
- In the palliative setting when treatment of the underlying malignancy is no longer appropriate, intravenous (IV) rehydration and bisphosphonates (most usually pamidronate 90 mg or zoledronic acid 4 mg) are the mainstays of treatment. Pamidronate can be given subcutaneously (SC) via hyperdermacolysis (e.g., 90 mg of pamidronate in 1 L of normal saline over 12–24 hours).
- Hypercalcaemia can become refractory to treatment and may be a mode of death. In a moribund patient with other biochemical abnormalities or irreversible pathologies, not treating may be appropriate.

Seizures and Status Epilepticus

GUIDELINE

Wilcock, A., Howard, P., & Charlsworth, S. (2021). *Palliative care formulary* (7th ed). London: Pharmaceutical Press.

Presenting Features

- Seizures can result in patients with primary or secondary brain tumour(s); they may be the initial presentation of these pathologies.
- They may also be a consequence of preexisting epilepsy (especially when a person becomes unable to take oral antiepileptic medication), other structural brain lesions (e.g., multiple sclerosis), metabolic abnormalities arising in advanced incurable disease, or alcohol withdrawal.
- Seizures may be of any type, but in patients with intracerebral malignancy, they are often focal with subsequent secondary generalisation.

Management

- *Acute emergency when further hospital management is considered appropriate and desirable.*
  a. Exclude hypoglycaemia.
  b. Hospitalisation for further investigation may be indicated, especially if this is the first seizure from an unknown cause or when seizure becomes prolonged.
  c. Diazepam may be given 10 mg per rectum or midazolam 10 mg buccal, SC, or intramuscular (IM) (repeated after 30 minutes if necessary).
- *When hospital admission is not appropriate* (e.g., at end of life or in a terminal event):
  - Control acute seizure.
    a. Diazepam 10 mg per rectum or midazolam 10 mg buccal, SC, or IM. This can be repeated every 20 to 30 minutes until seizure activity is controlled.
    b. If ineffective, consider phenobarbital IM, up to 10 mg/kg (seek specialist advice).
  - Prevent further seizures; ensure regular antiseizure medication:
    a. Continuous subcutaneous infusion (CSCI) midazolam 20 to 30 mg/24 h plus as needed (PRN) midazolam 5 to 10 mg SC/IM 1-hourly. The CSCI dose can be titrated every 24 hours according to PRN midazolam use *or*
    b. CSCI phenobarbital 200 mg CSCI/24 h. The CSCI dose can be titrated every 24 hours according to PRN use (see later) *or*
    c. CSCI levetiracetam starting at 1 g CSCI/24 h or at the equivalent to the current oral daily dose. The oral-to-CSCI conversion is 1:1.
  - If seizures remain poorly controlled despite 50 mg or more of midazolam CSCI, *add* phenobarbital 200 mg CSCI/24 h. This can be titrated by 100 mg/day to 400 mg CSCI/24 h.

- Longer term prevention: See 'Symptom Management Guidelines: Neurologic Symptoms: Seizures'.

Opioid Toxicity

GUIDELINE

National Institute for Health and Care Excellence. (n.d.). *Poisoning, emergency treatment: Treatment summaries.* Available at https://bnf.nice.org.uk/treatment-summaries/poisoning-emergency-treatment/#opioid-poisoning.

Presenting Features

- Signs and symptoms: Consider opioid toxicity if the patient has experienced:
  - A drug error (e.g., inadvertent dose increase) or rapid escalation of an opioid
  - Unexplained drowsiness or deterioration in any patient receiving an opioid
  - Confusion or hallucinations, myoclonic jerks, drowsiness, or pinpoint pupils
  - Reduced respiratory rate
- Important considerations include:
  - Management is dictated by level of respiratory depression.
  - Full reversal is not always necessary and can precipitate acute withdrawal reaction and pain in patients established on opioid analgesia.
  - Normal oxygen saturation does not exclude respiratory depression; a reduced respiratory rate occurs first, resulting in increased carbon dioxide levels. Low O_2 saturations (SaO_2) are a late sign.
  - If the drug has been given recently, the patient's condition may continue to deteriorate as the drug is absorbed.
  - Naloxone is removed from the body more quickly than many opioids. Repeat doses or hospitalisation may be required.

Management

- *Is there imminently life-threatening respiratory depression?*
  - Respiratory rate less than 4 breaths/min *and* semiconscious or unconscious.
  - Give full reversal. Naxalone 400 µg (IV: dilute to 4 mL with 0.9% NaCl or SC: use undiluted).
  - Repeat every 2 minutes until respiration is restored.
  - Consider transfer to acute hospital; call 999 because assisting ventilation via bag–valve–mask may be required.
  - If SaO_2 is less than 90%, give supplemental oxygen and attempt bag–valve–mask ventilation.
  - If there is no response to 2 to 4 mg of naloxone, consider an alternative diagnosis (e.g., other sedative, neurologic event, sepsis).
  - NB buprenorphine requires higher doses.

- *Is there respiratory depression?*
  - Respiratory rate less than 8 breaths/min.
  - Titrate partial reversal. Naloxone 100 µg (IV/SC: dilute to 4 mL with 0.9% NaCl). Give 1 mL (100 µg).
  - Repeat every 2 minutes until respiration is restored and sustained above 8 breaths/min to avoid complete reversal of analgesia.
  - Try other conservative methods to stimulate respiratory rate (i.e., oxygen, bag–valve–mask).
  - It is important to titrate against respiratory rate, not level of consciousness, because total antagonism will cause return of severe pain with hyperalgesia and physical withdrawal and agitation.
  - Further boluses may be necessary if the respiratory rate drops below 8 breaths/min because naloxone is shorter acting than many opioids; consider continuous SC infusion.
  - If SaO_2 is less than 90%, give supplemental oxygen; consider bag–valve–mask.
    Consider if transfer to hospital may be appropriate.
- *No respiratory depression*:
  - Monitor respiratory rate, level of consciousness, oxygen saturation, blood pressure, and pulse initially every 15 to 30 minutes.

Haemorrhage (Massive)

Risk Factors

- Tumour adjacent to or invading large blood vessels (e.g., head and neck cancers, bronchogenic carcinoma).
- Disorders of coagulation (e.g., thrombocytopenia, disseminated intravascular coagulation (DIC)).
- Sometimes (but not always) the patient will experience warning bleeding (e.g., minor haemoptysis).

Management

- Preparing the patient and family for this possibility is important.
- Midazolam 10 mg PRN should be available to administer in the event of distress caused by massive haemorrhage. This can be given as IM injection or buccal preparation because cutaneous circulation is often reduced.

Irreversible Airway Obstruction and Acute Respiratory Distress

Risk Factors and Causes

- Patients with a tumour encasing or involving a large airway (e.g., trachea or bronchus):
  - The tumour may be overgrowing a tracheostomy or causing intrinsic or extrinsic pressure on a large airway such as a thyroid malignancy or bronchial carcinoma.
- Massive pulmonary embolism.
- Advanced respiratory disease (e.g., chronic obstructive pulmonary disease (COPD), pulmonary fibrosis).
- Advanced heart failure.
- MND.

Management

- High-dose benzodiazepines are often required to manage respiratory and psychological distress (e.g., midazolam 5–10 mg SC or IM).
- Opioids may also be helpful (morphine 2.5–10 mg SC if opioid naïve or an appropriate PRN dose if already taking opioids; see 'Symptom Management Guidelines: Respiratory: Breathlessness').
- Both benzodiazepines and opioids may be required CSCI if obstruction happens over the course of hours or days.

Agitation (Terminal Agitation)

Presenting Features

- See also 'Symptom Management Guidelines: Neurologic Symptoms: Delirium.'
- Agitation at the end of life is often a combination of delirium, extreme physiological symptoms, and psychological distress in response to an irreversible problem(s) that is leading to death.
- Terminal agitation is often a diagnosis made in retrospect, but it can be heralded by:
  - Rapid escalation in physical symptoms which are not responding to management (e.g., intractable pain or breathlessness)
  - Rapid escalation in psychological distress
  - Worsening delirium

Management

- It is crucial to recognise and manage agitation as quickly as possible; sedation may be the most appropriate management in this situation.
- It is important to provide one-to-one care and regular review.
- The patient and those important to them require support and explanation.
- Sedatives and anxiolytics should be administered PRN as frequently as is necessary until the patient is settled and should be continued CSCI.
- Sedative and anxiolytics should be titrated in proportion to distress and agitation:
  a. Patient anxious or frightened but lucid:
     - Explore fears.
     - PRN: lorazepam 0.5 mg PO 4-hourly *or* midazolam 2.5 to 5 mg half-hourly SC.
  b. Patient has continuous or worsening anxiety:
     - Regular: diazepam 2 mg twice daily (titrated to 5 mg twice daily) *or* midazolam 10 mg CSCI/24 h.
     - Increase midazolam CSCI in steps of 30% to 50% daily (up to 100 mg); continue midazolam PRN.
  c. Patient has signs of delirium with distress (e.g., confusion, hallucinations):
     - PRN and regular haloperidol: 1 to 2 mg 4-hourly PRN SC + 5 mg CSCI/24 h

d. If worsening confusion or agitation:
- Increase haloperidol to 10 mg CSCI/24 h plus haloperidol PRN.
- Consider adding midazolam, as earlier.

e. If agitation or distress persists despite the above:
- PRN: levomepromazine 12.5 to 25 mg 4-hourly PRN SC.
- Regular: switch CSCI to a combination of levomepromazine (25–150 mg CSCI) and midazolam (20–100 mg CSCI).

f. If the above is ineffective, seek specialist advice.

Symptom Management Guidelines

Pain: General Considerations

> **GUIDELINES**
>
> British Pain Society. (n.d.). *BPS patient publications.* Available at https://www.britishpainsociety.org/people-with-pain/patient-publications.
>   CKS National Institute for Health and Care Excellence. (2021). *Palliative cancer care—pain.* Available at https://cks.nice.org.uk/topics/palliative-cancer-care-pain/.
>   Medications and Healthcare Products Regulatory Agency. (2014). *Off label or unlicensed use of medication: Prescribers' responsibilities.* Available at https://www.gov.uk/drug-safety-update/off-label-or-unlicensed-use-of-medicines-prescribers-responsibilities.
>   National Institute for Health and Care Excellence. (2016). *Palliative care for adults: Strong opioids for pain relief. NICE clinical guideline 140.* Available at https://www.nice.org.uk/Guidance/CG140.

Assessment of Pain

- Pain is a common problem in advanced LLIs. Its presence should be identified and its management reviewed regularly.
- Pain may be caused by:
  - Underlying LLI
  - Treatment for disease (e.g., radiotherapy)
  - Comorbidities and debility (e.g., arthritis, ulcers)
- Various means of scoring pain are available. Patients able to communicate can often provide a vivid description and rating using a visual analogue scale.
- For those unable to articulate or verbalise (e.g., in severe learning disability or advanced dementia), other pain scales are helpful such as the Abbey Pain Scale.
- Breakthrough and incident pain:
  - Breakthrough pain is a spontaneous and unpredictable increase in pain in a patient whose background pain is otherwise well controlled.
  - Incident pain is an increase in pain associated with an identifiable trigger such as movement.

Management: General Principles

- Consideration of the underlying cause (e.g., nociceptive, neuropathic, mixed, acute or chronic) should guide initial management. Start at the lowest effective analgesic dose and titrate gradually.
- In addition to pains caused directly by the LLI, pain may be functional or caused by concurrent problems. As such, approaches other than those used palliatively may be required.
- The most appropriate analgesia should be given:
  - Regularly, at the right dose, by the right route, at the right time and frequency.
  - A suitable analgesic should be available PRN to treat breakthrough or incident pain.
- The World Health Organization's pain ladder has been used for many years to guide management of cancer pain.
- If the nature of the pain is unclear, try simple analgesia and nonpharmacologic approaches before moving on to opioids and adjuvant analgesia.
- Consider the patient's ability to take and self-administer medication. Various preparations of analgesia are available to enable administration by mouth, including the transdermal (TD) patch, enteral tube, and CSCI.
- Review the efficacy of analgesia frequently (daily if necessary) and consider giving patients scope to escalate their own analgesia. If analgesia proves ineffective after escalation or has burdensome side effects, be prepared to stop it.
- Consider underlying causes which might be treatable:
  - Management of constipation or urinary retention
  - Spinal metastases or impending MSCC
  - Painful bone metastases that may respond to radiotherapy
  - Surgical fixation of pathological fractures
  - Infection or oedema around a tumour (often increases pain in head and neck tumours)
- If the source of pain has been managed and treated, be prepared to reduce analgesia (e.g., aim to reduce analgesia after painful metastasis treated with palliative radiotherapy).
- See the sections on end-stage neurologic disease and renal and heart failure for specific guidance on analgesia in these contexts.

Use of Medications Off Label

- In palliative care, many medications are used off label (i.e., outside the terms of the licence or marketing authorisation, such as amitriptyline for neuropathic pain).
- This should be explained to patients when starting these medications.

Opioid Side Effects

- When starting a regular opioid, anticipate common side effects such as constipation, dry mouth, drowsiness or sedation, and nausea.
- Consider starting:
  - A regular laxative (docusate sodium 100–200 mg twice daily with or without senna 7.5 mg at night).

- An antiemetic (haloperidol 1 mg at night/cyclizine 50 mg three times daily). This may only be required for 1 week or so and can then be stopped.
- Explain to the patient that tolerance to any drowsiness or sedation normally develops.
- To combat dry mouth, ensure good oral hygiene, encourage sips of fluid to keep the mouth moist, or use saliva replacements.

Tolerance, Dependence, and Addiction in Patients Taking Opioids

- Increasing pain in patients with LLIs may be caused by disease progression; however, there is increasing recognition of tolerance, dependence, and even addiction.
- These phenomena may be encountered in patients using opioids who have increasing life expectancy, made possible by newer palliative therapies in oncology, for example.
- Consider the potential for these problems in patients with LLIs but a prognosis of months to years.
- Tolerance (requiring increasing doses of analgesia to achieve the same reduction in pain) may respond to switching between opioids (e.g., switch from morphine to oxycodone).
- Dependence is seen in patients taking long-term opioids but is rarely a problem as long as they have sufficient prescribed medication.
- Addiction is rare but may be preexisting; if so, it deserves consideration when choosing appropriate opioid analgesia and when making prescribing arrangements for strong opioids (and other potentially addictive medication). It may lead to tolerance of opioids.

Patient Information

- Provide information to patients when starting strong opioids, including information on potential side effects and who to speak with for further advice.
- Ensure they are confident with how, when, and why to take their analgesia, dosing, what they should take regularly, and when required (PRN). Local palliative care services often have patient information leaflets, or they can be found online.

Legal Implications

Drugs and Driving
- Patients driving while taking strong medication should be made aware that:
  - Side effects from prescribed medications may affect their ability to drive.
  - Ultimately, patients themselves are responsible for making the assessment on their ability to drive safely; they should not drive if they think there may be any impairment in their ability to do so.
  - The law on drugs and driving in the United Kingdom (see https://www.gov.uk/drug-driving-law) states that it is illegal to drive if one of the following is present:
    a. You are unfit to do so because you are on legal or illegal drugs.

    b. You have certain levels of illegal drugs in your blood (even if they have not affected your driving).

For this second point, there is a statutory 'medical defence' to protect patients who may test positive for certain specified drugs taken in accordance with the advice of a healthcare professional. They must also be fit to drive when taking these medications. It may therefore be helpful for patients to keep some suitable documentation with them when they are driving that provides evidence that they are taking the controlled drug as a medicine prescribed or supplied by a healthcare professional.

Travelling Abroad
- When travelling outside the United Kingdom, UK residents taking prescribed medications (in particular controlled drugs) need to consider laws governing their use, as well as import into and export out of all countries to which they are travelling.
- The UK Home Office recommends patients carry a covering letter from their doctor or prescriber or a prescription as supporting evidence that the medication they are carrying was prescribed for their use.
- Medication should be kept in the original packaging.
- The requirements for prescriptions and controlled drug import and export for all countries in which the patient will pass through customs must also be fulfilled. Patients should be advised to check requirements with the relevant embassy and customs procedures before travelling. Current government guidance can be found at https://www.gov.uk/guidance/controlled-drugs-personal-licences#medicines-for-your-personal-use.

Pain: Nociceptive

GUIDELINE

National Institute for Health and Care Excellence. (2016). *Palliative care for adults: Strong opioids for pain relief. NICE clinical guideline 140.* Available at https://www.nice.org.uk/Guidance/CG140.

Presenting Features
- Nociceptive pain is associated with tissue damage. It is often well localised and described as sharp or dull in nature. Synonyms include *physiological* and *inflammatory pain*.
- It normally correlates with an area of known physical injury or disease.

Management: Nonopioids
- Simple analgesia such as paracetamol and nonsteroidal antiinflammatory drugs (NSAIDs) can be effective.
- When using NSAIDs:
  - Choose those with the fewest side effects and consider gastric protection in the form of a PPI (see notes on NSAIDs in renal and cardiac disease).

- Naproxen 250 to 500 mg PO twice daily is often the NSAID of first choice.
- Topical NSAIDs are proven to be effective in gel formulation.

Management: Opioids

- Opioids remain the mainstay of managing acute nociceptive pain in patients with LLI.
- Strong opioids in small doses are often preferred to weak opioids because they come in various preparations, dosing is flexible, they provide scope for titration without having to switch opioid, and they may have fewer side effects.
- When using opioids, as with any analgesia, consider:
  - *Right analgesia:* Most people tolerate morphine, so it is appropriate to begin with this.
  - *Right dose:* Start with the lowest possible dose in an opioid-naïve individual.
  - *Right route:* If possible, begin with a PO opioid to allow more accurate dose titration. If the PO route is unavailable, consider low-dose TD or CSCI.
  - *Right frequency:* Oral opioids are prescribed on a regular basis, with additional PRN doses available for breakthrough pain.
  - *Review:* Be prepared to increase the dose if analgesia is suboptimal or stop if there is no benefit.
- Anticipate common side effects (see previous discussion).
- When possible, use only one opioid at a time; there is no benefit in combining weak and strong opioids or two strong opioids.
- When given by injection, SC is preferred to IM or IV.
- Prescribers should be aware of the potential for *opioid-induced hyperalgesia.* This manifests when (often rapid) opioid escalation leads to increasing pain, which is often more diffuse and less well defined than the presenting pain. Patients exhibit hypersensitivity in the form of hyperalgesia or allodynia. Management requires a reduction in the opioid dose or switching to an alternative (and reduction in equivalent dose).
- See Appendix 32 for comparative doses of different opioids.
- The following opioids are used most often:
  - Codeine
    a. Most often used for moderate pain, often in combination formulation with paracetamol
    b. Starting dosage: 30 mg four times daily to 60 mg four times daily
    c. Maximum dosage: 240 mg/day is equivalent to approximately 20 mg of PO morphine in 24 hours
  - Tramadol
    a. Use for moderate to severe pain
    b. Has additional nonopioid analgesic effects
    c. Starting dosage: 50 to 100 mg four times daily
    d. Maximum dosage: 400 mg/day is equivalent to approximately 40 to 80 mg of PO morphine in 24 hours
  - Morphine
    a. First-choice strong opioid for moderate or severe pain
    b. Preparations include immediate-release (tablets, oral solution, orodispersible tablets, injection) and modified-release (tablets, capsules, granules—normally 12-hourly modified release) formulations.
    c. Can be given CSCI when patients are unable to swallow. Morphine's PO:SC potency ratio is 1:2, so the starting dose CSCI should be half the total 24-hour PO morphine dose.
    d. The PRN PO dose for breakthrough pain should be 1/6 of the 24-hour oral dose; the PRN dose for SC injection should be 1/6 of the total 24-hour CSCI dose. The PRN dose is normally prescribed 4-hourly.
    e. Starting dosage:
      1. Opioid-naïve patient: morphine immediate release 2.5 to 5 mg PO 4-hourly regularly and PRN *or* morphine 12-hourly modified release 10 mg twice daily plus morphine immediate release 2.5 to 5 mg PO 4-hourly PRN
      2. Patient taking a weak opioid (e.g., codeine 240 mg/day): morphine immediate release 5 mg 4-hourly and PRN *or* morphine 12-hourly modified release 10 mg twice daily plus 5 mg immediate release PO 4-hourly PRN
    f. Titration: Aim to establish the lowest effective regular (modified-release dose) as soon as possible to provide even analgesia over 24 hours.
    1. Ask the patient to complete a daily record of all morphine used.
    2. After 2 to 3 days, calculate the average daily (24-hour) total morphine dose required.
    3. Divide the total 24-hour dose by 2 and give this as a twice-daily 12-hourly modified-release preparation.
    4. Provide the PO PRN dose for breakthrough pain, equivalent to 1/6 of the oral 24-hour dose.
      For example, the patient uses 6×5-mg immediate-release morphine doses in 24 hours. Total 24 hours oral morphine dose = 30 mg.
      12-hourly modified-release morphine dose = 15 mg twice daily
      Oral PRN dose = 5 mg of immediate-release morphine PO 4-hourly
      For example, the patient takes 30-mg modified-release morphine twice daily. In addition, the patient uses four 10-mg PRN doses every day for 1 week. Total 24-hour oral morphine dose = 30 mg + 30 mg + 40 mg = 100 mg.
      Increase 12-hourly modified-release morphine to 50 mg twice daily.
      Increase oral PRN dose to 15 mg immediate-release morphine PO 4-hourly.
  - Oxycodone
    a. Indications:
      1. Useful for moderate to severe pain.
      2. Used if morphine is contraindicated or not tolerated.
      3. Most often used as second-line treatment for patients taking morphine who experience opioid neurotoxicity and suboptimal analgesia.

b. The PRN oral dose for breakthrough pain should be 1/6 of the 24-hour oral dose; the PRN dose for SC injection should be 1/6 of the total 24-hour CSCI dose.

c. Starting dose:

1. Estimates of potencies vary, but it is safe to consider it 1.5 to 2 times as potent as morphine (i.e., oral morphine:oral oxycodone potency ratio is 1:2.)

2. Based on this, it is usual practice to halve the previous morphine dose when switching to oxycodone. For example, morphine PO 30 mg in 24 hours = oxycodone PO 15 mg in 24 hours.

3. If oxycodone is the first opioid used, start with 1 to 2 mg 4-hourly and PRN PO.

d. Titration:

1. Use the same principle as for morphine.

As with morphine, it comes in a variety of formulations, and the oxycodone PO:SC potency ratio is approximately 1:2. (The SC dose is half the oral dose.)

- Diamorphine

a. Indications:

1. Useful for moderate to severe pain if SC or CSCI administration is required.

b. Available as powder for solution for injection in ampoules; it can be reconstituted to the desired volume. This is helpful in minimising volume of SC injections (or CSCI infusion) for patients requiring large doses of opioid.

c. PO morphine: SC:diamorphine potency ratio is 1:3. For example, morphine 30 mg PO in 24 hours = diamorphine 10 mg CSCI in 24 hours.

d. Diamorphine PRN dose (SC) should be 1/6 of the total daily diamorphine CSCI dose.

- Fentanyl (TD patch)

a. Indicated for chronic pain management in:

1. Patients who are unable to swallow or prefer not to take PO medications

2. Patients experiencing intolerable side effects from morphine (especially constipation, nausea or vomiting, hallucinations)

3. When there is a risk of tablet diversion or misuse

4. When it is safer, as in patients with severe renal impairment or failure (glomerular filtration rate (GFR) <30%)

b. For patients with a prognosis of months (because of the time required for titration).

c. Considered less constipating than morphine or oxycodone; reduce the laxative dose if switching from these opioids.

d. The TD dose is expressed in micrograms per hour. The smallest dosage is 12 μg/h. This is equivalent to at least 30 mg of oral morphine in 24 hours.

e. Equivalences to morphine and potencies vary, but Appendix 32 draws on several sources when estimating equivalence. TD absorption may be influenced by skin temperature, circulation, and patch adherence.

f. Starting dose:

1. It should not be used on opioid-naïve patients given the strength of the dose.

2. It is often more practical to titrate the patient on an alternative PO or CSCI strong opioid first and when satisfactory analgesia achieved to convert this to the equivalent fentanyl TD patch.

3. NB: When switching a patient from morphine or oxycodone to fentanyl, a temporary partial opioid withdrawal reaction can occur because fentanyl is predominantly centrally acting; gastric flulike signs of opioid withdrawal can occur (e.g., shivering, sweating, diarrhoea). These can be managed by giving a PRN dose of the previous opioid.

g. Titration:

1. Patches are reapplied to a fresh site every 3 days and may take 3 days or so to reach steady-state plasma concentrations and maximum therapeutic benefit.

2. Morphine or oxycodone PRN should be prescribed for breakthrough pain if the patient does not have severe renal failure.

3. If three or more PRN doses of breakthrough opioid analgesia are required every day, for several days, the strength of the next patch applied can be increased by between 12 and 25 μg/h.

4. Increase the TD patch no more often than every 3 days (preferably weekly), giving the patch time to reach maximum therapeutic benefit between increases. It is therefore unsuitable for acute pain requiring rapid titration of analgesia.

Buprenorphine (Transdermal Patch)

a. Indications: The patch is helpful in the same patient groups as fentanyl.

b. Given the partial agonist and antagonist action of buprenorphine on opioid receptors, there may be less tendency toward tolerance.

c. Reports of potency compared with other strong opioids vary: Appendix 32 has a cautious conversion, considering fentanyl TD 1.4 times more potent than buprenorphine TD.

d. Available in lower strength doses than fentanyl TD patches, so there is more scope for titration. Patch strengths of 5, 10, 15, and 20 μg/h are available as 7-day patches; 33-, 52.5-, and 70-μg/h patches can be changed every 3 to 4 days.

e. Starting dose:

1. Opioid-naïve patients: Start at the lowest dose (i.e., 5 μg/h); change it every 7 days.

2. Switching from another strong opioid:

Use a cautious conversion ratio based on the current opioid's dose (see Appendix 32).

Switching from another strong opioid to TD buprenorphine may cause opioid withdrawal (gastric flulike symptoms), which can be managed by PRN doses of the previous opioid.

f. Morphine and other μ-receptor agonists at an appropriate dose (buprenorphine TD 5 μg/h is equivalent to ~12 mg morphine PO in 24 hours) may be used for breakthrough pain.

g. Titration:
1. If over a period of several days, three or more PRN doses of breakthrough opioid analgesia are being used daily, increase buprenorphine TD patch strength.
2. Increase TD patch dose weekly; this makes it unsuitable for acute pain in which rapid titration is necessary.

Note that patches are available in various strengths formulations, which last for 3, 4, or 7 days.

- Other opioids are encountered less frequently.
  - Fentanyl (immediate-release transmucosal)
    a. Indications:
    1. Various preparations of transmucosal fentanyl are now available, including sublingual and buccal tablets, a lozenge, and a nasal spray.
    2. Transmucosal fentanyl products are designed to provide rapid onset pain relief for a short duration, which better fits the profile of breakthrough pain or incident pain.
    b. It is thought best practice to use PO strong opioids as first-line treatment for breakthrough pain and then switch to transmucosal fentanyl only if the patient experiences prolonged undesirable effects or the onset of action is too slow.
    c. Immediate-release fentanyl should be prescribed on the recommendation of a specialist in palliative care or multidisciplinary team (MDT). The starting dose and titration are as follows:
    1. The manufacturers of the various products publish guidelines on their use and titration.
    2. They should not be used in opioid-naïve patients or acute noncancer pain.
  - Fentanyl (SC or CSCI)
    a. Indications:
    1. Pain in severe or end-stage renal failure (ESRF; estimated GFR (eGFR) <30 mL/min)
    2. When rapid titration of analgesia is required (often at the end of life)
    b. Starting dose:
    1. Opioid-naïve patients: 12.5 to 25 μg 1-hourly PRN SC; 100 μg CSCI/24 h
    2. Switching from other opioids: See Appendix 32. (Fentanyl is considered approximately 100 times more potent than morphine.)
    c. Titration:
    1. On established fentanyl CSCI dose: Use PRN SC dose (1-hourly) equivalent to 1/8 to 1/10 of the fentanyl 24-hour CSCI dose.
    2. As with other strong opioids CSCI, if three or more PRN doses are required in 24 hours, increase CSCI by the equivalent amount:

For example, fentanyl 100 μg CSCI/24 h background analgesia plus 4 × 12.5 μg SC PRN in 24 hours: Increase CSCI fentanyl to 150 μg CSCI/24 h.

- Alfentanil (SC or CSCI)
  a. Indications:
  1. Pain in severe renal failure or ESRF (eGFR <30 mL/min)
  2. When morphine neurotoxicity develops
  3. When the volume required prevents use of fentanyl
  4. Alfentanil's duration of action is too short to be useful as an SC PRN analgesic. Use fentanyl for PRN dosing.
  b. Starting dose:
  1. Switching from other opioids: See Appendix 32. (Alfentanil is considered approximately 30 times more potent than PO morphine.)
  2. An SC PRN dose of an alternative opioid should be available. (The author recommends fentanyl.)
  c. Titration:
  1. As with other strong opioids CSCI, if three or more PRN doses are required in 24 hours, increase CSCI by the equivalent amount.
- Methadone
  a. Methadone is an opioid with mixed properties, including a μ-opioid receptor agonist and N-methyl-D-aspartate (NMDA) receptor channel blocker.
  b. It has a highly variable plasma half-life and should only be used under specialist supervision for analgesia.
  c. Indications:
  1. In palliative care, it is most often used when pain fails to respond to more conventional analgesia (i.e., regular opioids and nonopioids) and adjuvant (e.g., severe, mixed nociceptive or neuropathic pain).
  2. It can be used in ESRF.
  d. Starting dose:
  1. Switching from other opioids: This process is complicated, usually requiring supervision in a hospice inpatient unit.
  2. Ultimately, a regular dose is often administered twice daily.
  e. Titration:
  1. PRN dose is most often 1/6 to 1/10 of the total 24-hour oral methadone dose. This should be given no more frequently than every 3 hours (unlike other opioids).
  2. Patients requiring additional analgesia within 3 hours of a methadone dose may be prescribed the following PRN: nonopioid or previous opioid PRN (at half the previous dose).
  3. Increases in the regular dose should be undertaken no more frequently than once a week because of the accumulation of methadone.

Pain: Neuropathic

GUIDELINES

National Institute for Health and Care Excellence. (2020). *Neuropathic pain in adults: Pharmacological management in non-specialist settings. NICE clinical guideline CG173.* Available at https://www.nice.org.uk/Guidance/CG173.

Presenting Features

- Neuropathic pain results from a lesion or disease of the sensory nervous system.
- Its character is often described as burning, shooting, pins and needles, or numbness and is usually poorly localised (although it may be associated with a particular sensory dermatomal distribution).
- Abnormal sensation in the region of a pain is often a good indicator of a neuropathic cause.
- If it becomes chronic, indicators of chronic regional pain syndrome may develop (e.g., autonomic features with changes in the skin, hair, or nails; oedema; and motor function).

Management

- Opioids and NSAIDs may sometimes be effective at managing neuropathic pain, but specific neuropathic analgesics are often required. These are a diverse group, including:
  - Antidepressants
  - Antiepileptics
  - Anaesthetics (local: lidocaine; systemic: ketamine)
- Indications for neuropathic analgesia:
  - Monotherapy for neuropathic pain alone
  - Neuropathic pain unresponsive to opioid plus an NSAID
- Choice:
  - The most commonly used medications for long-term management are amitriptyline, duloxetine, gabapentin, and pregabalin.
  - Both antidepressants and antiepileptics have been shown to have similar tolerability and efficacy in patients with neuropathic pain.
  - Carbamazepine is normally used only for patients with trigeminal neuralgia.
  - Others such as nortriptyline, sodium valproate, and ketamine are usually started by a specialist.
  - Steroids (dexamethasone 8 mg) can be used in the short term (maximum, 2 weeks) for pain caused by nerve compression while waiting for neuropathic analgesia or definitive treatment (e.g., radiotherapy) to have an effect.
  - It is usual practice to start with either an antidepressant or antiepileptic:
    a. If the initial drug is poorly tolerated or ineffective, switch to a drug from the other category.
    b. If it has no benefit, try a combination of an antidepressant and an antiepileptic.

- Commonly used neuropathic analgesics:
  - *Amitriptyline* (a tricyclic antidepressant—serotonin and norepinephrine reuptake inhibitor (SNRI))
    a. Its sedative side effect can be useful in patients whose pain causes difficulty sleeping.
    b. Benefit in neuropathic pain is often seen in subantidepressant doses.
    c. Starting dosage: 10 mg PO at night.
    d. Titration: Can be increased weekly, often done stepwise from 10 to 25 mg; then by 25 mg weekly if required. The maximum dose is 75 to 150 mg.
  - Duloxetine (an SNRI)
    a. Similar efficacy and side effect profile to amitriptyline.
    b. Starting dosage: 30 mg/day.
    c. Titration: Increase after 1 week to 60 mg. Can be increased by a further 30 mg weekly. The maximum dose is 120 mg.
  - Gabapentin
    a. Starting dosage: typically 300 mg/day (100 mg three times daily or 300 mg once daily). This requires a dose reduction in patients with renal failure.
    b. Titration: Increase by 300 mg/day every 3 to 7 days. Benefit is usually experienced by 600 mg three times daily, but the maximum recommended dosage is 1200 mg three times daily.
  - Pregabalin
    a. The advantage over gabapentin is twice-daily dosing (rather than thrice), but there is no significant analgesic benefit.
    b. Starting dosage: 75 mg twice daily; requires dose reduction in patients with renal failure.
    c. Titration: Increase weekly by 150 mg/day in divided doses (i.e., to 150 mg twice daily; then 225 mg twice daily if required). The maximum dosage is 300 mg twice daily.
- Other neuropathic analgesics (used under specialist guidance)
  - Steroids
    a. May be helpful as a short course in managing pain caused by MSCC or nerve root compression while definitive treatment awaited or to manage pain flare after radiotherapy or when radiotherapy or surgery is not possible.
  - *Nortriptyline*
    a. Alternative to amitriptyline
  - *Ketamine*
    a. NMDA receptor channel blocker
    b. Used in patients with neuropathic pain unresponsive to other measures
    c. Potential for urinary tract, hepatobiliary, and neuropsychiatric side effects, so most often given as a short course
    d. May be given as CSCI (100–500 mg CSCI/24 h) or regular oral dose (10–100 mg four times daily)
  - *Methadone*
    a. May be used in complex mixed neuropathic–nociceptive pain (see 'Pain: Nociceptive: Management: Opioids').

- Lidocaine plasters
    a. These are increasingly used to treat localised neuropathic pain, but data on efficacy are limited.
    b. Consider only if systemic neuropathic analgesics have failed or are contradicted.
    c. If used, benefit over a 2-week period should be assessed and plasters stopped if no benefit is seen.

Pain: Other Types

Malignant Bone Pain

- *Presenting features*
  Pain is well localised to the bony skeleton in regions of known metastatic disease.
- *Management*
    - Radiotherapy: This is appropriate in patients with a prognosis of months because benefit can take 2 to 3 months. Pain flare may occur shortly after treatment and requires additional analgesia. Analgesics may need to be reduced if successful pain relief is achieved by radiotherapy.
    - IV bisphosphonates have a role in treating patients with painful metastatic disease.
    - Surgery: for painful osteolytic metastases at risk of fracture (or after pathological fracture) in patient fit enough to undergo surgical intervention.
    - Analgesia
        a. NSAIDs and strong opioids are most commonly used (see earlier).
        b. Steroids may provide short-term relief while titrating other analgesia but should not be used for more than 2 weeks.

Smooth Muscle Spasm

- Presenting features
    - Spasmodic pain in the oesophagus, bowel (including rectum), or bladder
- Management
    - Oesophageal spasm: nitrates (glycerol trinitrate) or nifedipine 5 mg three times daily PO (titrated to 20 mg TDS)
    - Bowel spasm: hyoscine butylbromide 20 mg PO/SC 4-hourly PRN or QDS
    - Bladder spasm: oxybutynin 5 mg PO twice daily (titrated to 5 mg PO QDS)

Skeletal Muscle Spasm

- Presenting features
    - Painful chronic spasm associated with nerve injury in advanced neurologic disease or malignancy
- Management (see also 'Advanced Neurologic Diseases')
    - Baclofen, tizanidine, dantrolene, and diazepam all have similar efficacies. Start with baclofen and use diazepam only if it is for a short course (<1 month).
        a. *Baclofen:* The starting dosage of 5 mg can be given once, twice, or three times daily (maximum starting dosage, 5 mg three times daily). Titration: Increase

the daily dosage by 5 mg to 15 g (in divided doses) every week to a maximum of 100 mg/day. Withdraw slowly over 2 weeks if discontinuing.
        b. *Tizanidine:* The starting dosage is 2 mg once daily. Titration: Increase by 2 mg every 4 days (divided doses). The maximum dosage is 9 mg four times a day.
        c. *Dantrolene:* The starting dosage is 25 mg once daily. Titration: Increase the daily dose by 25 mg once a week and give as divided doses. The maximum dosage is 100 mg four times a day. Monitor liver function.
        d. *Diazepam:* 2 to 5 mg at night and PRN for a maximum of 4 weeks

Tenesmus

- Presenting features
    - Painful sensation of rectal fullness, often caused by a local tumour
- Management
    - Manage aggravating factors such as constipation.
    - Use NSAIDs, amitriptyline, nifedipine, or antiepileptics (doses as detailed earlier; see 'Pain: Neuropathic and Pain: Other Types: Smooth Muscle Spasm').

Pain: Total Pain

> **GUIDELINE**
>
> Twycross, R. (2003). *Introducing palliative care* (4th ed.). London: Radcliffe Medical Press.

Definition

- Total pain is the concept that pain includes many contributing factors, notably:
    - Biological: disease, treatment, comorbidities, fatigue
    - Psychological: anxiety, depression, fear, experiences, change in body image
    - Social: loss of role, job, change in relationships, isolation
    - Spiritual: faith, loss, search for meaning, fear of the unknown

Presenting Features

- Patients often identify the factors that contribute to the pain (but not always, so they may need help exploring these).
- Pain resistant to management with analgesics often has a total component.
- It may manifest as overwhelming pain or be disproportionate to the degree of pain expected from known disease.

Management

- Consider holistic, individualised approaches to the management of pain (i.e., choose management options addressing the contributing factors as identified by the patient):

- Analgesics as for nociceptive or neuropathic pain. But be prepared to reduce or stop analgesics if no benefit is experienced.
- Helping the patient achieve sleep at night can be a particularly helpful initial step.
- Other approaches include physiotherapy, transcutaneous electrical nerve stimulation (TENS), complementary therapies, counselling and psychological therapies, management of anxiety or depression, addressing social issues, distraction, and relaxation.

Pain: Nonpharmacologic Interventions

- Consider nonpharmacologic interventions when possible or when patients are reluctant to try analgesia.

Options

- Radiotherapy for painful metastases
- Splints for fractured bones or braces for spinal stabilisation
- TENS: useful for localised neuropathic pain
- Physiotherapy: especially useful for pain associated with immobility or muscle spasm or contractures
- Complementary therapies: Evidence for these is inconsistent, but they may well address components of total pain (see earlier); examples are acupuncture, reflexology, aromatherapy, and art and music therapies.

Pain: Interventional Techniques

Presenting Features

- Pain resistant to systemic analgesia or when the effectiveness of analgesia limited by side effects
- Pain limited to one region or clear source (e.g., compression of specific nerve(s) by malignant tumour)

Management

- Consider referring patients for specialist advice if any of the following techniques may be helpful:
  - *Cordotomy:* for pain in one side (hemithorax), such as that caused by mesothelioma.
  - *Neurolysis:* indicated in patients with limited prognosis when pain fails to respond to other measures and a clear cause or pathway is evident. Effectiveness and tolerability are assessed with a local anaesthetic before proceeding to a neurolytic block or ablation. Regions that can be targeted include the coeliac plexus (often implicated in pancreatic or upper GI pain), superior hypogastric (pelvic pain), and ganglion of Impar (perineal pain).
  - *Neuraxial (intrathecal and epidural):* indications include intolerable neuropathic pain, especially with a sympathetically mediated component, when systemic analgesia is ineffective or limited by side effects. The challenges with this technique are provision of ongoing specialist monitoring and management in

the community because they need to be undertaken by experienced specialist teams.

Respiratory

Breathlessness

- Breathlessness is a very common symptom in palliative care, especially in patients with malignant, cardiac, respiratory, and neurologic disease.
  - Consider if there is a potentially reversible problem with an appropriate treatment acceptable to the patient (Table 24.1). As with all decisions in palliative

TABLE 24.1	Potentially Reversible Causes of Dyspnoea and Management Options
Cause	**Potential Management**
Large airway obstruction	Stent, laser or cryotherapy
Small airway obstruction	Optimise bronchodilator dose and delivery: salbutamol and ipratropium nebuliser, oral corticosteroids
Pulmonary embolus	Anticoagulation: LMWHs
Pulmonary oedema	Diuretics
Pulmonary fibrosis	Optimise treatment, oral corticosteroids
Pleural effusion	Pleural drain (temporary or indwelling PleurX drain), pleurodesis
Ascites	Paracentesis
Pain (in chest wall/pleura or elsewhere)	Analgesia
Infection	Antibiotics
Radiation pneumonitis (consequent to radiotherapy)	Dexamethasone (8 mg/day)
Anaemia	Blood transfusion
Anxiety	Beta-blocker, lorazepam
Acute type 2 respiratory failure (in acute exacerbation of COPD)	NIV if decompensated respiratory acidosis
Superior vena cava obstruction	Radiotherapy, stent

COPD, Chronic obstructive pulmonary disease; *LMWH,* low-molecular-weight heparin; *NIV,* noninvasive ventilation.

care, consider *appropriate* options for management in the context of the LLI and disease trajectory.
- When the underlying cause of dyspnoea cannot be treated, when a patient wishes, or when expected prognosis or performance status make it inappropriate to do so, management should be aimed at palliating symptoms.
- Mainstays of management are nonpharmacologic therapies, opioids, and benzodiazepines. Anxiolytic antidepressants may also have a role in patients who have sufficient prognosis to benefit.
- Choice of palliative management option should depend largely on the patient's estimated prognosis: breathlessness in patients expected to live months to years to live should use predominantly nonpharmacologic therapies initially, but severe breathlessness in patients with days to weeks to live should likely rely more on opioids and benzodiazepines (Fig. 24.1).
- Local palliative care centres may have specific breathlessness clinics.
- Management options include:
  a. Education
     Improving patient understanding of the physiology of breathing and breathlessness and providing techniques to optimise breathing can be very helpful. A useful resource is the Breathing, Thinking, Functioning approach designed at Cambridge University Hospitals' Breathlessness Intervention Service.
     The focus is on improving breathing technique, using positions to ease breathlessness, changing thought processes around breathlessness, and maintaining function and efficient use of energy.
     Cognitive-behavioural therapy (CBT) and relaxation are also helpful.
     Teaching patients simple techniques for recovering control over their breathing when they feel particularly breathlessness is valuable; examples

include the use of a fan, sitting forward, and focusing on breathing out (rather than in).
  b. Physiotherapy
     Maintaining activity helps maintain function and prevent muscle wasting and deconditioning.
     Physiotherapists are also crucial in optimising efficient breathing technique.
  c. Fans
     Air flow over the nose and mouth has been shown to be effective in reducing the sensation of breathlessness.
     A handheld fan is a simple, portable, and effective device for easing breathlessness.
     Similarly, air flow through an open window or larger fan is effective.
  d. Antidepressants
     Selective serotonin reuptake inhibitors (SSRIs) may benefit breathless patients, especially when anxiety is a contributing factor (e.g., sertraline, dosed as for anxiety or depression).
  e. Opioids
     These reduce the sensation of breathlessness and respiratory effort through reducing response to hypercapnia, hypoxia, and exercise.
     Morphine is the first-choice strong opioid, but if side effects limit the dose, oxycodone is an alternative and is titrated in the same way (although it is twice as potent as morphine).
     The starting dose depends on whether the patient is already using morphine (for pain or breathlessness) (Tables 24.2 and 24.3).
  f. Benzodiazepines
     Patients with a prognosis of months: Avoid.
     Patients with a prognosis of weeks: Use if there is a significant anxiety component to breathlessness. Use oral benzodiazepine with a shorter half-life (lorazepam) initially.
     Patients with a prognosis of days: Benzodiazepines are often used parenterally in combination with an opioid. The intent of benzodiazepine use is to

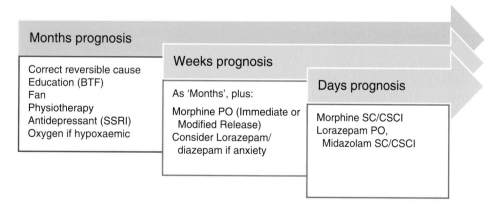

• **Fig. 24.1** Summary: management options for breathlessness according to likely prognosis. *BTF,* Breathing, Thinking, Functioning; *CSCI,* continuous subcutaneous infusion; *PO,* by mouth; *SC,* subcutaneous; *SSRI,* selective serotonin reuptake inhibitor.

TABLE 24.2	Starting Doses and Titration of Morphine for Breathlessness in Opioid-Naïve Patients[a]		
	Months Prognosis	**Weeks–Months Prognosis**	**Days Prognosis**
Morphine PO (immediate release)	1 mg twice daily → 1 mg four times daily → 1 mg q4h → 2 mg q4h → 3 mg q4h → 5 mg q4h → further increases by 30%–50% (increase weekly)		2.5–5 mg q4h
Morphine PO (modified release)	5 mg twice daily	5 mg twice daily. Titrate total daily dose once a week by 10 mg, i.e., to 10 mg twice daily → 15 mg twice daily. The maximum effective dose is usually 30 mg/day.	N/A
Morphine SC	N/A	N/A	2.5–5 mg q4h
Morphine CSCI/24 h	N/A	N/A	Start with 10 mg CSCI/24 h

[a]Oxycodone is an alternative in patients unable to tolerate morphine. Because morphine:oxycodone potency is approximately 1:2, start with half the equivalent morphine dose.

CSCI, Continuous subcutaneous infusion; *N/A*; not applicable; *PO*, by mouth; *q*, every; *SC*, subcutaneous.

TABLE 24.3	Starting Doses and Titration of Morphine for Breathlessness in Patients Already Taking Morphine		
	Months Prognosis	**Weeks Prognosis**	**Days Prognosis**
Morphine PO PRN (immediate release)	25%–100% of the 4-hourly analgesic dose (e.g., morphine total 60 mg PO in 24 h → 4-hourly analgesia dose = 1/6 of 24-h dose = 10 mg PO → breathlessness dose = 2.5–10 mg PO morphine)		
Morphine PO (modified release)	Titrate preexisting morphine MR dose according to *regular* PRN morphine IR use. (e.g., morphine MR 30 mg BD but taking 4 doses of morphine IR 5 mg every day for breathlessness → increase morphine MR to 40 mg twice daily).		N/A
Morphine SC PRN	N/A	N/A	Half of oral PRN dose (PO:SC 1:2), calculated as above
Morphine CSCI/24 h	N/A (unless vomiting and needs temporary replacement; then as for days prognosis)		Half the current PO 24-h dose

If established on oxycodone, the same principles apply.

CSCI, continuous subcutaneous infusion; *IR*, immediate release; *MR*, modified release; *N/A*, not applicable; *PO*, by mouth; *PRN*, as needed; *q*, every; *SC*, subcutaneous.

relieve distress. Sedation may be a consequence but is likely anyway because of the exhausting effects of dyspnoea and deteriorating condition. Doses are shown in Table 24.4.

g. Oxygen
Oxygen should only be started in the presence of hypoxaemia.

- Bear in mind that correcting oxygen saturations alone does not always alleviate breathlessness and that there are some conditions in which correction of hypoxaemia is not physiologically possible (e.g., end-stage COPD).
  This is used as long-term therapy for patients who are hypoxaemic because of LLI (e.g., COPD, interstitial lung disease, cardiac failure, cystic fibrosis, neuromuscular disorders, obstructive sleep apnoea, pulmonary hypertension).
  Ambulatory oxygen should be supplied to patients qualifying for long-term oxygen therapy who are mobile and wish to leave the home and in patients who desaturate on exercise.

Nocturnal oxygen can be used for patients with nocturnal hypoxaemia.

Oxygen's potential for psychological dependence and associated complications (drying or bleeding of the nasal mucosa, hazards of equipment and tubing, risks in hypercapnic respiratory failure) mean it should only be started if absolutely necessary.

Cough

- Management is guided by whether the cough is productive and whether the patient is able to expectorate.

Productive, Able to Expectorate

- Treat the cause or infection: antibiotics
- Loosen secretions: 0.9% saline nebulisers 2.5 to 5 mL four times daily; carbocisteine 375 to 750 mg three times daily

TABLE 24.4	Breathlessness: Benzodiazepine Dose and Choice		
	Months Prognosis	Weeks Prognosis	Days Prognosis
Lorazepam	Avoid	If significant anxiety: 500 µg q4h	If significant anxiety: 500 µg–1 mg q4h
Diazepam	Avoid	Avoid unless significant anxiety; minimal effective dose, e.g., 2 mg twice daily, titrated slowly	N/A
Midazolam SC	N/A	N/A	2.5–5 mg every hour
Midazolam CSCI	N/A	N/A	Minimum 10 mg CSCI/24 h

CSCI, Continuous subcutaneous infusion; *N/A,* not applicable; *q,* every; *SC,* subcutaneous.

- Physiotherapy
- Bronchospasm: salbutamol

Productive, Unable to Expectorate
- Antimuscarinics (e.g., glycopyrronium; see section on end-of-life symptom control); hyoscine TD patches may be helpful if the patient has a prognosis of weeks)
- Cough suppressants (see upcoming discussion)
- Cough-assist devices (often used in patients with neurologic disease; specialist initiation is needed)

Nonproductive
- If there is an irreversible cause, a dry cough should be suppressed.
  a. Peripheral suppressants: Simple linctus may help pharyngeal irritation.
  b. Central suppressants
     - Opioid-naïve patients: dextromethorphan; codeine 30 to 60 mg four times daily or morphine 2.5 to 5 mg PO every 4 hours. Titrate morphine as for pain.
     - Patients established on a strong opioid: The dose equivalent to the PRN analgesic dose can be tried.
     - Diazepam 5 mg PO daily can be given if other measures are ineffective.

Other Symptoms
Bronchorrhoea
- Bronchorrhoea is large-volume mucous production which is seen most often in patients with lung cancer and chronic nonmalignant lung conditions.
- Radiotherapy for patients with lung cancer should be considered, but if this is not possible or appropriate, the following can be tried:
  - Antimuscarinics: glycopyrronium (PO solution, SC, and CSCI), hyoscine (TD, SC, and CSCI)
  - Corticosteroids PO: dexamethasone 4 to 8 mg/day PO
  - Octreotide CSCI 300 µg CSCI/24 h

Haemoptysis
- Consider using antibiotics (if caused by infection), low-molecular-weight heparin (LMWH) (if caused by pulmonary embolism), or radiotherapy (for bleeding tumour).

- Tranexamic acid 1 g PO three times daily can be used to improve coagulation; reduce the dosage to 500 mg three times daily 1 week after bleeding stops. Alternatively, it can be stopped 1 week after bleeding ceases but should be resumed if bleeding recurs.
- Minor to moderate haemoptysis may herald a massive haemorrhage. For management of massive haemoptysis, see 'Emergencies: Haemorrhage (Massive)'.

Lymphangitis Carcinomatosis
- Corticosteroids (dexamethasone 8 mg PO daily) may improve symptoms.
- Diuretics may have some benefit (furosemide 40 mg daily).

Gastrointestinal Symptoms

> **GUIDELINES**
>
> NHS Scotland. (n.d.). *Scottish palliative care guidelines*. Available at https://rightdecisions.scot.nhs.uk/scottish-palliative-care-guidelines.
>   Watson, M., Lucas, C., Hoy, A., et al. (2019). *Oxford handbook of palliative care* (3rd ed.). Oxford: Oxford University Press.

Nausea, Vomiting, and Regurgitation
- Nausea and vomiting should be assessed separately. They can occur independently or together.
- When considering vomiting, it is important to distinguish it from expectoration and true regurgitation.
  - Expectoration should be managed as for cough.
  - Regurgitation is often caused by intrinsic or extrinsic compression of the oesophagus by tumour. If caused by an oesophageal mass, it may be amenable to stenting or balloon dilatation (if the patient can tolerate the procedure).

Potential Causes
- Drugs: opioids, NSAIDs, antibiotics, iron supplements
- Metabolic: hypercalcaemia, uraemia
- Treatments: radiotherapy, chemotherapy
- Intracerebral malignancy (primary or secondary)

- Gastrointestinal (GI) stasis, constipation
- Bowel obstruction
- Vestibular dysfunction
- Psychological factors: anxiety, fear
- Paraneoplastic
- Infection

Potentially Reversible Causes
- Constipation, pain, infection, hypercalcaemia, ascites, increased intracranial pressure (ICP), medications

Management
Based on the following principles:
1. Identify the underlying cause.
2. Treat or manage the cause if it is reversible.
3. Have a clear rationale for pharmacologic management: Choose an antiemetic or antinausea medication based on the likely cause.
4. Administer the antiemetic:
   a. Regularly: Give a stat dose before starting a regular antiemetic.
   b. Give it by the appropriate route (often parenteral, especially if vomiting).
   c. Be prepared to titrate the regular dose after 24 hours.
   d. Rotate antiemetics if the initial choice is ineffective after 24 to 48 hours.
   Table 24.5 summarises antiemetic choice by underlying cause.
- Specific considerations:
  - Some nausea and vomiting may require combinations of antiemetics. When choosing combinations, use antiemetics with different (complementary) central

actions. Be aware that some combinations are antagonistic (e.g., cyclizine + metoclopramide antagonise one another's actions peripherally).
- Ondansetron is very specific in its mode of action and very constipating. Aside from its use in cytotoxic chemotherapy and radiotherapy, the only other main indication is disseminated abdominal or GI malignancy (which can release large amounts of serotonin). Generally, it should be for short-term use (days).
- Route of administration and dosing:
  - Antiemetics should be given parenterally if vomiting is persistent or severe because this will impair absorption of oral medications.
  - If an antiemetic is given CSCI, the regular opioid dose can also be replaced in this way until nausea or vomiting is controlled.
  - After nausea or vomiting is settled for more than 48 hours on CSCI medication, switch to the equivalent oral antiemetic dose.
  - Unless the underlying cause resolves, antiemetics will likely be required for the long term. The exception is when starting an opioid because tolerance to nausea may develop in 1 week or so.
- Table 24.6 summarises dosing and routes of administration.

Constipation
- Constipation is a common problem in patients with LLI.
- Patients may experience infrequent or irregular bowel evacuations and difficulty in defecating. The stools may be hard.

TABLE 24.5	Antiemetic Choice According to Underlying Cause		
Stimulus or Cause of Nausea or Vomiting	**Central Receptor**	**Antagonist—Appropriate Antiemetic Choice**	**Peripheral Action**
Drugs (morphine), metabolites, toxins, uraemia, hypercalcaemia	D2 (CTZ)	Haloperidol	None
Gastric stasis	D2 (CTZ)	Metoclopramide	Cholinergic; blocks dopamine brake in gut; prokinetic effect
Raised intracranial pressure	H1 (VC)	Cyclizine	Antimuscarinic (slows bowel)
Motion	Achm (VC)	Hyoscine hydrobromide	Anticholinergic; reduces secretions and spasm
Vestibular	D2, 5HT2, H1	Prochlorperazine	
Various	D2, 5HT2, Achm, H1 (VC and CTZ)	Levomepromazine	
Cytotoxic chemo, Radiotherapy (RT)	5HT3	Ondansetron (metoclopramide)	5HT3 receptors in bowel; ondansetron is very constipating
Anxiety, fear	GABA mimetic (cerebral cortex)	Lorazepam	

Receptors: *5HT2/3,* serotonin; *Achm,* acetylcholine; *D2,* dopamine; *H1,* histamine.
Locations of receptors: *CTZ,* Chemoreceptor trigger zone; *VC,* vomiting centre.

TABLE 24.6   Antiemetics: Dosing by Route of Administration

| Antiemetic | Dose and Frequency | | | Notes |
	PO	SC	CSCI	
Haloperidol[a]	500 µg–1.5 mg at night and q4h PRN		2–5 mg/24 h	Good at end of life when anxiolytic and antipsychotic properties may also be beneficial
Metoclopramide[a]	10 mg three times daily to 20 mg four times daily (10 mg q4h PRN with maximum 24-h dose of 100 mg)		30–100 mg/24 h	Good prokinetic, comparatively large volume for SC injection
Cyclizine	50 mg twice/thrice daily or q8h PRN		100–150 mg/24 h	Can cause cutaneous irritation
Levomepromazine[a]	6.25 mg at night and q4h PRN (up to 25 mg in 24 h)		12.5–25 mg/24 h	Broad-spectrum, second-line antiemetic; useful PRN in addition to another regular antiemetic
Ondansetron	4–8 mg twice or thrice daily		8–16 mg/24 h	Very constipating: short-term (days) use when possible
Domperidone	10 mg thrice daily	Unavailable	Unavailable	Good prokinetic which does not cross the blood–brain barrier (no antidopaminergic effects) but only available PO and PR
Lorazepam	500 µg–1 mg once daily and q4h PRN	N/A		Useful for anticipatory nausea or vomiting

[a]Avoid in patients with Parkinson disease or Lewy body dementia.
CSCI, Continuous subcutaneous infusion; *N/A,* not applicable; *PO,* by mouth; *PR,* per rectum; *PRN,* as needed; *SC,* subcutaneous.

- Causes include debility, diet (reduced intake, low residue), poor fluid intake, medications (opioids, antimuscarinics, diuretics, 5-hydroxytryptamine (5HT3) receptor antagonists), and biochemical abnormalities (hypercalcaemia, hypokalaemia).
- Consequences include pain, urinary retention, confusion, and overflow diarrhoea.
- Many laxatives are available, and they are often classified by action, although there is much overlap.
- Laxative choice should be based on patient preference and ability; almost all work if given in sufficient doses.

Management
- Anticipate constipation (e.g., when starting an opioid prescribe prophylactic laxatives) and manage it proactively.
- Encourage general measures to aid regular bowel habits (e.g., fluid intake, fibre in diet, mobility, good access to a toilet).
- Use an oral laxative first (rather than rectal).
  - A combination of a stimulant and softener and osmotic is usual.
  - Titrate the dose until the desired stool consistency and frequency are achieved.
- Patients with spinal cord compression or cauda equina or neurologic disease may need a bowel regimen to aid defecation. This often consists of senna taken 3 nights per week, with a glycerol or bisacodyl suppository given the next morning to empty the rectum and sigmoid colon.
- Table 24.7 classifies laxatives by their modes of action and doses.

Diarrhoea
- Ensure adequate fluid intake while managing the cause.
- Causes include:
  - Laxatives
  - Other medications (e.g., antibiotics)
  - Infection
  - Faecal impaction: sudden-onset diarrhoea after a period of constipation
  - Radiotherapy (colitis)
  - Malabsorption
    a. Pancreatic exocrine insufficiency (cystic fibrosis, pancreatic cancer, pancreatectomy): steatorrhoea (i.e., pale, fatty stools with an offensive odour)
    b. Gastrectomy: steatorrhoea
    c. Colectomy: profuse, watery stools
  - Carcinoid tumour: profuse diarrhoea

Management
- Laxatives: Stop and review doses.
- Antibiotics: Check for and treat *Clostridioides difficile* infection.
- Faecal impaction: Give appropriate laxatives, often macrogols.
- Radiotherapy (colitis): Give steroids (dexamethasone 8 mg/day for 1–2 weeks).
- Malabsorption—steatorrhoea: Replace pancreatic enzymes with every meal, snack, and drink that is not clear fluid; give a PPI.

TABLE 24.7	**Laxatives Classified by Mode of Action and Dose**	
Stimulants	• Senna 15 mg at night (prophylaxis); 15–30 mg twice daily (established constipation) • Sodium picosulphate 5–10 mL twice daily • Bisacodyl 5–10 mg at night (prophylactic); 20 mg at night to 20 mg twice daily (established constipation)	Avoid in bowel obstruction
Softeners	• Docusate 100–200 mg twice daily	May be useful in partial bowel obstruction
Osmotic	• Macrogols	Avoid lactulose unless indicated in hepatic impairment (requires a large volume of fluid, causes bloating or flatus and abdominal cramps)
Bulk forming	• Ispaghula husk, methylcellulose	Generally avoided because it may worsen constipation if the patient is unable to take in sufficient fluids
Rectal agents	• Glycerol suppository (lubricates and softens stool) • Bisacodyl suppository (stimulates rectal mucosa) • Microenema • Phosphate enema	Avoid in patients at risk of bleeding (e.g., thrombocytopenia) or infection (neutropenia)
Peripheral opioid antagonists	• Methylnaltrexone bromide (injection) • Naloxegol (oral)	For opioid-induced constipation when other measures have failed

• Carcinoid tumour: 5HT3 receptor antagonist (ondansetron), octreotide
• Nonspecific: loperamide or opioids (e.g., codeine, morphine)

Acid Reflux, Gastritis, and Oesophagitis
• These can be problems in patients with tumours affecting the stomach and oesophagus.

Management
• PPIs can be used at up to double the dose (e.g., lansoprazole 30 mg twice a day, omeprazole 40 mg/day).
• The H_2-antagonist famotidine can be used in dosages of 40 to 80 mg/day (in divided doses twice daily). It can also be given CSCI (20–40 mg CSCI/24 h) under specialist advice. (Supply can be an issue.)

Hiccup
• Diaphragmatic spasms, often caused by irritation from gastric distension or hepatomegaly. Renal failure and steroids are other potential causes in patients with LLIs.

Management
• Antiflatulent, prokinetic, PPI, such as one of the following:
  • Peppermint water 10 mL PRN
  • Metoclopramide 10 mg three times daily PO
  • Lansoprazole 30 mg/day
• Smooth muscle relaxant (e.g., nifedipine 5 mg three times daily)
• Suppression of central hiccup reflex, for example:
  • Baclofen 5 to 10 mg three times daily PO
  • Haloperidol 1 to 3 mg twice daily
  • Midazolam 10 mg + CSCI/24 h for severe hiccup in patients in the last days of life

Ascites
• This may be from a malignant or nonmalignant cause.
• If the patient is too frail for either diuretics or invasive procedures, symptom management with analgesia and antiemetics should be maximised.

Causes
• *Nonmalignant:* advanced hepatic disease with portal hypertension, cardiac failure
• *Malignant:* tumours of the ovary, endometrium, bowel, or liver (primary or secondary); peritoneal metastases from other tumours (e.g., breast)

Management
• *Nonmalignant:* Diuretics (spironolactone and furosemide) are especially valuable in patients with portal hypertension. Expect 0.5 to 1 kg/24 h weight loss; may take 2 to 4 weeks to achieve a significant reduction in ascites:
  a. Monitor for electrolyte disturbance, hypotension, and renal function. Monitor urea and electrolytes weekly or before changing dose.
  b. Dose and titration:
    • Start spironolactone 100 to 200 mg every morning. Increase by 100 mg every 3 to 7 days (maximum response after 2–3 days). The usual maintenance dosage is 300 mg every morning. The maximum dosage is 400 mg every morning or 200 mg every morning in patients who are frail, older, or renally impaired.
    • If there is no change after 2 weeks, consider adding furosemide 40 mg for a few days. This can be increased by 40 mg every 3 to 7 days to a maximum of 160 mg/day.

c. Monitoring: Monitor renal function.

d. Stop diuretics if not tolerated, ascites is unchanged, or renal function is impaired.

- *Malignant:*
    a. Diuretics can be tried but are likely to be less successful than in nonmalignant ascites because ascites is often caused by factors other than portal hypertension alone.
    b. Paracentesis provides effective relief of symptoms, but fluid may reaccumulate within weeks and may require repeat drainage.
    c. Indwelling, tunneled ascitic drains (PleurX peritoneal catheter drainage system) are recommended for patients with recurrent ascites resistant to treatment. Patients can empty these themselves every few days PRN.

Anorexia, Cachexia, and Dysphagia

- All three of these conditions can cause significant distress to patients and those important to them. Managing these symptoms is important, but consideration needs to be given to the fact that they are often inevitable consequences of advanced disease in the final days of life, so this should be communicated to the patient and those important to them.

Anorexia

- This is a loss of appetite for food.
    - Manage underlying or contributing factors if possible (e.g., nausea, constipation, oral problems, ascites).
    - Encourage patients to eat what they like rather than specific foods or supplements.
    - Steroids (e.g., dexamethasone 2–4 mg/day PO) may help improve appetite, but the effects are often short lasting.
    - Megestrol acetate 80 to 160 mg/day may be better for longer term appetite stimulation, but there are numerous contraindication and risks, such as thromboembolism.
    - Both steroids and progestogens increase catabolism of skeletal muscle.
    - Prokinetics may improve early satiety.

Cachexia

- This is a common but complex problem seen in patients with advanced LLIs, including those with heart failure, respiratory disease, and cancer.
- It is likely related to factors such as development of a chronic inflammatory state (caused by cytokine production), abnormal metabolism, and anorexia.
- The consequence is a loss of fat and skeletal muscle, which is not improved by increasing nutritional intake alone.
- Management: Manage anorexia and optimise nutrition.

Dysphagia

- Look for a reversible cause (e.g., oesophageal tumour) amenable to stent or balloon dilatation.
- Prokinetics may be helpful.

Malignant Bowel Obstruction

- This is most often associated with cancer of the bowel or ovary. Intrinsic or extrinsic compression of the bowel by tumour (e.g., peritoneal metastases) can cause obstruction in multiple sites.
- It is often a clinical diagnosis. Investigations may show the site of obstruction but not always (i.e., functional obstruction).
- Symptoms may wax and wane for many months before complete obstruction develops.
- Symptoms depend on the site of obstruction.
    - *High obstruction of the gastric outlet and small bowel:* Large-volume vomiting is the predominant feature, often faeculent after being established.
    - *Low obstruction of the colon:* Constipation is the predominant feature with vomiting coming later.
    - Both can cause colicky abdominal pain and vomiting with or without nausea.

Management

- Consider surgical or interventional options.
    - In patients with advanced malignancy with peritoneal disease, obstruction is likely to be at several sites, and patients are likely to be unfit for surgery. However, suspected obstruction at a single site may be amenable to surgery (e.g., colostomy for obstructing rectal mass, stent to the gastric outlet or duodenum).
    - Parenteral fluid and nutritional support may be appropriate temporary bridging measures for patients in whom there is potential for intervention by surgery or stent or disease-modifying therapies (e.g., chemotherapy).
- Symptomatic treatment for patients unsuitable for surgery:
    - On initial presentation, management is aimed at encouraging peristalsis (prokinetic (e.g., metoclopramide 30–120 mg/day CSCI); stop if it causes colic), reducing peritumour oedema and compression (dexamethasone 8 mg/day PO or SC), and softening stool (docusate 100–200 mg twice daily).
    - Stop steroids if there is no improvement within 2 to 3 days to avoid stimulating the appetite and other side effects.
    - If symptoms do not resolve in 2 to 3 days or obstruction is thought to be complete, treat nausea (cyclizine 150 mg CSCI/24 h), colic (hyoscine butylbromide 60–120 mg CSCI/24 h), and pain (CSCI opioids). In patients with complete bowel obstruction, the aim is to reduce the volume and frequency of vomits and associated symptoms.
    - If the patient has high-volume vomiting, consider placing a Ryle tube for drainage or pharmacologic management (hyoscine butylbromide as above or octreotide 300 µg CSCI/24 h or famotidine 20–40 mg CSCI/24 h).

Oral Symptoms

Oral Candidiasis

- The typical presentation is with altered taste and adherent white *Candida* plaques, but it may also present with redness or soreness.
- When diagnosing oral candidiasis, consider if oesophageal extension is likely.

Management

- Good denture hygiene and mouth care
- Oropharyngeal: nystatin 100,000 units/mL (1 mL four times daily for 7 days) or miconazole gel (5–10 mL four times daily for 7 days) for mild infections; fluconazole (50 mg once daily for 7 days minimum) for moderate to severe infections
- Oesophageal candidiasis: fluconazole 50 mg/day for 7 to 14 days
- In immunocompromised patients, longer courses of fluconazole may be necessary.

Mouth Ulcers and Oral Stomatitis

Mouth Ulcers: Treatment

- Corticosteroids (e.g., hydrocortisone oromucosal tablets 2.5 mg four times daily)

Oral Inflammation and Stomatitis: Treatment

- Correct reversible causes such as badly fitting dentures.
- Maintain oral hygiene with mouthwashes if brushing is too painful (e.g., sodium chloride, sodium bicarbonate, or chlorhexidine (alcohol free)).
- Coating agents can help in oral mucositis caused by chemotherapy or radiotherapy (e.g., GelClair and Orabase).
- Local anaesthetics may help (e.g., lidocaine ointment 5%, cocaine hydrochloride 2%).
- NSAIDs may help (e.g., benzydamine 0.15% mouthwash).
- Systemic analgesics (opioids and nonopioids) may be helpful but may need to be given parenterally (CSCI).
- Treat all secondary infections.

Xerostomia

- This is often the consequence of medications (e.g., morphine, antimuscarinics) or treatment for cancer (e.g., radiotherapy).

Management

- Stimulate natural saliva (e.g., using sugar-free chewing gum).
- Use artificial saliva (e.g., Biotene Oral Balance gel, AS Saliva Orthana).
- Pilocarpine:
  - Particularly useful after radiotherapy for head and neck cancer
  - 5 to 10 mg PO four times daily (pilocarpine 4% eyedrop solution is an alternative; use three drops PO four times daily)

Sialorrhoea

- This is seen most often in patients with advanced neurologic disease.

Management

- Tricyclic antidepressants (e.g., amitriptyline 10 mg at night)
- Hyoscine hydrobromide TD patch 1 mg/72 h; up to two patches can be applied at one time
- Propantheline 15 mg three times daily
- Atropine (1% eye drops) two to three drops three times daily

Neurologic Symptoms (See Also 'Advanced Neurologic Diseases')

Seizures

- Seizures may be caused by preexisting epilepsy or a presenting or later feature of intracerebral malignancy or neurodegenerative disease.

Management

- For acute management see 'Emergencies: Seizures'.
- If there is known epilepsy in a patient on established therapy:
  - Consider an increase in the current antiepileptic drug (AED) dose.
  - Consider addition of levetiracetam.
- If initiating AED for new seizure in patients with irreversible intracerebral lesion or malignancy:
  a. In patient with intracerebral mass or metastases with peritumour oedema, consider dexamethasone 16 mg/day PO (temporary measure); this requires titration downward to the lowest tolerated dose.
  b. Antiepileptics:
    - Sodium valproate 200 mg PO twice daily (modified release); titrate by 200 mg twice daily every 3 days to a maximum 2.5 g/day *or*
    - Levetiracetam 250 mg PO twice daily; titrate by 250 mg twice daily every 2 weeks to a maximum of 3 g/day
- Second-line treatment (e.g., uncontrolled seizures currently taking an oral AED or when other AED is contraindicated or not tolerated): levetiracetam, dosed as above
Note: Levetiracetam can be administered via CSCI. Conversion of the daily PO dose to CSCI of levetiracetam is 1:1.

Intracerebral Malignancy

- Intracerebral malignancy may cause a variety of symptoms, but most usually:
  - Weakness, incoordination, dysphasia
  - Headache
  - Seizures
  - Nausea or vomiting
  - Reduced consciousness
- Radiotherapy may exacerbate symptoms.
- Dexamethasone may reduce any symptoms related to intracerebral oedema.

Management With Steroids

- Consider a high-dose dexamethasone trial (e.g., 8–16 mg/day PO).
- Symptomatic improvement should be seen in 2 to 3 days.
- Monitor for hyperglycaemia, measuring capillary blood glucose (CBG) a minimum of twice weekly in patients with no known diabetes or daily in patients with diabetes.
- If the patient is unable to swallow, dexamethasone can be given SC (best given once to twice daily in doses before lunchtime to reduce the risk of insomnia).
- Discontinue dexamethasone if:
  - There is no improvement after 1 week.
  - Side effects result from steroids (e.g., uncontrolled hyperglycaemia, restlessness).
- If there is improvement in symptoms after 1 week, titrate the dose down to the lowest dose tolerated. Typical reduction of daily dose by 2 to 4 mg, reduced weekly (see Table 24.10).
- After cerebral radiotherapy, the steroid dose should not be reduced until 1 week after radiotherapy is completed. Reduce as above.

Fatigue

- Fatigue is a common symptom in patients with advanced LLIs, especially cancer and its treatment.
- It is often related to cachexia (see the discussion of GI symptoms management).

Management

- Check for symptomatic anaemia.
- Perform thyroid function tests.
- Manage other symptoms (e.g., uncontrolled pain, insomnia, mood disturbance).
- Review concurrent medications.
- Recommend:
  - Regular exercise
  - Sleep hygiene
  - Pacing or prioritisation of activities
- For fatigue refractory to these measures, consider a psychostimulant (e.g., methylphenidate or modafinil).

Delirium

GUIDELINES

Inouye, S. K., van Dyck, C. H., Alessi, C. A., Balkin, S., Siegal, A. P., & Horwitz, R. I. (1990). Clarifying confusion: The confusion assessment method. A new method for detection of delirium. *Annals of Internal Medicine, 113,* 941–948.

National Institute for Health and Care Excellence (2010). *Guideline on the care of dying adults in the last days of life.* Available at https://www.nice.org.uk/guidance/ng31.

National Institute for Health and Care Excellence. (2023). *Delirium: Diagnosis, prevention and management in hospital and long-term care. NICE clinical guideline 103.* Available at https://www.nice.org.uk/Guidance/CG103.

Diagnosis and Presenting Features

- Several tools for identifying and diagnosing delirium are available. The key is to suspect delirium, especially in patients who may present with the hypoactive type. Consider use of the Confusion Assessment Method (Box 24.1).
- The onset is typically acute (within hours or days) and fluctuates hourly or daily.
- Cognitive function is impaired (e.g., worsened concentration, slow responses, and disorientation).
- Perception is altered (e.g., visual or auditory hallucinations).
- Physical function is impaired (e.g., reduced mobility, reduced movement, restlessness, agitation, changes in appetite, sleep disturbance).
- Social behaviour changes are present (e.g., lack of cooperation with reasonable requests; withdrawal; or alterations in communication, mood, or attitude).
- Be particularly vigilant for signs of hypoactive delirium.

Management

1. Identify and treat reversible underlying causes (if appropriate), for example:
   - Infection (e.g., urinary tract infection (UTI), lower respiratory tract infection)
   - Medications: morphine, sedatives, steroids, anticholinergics, tricyclics, neuroleptics, dopaminergics
   - Metabolic: hyperosmolar hyperglycaemic state or hypoglycaemia, hepatic failure, hypercalcaemia, uraemia, hyponatraemia
   - Hypoxia
   - Dehydration
   - Urinary retention, constipation
   - Drug or alcohol withdrawal, including withdrawal of nicotine, antidepressants
   - Psychological distress
2. Provide constant environment and deescalate the situation:
   - Quiet room with subdued lighting
   - Ensure access to sensory aids (i.e., glasses, hearing aids)

• BOX 24.1 Four-Item Confusion Assessment Method

1. Acute onset and fluctuating course
   a. Is there evidence of an acute change in mental status from the patient's baseline?
   b. Did the abnormal behaviours fluctuate during the day or change in severity?
2. Inattention
   a. Did the patient have difficulty focusing attention (e.g., being easily distractible) or have difficulty keeping track of what was being said?
3. Disorganised thinking
   a. Rambling or irrelevant conversation, unclear or illogical flow of ideas, unpredictable switching from one subject to another
4. Altered level of consciousness
   a. Vigilant (hyperalert), lethargic (drowsy, easily roused), stupor (difficult to rouse), unrousable

If YES to 1 + 2 + 3 or 4, a diagnosis of delirium is suggested.

- Clock, calendar, and routine should be on clear display to the patient in the room
- Familiar objects and people (involve family, friends, carers)
- Few interruptions
- Repeated reassurance and explanation (use lucid intervals)
- Simple, respectful communication (use short sentences, calm manner, allow thinking time for patient)
- Avoid moving the patient between rooms
3. Ensure the safety of patient and others.
4. Medications:
   Medications may be used when a person is very distressed, nonpharmacologic measures have failed, and they are a risk to themselves or others.
   - Chronic or mild delirium:
     i. Haloperidol only (benzodiazepines do not improve cognition; they may worsen it). The dosage is 1 to 5 mg SC or 500 µg to 5 mg PO stat and PRN, with a typical maintenance dose of 2.5 to 10 mg CSCI/24 h or 0.5 to 3 mg twice daily PO.
   - Acute or severe delirium (with or without agitation):
     i. First-line treatment: haloperidol only. The dosage is 2.5 to 5 mg PO, SC, or IM hourly. The maximum is 20 mg/24 h, with the maintenance dose typically half of the first 24-hour dose or based on stat doses used.
     ii. Second-line treatment: Add benzodiazepines; use only if sedation is needed or alcohol or benzodiazepine withdrawal is a factor.
   Chronic confusion, dementia (behaviour that challenges), and other symptoms specific to neurodegenerative disease are included in additional sections.

Chronic Confusion

- Presenting features:
  - The onset or course is typically chronic (days to weeks).
  - The pattern is constant: little to no fluctuation; may be progressive.
  - Cognitive function may be normal or impaired (disorientated), but consciousness is not altered.
  - Hallucinations are unusual.
  - Physical impairment is rare; health is generally good.
  - Memory loss is prominent in confusion caused by dementia; mood may be depressed.
  - Confusion caused by dementia gradually worsens over months.

Management

1. Exclude depression.
2. General measures as for delirium (see Delirium).
3. Medications:
   - Chronic confusion: risperidone 0.25 to 1 mg at night (gradually increase to 1 mg twice daily)

- Acute-on-chronic confusion with delirium: haloperidol as for delirium (see 'Delirium')
- Insomnia: trazodone 50 to 100 mg at night

Skin Symptoms

> **GUIDELINES**
>
> British Lymphology Society and Lymphoedema Support Network. (2016). *Consensus document on the management of cellulitis in lymphoedema.* Available at https://www.thebls.com/public/uploads/documents/document-75091530863967.pdf
>   International Lymphoedema Framework and Canadian Lymphedema Framework. (2010). *International Lymphoedema Framework position document: The management of lymphoedema in advanced cancer and oedema at the end of life.* Available at http://ww.lympho.org.

Lymphoedema and Oedema

Classification of Oedema in Patients With Life-Limiting Illnesses

- Oedema in advanced disease is common and often multifactorial in nature, occurring when net capillary filtration exceeds lymphatic drainage. It may or may not have impaired lymphatic drainage (lymphoedema) as a component.
- *Causes of impaired lymphatic drainage (lymphoedema):* metastatic lymphadenopathy, surgery (especially when lymph nodes removed), radiotherapy, immobility, long-standing increased flow.
- *Causes of increased capillary filtration:* hypoalbuminaemia, venous hypertension (cardiac failure, extrinsic compression from tumour, inferior vena cava obstruction or SVCO, venous thrombosis), medications (e.g., corticosteroids, NSAIDs, hormones, chemotherapy).
- Oedema and lymphoedema may present in patients with advanced cancer, heart failure, respiratory disease, renal failure, neurologic disease, or liver disease. As oedema becomes chronic, inflammatory and fibrotic changes develop.
- Lymphoedema services are often part of local palliative care provision and normally manage patients with primary (congenital) lymphoedema and secondary lymphoedema caused by the effects of disease or its treatment. They are also a useful source of reference for patients with more general oedema at the end of life.

Signs and Symptoms

- Oedema may be a well-recognised complication of the underlying diagnosis (e.g., in cardiac or hepatic failure).
- Consider underlying venous thrombosis if asymmetric oedema develops acutely in a limb.
- Lymphoedema classically presents as follows:
  - In a discrete anatomic location from an underlying cause (e.g., arm lymphoedema after axillary node clearance)

- Skin indurates or pits when pressure is applied.
- Skin becomes thickened, and changes become chronic; hyperkeratosis, papillomata, and lymphangiectasia develop.
- Cellulitis and lymphorrhoea (leakage of lymph fluid caused by breaks in the skin) are recognised complications.

Management

- *Of lymphoedema:* Management is aimed at reducing swelling and thereby restoring function and reducing discomfort. It is tailored to the individual and their stage of underlying illness; early intervention is important to prevent chronic changes. Contraindications are unusual but include uncontrolled cardiac failure. Patients diagnosed with acute deep vein thrombosis must wait 8 weeks before receiving intensive lymphoedema intervention, and those with arterial insufficiency (Ankle–brachial pressure index (ABPI) <0.5) should not have compression.
- Consider investigation or treatment for underlying or exacerbating causes (e.g., for malignancy, venous thrombosis, cardiac failure, anaemia, or management of medications exacerbating oedema).
- Complete or complex decongestive therapy (CDT) is the mainstay of management. Management is initiated by specialist lymphoedema practitioners, and when possible, self-care is taught to the patient or family. CDT involves:
  - Manual lymphatic drainage (MLD). This stimulates lymphatic tissues, decongesting deep lymphatics and increasing drainage of lymph from the affected site. MLD is undertaken by specialised professionals who can teach a simplified version (simple lymphatic drainage) to patients or carers.
  - Compression bandaging, hosiery, or Velcro compression devices are used. These increase tissue pressure to reduce oedema and promote drainage of lymph (when used with MLD) while preventing backflow or evacuated lymph. Multilayered compression can contain dressings to absorb lymphorrhoea.
  - Skin care and infection prevention: Skin care with the intent of avoiding infection or cellulitis includes maintaining skin hydration (using emollients daily), careful hygiene, and avoidance of skin trauma.
  - Exercise is undertaken under compression to improve venous drainage and uptake of lymph and to soften fibrosis. It may be active or passive.
  - Elevation of the affected limb (to a level above the heart) can be helpful in patients with advanced disease who are unable to exercise.
- *Of cellulitis associated with lymphoedema:*
  - First-line treatment:
    a. Oral amoxicillin 500 mg 8-hourly is the treatment of choice.
    b. If there is evidence of *Staphylococcus aureus* infection: flucloxacillin 500 mg four times daily in addition to or as alternative to amoxicillin.

    c. In patients with confirmed penicillin allergy: erythromycin 500 mg four times daily or clarithromycin 500 mg twice daily.
    d. If there are complicating factors (e.g., animal scratch/bite): discuss with a microbiologist.
  - Second-line treatment (if there is a poor response to amoxicillin or flucloxacillin after 48 hours): clindamycin 300 mg four times daily
- *Duration of antibiotics.* Continue antibiotics until all signs of acute infection have resolved. This often means treatment for a minimum of 2 weeks but may be as long as 1 to 2 months. Note that skin changes or discolouration may persist after infection resolves.
- *Other measures.* Do not use compression garments in the acute attack but replace them as soon as the affected area is able to tolerate them. Elevation of affected limb and bed rest are important. Exercise can be resumed after inflammation subsides.

Sweating (Paraneoplastic)

Presenting Features

- Uncontrolled sweating is often associated with malignancy.
- It may be associated with paraneoplastic pyrexia (i.e., pyrexia in absence of infective cause).
- Sweating may affect one specific part of the body or be more generalised.

Management

- Antipyretics:
  - Paracetamol 500 mg to 1 g four times daily
  - Naproxen 250 to 500 mg twice daily (or an alternative NSAID)
- Antimuscarinics:
  - Amitriptyline 10 to 50 mg at night
  - Propantheline 15 to 30 mg twice daily
  - Hyoscine hydrobromide or glycopyrronium
- Other:
  - Propranolol 10 to 20 mg twice daily, gabapentin

Pruritus

Causes

- A relatively common symptom in advanced LLIs, pruritus may have a wide variety of causes.

Management

1. *General:*
   - Establish, treat, and remove all causes (e.g., skin infection, medication).
   - Keep the skin moisturised: Use emollient daily, use aqueous cream instead of soap, avoid hot baths, and dry skin by patting.
   - Avoid sweating (see the section on managing sweating) and keep the skin cool.
   - Macerated skin should be dried and hydrocortisone 1% used if localised inflammation (dermatitis) is present.

- Topical antipruritics include menthol 0.5% to 2%, phenol 0.5% to 3%, and camphor 0.5% to 3%.
- Use sedative antihistamines at bedtime or regularly (e.g., chlorphenamine 4 mg three times daily).
2. *Cause specific:*
   - Rashes: antihistamines (topical cream or systemic), menthol in aqueous cream, hydrocortisone 1% cream
   - Opioids: chlorphenamine 4 mg three times daily or cetirizine 10 mg/day; switch to an alternative opioid; ondansetron (4–8 mg twice daily)
   - Cholestasis: measures to resolve cholestasis if appropriate (e.g., biliary stent); cholestyramine (often poorly tolerated), sertraline 50 to 100 mg once daily, rifampicin 150 to 600 mg once daily, naltrexone 12.5 to 25 mg once daily (if not taking opioid analgesia)
   - Uraemia: localised itch can respond to topical capsaicin cream, ultraviolet B phototherapy, gabapentin 100 mg after haemodialysis or doxepin 10 mg twice daily
   - Hodgkin lymphoma: prednisolone 10 to 20 mg three times daily
   - Paraneoplastic or other causes: paroxetine 5 to 20 mg once daily or sertraline 50 to 100 mg once daily, mirtazapine 15 mg/day

Malignant Wound Management (Bleeding From Wounds, Odour and Infection, Fistulae)

- Wounds from cancer can cause a variety of problems.
- Ideally, palliative radiotherapy, surgery, or even chemotherapy may help their management, but in advanced disease, these are not always possible.
   - In all cases, aim to make dressings as unobtrusive and comfortable as possible, change dressings as infrequently as possible, and protect surrounding healthy tissues.
   - Pain should be managed using approaches as outlined in 'Symptom Management: Pain'. If wounds are significantly painful, systemic analgesia is often required:
      - It is advisable to make PRN analgesia available, which can be given before changing dressings on malignant wounds.
      - If changing of dressings causes significant distress, lorazepam 500 µg to 1 mg PO can also be given before dressing change.
- An increase in pain in a wound may be a sign of infection (see upcoming discussion).

Bleeding

- Haemostatic can be used topically or systemically:
   - Topical: tranexamic acid 10% (500-mg/5-mL ampoule) applied to gauze and held against the bleeding surface of the wound
   - Systemic: tranexamic acid 1 g PO three times daily. Because of potential side effects, halve the dose or stop 1 week after bleeding is stopped. Resume if bleeding recurs.

- Other options:
   - Gauze soaked in adrenaline 1:1000 solution (1 mg in 1 mL) and applied to areas of bleeding (prolonged or repeated use may cause further ischaemia and further bleeding)
   - Alginate dressings

Odour and Infection

- Tumours breaching the skin surface (whether primary or metastatic) are liable to ischaemia, necrosis, and anaerobic infection.
   - Infection may be acute or chronic. If evidence of infection develops, treat as for cellulitis (e.g., flucloxacillin or erythromycin).
   - Odour is often caused by the presence of anaerobic bacteria. Options for managing odour include metronidazole topical gel 0.75% applied to the wound or dressing daily or metronidazole PO 400 mg three times daily for 1 week. If odour improves, metronidazole may be reduced to 200 mg once daily (indefinitely).

Exudate and Enterocutaneous Fistulae

- Exudate requires containment with highly absorbent dressings. Undamaged skin around the wound should be protected with a barrier cream such as Cavilon.
- When fistulae develop, management should include:
   - Protecting surrounding skin (see earlier)
   - Containing any effluent using ostomy collection bags if necessary
   - Reducing fistula output. Octreotide may be given SC (e.g., 100 µg SC twice or thrice daily).

Depression and Anxiety

Depression

- Depression is a significant problem in patients with LLIs of all types.
- Its presence should be actively sought, and it should not be assumed that low mood or depression in patients with LLIs is inevitable.

Diagnosis

- Many physical symptoms of depression are common in LLIs, such as loss of appetite, disturbed sleep, fatigue, and psychomotor slowing.
- In palliative care patients, withdrawal, anhedonia, feelings of guilt, hopelessness, or wishes for death or suicide may suggest depression.
- The simple question 'Are you feeling depressed'? can be helpful in identifying depression.
- A variety of screening tools are available; those that have fewer questions are often more appropriate for the palliative population (e.g., Edinburgh Depression Scale).
- Use of the distress thermometer can assist in identification of factors contributing to distress.

Management

- Assess for medications that may affect mood, delirium, hypothyroidism, and dementia.
- Ensure good palliative care is provided, including adequate management of any physical symptoms, spiritual needs, and social support needs. Review depressive symptoms after these have been addressed.
- As for any depressive episode, mild to moderate depression may be managed with psychological support and CBT.
- If an antidepressant is indicated (moderate to severe depression) and the patient's anticipated prognosis long enough to benefit (i.e., >1 month), then the choice can be based on side effects, safety profiles, and patient comorbidities:
  a. The first choice is usually an SSRI. If it is partially effective, titrate the dose. If it is ineffective, switch to an alternative SSRI or mirtazapine.
  b. Sertraline (an SSRI; 50-mg starting dose in depression; 25 mg starting dose in anxiety). It is safer in chronic renal failure and after myocardial infarction (MI).
  c. Citalopram (an SSRI; 10-mg starting dose). It is good in anxiety and safer in patients with seizures and taking AEDs. An oral suspension is available.
  d. Mirtazapine (15-mg starting dose). It possibly has a faster mode of action than other antidepressants. Sedative effect and appetite stimulation may be helpful. It is safe in patients with cardiac failure and diabetes.
  e. Amitriptyline: useful for patients with concurrent pain or insomnia. Avoid if the patient has significant cardiac disease or after MI, in hepatic failure, and in patients with glaucoma. There is a greater risk in overdose.
  f. Duloxetine (an SNRI) may be useful when patients have concurrent neuropathic pain.
  g. Methylphenidate may be used in patients whose prognosis is thought to be weeks at most, when time is insufficient for conventional antidepressant. It may have an onset of action within days. The dosage is 5 mg PO twice daily (maximum, 40 mg/day).

Anxiety

- May present with depression or alone
  - In patients with days to live, manage with benzodiazepines.
  - For patients with longer prognoses:
    a. Venlafaxine (an SNRI) can be helpful. Start with 37.5 mg PO twice daily.
    b. Sertraline (start with 25mg/day PO) and citalopram are alternatives.
    c. Pregabalin is useful in patients with concurrent neuropathic pain.
    d. Benzodiazepine may also be required.

Bleeding

- For massive haemorrhage, see 'Emergencies'.
- For haemoptysis, see 'Symptom Management: Respiratory'.
- For bleeding wounds, see 'Symptom Management: Skin'.
- Bleeding can occur from a number of anatomic sites; management may be directed at the bleeding site or via systemic therapy.
- Ensure that any medications that may encourage bleeding have been reviewed and stopped if necessary (e.g., LMWH (check for heparin-induced thrombocytopenia), warfarin, aspirin, clopidogrel, NSAIDs).
- Treat for any infection which may exacerbate bleeding or cause DIC (e.g., UTI, chest infection).
- Consider referring for radiotherapy to bleeding tumours (e.g., to bladder, lung) or local coagulation (e.g., cryotherapy or diathermy) if appropriate.
- *Systemic treatment* (for any bleeding site):
  - Tranexamic acid PO: 1 g three times daily initially. One week after bleeding stops, it may be stopped completely or reduced to 500 mg three times daily. If bleeding recurs, resume 1 g three times daily and continue indefinitely.
  - Note: There is risk of clot retention if used for haematuria.
- *Local treatment:*
  - Topical tranexamic acid: 10% solution (500 mg/5 mL applied on gauze) for cutaneous bleeding or epistaxis; 5% solution (500 mg/10 mL) as mouthwash or for rectal bleeding
  - Silver nitrate stick applied to bleeding points
  - Sucralfate paste or suspension

Special Notes on Steroids

GUIDELINES

Diabetes UK. (2021). *End of life care.* Available at https://www.diabetes.org.uk/for-professionals/improving-care/clinical-recommendations-for-professionals/diagnosis-ongoing-management-monitoring/end-of-life-care.

National Institute of Clinical Excellence. (2020). *Clinical Knowledge Summary: Corticosteroids—oral.* Available at https://cks.nice.org.uk/topics/corticosteroids-oral.

Indications for and Use of Steroids (Dexamethasone)

- Steroids are indicated in the palliative management of patients with various conditions. The most commonly used in palliative care is dexamethasone; the dosage varies depending on the condition and symptom being managed (Table 24.8).
- When used, consideration should be given to their side effects, notably hyperglycaemia, muscle wasting (proximal myopathy), mood disturbance, osteoporosis, and adrenal suppression.
- Corticosteroids vary in their ratio of mineralocorticoid-to-glucocorticoid properties (Table 24.9). This determines their therapeutic action, with glucocorticoid properties being used in palliative care for antiinflammatory action. High mineralocorticoid action is generally

TABLE 24.8 Oral Dexamethasone Starting Doses

Indication	Daily Dose (Daily Dose >4 mg Usually Given in Two Divided Doses, Before Lunchtime)
Appetite (anorexia)	4 mg
Liver capsule pain	4–8 mg
Pain due to nerve compression	4–8 mg
Bowel obstruction	8 mg Note: Often given as a trial SC. Ensure that the steroid is reviewed daily because it may stimulate appetite, which can cause significant distress in patients with irreversible obstruction.
Intracerebral oedema, increased ICP, nausea and vomiting caused by increased ICP	8–16 mg Note: If for nausea or vomiting in increased ICP, give in combination with an antiemetic SC or CSCI.
Superior vena cava obstruction	16 mg
Metastatic spinal cord compression	16 mg

Subcutaneous Dexamethasone

Dexamethasone can be given by SC injection. The injectable formulation varies, most often either 3.3 or 3.8 mg/mL. For practical purposes, consider dexamethasone 4 mg PO equivalent to either 3.3 or 3.8 mg SC.

CSCI, Continuous subcutaneous infusion; *ICP,* intracranial pressure; *PO,* by mouth; *SC,* subcutaneous.

TABLE 24.9 Steroids: Approximate Equivalent Antiinflammatory, Glucocorticoid, and Mineralocorticoid Properties

Steroid	Dexamethasone	Prednisolone	Hydrocortisone
Equivalent antiinflammatory dose	1 mg	7.5 mg	25 mg
Relative glucocorticoid activity	30	4	1
Relative mineralocorticoid activity	Minimal mineralocorticoid action	0.8	1

undesirable (because of resulting water retention) but useful in adrenal replacement.

- Generally, just one corticosteroid should be prescribed. See Table 24.9 for equivalent antiinflammatory doses.
- Dexamethasone should be started at an appropriate dose (see Table 24.8), and a reduction in the dose should be attempted when symptoms improve (or after 2 weeks at most).
- Gastric protection in the form of lansoprazole (or similar) should be given, especially to patients also taking NSAIDs.
- Check CBG in all patients before commencing corticosteroids.
- To avoid insomnia, steroids should be given in divided doses with the latest dose at lunchtime.
- Steroids may be given by SC injection. This may be helpful as a temporary measure in a patient with dysphagia or vomiting (e.g., caused by intracerebral mass or oedema), but steroids should not be routinely

continued when a patient is in the last days of life (discussion to come).

Monitoring Patients Taking Corticosteroids

- CBG should be monitored in all patients: daily in patients with known diabetes (to enable titration of oral hypoglycaemic medications/insulin) and twice weekly in those not known to have diabetes.
- Monitor symptom benefit and reassess after 1 week.
- See management of steroid-induced diabetes (later).

Stopping or Withdrawing Steroids

- At the time of starting steroids, a plan should be made for review and reducing the dose.
- Monitor patients for signs of hypoadrenal crisis when steroids are withdrawn.
- Stop steroids abruptly if:
  - Steroids bring no symptomatic benefit after 1 week.
  - Unacceptable side effects occur less than 1 week after starting.

- A patient enters the last days of life (stop steroids when a patient is dying and no longer responsive). In this situation, steroids can be stopped abruptly, however long the duration. But if steroids are potentially managing significant symptoms (e.g., increased ICP or SVCO), consider alternative symptom management options (e.g., prophylactic midazolam CSCI) to prevent seizures.
- Taper steroids gradually when:
  - The patient has been taking more than 4 mg of dexamethasone for over 1 week or a lower dose for over 2 weeks in total (because this may have suppressed endogenous production).
  - The risk of rebound symptoms exists (e.g., significant cerebral oedema).
- The aim is to stop all courses of steroids completely unless the patient has a significant recurrence of symptoms. In this case, maintain the patient on the minimal effective dose.
- Table 24.10 provides guidance on how to taper the steroid dose.

Management of New-Onset Steroid-Induced Diabetes

- Steroid-induced diabetes can occur in patients previously not known to have diabetes. It can occur with any corticosteroid taken for more than a few days.
- Steroids taken in the morning tend to cause an increase in blood glucose around late afternoon to early evening. This can be managed by giving gliclazide or isophane insulin in the morning.
- CBG should be checked before starting steroids in all patients. If CBG is above 8 mmol/L, check with a venous sample and manage accordingly before starting steroids.
- In patients with LLIs, aim for CBG in the range of 6 to 15 mmol/L to minimise symptoms of hyperglycaemia (although 10–15 mmol/L is acceptable).
- When discontinuing steroids, reduce hypoglycaemic medications.
- Patients already known to have diabetes should have their medications titrated according to any changes in CBG exacerbated by steroids.

TABLE 24.10	Tapering Dexamethasone Dose	
Starting Dose	Weekly Reduction in Daily Dose by	If Recurrent Symptoms
>8 mg/day	4 mg; then once <8 mg/day as below	Increase back to lowest effective dose; then try more cautious reduction (e.g., 1–2 mg weekly)
<8 mg/day	2 mg	

- *Management of new steroid-induced diabetes when steroids are given once daily (mornings):*
  - Check the CBG before the evening meal.
  - If the CBG is consistently above 15 mmol/L, start gliclazide 40 mg with breakfast.
  - Titrate gliclazide by increments of 40 mg/day until the CBG is 6 to 15 mmol/L. The maximum morning dosage is 240 mg/day.
  - If gliclazide is ineffective, switch to morning insulin and seek specialist advice.

Care in the Last Days of Life

Prognostication

GUIDELINES

Leadership Alliance for the Care of Dying People. (2014). *One chance to get it right: Improving people's experience of care in the last few days and hours of life.* Available at http://www.gov.uk/government/uploads/system/uploads/attachment_data/file/323188/One_chance_to_get_it_right.pdf.

National Institute for Health and Care Excellence. (2015). *Care of dying adults in the last days of life. NICE clinical guideline 31.* Available at https://www.nice.org.uk/guidance/ng31.

Thomas, K., Wilson, J. A., & GSF Team. (2022). *2022 GSF PIG . National Gold Standards Framework Centre in End of Life Care.* Available at https://goldstandardsframework.org.uk/how-to-use-the-new-2022-gsf-pig-in-your-practice.

- Judging whether a person is entering the last few days of life can be challenging.
- Regardless of how much experience a professional has, there always remains some uncertainty. It is important to openly acknowledge this, especially to patients and those caring for them.
- The following clinical signs may suggest a person is dying:
  - Global clinical deterioration despite optimal management of underlying LLI or concurrent problems
  - Daily deterioration in performance status
  - Profound fatigue, minimal oral intake (sips of fluid only), and difficulty swallowing oral medications
  - Signs such as agitation, Cheyne–Stokes breathing, significant deterioration in level of consciousness, mottled skin, and noisy respiratory secretions
    - In this situation, ensure that the patient's symptomatic and physical care needs are anticipated and that measures are put in place to address their holistic care.
  - Involve the patient as much as they are able or desire. When they are no longer able to contribute, consider any advance decisions they made and recorded.
  - Attending to the understanding, wishes, and needs of those important to them, especially any carers, is crucial in providing successful care in the last days of life.

Stopping Treatments

GUIDELINES

General Medical Council. (2022). *Treatment and care towards the end of life: Good practice in decision making.* Available at https://www.gmc-uk.org/ethical-guidance/ethical-guidance-for-doctors/treatment-and-care-towards-the-end-of-life.
National Institute for Health and Care Excellence. (2017). *Nutrition support for adults: Oral nutrition support, enteral tube feeding and parenteral nutrition. NICE clinical guideline 32.* Available at https://www.nice.org.uk/guidance/cg32.

- As death approaches, it is appropriate to rationalise medications and treatment, stopping them when appropriate.
- An informed decision to stop any treatment can be made by any patient with capacity.
- If a medication or treatment is stopped, either intentionally or because it is no longer possible to administer it, thought should be given to ensure ongoing symptom control is unaffected.
- When needed, medications for symptom control should be provided by effective and accessible means (see later).

Medications

- Medications that can be stopped:
  - Oral medications for which there is no parenteral replacement after a patient loses the ability to swallow
  - Oral medications not contributing to symptom control (e.g., prophylactic medications such as statins)
- Medications that should be continued or alternative:
  - Medications required for symptom control (e.g., long-term opioids for pain)
  - Medications whose withdrawal may cause severe symptoms (e.g., long-term antiepileptic medications or benzodiazepines)
- Means of continuing medications:
  - When the oral route is no longer viable, consider liquid formulation that can be given via percutaneous endoscopic gastrostomy (PEG) or radiologically inserted gastrostomy (RIG) (if available). Only continue medications considered necessary for ongoing symptom relief.
  - Most medications for symptom control at end of life can be given CSCI via a syringe driver (see 'Syringe Drivers').

Nutrition and Hydration

- A patient with capacity to do so may choose to stop clinically assisted nutrition and hydration at any point.
- Consider the benefits, burdens, and risks of nutrition and hydration separately.
- Nutrition and hydration administered by tube or drip are considered as medical treatment.
- For a person considered to be in the last hours to days of life, the burdens and risk of clinically assisted nutrition and hydration often outweigh the benefits. But it is important to consider any previous request of the patient (including any valid ADRT), those appointed as a legal proxy, and those important to the patient. Guidance from the General Medical Council is available to assist decision making.
- Both should be reviewed regularly, particularly if the patient exceeds their anticipated prognosis.
- Nutrition:
  - Most people in the last days to week of life gradually stop eating.
  - Clinically assisted nutrition (administered by tube or drip) may be stopped by any patient with capacity to make this decision or in the patient's best interests if they are not competent to give consent (if those responsible for a best interests decision conclude that the burdens and risks outweigh benefits).
- Hydration:
  - In most circumstances, the dying process entails a person gradually ceasing to take oral fluids, and when in the last hours to days of life, parenteral replacement is unlikely to be appropriate.
  - A person's hydration status and needs should be assessed as they enter the last few days of life.
  - Clinically assisted fluids (administered via tube or drip) can be stopped by any patient with capacity to do so or in the patient's best interests if they are not competent to consent (if those responsible for a best interests decision conclude that the burdens and risks outweigh the benefits).
  - Regular mouth care should be provided to patients in the final days to week of life.

Noninvasive Ventilation

- As with other treatments, noninvasive ventilation (NIV) can be stopped at any time by a patient competent to make the decision to do so.
- Specialist support from palliative care teams or professionals with working knowledge of the legal and ethical guidelines and practicalities around stopping NIV should be available to healthcare professionals and patients in this situation.
- When stopping, medication may be given to alleviate any symptoms experienced, particularly for patients requiring NIV 24 hours a day:
  - For example, SC or CSCI opioids for breathlessness, with SC or CSCI benzodiazepines for breathlessness and anxiety. See 'Symptom Control: Breathlessness', 'Care in the Last Days of Life: Anticipatory Medications', and 'Syringe Driver' for dosages and guidance.

Anticipatory Medications and Care

For guidance on dosages of CSCI medications at end of life, see 'Syringe Driver'.

- Everything possible should be done to anticipate symptoms, care, and support needs of people in the last days of life and those important to them.

- Equipment needed to manage a patient at home (e.g., hospital bed, commode, hoist) should be anticipated whenever possible and adequate support by professional carers arranged.
- Anticipatory medications should be readily available for SC administration:
  - Medications should have appropriate community administration instructions or record.
  - A minimal number of medications should be available to avoid confusion (for more options, see relevant symptom control sections).
- Commonly used anticipatory medications are listed in Tables 24.11 and 24.12, along with appropriate indications for their use and doses. All injections should be administered SC. There may be variation to this in local guidance; local guidance should be followed whenever possible.
- Anticipatory medications should be selected based not simply on local policy or availability but also considering the symptoms that specific person is likely to experience, any intolerances or contraindications (e.g., haloperidol in Parkinson disease), and established medications (e.g., oxycodone rather than morphine).
- If patients regularly require PRN doses (e.g., three or more PRN doses of analgesia daily), their regular (CSCI) dose should be increased accordingly.
- Guidance around opioid use in renal failure varies according to local policy. See 'End-Stage Renal Failure' for guidance.

Syringe Driver

GUIDELINES

MIMS Online. (2016). *Syringe driver compatibility*. Available at http:/ww.mims.co.uk.

Right Decisions for Health and Care. (n.d.). Scottish Palliative Care guidelines. *Compatibility and stability tables for SC infusion*. Available at https://rightdecisions.scot.nhs.uk/scottish-palliative-care-guidelines/symptom-control/syringe-pumps/assessment/compatibility-and-stability-tables-for-subcutaneous-infusion-2a-to-7.

Indications and Practicalities

- Syringe drivers are used to enable delivery of symptom-control medications when an alternative to the oral route is required, for example:
  - At the end of life when the patient is no longer able to swallow
  - As a temporary measure in a patient with vomiting or dysphagia
- They are battery-powered devices that enable the administration of medications by CSCI. The most common in current use is the CME McKinley T34.
- Infusion through the skin is achieved by plastic or Teflon cannula:
  - The best sites for these are the upper arms and anterior chest wall and suprascapular region, but the abdominal wall and thighs can also be used.

TABLE 24.11   Anticipatory As-Needed Medications for Symptom Control in Opioid-Naïve Patients

Symptom or Indication	Medication	PRN Dose (SC Unless Stated Otherwise)
Pain	Morphine (opioid naïve patient)	2.5–5 mg 1-hourly
	Diamorphine (opioid naïve patient)	2.5–5 mg 1-hourly
Nausea or vomiting	Haloperidol	1–2 mg 4-hourly
	Levomepromazine	6.25–12.5 mg 4-hourly
Secretions	Glycopyrronium	200–400 µg 4-hourly
	Hyoscine butylbromide	20 mg 4-hourly
Delirium	Haloperidol	1–5 mg SC 4-hourly (see also section on delirium)
Agitation	Midazolam	2.5–5 mg 1-hourly
Seizures	Midazolam PO	10 mg for prolonged or distressing seizures (may also be given in buccal formulation; see also section on seizures)
	Diazepam	10 mg PR
Risk of distressing life-threatening event (e.g., massive haemorrhage, airway obstruction)	Midazolam	10 mg IM (if haemorrhage)

IM, Intramuscular; *PO,* per oral; *PR,* per rectum; *PRN,* as needed; *SC,* subcutaneous.

TABLE 24.12 Anticipatory As-Needed Opioid Analgesia for Patients Taking Regular or Established Opioids[a]

Regular Opioid	PRN SC Opioid	Additional Information
Morphine or oxycodone PO	1/12 of patient's current daily (24 h) oral dose	Replace regular PO opioid with CSCI dose when patient is unable to swallow
Morphine or oxycodone CSCI	1/6 of total daily CSCI dose	—
Diamorphine CSCI	1/6 of patient's current CSCI dose	—
TD opioid patch (e.g., buprenorphine or fentanyl)	Provide PRN medication at appropriate dose (see approximate equivalences in the 'Pain' section or Appendix 32 or seek specialist advice)	Continue TD opioid patch until death; titrate analgesia by adding in a regular CSCI opioid if indicated
Methadone	Seek specialist guidance	—

[a]Ensure the patient has anticipatory medications for other symptoms; see also Table 24.11.
CSCI, Continuous subcutaneous infusion; *PO,* by mouth; *PRN*, as needed; *TD*, transdermal.

- Sites should be inspected regularly for signs of reaction or irritation. They should be rotated every 3 to 5 days.
- CSCI administration is off-label use for most medications.
- The conventional infusion period is 24 hours, which helps ensure contents remain stable and sterile and achieves more even plasma concentration of medication than repeated SC injections:
  - Contents are changed (and adjusted as necessary) once daily.
- Combinations of medications (e.g., analgesia plus antiemetic) can be used. When using combinations of medications:
  - Check compatibility data because some do not mix and may precipitate, affecting symptom control (see Appendix 30).
  - Water for injection is the normal diluent, with a few exceptions.
  - Dilute contents to the maximum volume possible to reduce the risk of skin reactions at the infusion site.
  - Usually up to three drugs are combined.
  - Combination and dosing are limited by volume: The maximum fill volume of a McKinley T34 is 34 mL in a 50-mL syringe, although 22 mL in a 30-mL syringe is more commonly used.
- It is good practice to ensure patients have additional PRN medications available for symptom control. It can take hours to appreciate the benefit of starting CSCI medications, and SC alternatives should be available for symptoms such as breakthrough pain or nausea.

Starting Doses

See also 'Symptom Management Specific to Advanced Chronic Kidney Disease: End-Stage Renal Failure' for patients with known renal impairment.
- Syringe driver starting doses: Table 24.13 gives common starting doses for CSCI medications.

TABLE 24.13 Starting Doses for Continuous Subcutaneous Infusion Medications in the Last Days to Week of Life

Symptom	CSCI Medication/24 h
Pain (opioid naïve)	Morphine 10 mg CSCI/24 h *or* Oxycodone 5–10 mg CSCI/24 h *or* Diamorphine 10 mg CSCI/24 h
Agitation	Midazolam 10–20 mg CSCI/24 h
Nausea or vomiting	Haloperidol 3–5 mg/24 h *or* CSCI equivalent of alternative antiemetic
Secretions	Glycopyrronium 600 μg–1.2 mg/24 h
Risk of seizures	Midazolam 20 mg+/24 h

CSCI, Continuous subcutaneous infusion.

- See the section on symptom control of nausea and vomiting for CSCI doses of antiemetics (see Table 24.6).
- *Patients taking established medications.* Remember to stop the equivalent PO medications (e.g., modified-release opioid) if switching to CSCI delivery (Table 24.14):
- Converting from PO to CSCI and vice versa:
  a. Medications are normally more potent SC (CSCI) than PO; as such, dose reductions are usual.
  b. Refer to local guidelines on dose conversion; seek specialist advice and refer to opioid equivalence tables (see Appendix 32) and the antiemetic dosing table in symptom control section (see Table 24.6).
  c. If symptoms are controlled and a switchback from CSCI to PO is indicated, remember to increase doses when necessary. CSCI is usually stopped when the first PO dose is given.
  - Converting from TD to CSCI: When a patient is in the last days to week of life, TD opioids should be continued. Any additional analgesic requirements are supplemented by a PRN SC and CSCI strong opioid.

Symptom and Medication	CSCI/24 h
TABLE 24.14 Guidance on Switching From Established Oral and Transdermal to Continuous Subcutaneous Infusion Medications	
Pain: Morphine or oxycodone PO regular dose (IR or MR) continuing as CSCI equivalent	PO:SC potency ratio for both morphine and oxycodone is ~1:2, so halve the total oral 24-h dose and administer CSCI. For example, morphine 100 mg total PO/24 h = morphine 50 mg CSCI/24 h. For example, oxycodone 40 mg total PO/24 h = oxycodone 20 mg CSCI/24 h.
Pain: Morphine PO regular dose switching to equivalent CSCI diamorphine (see 'Symptom Control: Pain' and Appendix 32 for guidance)	PO morphine: SC diamorphine potency ratio is ~1:3. For example, morphine 30 mg total PO/24 h = diamorphine 10 mg CSCI/24 h.
Pain: TD buprenorphine or fentanyl patches	Continue TD patch and supplement with SC PRN strong opioid (morphine, diamorphine, or oxycodone if no renal impairment). If requiring three or more PRN SC opioid doses daily, supplement with CSCI opioid. For example, additional three doses of morphine 5 mg SC in 24 h. Start morphine 15 mg CSCI/24 h in addition to TD patch. Seek specialist advice on dosing.
If nausea or vomiting:	CSCI equivalent of previous antiemetic. See Table 24.6 in 'Symptom Management Guidelines: Gastrointestinal Symptoms'.
Established antiepileptic medication	Midazolam 20 mg+/24 h Levetiracetam and sodium valproate are used CSCI in some regions; seek specialist advice.
For renal failure, seek specialist advice and refer to 'End-Stage Renal Failure'.	

CSCI, Continuous subcutaneous infusion; *IR*, immediate release; *MR*, modified release; *PO*, by mouth; *PRN*, as needed; *SC*, subcutaneous; *TD*, transdermal.

Advanced Neurologic Disease

- See also sections:
  - 'Symptom Management Guidelines: Pain: Other Types: Skeletal Muscle Spasm'
  - 'Symptom Management Guidelines: Neurologic Symptoms: Seizures, Fatigue, and Delirium'

General Problems

GUIDELINE

National Institute for Health and Care Excellence. (2018). *Dementia: Assessment, Management and support for people living with dementia and their carers.* NICE clinical guideline 97. Available at https://www.nice.org.uk/guidance/ng97.

- Most symptoms can be managed successfully using the general guidelines already discussed (see the section on symptom control).
- Needs can change rapidly, so they require ongoing assessment and specialist input.
- In addition to local palliative care services, local specialist services for people with advanced neurologic diseases often exist (e.g., specialist nurses or teams to support people with motor neurone disease, multiple sclerosis, or Parkinson disease).

- A few specific considerations and medications are outlined in this section.

Communication

- Patients should be reviewed by a speech and language therapist.
- They should have access to both low-level (e.g., alphabet board) and high-level (e.g., eye-gaze computer systems) augmentative and alternative communication technologies.
- Deteriorating communication ability should be a trigger for advance care planning (see 'Basic Principles', i.e., the initial section of the chapter).

Nutrition, Hydration, and Poor Swallow

- Management of reduced oral intake should be considered early in the course of disease. If appropriate and desired, procedures to provide long-term enteral access (e.g., PEG) should be planned and undertaken while the patient remains well enough to undergo the procedure.
- Poor nutrition, anorexia or cachexia, and aspiration may be inevitable consequences of the end stage of advanced neurologic disease, and when reversal of the underlying cause is not possible, symptomatic treatment should be provided (see 'Care in the Last Days of Life').
- Similarly, hydration needs must be assessed in context and managed according to individual risk and benefit.

- Decision may be reached to continue giving food and fluids orally, accepting the risk of aspiration, and to manage complications symptomatically if they occur.
- Mouth care should always be provided to patients when they are no longer able to swallow.

Recurrent Infection

- Infections, such as UTIs or chest infections, or aspiration are seen in patients with advanced respiratory disease because of the consequences of the disease itself (recurrent aspiration from impaired swallow or interventions to manage symptoms, e.g., UTI associated with catheterisation).
- When treating infection, consider general principles (see 'Basic Principles'), the routes available to administer medication (PO, PEG, RIG), and the likelihood of treatment success (may be reduced if multidrug-resistant infection or irreversible underlying cause such as aspiration from at-risk feeding).
- If treatment of underlying infection is not desired or indicated, symptoms should be managed.

Muscle Spasms and Spasticity

- In addition to pain-relieving measures as described previously, the following may be considered in people with neurodegenerative disease causing painful muscle spasms:
  - Gabapentin and clonazepam may also be used if other medications are poorly tolerated.
  - Botulinum toxin injections can be used for isolated muscle spasm.
  - Physiotherapy input and specialist spasticity services are usually available locally.
  - Midazolam CSCI may be required as the end of life approaches.
- See also the section on pain.

Activities of Daily Living

- Equipment is available (usually via physiotherapy, occupational therapy, or specialist services for people with advanced neurologic disease) and should be provided to aid activities of daily living and mobility.

Dementia

- Dementia may be the primary diagnosis or comorbidity in a patient with LLI.
- As with all illnesses, medications to address the underlying pathology are the mainstays of management.
- Advanced dementia may have associated complications, including:
  - Reduced nutritional intake and weight loss (forgetting to eat or poor swallowing)
  - Recurrent infections (aspiration, debility, reduced fluid intake)
  - Behaviour that challenges and makes the patient at risk to self or others

Management of Behaviour That Challenges

Drug treatments for the control of violence, aggression, and extreme agitation should be used to calm the person with dementia and reduce the risk of violence and harm rather than treat any underlying psychiatric condition. Aim to reduce agitation or aggression without causing unnecessary sedation.

- If required, give medications for behaviour that challenges; give PO preparations as first-line treatment and SC preparations as second-line treatment. However, IM injections may be used if required.
- If SC or IM preparations are needed, lorazepam, haloperidol, or olanzapine should be used. Whenever possible, a single agent should be used in preference to a combination.
- If a patient exhibiting agitation or delirium is at the end of life, manage as for agitation (see 'Emergencies').
- Quetiapine and clozapine are options for managing psychotic symptoms in people with Parkinson disease. (See also 'Parkinson Disease and Parkinsonism (Parkinson-Plus Syndromes)'):
  - Agitation, severe distress, and psychosis in people with dementia can be managed with antipsychotics if there is a risk of harm to the self or others or distress from hallucinations or delusions.
  - Target symptoms for treatment should be identified and individual risk to benefit considered. Treatment should be discussed with patients and those important to them.
  - The antipsychotic should be commenced at a low dose and reviewed regularly (monthly). Monitor for neuroleptic sensitivity (i.e., changes in cognition and physical function).

Management of Reduced Oral Intake and Infection

- Managing these complications of advanced dementia should always be undertaken in context (i.e., with involvement of the patient and those important to the patient and with due consideration to the stage of underlying disease) (see 'Basic Principles').
- Also see the earlier discussion under 'Nutrition, Hydration, and Poor Swallow'.

Parkinson Disease and Parkinsonism (Parkinson-Plus Syndromes)

GUIDELINE

National Institute for Health and Care Excellence. (2017). *Parkinson disease in adults*. Available at https://www.nice.org.uk/guidance/ng71.

- Advanced end-stage Parkinson disease may cause specific symptomatic problems; bradykinesia, rigidity, tremor, and pain are possible.

- The goal of management is to optimise dopamine treatment and administration while avoiding dopamine antagonists.
- Worsening of symptoms may be caused by loss of dopaminergic response. Optimise administration and regular dosing of dopaminergic medications but consider stopping these at the end of life or when they are of no benefit.
- Difficulty with swallowing may cause problems with administration of PO dopaminergic medications:
  - Madopar is available in dispersible formulations, or other dopaminergic medications can be given via PEG if present.
  - Rotigotine TD patches are available and can be used under specialist guidance.
  - Pain: Optimise analgesia (see 'Symptom Control: Pain'). Skeletal muscle relaxants (e.g., midazolam CSCI) may be necessary, especially when dopaminergic medications can no longer be taken or are of little benefit.
  - Nausea and vomiting: Domperidone and cyclizine are preferred antiemetics (see the section on symptom control related to nausea and vomiting).
  - Hallucinations and delirium:
    - Exclude all potentially reversible causes.
    - Dopaminergic drugs are a potential cause.
    - Quetiapine (minimum, 12.5 mg at night) is the only recommended antipsychotic.
    - In advanced disease, when a parenteral route is required, levomepromazine with or without midazolam may be more appropriate (see 'Emergencies: Agitation').

Motor Neurone Disease and Amyotrophic Lateral Sclerosis

> **GUIDELINE**
>
> National Institute for Health and Care Excellence. (2016). *Motor neurone disease—assessment & management. NICE clinical guideline 42*. Available at http:/www.nice.org.uk.

- Many principles of symptom management in MND are common to other advanced LLIs, as already discussed, but those in this section pertain specifically to MND.

Ventilatory Support

- *NIV.* Patients can be offered NIV if they develop signs and symptoms of respiratory impairment (e.g., breathlessness, weak cough or sniff, disturbed or nonrefreshing sleep, nightmares, daytime drowsiness, morning headache, fatigue, shallow breathing, recurrent chest infection, accessory muscle use, abdominal paradox, orthopnoea, increased respiratory rate).
- This is set up and monitored according to patient wishes with the local specialist MDT or respiratory ventilation service. It can be stopped by a patient with capacity at any time (see 'Care in the Last Days of Life').

Cough

- Breath stacking (manual or assisted) and mechanical cough-assist devices can be used to improve the effectiveness of cough. This may be particularly helpful in clearing secretions associated with infection.

End-Stage Renal Failure

> **GUIDELINE**
>
> Scottish Palliative Care Guidelines. (2015). *Renal disease in the last days of life*. Available at https://rightdecisions.scot.nhs.uk/scottish-palliative-care-guidelines/end-of-life-care/renal-disease-in-the-last-days-of-life.

- Renal failure is considered end stage when the eGFR decreases to below 15 mL/min/1.73 m^2 (stage 5 chronic kidney disease (CKD)).
- However, symptoms are common in patients with stage 4 CKD (eGFR 15–29 mL/min/1.73 m^2), and symptom control or pharmacologic considerations mentioned later are appropriate for all patients with an eGFR below 30 mL/min.
- *Note on eGFR and creatinine clearance:* Most pharmacokinetic studies used an estimate of creatinine clearance based on Cockcroft-Gault equation. Dose adjustments of drugs were therefore based on this. eGFR, most often based on modification of diet in renal disease (MDRD) calculation, is not the same as creatinine clearance but is an acceptable substitute when considering whether adjustments need to be made in the dosing of medications in the context of palliative symptom management. eGFR is adjusted to body surface area and as such should be used with caution if body size is unusually low or high. eGFR should be taken as an indication of the need to modify drug doses.
- CKD may be the underlying LLI or a comorbidity. It is most often caused by:
  - Diabetes
  - Hypertension or cardiovascular disease
  - Renal disease (e.g., glomerulonephritis, polycystic kidney disease), infection, or obstructive uropathy
  - Malignancy (e.g., myeloma, tumour causing obstructive uropathy, effects of chemotherapy)
  - Medications (e.g., lithium, long-term NSAIDs)
- Patients with ESRF may be managed in a variety of ways, either conservatively or with a form of renal replacement therapy (peritoneal dialysis or haemodialysis).

Symptoms

- Patients with ESRF have at least as many symptoms as patients with advanced cancer, possibly more.
- Many similarities exist between symptoms experienced in ESRF and other LLIs toward the end of life (e.g., pain, fatigue or lethargy, nausea or vomiting, anorexia).

- However, there are some symptoms specific to ESRF that are often the consequences of uraemia or drug toxicity. For example:
  - Pain caused by renal disease, renal osteodystrophy, carpal tunnel syndrome, osteoporosis, osteomyelitis, or renal neuropathy
  - Calciphylaxis (painful tissue ischaemia caused by calcification of small blood vessels)
  - Itch
  - Fluid overload
  - Restless legs or muscle cramps
- In addition to symptoms from disease, the demands of treatment can be a significant source of distress for patients with advanced renal disease; these can be a significant factor in patients choosing to withdraw from dialysis.

Indicators of Poor Prognosis (Being in the Final Months to Year of Life) in Advanced and End-Stage Renal Failure (Stage 4 or 5 Chronic Kidney Disease)

- Symptomatic renal failure (e.g., nausea or vomiting, fluid overload, anorexia, pruritus, declining performance status) in patients having conservative management
- Patients choosing conservative management
- Poor tolerance of dialysis (e.g., hypotension preventing haemodialysis)
- Progressive cachexia and decline in performance status and increasing symptom burden despite dialysis
- Patients declining or withdrawing from dialysis (Note: The average survival time for patients discontinuing haemodialysis varies but is likely in the range of several days to 2 weeks.)

Pharmacologic Considerations in Stage 4 and 5 Chronic Kidney Disease

NB: Modifications to medications are appropriate in all patients with established acute kidney injury (AKI; eGFR <30 mL/min) as well as those with CKD.

General Considerations

- Renal failure can reduce the oral absorption, alter the distribution, and reduce the excretion of many different drugs (and their metabolites):
  - When possible, use medications that do not rely on renal excretion.
  - Nephrotoxic medications should be avoided if there is some residual renal function.
  - Medications that rely on renal excretion should be reduced in dose.
- Some medications are removed by dialysis. In patients having dialysis, seek advice on medications from specialist teams.
- Detailed guidance on dose adjustment of medications in renal failure can be found in the British National

Formulary, Palliative Care Formulary, or Summary of Product Characteristics (available online).
- *In patients with ESRF estimated to be in their final hours to days of life:*
  - Side effects from potential accumulation of medications and their metabolites need to be weighed carefully against the need to achieve timely symptom control, comfort, and dignity.
  - If there is a delay or difficulty in sourcing preferred 'renally safe' medications and patients are experiencing uncontrolled symptoms or distress, the priority should be to provide symptom control with the medications available.
  - In this situation, smaller doses of less ideal medication (e.g., morphine, diamorphine) can be given less frequently.
  - Patients with a previously normal renal function dying from any cause may well develop renal failure or AKI because of the physiologic processes that occur as death approaches (e.g., reduced fluid intake). In this patient group, modifications to well-tolerated, established medications for symptom control (e.g., morphine) are generally not needed. It is not appropriate to monitor renal function in the final days of life.

Symptom Management Specific to Advanced Chronic Kidney Disease or End-Stage Renal Failure

- As with most advanced LLIs, maximising therapy aimed at managing the disease and its complications is an important part of symptom management.
- As disease progresses and the prognosis deteriorates, it is important to review these medications and discontinue them when possible.

Medications Used to Manage Advanced Chronic Kidney Disease or End-Stage Renal Failure (and Its Complications)

- Calcium and vitamin D
- Phosphate binders
- Diuretics
- Iron, erythropoietin: for anaemia
- Antihypertensives
- Secondary prevention of cardiovascular disease (e.g., statins, antiplatelet therapy)
- Fluid restrictions

Managing Medications Used in Advanced Chronic Kidney Disease or End-Stage Renal Failure

- Medications for patients with advanced CKD and its complications should be reviewed when it becomes clear that a patient is deteriorating.
- Table 24.15 provides a guide as to when it may be appropriate to discontinue these medications.

TABLE 24.15   Management of Medications in Advanced Chronic Kidney Disease or End-Stage Renal Failure

Medication	When to Consider Stopping
Medications for anaemia: iron, erythropoietin	Stop in final weeks of life.
Medications to maintain dialysis access (e.g., warfarin)	Stop when dialysis stops.
Medications to reduce cardiovascular risk (e.g., statin, aspirin)	Stop when dialysis stops or the tablet burden is thought to be too great.
Calcium, vitamin D	Stop when dialysis stops or when the patient is no longer swallowing.
Phosphate binders	Stop when the patient is no longer eating.
Diuretics	Continue for as long as possible.
Medications for symptom control (e.g., long-term analgesia, antiemetics)	Continue while the patient is able to swallow and replace when possible with equivalent continuous subcutaneous infusion medication until death.

Management of Symptoms Specific to Advanced Chronic Kidney Disease or End-Stage Renal Failure

- The following guidance is appropriate for all patients with eGFR below 30 mL/min/1.73 m² (stage 4 or 5 CKD). It suggests alternative medications for symptom management for those with advanced renal disease. The general principles guiding use of these medications are mostly described under the general symptom control section. Please also refer to this section.
- Local practice may vary. Seek advice of local specialist palliative care team.
- Patients undergoing dialysis: Seek specialist advice for these patients because some medications (e.g., gabapentin and pregabalin) are cleared by dialysis.
- Table 24.16 summarises the medications most appropriate to use and those best avoided.

Pain

- Paracetamol: 500 mg to 1 g four times daily
- NSAIDs: *Only* for use in patients undergoing dialysis if they have no residual renal function
- Opioids:

TABLE 24.16   Summary of Medications for Symptom Control When Estimated Glomerular Filtration Rate Is Below 30 mL/min/1.73 m²

Symptom	Avoid	Manage With[a]
Pain	Codeine, tramadol, NSAIDs (if any remaining renal function), morphine, diamorphine, oxycodone (used in some centres; use with caution)	Paracetamol, buprenorphine TD, fentanyl TD, fentanyl SC or CSCI, alfentanil CSCI, methadone, amitriptyline (titrate slowly), gabapentin (reduce dose), pregabalin (reduce dose), ketamine (specialist use)
Anxiety, depression	Venlafaxine, mirtazapine, duloxetine	Sertraline, lorazepam or diazepam (reduced dose)
Nausea or vomiting	Metoclopramide (long term)	Domperidone, haloperidol (reduce dose), cyclizine (reduce dose), ondansetron, levomepromazine (reduce dose)
Restless legs	—	Clonazepam, gabapentin (reduced dose)
Muscle jerks (myoclonic)	Diazepam (if possible)	Lorazepam, clonazepam
Breathlessness	Diazepam (if possible)	Fentanyl SC PRN or CSCI, alfentanil CSCI, lorazepam, midazolam PRN (reduced dose)
Delirium	—	Olanzapine, haloperidol (reduced dose)
Agitation	—	Midazolam (reduce doses), levomepromazine (reduce doses)
Respiratory secretions	Hyoscine hydrobromide	Glycopyrronium, hyoscine butylbromide
Pruritus	—	Capsaicin, gabapentin
Seizures	Phenobarbital	Sodium valproate, midazolam CSCI

[a]For doses of medications in the table, please see the main text.
CSCI, Continuous subcutaneous infusion; *NSAID,* nonsteroidal antiinflammatory drug; *PRN,* as needed; *SC,* subcutaneous; *TD,* transdermal.

- Buprenorphine TD patches: no dose reduction required. Useful for chronic, stable pain. Consider the time taken to titrate dose; use in patients with weeks to months to live to give time for titration.
- Fentanyl TD patches: may require dose reduction; titrate slowly. Useful for chronic, stable pain. Consider the time taken to titrate dose; use in patients with weeks to months to live to give time for titration.
- Fentanyl injection SC PRN or CSCI: useful for opioid-naïve patients with severe renal failure in the last days to week of life requiring rapid titration. Starting dosages are typically 12.5 to 25 µg SC 1-hourly PRN and 100 µg CSCI/24 h.
- Alfentanil injection CSCI: useful for replacing other opioids via CSCI at end of life and those requiring rapid opioid titration. Alfentanil SC is 10 times as potent as diamorphine SC (i.e., 10 mg diamorphine SC is approximately equivalent to 1 mg SC alfentanil). It is too short acting to use as SC PRN.
- Methadone: specialist use. May be used PO or converted to CSCI at the end of life (halve the PO dose if starting CSCI because it is considered twice as potent SC compared with PO); it may require dose reduction in severe renal failure.
- Others:
  - Amitriptyline: Start with a low dose (10 mg at night) and titrate slowly.
  - Gabapentin: requires dose reduction. Creatinine clearance 15 to 29 mL/min: 100 to 600 mg/day, titrated slowly. Creatinine clearance below 15 mL/min: 100 mg alternate days to 300 mg/day. (See the manufacturer's summary of product characteristics for guidance; these doses are both lower than the manufacturer's guidance.)
  - Pregabalin: requires dose reduction. Creatinine clearance 15 to 29 mL/min: 25 to 150 mg once daily. Creatinine clearance below 15 mL/min: 25 to 75 mg once daily.
  - Clonazepam: specialist use. May be helpful for nerve pain. Dosage: 500 µg to 2 mg at night.
  - Ketamine: specialist use. The typical starting dosage is 5 to 10 mg PO four times daily.

Anxiety and Depression
- Sertraline: no dose reduction required
- Lorazepam (severe anxiety): 500 µg 6-hourly
- Diazepam (severe anxiety): avoid if possible. If necessary, start with a reduced dose (e.g., 2.5 to 5 mg at night) and titrate slowly.

Nausea and Vomiting
- Manage according to the likely cause (see section 'Symptom Management Guidelines: Gastrointestinal: Nausea')

- Ondansetron: no dose reduction required (i.e., 4–8 mg PO/SC twice daily)
- Cyclizine: no dose reduction required but may exacerbate dry mouth, so start with 25 to 50 mg PO/SC thrice daily
- Haloperidol: reduce dose by 50%; start with 500 µg at night
- Metoclopramide: reduce dose by 50%; start with 5 mg PO or SC thrice daily
- Domperidone: start with low dose (e.g., 10 mg PO once or twice daily)
- Levomepromazine: start with low dose (i.e., 6.25 mg PO or SC at night and/or 6-hourly PRN)

Restless Legs
- Clonazepam: 500 µg PO at night; titrate slowly
- Gabapentin: dose reduced according to renal function as mentioned earlier under 'Pain'

Muscle Jerks (Myoclonic)
- Lorazepam or clonazepam (doses as mentioned earlier)

Breathlessness
- Opioids: fentanyl or alfentanil (doses as mentioned earlier under 'Pain')
- Benzodiazepines: lorazepam (doses as mentioned earlier) or midazolam starting at 2.5 mg SC 1-hourly PRN (at the end of life)

Delirium
- See the section on symptom management of neurologic symptoms and delirium.
- Olanzapine is an alternative, starting at 5 mg/day.

Agitation
- See the section 'Emergencies: Agitation'.
- Lower doses of midazolam (starting at 2.5 mg SC 1-hourly) and levomepromazine (6.25 mg SC 4-hourly) may be effective.

Respiratory Secretions
- Glycopyrronium 200 µg SC 4-hourly or hyoscine butylbromide 20 mg SC 4-hourly

Pruritus
- See the section 'Symptom Management: Skin and Pruritus'.

Seizures at End of Life
- See the section 'Emergencies: Seizures'.
- If CSCI is required, midazolam is preferred. Phenobarbital should be avoided unless the patient has intractable seizures in the last hours to days of life.
- Sodium valproate is preferred if a PO antiepileptic is appropriate; the dose is unchanged.

End-Stage Respiratory Disease

GUIDELINES

Gold Standards Framework. (2022). *Proactive identification guidance.* Available at https://goldstandardsframework.org.uk/proactive-identification-guidance-pig.

National Institute for Health and Care Excellence. (2015). *Care of dying adults in the last days of life. NG 31.* Available at https://www.nice.org.uk/guidance/ng31.

National Institute for Health and Care Excellence. (2019). *Chronic obstructive pulmonary disease in over 16s: Diagnosis and management. NICE clinical guideline 115.* Available at https://www.nice.org.uk/guidance/NG115.

- The end stage of respiratory disease is not clearly defined.
- However, when the underlying disease becomes unresponsive to usual medical treatment (resulting in persistent or worsening symptoms) and the estimated prognosis is less than 1 year, these factors suggest that the patient is in the 'end stages' and approaching the end of life.

Indicators of Poor Prognosis (Being in the Final Months to Year of Life) in Advanced Respiratory Disease

- Frequent exacerbations and hospital admissions
- Patient too unwell for pulmonary rehabilitation
- Patient qualifies for long-term oxygen therapy (LTOT)
- COPD with forced expiratory volume in 1second less than 30% predicted
- Medical Research Council Dyspnoea Scale grade 4 of 5 (i.e., breathless on walking 100 yards or on minimal exertion)
- Cachexia, weight loss, low body mass index
- Comorbidities such as heart failure

Symptom Management Specific to End-Stage Respiratory Disease

- Many symptoms experienced in end-stage respiratory disease can be managed according to general symptom management guidelines for pain, breathlessness, cough, secretions, anxiety, and depression (as detailed earlier).
- It is important to always consider whether symptoms in end-stage respiratory disease are reversible, for example:
  - Treating infection with antibiotics
  - Treating inflammation with steroids
  - Managing bronchospasm with salbutamol and ipratropium.
- Management options specific to the underlying cause of the respiratory disease should always be optimised (e.g., β_2-agonists and muscarinic antagonists, antifibrotics, corticosteroids).
- When symptoms are no longer controlled by optimal medical treatment, palliative approaches should be used. It is appropriate to manage uncontrolled symptoms with opioids or benzodiazepines. Anxiety about causing respiratory depression should not prevent use of these medications when needed.
- Local specialist teams (respiratory, palliative care) should remain involved in supporting patients and their needs.

Oxygen in End-Stage Respiratory Disease

- Oxygen may be helpful in the palliation of breathlessness caused by hypoxia (see section 'Symptom Management Guidelines: Respiratory: Breathlessness').
- Appropriate use of oxygen:
  - Many patients are on LTOT (PaO_2 <7.3 kPa).
  - If not, short-burst oxygen therapy (oxygen given intermittently for 10–20 minutes at a time) can be considered for breathlessness not responding to other measures.
  - Use a 24% or 28% Venturi mask at a flow rate of 2 to 4 L/min.
  - Use oxygen with caution if there are symptoms of CO_2 retention such as headache, lethargy, hand flap, or confusion.
- As disease progresses, routine measurement of oxygen saturations becomes less appropriate. In fact, it may cause undue concern to patients for whom no remedial measures are possible.
- The focus should switch to managing symptoms of breathlessness regardless of measured oxygen saturations.

Anticipating Care Needs and Management

- Patients often have extensive experience of hospitalisation for management of exacerbations with their conditions and may well have strong opinions on the treatment they would or would not want. If so, they should be encouraged to record an ACP or ADRT.
- For patients with respiratory disease, opportunity should be created to discuss future treatment or care, such as whether they want further hospital admission, antibiotics (at home or in hospital or not at all), and ventilation (if this is considered appropriate).
- Clinical condition and symptom burden can deteriorate rapidly in patients with advanced respiratory disease. For patients who choose to have their symptoms managed in the community, arrangements should be made to ensure anticipatory medication for symptom control and end-of-life care is readily available to them at home.

End-Stage Heart Failure

GUIDELINES

National Institute for Health and Care Excellence. (2018). *Chronic heart failure in adults. NICE clinical guideline 106.* Available at https://www.nice.org.uk/guidance/ng106.

Resuscitation Council UK. (2015). *Cardiovascular implanted electronic devices in people towards the end of life, during cardiopulmonary resuscitation and after death.* Available at https://www.resus.org.uk/library/publications/publication-cardiovascular-implanted-electronic-devices

- Heart failure may be the sole underlying LLI, but it is often encountered as a comorbidity or consequence of another condition (e.g., cardiomyopathy secondary to effects of chemotherapy or cor pulmonale).
- All management options for patients with heart failure are designed to improve symptoms; some will improve survival, but none cures the disease.
- The severity of heart failure is classified according to the New York Heart Association (NYHA) functional system:
  - These are class I (no limitation of physical activity or symptoms but heart failure symptoms in the past) to class IV (symptomatic at rest and discomfort from any physical activity).
  - NYHA grading allows assessment of symptomatic response to treatment.
  - Further classification can be based on which side of the heart is predominantly affected. Treatment is based on whether left ventricular systolic dysfunction (reduced left ventricular ejection fraction) is present or not.

Symptoms

- Many patients with heart failure experience symptoms that are similar to those with advanced malignant disease, such as breathlessness, pain, fatigue, and depression.
- However, some symptoms of heart failure (e.g., fluid retention) require disease-specific management. Disease-specific treatments are the mainstays of symptom control.
- Consequently, some modifications to general palliative symptom management are required to address the differing aetiology of symptoms in heart failure (described later).
- The risk of sudden death in patients with heart failure has declined, but this potential may still cause anxiety and underlines the need for advance care planning.
- Patients should be screened for depression.
- Initial management is pharmacologic. However, cardiac resynchronisation therapy pacing (CRT-P) or defibrillator (CRT-D) devices may improve cardiac function and symptoms.

Indicators of Poor Prognosis (Being in the Final Months to Year of Life) in Advanced Heart Failure

- NYHA grade III or IV with symptoms becoming resistant to maximum tolerated medications
- Increasing frequency of episodes of decompensation or hospitalisation
- No further possible interventions
- Complications of heart failure or medications used to manage it (e.g., renal failure, hypotension at rest, hyponatraemia)
- Anaemia
- Life-limiting comorbidity
- Factors common to other LLIs (i.e., cachexia, declining performance status)

Symptom Management Specific to End-Stage Heart Failure

- Medications designed to manage disease should be continued for as long as possible because they all have symptomatic benefit.

Medications Used to Manage Heart Failure (and Its Symptoms)

- *In patients with left ventricular systolic dysfunction (and eGFR of ≥30 mL/min/1.73 m²):*
  - First-line treatment: Angiotensin-converting enzyme inhibitors and beta-blockers
  - Second-line treatment (if the patient has symptoms despite first-line medications): a mineralocorticoid receptor antagonist or an angiotensin II receptor blocker
  - Ivabradine and sacubitril valsartan (Entresto)
  - Digoxin if the patient has worsening heart failure despite first- and second-line treatment
- *In all types of heart failure:*
  - Diuretics for relief of fluid retention and congestive symptoms
  - Amiodarone; anticoagulants may be used

Managing Cardiac Medications to Improve Symptoms in Advanced End-Stage Heart Failure (Table 24.17)

- *Medications that improve survival and symptoms:*
  - Aldosterone antagonists, ACE inhibitors, angiotensin receptor blockers, beta-blockers, sacubitril valsartan.
  - Continue these for as long as possible.
  - Consider a dose reduction if the patient has symptomatic hypotension, worsening renal impairment, or tablet burden.
- *Medications that improve symptoms:*
  - Loop diuretics: Continue unless patients become clinically hypovolaemic or anuric. To symptomatically manage fluid overload at the end of life, furosemide

TABLE 24.17	Management of Medications in Advanced Cardiac Failure	
Medications That Can Be Stopped Early	**Medications to Continue as Long as Possible**
Cholesterol-lowering drugs	Loop diuretics Note: Furosemide can be continued continuous subcutaneous infusion if required (see text).
Antihypertensives	Angiotensin-converting enzyme inhibitors
Digoxin (if in sinus rhythm or renal failure)	Beta-blockers
Antiarrhythmic (if no symptomatic arrythmia)	Angiotensin receptor blockers Aldosterone antagonists

may be given CSCI, starting at a CSCI dose over 24 hours identical to the previous PO dose.

- Antiarrhythmic: Continue if symptomatic tachycardia is present. Otherwise, these can be discontinued relatively early.
- Antianginals can be stopped if the patient does not have angina.
- Antihypertensives become less important in patients with advanced cardiac failure. Stop if the patient has symptomatic hypotension.
- Digoxin should be stopped in patients with renal failure and in those with sinus rhythm.

Secondary Prevention

- Cholesterol-lowering drugs can be discontinued early.

Pharmacologic Considerations in End-Stage Heart Failure

Medications to Avoid

- Some medications may worsen symptoms and are best avoided, but a pragmatic approach must also be applied to symptom control, particularly for patients believed to be in the last days to week(s) of life.
- Concurrent renal failure may necessitate careful consideration of medications used to control symptoms, such as opioids (see the section on renal failure).
- Medications to avoid when possible:
  - NSAIDs and cyclooxygenase-2 inhibitors: can exacerbate heart failure and fluid retention and may cause renal toxicity
  - Antimuscarinic medications, including cyclizine
  - Tricyclics: may exacerbate arrhythmias
  - Corticosteroids, progestogens
  - Medications that prolong the QT interval

Managing Cardiac Devices

Types of Implantable Cardioverter Defibrillators and Cardiac Resynchronisation Therapy

- Patients with heart disease or heart failure may have one of several implantable devices. It is important to consider which type of device a patient has because they are managed differently at the end of life.
- Commonly encountered devices can be categorised as follows:
  - Pacemakers for bradycardia.
  - Cardiac resynchronisation therapy devices: These are biventricular pacemakers used primarily for managing cardiac failure. If purely for pacing, it is termed CRT-P. If it includes an additional defibrillator component for patients at risk of ventricular arrhythmia causing sudden death, it is termed CRT-D.
  - Implantable cardioverter defibrillator (ICD): for treatment of patients with ventricular arrhythmia.
- Patients with cardiac failure may have CRT-P, CRT-D, or ICD.

- More unusually, other devices with external components such as a left ventricular assist device may be present. Specialist advice should be sought on the management of these in patients at the end of life.

Deactivation of Defibrillator Component of Devices at the End of Life

- The aim of deactivating the defibrillator function is to prevent distress and the indignity of inappropriate ICD shocks that have no useful or desirable purpose.
- Defibrillation shocks may be delivered by ICD or CRT-D devices.
- When the defibrillator function is deactivated, any pacing function is normally left unchanged.
- Deactivation of a defibrillator is not the same as a DNACPR decision. Both require full discussion when possible.
- Discussion about the circumstances in which the defibrillator function of a device may be turned off should be started before implantation:
  - This should be revisited as a patient's condition deteriorates.
  - A competent patient can make a decision for deactivation at any stage.
  - The decision may be recorded in an ACP.
- It should be explained to patients that deactivation is not painful, death is not likely to be immediate, and the pacemaker function will not be deactivated. The ICD can be reactivated if the person's condition or opinion changes.

Practicalities of Defibrillator Deactivation

- *Planned deactivation (in the community):*
  - This should come as a shared, informed decision, often after several discussions with the patient, those important to the patient, and healthcare professionals or MDTs closely involved in the patient's care.
  - The patient's informed consent should be recorded (or if made in the patient's best interests, appropriate people involved) and documentation completed.
  - The general practitioner, specialist nurse, or palliative care team should liaise with local cardiac services to arrange deactivation.
  - Deactivation itself is undertaken by a cardiac physiologist who should be able to see the patient in the patient's home if necessary.
- *Emergency deactivation:*
  - When there is no time to arrange a cardiac physiologist, temporary defibrillator deactivation can be achieved by placing a doughnut-shaped magnet over the device and taping it securely in place.
  - This should only be used only as a temporary measure while full deactivation is being arranged.
  - The magnet will not deactivate the pacemaker function. For some devices, the magnet will inhibit the device for only a few hours at a time; it will need to be removed (for a few seconds) and reapplied every few hours.

Deactivation of Other Pacemaker Function at the End of Life

- *Pacemakers for bradycardia:* These are not normally deactivated (because they aid symptom control) unless specifically requested by the patient.
- *CRT-P:* These are not normally deactivated because they are beneficial in symptom control.
- In rare circumstances, the patient may request deactivation of their pacemaker. This should be a shared, informed decision, and deactivation should be undertaken by a cardiac physiologist as for a defibrillator.
- CRT-P and pacemakers are not deactivated by magnets.

After Death

- An active pacemaker (including CRT-P) needs no immediate management.

- If still active, an ICD or CRT-D should be fully deactivated by a cardiac physiologist as soon as possible after death and before attempts are made to remove the device.
- All cardiovascular implanted electronic devices should be explanted before cremation. They are usually then returned to local device services for safe disposal.
- There are legal ambiguities over device ownership. Consequently, if a patient's consent to remove and retain the device after death has not already been gained, consent should be obtained from the executor(s) of their estate for removal, retention, or disposal of the device after death.

Appendix 1

UK Routine Schedule of Immunisations

Age	Immunisations
8 weeks	DTaP, IPV, Hib, and Hep B (6-in-1 vaccine) Men B Rotavirus (oral drops)
12 weeks	DTaP, IPV, Hib, and Hep B (6-in-1 vaccine) Rotavirus (oral drops) PCV
16 weeks	DTaP, IPV, Hib, and Hep B (6-in-1 vaccine) Men B
12–13 months	Hib/Men C, MMR, PCV, and Men B
2–8 (up to 18 for children in clinical risk groups) years annually; given at school to children from reception to year 4	Nasal flu spray
3 years–4 months (preschool)	MMR DTaP/IPV (4-in-1 vaccine)
12–13 years	HPV (two doses given 6–24 months apart)
14 years (school year 9)	Td and IPV (3-in-1 vaccine) Men ACWY
50 years (and severely immunosuppressed) Shingles 65 years PCV once, Flu annually, shingles	Flu PCV once
70–80 years ongoing catchup programme for shingles	Shingles

aP, Acellular pertussis; *d,* low-dose diphtheria; *D,* diphtheria; *DTaP,* diphtheria, tetanus, and acellular pertussis; *flu,* influenza; *Hep B,* hepatitis B; *Hib, Haemophilus influenzae* type b; *HPV,* human papillomavirus; *IPV,* inactivated polio vaccine; *Men ACWY,* meningitis A, C, W, and Y; *Men B,* meningitis B; *Men C,* meningococcal C; *MMR,* mumps, measles and rubella; *PCV,* pneumococcal vaccine; *T,* tetanus.

Incubation Periods and Infectivities of Common Diseases

Disease	Incubation Period	Period of Infectivity	Exclusion From School or Nursery (UK Guidance)
Bacillary dysentery (shigellosis)	1–7 days	Mean, 7 days	For 48 hours after last diarrhoea
Campylobacter spp.	1–10 days	1–3 weeks	For 48 hours after last diarrhoea
Cryptosporidiosis	1–14 days	2–4 weeks	For 48 hours after last diarrhoea
Enteroviral infection	2–3 days	1–2 weeks	None
Escherichia coli enteritis	2–48 hours or longer	≥12 days	For 48 hours after last diarrhoea
Gastroenteritis (rotaviral)	2–4 days	6–10 days	48 hours from last diarrhoea or vomiting
Gastroenteritis (adenoviral)	8–10 days	7–14 days	48 hours from last diarrhoea or vomiting
Gastroenteritis (Norwalk virus)	4–77 hours	0–3 days	3 days after onset
Gastroenteritis (unidentified)	N/A	N/A	48 hours from last diarrhoea or vomiting
Giardiasis	5–20 days	2 weeks	24 hours from last diarrhoea
Salmonellosis	4 hours–5 days	Adults, 4 weeks (median)	For 24 hours after last diarrhoea
Typhoid and paratyphoid	3–56 days	2 weeks to indefinite	Until 24 hours after last diarrhoea
Other Diseases			
Chickenpox	11–20 days	–4 to +5 days	5 days from start of rash
Conjunctivitis	3–29 days	2 weeks	None
Haemophilus influenzae	4–5 days	Indefinite (untreated)	24 hours from start of antibiotics
Head lice	N/A	Indefinite (untreated)	None
Hand, foot, and mouth disease	3–5 days	7 days	None
Hepatitis A	2–6 weeks	–17 days to +2 weeks	Exclude until 7 days after onset of jaundice or symptom onset if there is no jaundice
Hepatitis B	6 weeks–6 months or longer		None (although may be too ill to attend during acute infection)
Hepatitis C	2 weeks–6 months		None
Herpes simplex	1–6 days	1–8 weeks (primary infection) 1–3 days (recurrence)	None

Disease	Incubation Period	Period of Infectivity	Exclusion From School or Nursery (UK Guidance)
Impetigo	N/A	N/A	Until lesions crusted or 48 hours after starting antibiotics
Infectious mononucleosis	33–49 days	≥2 months	None
Influenza	1–3 days	? 1–3 weeks	None
Measles	9–18 days	–2 to +3 days	From prodromal symptoms to 4 days after the onset of the rash
Meningococcal disease	N/A	Indefinite (untreated) <2 days (treated)	For the duration of the illness
Meningococcal infection	2–10 days		Until 48 hours after starting treatment
Mumps	15–24 days	Days –6 to +4	3 days before to 5 days after the start of the swelling
Pertussis	5–21 days	≥6 weeks or 1 week if given a macrolide	48 hours after starting antibiotic treatment if they feel well enough to attend or 21 days after onset of illness if no antibiotics were given
Rabies	9 days–9 weeks (possibly ≤years)	Until death	N/A
Rubella	15–20 days	1–6 days	1 week before the rash appears to 6 days after
Scabies	7–27 days	Indefinite until treated	Until after first treatment
Scarlet fever	½–5 days	3 days if treated	24 hours after starting antibiotics
Slapped cheek disease	13–18 days	–6 to –3 (i.e., prodrome only)	None
Streptococcal pharyngitis	½–5 days	Indefinite (untreated)	None
Tetanus	4–21 days	Not contagious	None
Threadworms	2–4 weeks	Indefinite	None
Tinea	2–4 weeks	Indefinite	None
Tuberculosis	4 weeks to years	Smear positive: until 2 weeks after starting treatment	Until 2 weeks after starting treatment; no exclusion necessary for nonpulmonary tuberculosis
Warts	1–24 months	While present	None

N/A, Not applicable.

Appendix 3

Suggested Immunisations for Travel

This schedule is for an adult who has been fully immunised as a child according to the UK recommendations. Few travellers need all the immunisations listed; they should only be given if appropriate to the travel planned. Individual health problems and exposure risks should always be taken into account. Other vaccines such as those for tuberculosis, COVID-19, and chickenpox may be needed.

Day	Immunisations
Day 0	Rabies, Japanese encephalitis, tick-borne encephalitis, hepatitis B
Day 7	Rabies, Japanese encephalitis
Day 14	Tick-borne encephalitis
Day 28	Rabies, Japanese encephalitis, hepatitis B
At some point in this schedule (either together or spread out over the month), immunisation early in the month (≥1 week before departure) allows time for immunity to develop.	BCG, cholera, hepatitis A, Men ACWY, polio, tetanus and diphtheria (as Td), typhoid, and yellow fever

If exposure to risk continues, further immunisations against hepatitis B are needed at 2 months and at 1 year from the first dose, and against tick-borne encephalitis at 9 months to 1 year after the last dose.

BCG, Bacillus Calmette–Guérin; *Men ACWY,* meningitis A,C, W, and Y.

Appendix 4

Notification of Infectious Diseases

The notification of the following diseases is required by law in the United Kingdom, and the doctor is not excused from notification by considerations of confidentiality. The following list applies to England and Wales, with variations for Scotland and Northern Ireland indicated.

Acute encephalitis	Malaria[a]
Acute infectious hepatitis[a]	Measles
Acute meningitis	Meningococcal septicaemia
Acute poliomyelitis	Mumps
Anthrax	Plague
Botulism[b]	Rabies
Brucellosis[b]	Rubella
Cholera	Scarlet fever[a]
Diphtheria	Severe acute respiratory syndrome[b]
Enteric fever (typhoid or paratyphoid fever)	Smallpox
Food poisoning[a]	Tetanus
Haemolytic uraemic syndrome[b]	Tuberculosis
Infectious bloody diarrhoea[a,b]	Typhus[a]
Invasive group A Streptococcal Disease[a,b]	Viral haemorrhagic fever
Legionnaires disease[a]	Whooping cough
Leprosy[a,b]	Yellow fever

[a]Not in Scotland.
[b]Not in Northern Ireland.
Also notifiable in Scotland are clinical syndrome caused by *Escherichia coli* 0157 infection, *Haemophilus* influenza B, necrotising fasciitis, tularaemia, and West Nile fever.
Also notifiable in Northern Ireland are chickenpox, dysentery, gastroenteritis for less than 2 years, leptospirosis, and relapsing fever.

Appendix 5

Child Health Promotion

History and Examination	Health Education
Neonatal examination	
a. Elicit and consider concerns expressed by the parents.	a. Feeding and nutrition
b. Review the family history, pregnancy, and birth.	b. Sleeping position
c. Assess the risk of hearing defect and refer accordingly.	c. Baby care
d. Perform a full physical examination, including weight and head circumference.	d. Sibling management
e. Check for CDH and testicular descent.	e. Crying and sleep problems
f. Inspect the eyes and check red reflex.	f. Transport in a car
g. Check that PKU, thyroid tests, cystic fibrosis, and medium-chain acyl-coA deficiency rests have been done or are scheduled.	g. Advice on reducing risk of SIDS
h. Screen for haemoglobinopathy, if relevant.	
i. Check vitamin K according to protocol.	
j. Consider need for BCG and Hep B immunisations.	
First 2 Weeks	
In addition to the neonatal examination:	a. Nutrition
a. Assess the level of support and assistance that each new parent is likely to require	b. The effects of passive smoking
b. Perform a newborn hearing test	c. Accident prevention: bathing, scalding by feeds, fires
	d. Immunisation
6–8 Weeks	
a. Check history, review growth and development, and ask about parental concerns.	a. Immunisation
	b. Nutrition
b. Perform physical examination and check weight, head circumference (and length, if indicated), and testes (in males).	c. Dangers of fires, falls, overheating, and scalds
c. Check for CDH.	d. Recognition of illness and what to do
d. Enquire about concerns regarding vision, squinting and hearing.	
e. Check whether the baby is in the high-risk category for hearing loss and refer if necessary.	
f. Discuss and perform immunisations.	
2, 3 and 4 Months and 13 Months	
a. Give primary immunisations.	

History and Examination	Health Education

6–9 Months

a. Enquire about parental concerns regarding health and development, vision, and hearing

b. Look for evidence of CDH.
c. Check for testicular descent

d. Observe visual behaviour and look for squinting

e. Perform a distraction test for hearing (HV)
f. Assess infant feeding and obesity risk

a. Accident prevention: choking, scalds and burns (including sunburn), falls

b. Anticipate increased mobility (e.g., safety gates, guards)

c. Nutrition
d. Dental prophylaxis

e. Reinforcement of advice about safety in cars and passive smoking

f. Developmental needs

18–24 Months

a. Enquire about parental concerns, particularly regarding behaviour, vision, and hearing

b. Confirm that the child is walking with a normal gait and that speech and comprehension are appropriate for age
c. Arrange detailed vision, hearing, or language assessment if indicated.
d. Remember the prevalence of iron-deficiency anaemia

e. Measure height

Note: Inform the community paediatric services if there is any anxiety about a child's educational potential.

a. Accident prevention: falls from heights, drowning, poisoning, road safety

b. Nutrition
c. Developmental needs: language and play
d. Need to mix with other children: playgroup and so on
e. Avoidance and management of behaviour problems

36–54 Months

a. Ask about and discuss vision, squinting, hearing and behaviour, language acquisition, and development

b. Discuss, if appropriate, whether the child is likely to have special educational problems and refer as appropriate

c. Measure the child's height and chart it

d. Refer for a hearing test if concerned

a. Accidents: fires, roads, drowning
b. Road safety

c. Preparation for school
d. Nutrition and dental care

BCG, Bacillus Calmette–Guérin; *CDH*, Congenital Dysplasia of the Hip; *HV*, Health Visitor; *Hep B*, hepatitis B; *PKU*, phenylketonuria; *SIDS*, sudden infant deaths syndrome.
From Department of Health. (2004). *National service framework for children, young people, and maternity services*. https://www.gov.uk/government/publications/national-service-framework-children-young-people-and-maternity-services.

Stages of Child Development

Summary of Development: Birth to 16 Weeks

	0–4 Weeks	6–8 Weeks	12–16 Weeks
Social	Watches mother and may smile	Responsive smile by 6 weeks and vocalises	Recognises family Shows pleasure
Motor			
Ventral suspension	Head hangs down until 3–4 weeks; then up momentarily	Head held in horizontal plane and briefly up by 8 weeks	Head maintained well above plane of body by 12 weeks
Prone	Head to side, pelvis high, knees drawn up under abdomen	Chin up intermittently at 6 weeks; well up at 8 weeks Pelvis flat	Head, shoulders, and chest up by 16 weeks Weight on forearms
Supine	Head to side, limbs flexed or ATNR posture	ATNR posture common but head to midline by 8 weeks	ATNR declining Head and hands now to midline
Pull to sit	Complete head lag	Less head lag	Slight head lag
Held sitting	Very round back Head drops forward	Back rounded Head briefly up	Back straighter and head up
Held standing	Walking and placing reflexes present until 6 weeks	Sags at hips and knees Getting head up by 8 weeks	Increasingly bears weight on legs
Hands	Strong grasp reflex Hands often closed	Grasp reflex present but slight by 8 weeks Fingers extend more often	Grasp reflex fades between 12 and 16 weeks Can hold rattle briefly
Vision	Blink and pupil reflexes Eye-righting reflex Random movements but can fixate	Smoother conjugate eye movements Fixates on faces and objects and follows through 45–90 degrees	Follows through 130 degrees Hand regard common (12–20 weeks)
Vocalisation and hearing	Cries, stills, or startles to sounds	Eyes turn to sounds Starts vocalising	Varied coos, squeals and laughs Turns to sounds

ATNR, Asymmetric tonic neck reflex.

Summary of Development: 4–10 Months

	4–6 Months	6–8 Months	8–10 Months
Personal and social behaviour	Responsive to all comers Smiles at self in mirror Excited at approach of food	Discriminates between family and strangers Attracts attention Hand feeds biscuit	Wary of strangers Waves bye-bye Attempts to use spoon
Gross motor	No head lag in traction Rolls prone to supine Back straight in supported sitting	Lifts head up in supine Rolls supine to prone; creeps Sits without lateral support Bears weight on feet (5–8 months)	Sits steadily; pivots and leans Can get from prone to sitting Pulls self to stand and crawls
Fine motor and vision	Reaches and grasps toys (4–6 months) Plays with toes Very alert visually	Transfers cube hand to hand (5–7 months) Can hold two cubes Any squint reported after 6 months is abnormal	Pincer grasp of pellet (8–12 months) Releases object and looks for it (7–11 months) Points at 1 mm sweet
Language and hearing	Varied sounds and squeals Says consonants such as 'ba' or 'da'	Starts to babble 'da-da' Turns to sounds (4–8 months)	Varied babble 'ma-ma', 'ba-ba', and 'da-da' Indicates and understands 'no' Locates sounds well

Summary of Development: 12–24 Months

	12–15 Months	18–24 Months
Personal and social behaviour	Shows affection and may be shy Indicates wants, points, and claps hands (10–18 months)	Becoming egocentric, clinging, and resistant Loves domestic mimicry
	Mouthing stops (12–15 months) Enjoys casting (12–15 months)	Definitely stopped mouthing and casting (by 18 months)
	May manage cup and spoon with spills (10–17 months)	Helps undress Independent with cup and spoon (15–24 months)
Gross motor	Walks holding on (8–12 months) Walks alone (11–15 months)	Walks well (12–18 months) Climbs stairs, kneels (14–22 months)
Fine motor and vision	Fine pincer grasp Bangs bricks together (8–14 months) Holds two cubes Scribbles (12–18 months)	May show hand preference (after 15 months) Builds two to three cubes Turns pages (15–24 months)
Language and hearing	'Mama', 'dada' with meaning (9–15 months) Three to four clear words (12–18 months)	Can point to three parts of body Says 6 to 20 words and jargon (15–24 months)

Summary of Development: 2–5 Years

	2–3 Years	3–4 Years	5 Years
Personal and social skills	Enjoys solitary play alongside peers, not sharing Possessive: tantrums if thwarted Feeds quite neatly using spoon and fork or fingers May be clean and dry by day, with supervision, or may refuse to cooperate	Plays with peers, sharing toys Enjoys make-believe play Shows concern and sympathy for others and able to take turns by 4 years Easily manages spoon and fork and then knife Mostly dry day and night Can wash hands and dress and undress by 4 years, except fastenings	Plays complicated cooperative games Makes friends Comforts playmates and siblings in distress Almost completely independent in self-help skills now Can carry out simple domestic tasks and run errands
Gross motor	Now very mobile Runs, kicks ball, tries to throw Walks up and down stairs two feet to a step Propels tricycle by pushing with feet on floor	Goes up stairs one foot per step at 3 years and down by 4 years Can walk and then run on tiptoe and hop by 4 years Enjoys climbing; pedals a tricycle skilfully	Enjoys running, jumping, climbing, swings and slides, and starting to play ball games Can stand on one leg, hop 10 times, and heel–toe walk a narrow line
Fine motor and vision	Neat prehension and controlled release Builds tower of six to eight bricks Holds pencil in fist Circular scribble (24 months) Copies vertical line, imitates circle (30 months) Can do simple puzzles and thread large beads Difficult age to test vision Recognises two-dimensional symbols and may match letters at 30 months	Builds tower of 9–10 and imitates a three-cube bridge at 3 years; Can build steps by 4 years Awkward tripod grasp of pencil at 3 years; copies circle and imitates cross Dynamic tripod after 4 years; draws an adult male with a head, trunk, and legs Can do letter-matching vision tests using linear charts with each eye separately, by 3.5–4 years	Can write name and copy a square and a triangle Draws an adult male with detailed features and limbs Can fold paper and use scissors to cut out shapes Performs Snellen chart type of vision test
Language and hearing	Listens to simple stories and understands two-part instructions Can say 50–100 single words and join 2–3 (e.g., Daddy gone car) Asks many questions, including what? and who? Talks in long monologues; still uses some jargon; enjoys nursery rhymes and jingles Toy tests of hearing or may point to named pictures	Intelligible but immature speech; talks in three- to five-word sentences; knows name and sex at 3 years Tells long stories, asks constant more abstract questions, grammar mostly correct, and speech clear by 4 years Knows age and address, knows six or more colours, and can count to 4 or higher Can do cooperative (conditioned) hearing tests	Enjoys riddles and jokes Understands negatives and complex questions and instructions Gives long descriptions and explanations Speech easily intelligible with few errors Manages full audiometry and speech discrimination now

Appendix 7

Stages of Puberty

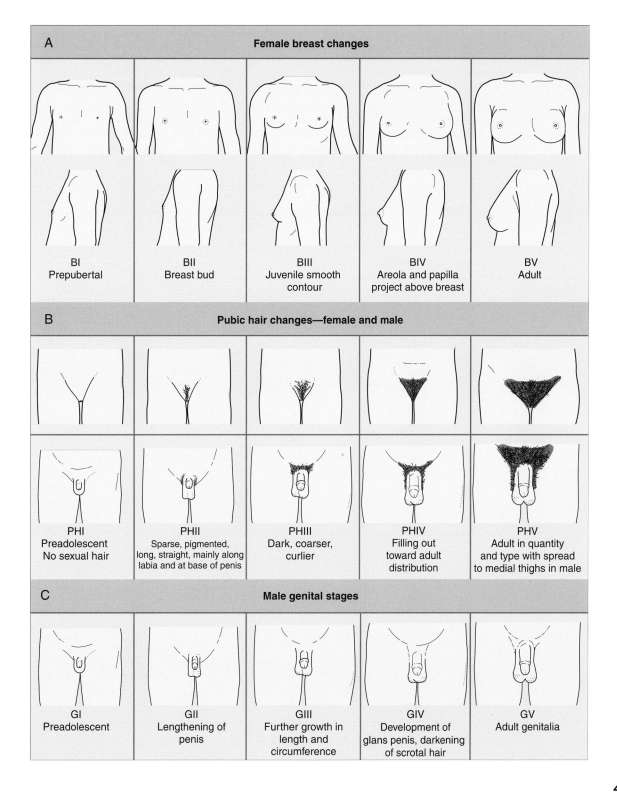

A   **Female breast changes**

- BI — Prepubertal
- BII — Breast bud
- BIII — Juvenile smooth contour
- BIV — Areola and papilla project above breast
- BV — Adult

B   **Pubic hair changes—female and male**

- PHI — Preadolescent No sexual hair
- PHII — Sparse, pigmented, long, straight, mainly along labia and at base of penis
- PHIII — Dark, coarser, curlier
- PHIV — Filling out toward adult distribution
- PHV — Adult in quantity and type with spread to medial thighs in male

C   **Male genital stages**

- GI — Preadolescent
- GII — Lengthening of penis
- GIII — Further growth in length and circumference
- GIV — Development of glans penis, darkening of scrotal hair
- GV — Adult genitalia

A. Stages of breast development in a female
  Stage 1 (BI): preadolescent: elevation in papilla only
  Stage 2 (BII): breast bud stage: elevation of breast and papilla as a small mound. Enlargement of areolar diameter
  Stage 3 (BIII): further enlargement and elevation of breast and areola, with no separation of their contours
  Stage 4 (BIV): projection of areola and papilla to form a secondary mound above the level of the breast
  Stage 5 (BV): mature stage; projection of papilla only caused by recession of the areola to the general contour of the breast
    (This last stage may not be reached in females until after their first pregnancy.)

B. Pubic hair development: male and female
  Stage 1 (PHI): preadolescent. The vellus over the pubes is not further developed than that over the abdominal wall (i.e., no pubic hair).
  Stage 2 (PHII): sparse growth of long, slightly pigmented downy hair, straight or slightly curled, chiefly at the base of the penis or along the labia
  Stage 3 (PHIII): considerably darker, coarser, and more curled. The hair spreads sparsely over the junction of the pubes
  Stage 4 (PHIV): hair now adult in type, but area covered is still considerably smaller than in the adult. No spread to the medial surface of the thighs
  Stage 5 (PHV): adult in quantity and type with distribution of the horizontal (or classically feminine) pattern. Spread to the medial surface of the thighs but not up the linea alba or elsewhere above the base of the inverse triangle (spread up linea alba occurs later and is rated stage 6)

C. Male genital development:
  Stage 1 (GI): preadolescent: testes, scrotum, and penis are of about the same size and proportion as in early childhood
  Stage 2 (GII): enlargement of the scrotum and testes. The skin of the scrotum reddens and changes in texture. There is little or no enlargement of penis at this stage
  Stage 3 (GIII): enlargement of the penis, which occurs at first mainly in length; further growth of testes and scrotum
  Stage 4 (GIV): increased size of penis with growth in breadth and development of the glans; testes and scrotum larger; scrotal skin darkened
  Stage 5 (GV): genitalia adult in size and shape. (The volume of the adult testis varies in size from 12–25 mL.)

Both sexes: axillary hair
  Stage 1: preadolescent: no axillary hair
  Stage 2: scanty growth of slightly pigmented hair
  Stage 3: hair adult in quality and quantity

With permission from Lissauer, T., & Clayden, G. (2005). *Illustrated textbook of paediatrics* (3rd ed.). Mosby.

Predicted Normal Peak Flow Values in Children (Younger Than 15 Years of Age)

Height		Peak Flow (L/min)
(cm)	(ft–in)	
91	3–0	100
99	3–3	120
107	3–6	140
114	3–9	170
122	4–0	210
130	4–3	250
137	4–6	285
145	4–9	325
152	5–0	360
160	5–3	400
168	5–6	440
175	5–9	480

Appendix 9

Peak Expiratory Flow (PEF) in Normal Subjects

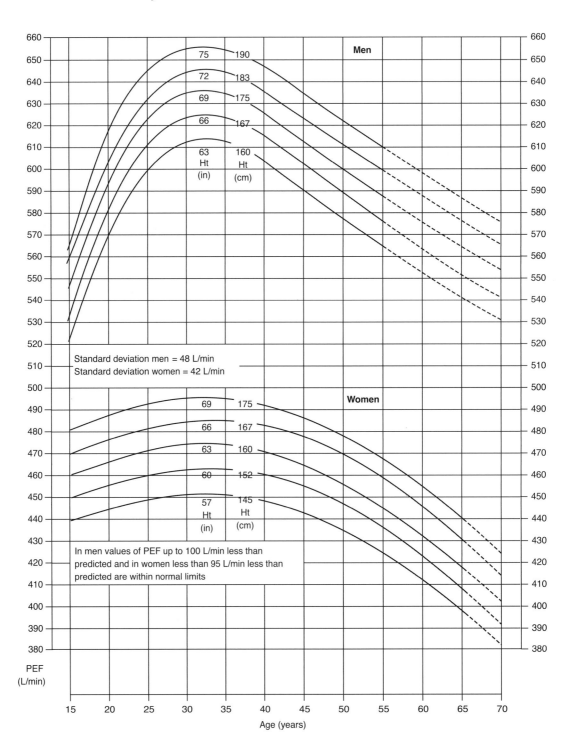

Standard deviation men = 48 L/min
Standard deviation women = 42 L/min

In men values of PEF up to 100 L/min less than predicted and in women less than 95 L/min less than predicted are within normal limits

Forced Expiratory Volume in 1 Second (FEV$_1$) and Forced Vital Capacity (FVC)

Females

Age (years)		Height (m)							
		1.45	1.50	1.55	1.60	1.65	1.70	1.75	1.80
25	FEV$_1$	2.5	2.7	2.9	3.1	3.4	3.6	3.8	4.0
	FVC	2.9	3.1	3.3	3.6	3.8	4.0	4.2	4.4
30	FEV$_1$	2.4	2.6	2.8	3.0	3.2	3.4	3.7	3.9
	FVC	2.8	3.0	3.2	3.4	3.6	3.9	4.1	4.3
35	FEV$_1$	2.3	2.5	2.7	2.9	3.1	3.3	3.5	3.7
	FVC	2.6	2.9	3.1	3.3	3.5	3.7	4.0	4.2
40	FEV$_1$	2.1	2.3	2.6	2.8	3.0	3.2	3.4	3.6
	FVC	2.5	2.7	2.9	3.2	3.4	3.6	3.8	4.0
45	FEV$_1$	2.0	2.2	2.4	2.6	2.9	3.1	3.3	3.5
	FVC	2.4	2.6	2.8	3.0	3.3	3.5	3.7	3.9
50	FEV$_1$	1.9	2.1	2.3	2.5	2.7	2.9	3.2	3.4
	FVC	2.2	2.5	2.7	2.9	3.1	3.3	3.6	3.8
55	FEV$_1$	1.8	2.0	2.2	2.4	2.6	2.8	3.0	3.2
	FVC	2.1	2.3	2.6	2.8	3.0	3.2	3.4	3.7
60	FEV$_1$	1.6	1.8	2.1	2.3	2.5	2.7	2.9	3.1
	FVC	2.0	2.2	2.4	2.6	2.9	3.1	3.3	3.5
65	FEV$_1$	1.5	1.7	1.9	2.1	2.4	2.6	2.8	3.0
	FVC	1.8	2.1	2.3	2.5	2.7	3.0	3.2	3.4
70	FEV$_1$	1.4	1.6	1.8	2.0	2.2	2.4	2.7	2.9
	FVC	1.7	1.9	2.2	2.4	2.6	2.8	3.0	3.3

Males

Age (years)		Height (m)							
		1.55	**1.60**	**1.65**	**1.70**	**1.75**	**1.80**	**1.85**	**1.90**
25	FEV_1	3.4	3.6	3.8	4.1	4.3	4.5	4.7	5.0
	FVC	3.9	4.2	4.5	4.8	5.1	5.4	5.7	6.0
30	FEV_1	3.3	3.5	3.7	3.9	4.2	4.4	4.6	4.8
	FVC	3.8	4.1	4.4	4.7	5.0	5.3	5.5	5.8
35	FEV_1	3.1	3.3	3.6	3.8	4.0	4.2	4.5	4.7
	FVC	3.7	4.0	4.3	4.5	4.8	5.1	5.4	5.7
40	FEV_1	3.0	3.2	3.4	3.6	3.9	4.1	4.3	4.5
	FVC	3.6	3.8	4.1	4.4	4.7	5.0	5.3	5.6
45	FEV_1	2.8	3.0	3.3	3.5	3.7	3.9	4.2	4.4
	FVC	3.4	3.7	4.0	4.3	4.6	4.9	5.2	5.4
50	FEV_1	2.7	2.9	3.1	3.3	3.6	3.8	4.0	4.2
	FVC	3.3	3.6	3.9	4.2	4.4	4.7	5.0	5.3
55	FEV_1	2.5	2.8	3.0	3.2	3.4	3.7	3.9	4.1
	FVC	3.2	3.5	3.7	4.0	4.3	4.6	4.9	5.2
60	FEV_1	2.4	2.6	2.8	3.1	3.3	3.5	3.7	4.0
	FVC	3.0	3.3	3.6	3.9	4.2	4.5	4.8	5.0
65	FEV_1	2.2	2.5	2.7	2.9	3.1	3.4	3.6	3.8
	FVC	2.9	3.2	3.5	3.8	4.1	4.3	4.6	4.9
70	FEV_1	2.1	2.3	2.5	2.8	3.0	3.2	3.4	3.7
	FVC	2.8	3.1	3.3	3.6	3.9	4.2	4.4	4.8

Female Children

Height			
(m)	**(in)**	**FEV_1**	**FVC**
0.80	32	0.41	0.46
0.90	35	0.56	0.64
1.00	39	0.75	0.86
1.10	43	0.98	1.11
1.20	47	1.24	1.43
1.30	51	1.55	1.79
1.40	55	1.90	2.20
1.50	59	2.29	2.68
1.60	63	2.73	3.22
1.70	67	3.23	3.82
1.80	71	3.77	4.48

Male Children

Height			
(m)	**(in)**	**FEV_1**	**FVC**
0.80	32	0.40	0.46
0.90	35	0.56	0.65
1.00	39	0.76	0.89
1.10	43	1.00	1.17
1.20	47	1.28	1.52
1.30	51	1.61	1.92
1.40	55	2.00	2.38
1.50	59	2.43	2.92
1.60	63	2.93	3.53
1.70	67	3.49	4.22
1.80	71	4.11	4.99

Appendix 11A

Summary of Management of Asthma in Adults

Reproduced from Scottish Intercollegiate Guidelines Network and British Thoracic Society. (2019). *British guideline on the management of asthma.*

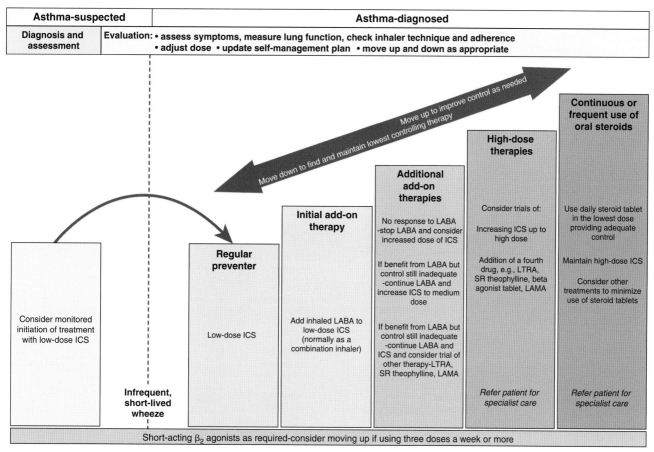

Asthma-suspected	Asthma-diagnosed
Diagnosis and assessment	**Evaluation:** • assess symptoms, measure lung function, check inhaler technique and adherence • adjust dose • update self-management plan • move up and down as appropriate

Move up to improve control as needed

Move down to find and maintain lowest controlling therapy

Continuous or frequent use of oral steroids

Use daily steroid tablet in the lowest dose providing adequate control

Maintain high-dose ICS

Consider other treatments to minimize use of steroid tablets

Refer patient for specialist care

High-dose therapies

Consider trials of:

Increasing ICS up to high dose

Addition of a fourth drug, e.g., LTRA, SR theophylline, beta agonist tablet, LAMA

Refer patient for specialist care

Additional add-on therapies

No response to LABA -stop LABA and consider increased dose of ICS

If benefit from LABA but control still inadequate -continue LABA and increase ICS to medium dose

If benefit from LABA but control still inadequate -continue LABA and ICS and consider trial of other therapy-LTRA, SR theophylline, LAMA

Initial add-on therapy

Add inhaled LABA to low-dose ICS (normally as a combination inhaler)

Regular preventer

Low-dose ICS

Consider monitored initiation of treatment with low-dose ICS

Infrequent, short-lived wheeze

Short-acting β₂ agonists as required-consider moving up if using three doses a week or more

ICS, Inhaled corticosteroids; *LABA,* long-acting beta-agonist; *LTRA,* leukotriene receptor antagonist; *MART,* maintenance and reliever therapy.

Appendix 11B

Summary of Management of Asthma in Children

Reproduced from Scottish Intercollegiate Guidelines Network and British Thoracic Society. (2019). *British guideline on the management of asthma.*

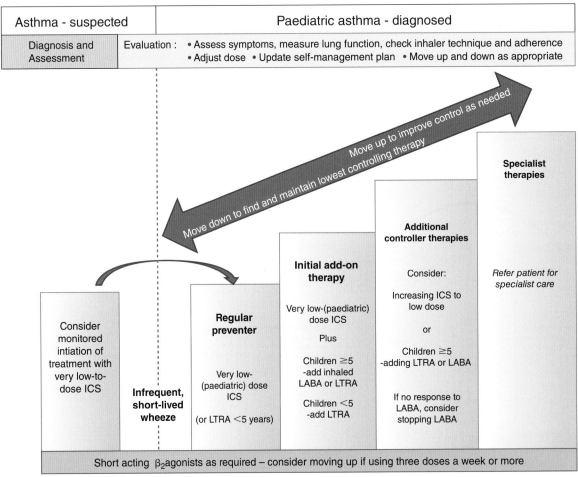

Asthma - suspected	Paediatric asthma - diagnosed	
Diagnosis and Assessment	Evaluation : • Assess symptoms, measure lung function, check inhaler technique and adherence • Adjust dose • Update self-management plan • Move up and down as appropriate	

Move up to improve control as needed

Move down to find and maintain lowest controlling therapy

Specialist therapies

Refer patient for specialist care

Additional controller therapies

Consider:

Increasing ICS to low dose

or

Children ≥5 -adding LTRA or LABA

If no response to LABA, consider stopping LABA

Initial add-on therapy

Very low-(paediatric) dose ICS

Plus

Children ≥5 -add inhaled LABA or LTRA

Children <5 -add LTRA

Regular preventer

Very low-(paediatric) dose ICS

(or LTRA <5 years)

Consider monitored intiation of treatment with very low-to-dose ICS

Infrequent, short-lived wheeze

Short acting β₂agonists as required – consider moving up if using three doses a week or more

ICS, Inhaled corticosteroids; *LABA*, long-acting beta-agonist; *LTRA*, leukotriene receptor antagonist; *MART*, maintenance and reliever therapy.

Management of Acute Asthma in Adults in General Practice

Reproduced from Scottish Intercollegiate Guidelines Network and British Thoracic Society. (2019). *British guideline on the management of asthma.*

Management of acute severe asthma in adults in general practice

Many deaths from asthma are preventable. Delay can be fatal. Factors leading to poor outcome include:

- Clinical staff failing to assess severity by objective measurement
- Patients or relatives failing to appreciate severity
- Underuse of corticosteroids

Regard each emergency asthma consultation as for acute severe asthma until shown otherwise.

Assess and record:

- Peak expiratory flow (PEF)
- Symptoms and response to self treatment
- Heart and respiratory rates
- Oxygen saturation (by pulse oximetry)

Caution: Patients with severe or life-threatening attacks may not be distressed and may not have all the abnormalities listed below. The presence of any should alert the doctor.

Moderate asthma	Acute severe asthma	Life-threatening asthma

INITIAL ASSESSMENT

PEF >50%–75% best or predicted	PEF 33%–50% best or predicted	PEF <33% best or predicted

FURTHER ASSESSMENT

• SpO$_2$ ≥92% • Speech normal • Respiration <25 breaths/min • Pulse <110 beats/min	• SpO$_2$ ≥92% • Can't complete sentences • Respiration ≥25 breaths/min • Pulse ≥110 beats/min	• SpO$_2$ <92% • Silent chest, cyanosis or poor respiratory effort • Arrhythmia or hypotension • Exhaustion, altered consciousness

MANAGEMENT

Treat at home or in surgery and **ASSESS RESPONSE TO TREATMENT**	**Consider admission**	**Arrange immediate ADMISSION**

TREATMENT

• β$_2$ Bronchodilator:
  – via spacer (give 4 puffs initially and give a further 2 puffs every 2 minutes according to response up to maximum of 10 puffs)
 	
If PEF >50%–75% predicted/best:
• Nebulizer (preferably oxygen driven) (salbutamol 5 mg)
• Give prednisolone 40–50 mg
• Continue or increase usual treatment
 	
If good response to first treatment (symptoms improved, respiration and pulse settling and PEF >50%) continue or increase usual treatment and continue prednisolone
	• Oxygen to maintain SpO$_2$ 94%–98% if available
	• β$_2$ Bronchodilator:
	  – nebulizer (preferably oxygen driven) (salbutamol 5 mg)
	  – or via spacer (give 4 puffs initially and give a further 2 puffs every 2 minutes according to response up to maximum of 10 puffs)
	• Prednisolone 40–50 mg or IV hydrocortisone 100 mg
	• **If no response in acute severe asthma: ADMIT**
		• Oxygen to maintain SpO$_2$ 94%–98%
		• β$_2$ Bronchodilator and ipratropium:
		  – nebulizer (preferably oxygen driven) (salbutamol 5 mg and ipratropium 0.5 mg)
		  – or via spacer (give 4 puffs initially and give a further 2 puffs every 2 minutes according to response up to maximum of 10 puffs)
		• Prednisolone 40–50 mg or IV hydrocortisone 100 mg immediately

Admit to hospital if any: • Life-threatening features • Features of acute severe asthma present after initial treatment • Previous near-fatal asthma Lower threshold for admission if afternoon or evening attack, recent nocturnal symptoms or hospital admission, previous severe attacks, patient unable to assess own condition, or concern over social circumstances	**If admitting the patient to hospital:** • Stay with patient until ambulance arrives • Send written assessment and referral details to hospital • β$_2$ bronchodilator via oxygen-driven **nebulizer in ambulance**	**Follow up after treatment or discharge from hospital:** • **GP review within 2 working days** • Monitor symptoms and PEF • Check inhaler technique • **Written asthma action plan** • Modify treatment according to guidelines for chronic persistent asthma • Address potentially preventable contributors to admission

Appendix 11D

Management of Acute Asthma in Children in General Practice

Reproduced from Scottish Intercollegiate Guidelines Network and British Thoracic Society. (2019). *British guideline on the management of asthma*.

Management of acute asthma in children in general practice

Age 2–5 years

ASSESS AND RECORD ASTHMA SEVERITY

Moderate asthma
- SpO_2 ≥92%
- Able to talk
- Heart rate ≤140/min
- Respiratory rate ≤40/min

Acute severe asthma
- SpO_2 <92%
- Too breathless to talk
- Heart rate >140/min
- Respiratory rate >40/min
- Use of accessory neck muscles

Life-threatening asthma
SpO_2 <92% plus any of:
- Silent chest
- Poor respiratory effort
- Agitation
- Confusion
- Cyanosis

Moderate asthma:
- β_2 agonist 2–10 puffs via spacer and facemask (given one puff at a time inhaled separately using tidal breathing)
- Give one puff of β_2 agonist every 30–60 seconds up to 10 puffs according to response
- Consider oral prednisolone 20 mg

Acute severe / Life-threatening:
- Oxygen via face mask
- 10 puffs of β_2 agonist or nebulized salbutamol 2.5 mg
- Oral prednisolone 20 mg

Life-threatening:
- Oxygen via face mask
- Nebulize every 20 minutes with:
  - salbutamol 2.5 mg
    +
  - ipratropium 0.25 mg
- Oral prednisolone 20 mg
  or
- IV hydrocortisone 50 mg if vomiting

Assess response to treatment 15 min after β_2 agonist

IF POOR RESPONSE REPEAT β_2 AGONIST AND ARRANGE ADMISSION

REPEAT β_2 AGONIST VIA OXYGEN-DRIVEN NEBULIZER WHILST ARRANGING IMMEDIATE HOSPITAL ADMISSION

IF POOR RESPONSE ARRANGE ADMISSION

GOOD RESPONSE
- Continue β_2 agonist via spacer or nebulizer, as needed but not exceeding 4 hourly
- **If symptoms are not controlled repeat β_2 agonist and refer to hospital**
- Continue prednisolone for up to 3 days
- Arrange follow-up clinic visit within 48 hours
- Consider referral to secondary care asthma clinic if 2nd attack within 12 months

POOR RESPONSE
- Stay with patient until ambulance arrives
- Send written assessment and referral details
- Repeat β_2 agonist via oxygen-driven nebulizer in ambulance

---

LOWER THRESHOLD FOR ADMISSION IF:
- Attack in late afternoon or at night
- Recent hospital admission or previous severe attack
- Concern over social circumstances or ability to cope at home

NB: If a patient has signs and symptoms across categories, always treat according to their most severe features

---

Age >5 years

ASSESS AND RECORD ASTHMA SEVERITY

Moderate asthma
- SpO_2 ≥92%
- Able to talk
- Heart rate ≤125/min
- Respiratory rate ≤30/min
- PEF ≥50% best or predicted

Acute severe asthma
- SpO_2 <92%
- Too breathless to talk
- Heart rate >125/min
- Respiratory rate >30/min
- Use of accessory neck muscles
- PEF 33%–50% best or predicted

Life-threatening asthma
SpO_2 <92% plus any of:
- Silent chest
- Poor respiratory effort
- Agitation
- Confusion
- Cyanosis
- PEF <33% best or predicted

Moderate asthma:
- β_2 agonist 2–10 puffs via spacer and mouthpiece (given one puff at a time inhaled separately using tidal breathing)
- Give one puff of β_2 agonist every 30–60 seconds up to 10 puffs according to response
- Consider oral prednisolone 30–40 mg

Acute severe:
- Oxygen via face mask
- 10 puffs of β_2 agonist or nebulized salbutamol 5 mg
- Oral prednisolone 30–40 mg

Life-threatening:
- Oxygen via face mask
- Nebulize every 20 minutes with:
  - salbutamol 5 mg
    +
  - ipratropium 0.25 mg
- Oral prednisolone 30–40 mg
  or
- IV hydrocortisone 100 mg if vomiting

Assess response to treatment 15 min after β_2 agonist

IF POOR RESPONSE REPEAT β_2 AGONIST AND ARRANGE ADMISSION

REPEAT β_2 AGONIST VIA OXYGEN-DRIVEN NEBULIZER WHILST ARRANGING IMMEDIATE HOSPITAL ADMISSION

IF POOR RESPONSE ARRANGE ADMISSION

GOOD RESPONSE
- Continue β_2 agonist via spacer or nebulizer, as needed but not exceeding 4 hourly
- **If symptoms are not controlled repeat β_2 agonist and refer to hospital**
- Continue prednisolone for up to 3 days
- Arrange follow-up clinic visit within 48 hours
- Consider referral to secondary care asthma clinic if 2nd attack within 12 months

POOR RESPONSE
- Stay with patient until ambulance arrives
- Send written assessment and referral details
- Repeat β_2 agonist via oxygen-driven nebulizer in ambulance

---

LOWER THRESHOLD FOR ADMISSION IF:
- Attack in late afternoon or at night
- Recent hospital admission or previous severe attack
- Concern over social circumstances or ability to cope at home

NB: If a patient has signs and symptoms across categories, always treat according to their most severe features

---

PEF, Peak expiratory flow; *SpO₂,* peripheral capillary oxygen saturation.

Guidance for Disease-Modifying Antirheumatic Drug Prescribing

GUIDELINES

British Society of Rheumatology. (2017). BSR and BHPR guideline for the prescription and monitoring of non-biologic disease-modifying anti-rheumatic drugs. *Rheumatology, 56*(6), 865–868.

National Institute for Health and Care Excellence. (2021). *DMARDs*. Available at http://cks.nice.org.uk.

Generic Recommendations Before Commencing Any Disease-Modifying Antirheumatic Drug

a. The decision to initiate Disease-Modifying Antirheumatic Drugs (DMARDs) should be made in conjunction with the patient or carer and be supervised by an expert in the management of rheumatic diseases.
b. Patients should be provided with education about their treatment to promote self-management.
c. When appropriate, patients should be advised about the impact of DMARD therapy upon fertility, pregnancy and breastfeeding.
d. Baseline assessment should include height, weight, blood pressure and laboratory evaluation; full blood count (FBC), estimated glomerular filtration rate (GFR), alanine aminotransferase (ALT) and/or aspartate aminotransferase (AST), and albumin.
e. Patients should be assessed for comorbidities because they may influence DMARD choice, including evaluation for respiratory disease and screening for occult viral infection.
f. Vaccinations against pneumococcus and influenza are recommended.

Drug-Specific Recommendations

- *Methotrexate.* All patients should be coprescribed folic acid supplementation at a minimal dose of 5 mg once weekly to be taken on a different day to the methotrexate.
- *Azathioprine.* Patients should have baseline thiopurine methyltransferase status assessed.
- *Hydroxychloroquine.* Patients should have baseline formal ophthalmic examination, ideally including objective retinal assessment, for example, using optical coherence tomography, within 1 year of commencing an antimalarial drug.

Prescribing Disease-Modifying Antirheumatic Drugs in Patients With Comorbidities

- Preexisting lung disease is not a specific contraindication to DMARD therapy; however, caution is advised when using drugs associated with pneumonitis in patients with poor respiratory reserve.
- In patients with deranged liver biochemistry, hepatotoxic DMARDs should be used with caution, with careful attention to trends in test results.
- In patients with impaired liver synthetic function (e.g., cirrhosis), DMARD therapy should be used with extreme caution.
- Patients with chronic viral hepatitis infection should be considered for antiviral treatment before immunosuppressive DMARD initiation.
- DMARDs must be used with caution in chronic kidney disease, with appropriate dose reduction and increased frequency of monitoring.
- Cardiovascular disease and prior malignancy are not considered contraindications to DMARD therapy.

Drug Monitoring

Recommended Disease-Modifying Antirheumatic Drug Blood Monitoring Schedule When Starting or Adding a New Disease-Modifying Antirheumatic Drug

1. Check FBC, creatinine or calculated GFR, ALT and/or AST, and albumin every 2 weeks until on stable dose for 6 weeks; then when on a stable dose, check monthly FBC, creatinine or calculated GFR, ALT and/or AST, and albumin for 3 months; thereafter, check FBC, creatinine or calculated GFR, ALT and/or AST, and albumin at least every 12 weeks. More frequent monitoring is appropriate in patients at higher risk of toxicity.

2. Dose increases should be monitored by FBC, creatinine or calculated GFR, ALT and/or AST, and albumin every 2 weeks until the patient is on a stable dose for 6 weeks; then revert to the previous schedule.

3. Note: If a patient is taking combinations of DMARDs, monitor according to the drug with the highest risk of toxicity.

Drug-Specific Monitoring Recommendations

TABLE Appendix 12.1   Summary of Monitoring Requirements

Drug	Laboratory Monitoring	Other Monitoring
Apremilast	No routine laboratory monitoring	None
Azathioprine	Standard monitoring schedule[a]	None
Ciclosporin	Extend monthly monitoring longer term	Blood pressure and glucose at each monitoring visit
Gold	Standard monitoring schedule[a]	Urinalysis for blood and protein before each dose
Hydroxychloroquine	No routine laboratory monitoring	Annual eye assessment (ideally including optical coherence tomography) if continued for >5 years
Leflunomide	Standard monitoring schedule[a]	Blood pressure and weight at each monitoring visit
Mepacrine	No routine laboratory monitoring	None
Methotrexate	Standard monitoring schedule	None
Methotrexate and leflunomide combined	Extend monthly monitoring longer term	None
Minocycline	No routine laboratory monitoring	None
Mycophenolate	Standard monitoring schedule	None
Sulfasalazine	Standard monitoring schedule for 12 months; then no routine monitoring needed	None
Tacrolimus	Extend monthly monitoring longer term	Blood pressure and glucose at each monitoring visit

Perioperative Disease-Modifying Antirheumatic Drug Management

- Steroid exposure should be minimised before surgical procedures, and increases in steroid dose to prevent adrenal insufficiency are not routinely required.
- DMARD therapy should not routinely be stopped in the perioperative period, though individualised decisions should be made for high-risk procedures.

Intercurrent Infections

- During a serious infection, methotrexate, leflunomide, sulfasalazine, azathioprine, apremilast, mycophenolate mofetil, ciclosporin, and tacrolimus should be temporarily discontinued until the patient has recovered from the infection.

Recommendations for Shared Care Agreements

a. The prescriber has responsibility for ensuring patients are adhering to monitoring guidance.

b. When prescribing takes place in primary care, it should be supported by local written shared care agreements, highlighting responsibilities of each party (patient, secondary care, primary care).

c. Contact the rheumatology team urgently and consider interruption in treatment if any of the following develop: white cell count less than 3.5×10^9/L; mean cell volume greater than 105 fL; neutrophils less than 1.6×10^9/L; creatinine increase greater than 30% over 12 months and/or calculated GFR less than 60 mL/min; unexplained eosinophilia greater than 0.5×10^9/L; ALT and/or AST greater than 100 U/L; platelet count less than 140×10^9/L; or unexplained reduction in albumin less than 30 g/L.

d. As well as responding to absolute values in laboratory tests, it is also relevant to observe trends in results (e.g., gradual decreases in white blood cells or albumin or increasing liver enzymes).

e. For clinically urgent abnormalities, emergency access to specialist rheumatology advice, with response within 1 working day, should be available as per National Institute for Health and Care Excellence guidelines.

Dermatomes and Myotomes

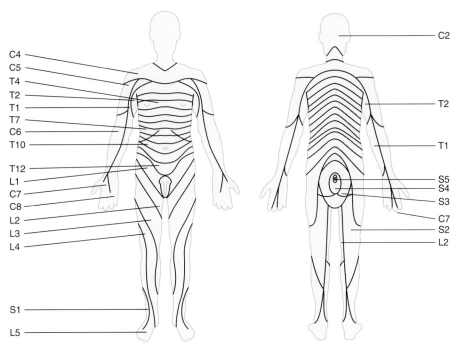

Muscle Group	Nerve Supply	Reflexes
Diaphragm	C3, C4, C5	
Shoulder abductors	C5	
Elbow flexors	C5, C6	Biceps jerk: C5, C6
Supinators and pronators	C6	Supinator jerk: C6
Wrist extensors	C6	
Wrist flexors	C7	
Elbow extensors	C7	Triceps jerk: C7
Finger extensors	C7	
Finger flexors	C8	
Intrinsic hand muscles	T1	Abdominal reflex: T8–T12
Hip flexors	L1, L2	
Hip adductors	L2, L3	
Knee extensors	L3, L4	Knee jerk: L3, L4
Ankle dorsiflexors	L4, L5	
Toe extensors	L5	
Knee flexors	L4, L5, S1	
Ankle plantar flexors	S1, S2	Ankle jerk: S1, S2
Toe flexors	S1, S2	
Anal sphincter	S2, S3, S4	Bulbocavernosus reflex: S3, S4 Anal reflex: S2-4 Plantar reflex

Testing Peripheral Nerves

Nerve Root	Muscle	Test by Asking the Patient to
C3, C4	Trapezius	Shrug shoulder, adduct scapula
C4, C5	Rhomboids	Brace shoulder back
C5, C6, C7	Serratus anterior	Push forward against resistance
C5, C6, C7,C 8	Pectoralis major (clavicular head)	Adduct arm from above horizontal and forward
C6, C7, C8, T1	Pectoralis major (sternocostal head)	Adduct arm below horizontal
C5	Supraspinatus	Abduct arm the first 15 degrees
C5, C6	Infraspinatus	Externally rotate arm, elbow at side
C6, C7, C8	Latissimus dorsi	Adduct horizontal and lateral arm
C5, C6	Biceps	Flex supinated forearm
C5, C6	Deltoid	Abduct arm between 15 and 90 degrees
Radial Nerve		
C7, C8	Triceps	Extend elbow against resistance
C5, C6	Brachioradialis	Flex elbow with forearm halfway between pronation and supination
C6, C7	Extensor carpi radialis longus	Extend wrist to radial side with fingers extended
C5, C6	Supinator	Arm by side, resist hand pronation
C7, C8	Extensor digitorum	Keep fingers extended at MCP joint
C7, C8	Extensor carpi ulnaris	Extend wrist to ulnar side
C7, C8	Abductor pollicis longus	Abduct thumb at 90 degrees to palm
C7, C8	Extensor pollicis brevis	Extend thumb at MCP joint
C7, C8	Extensor pollicis longus	Resist thumb flexion at IP joint
Median Nerve		
C6, C7	Pronator teres	Keep arm pronated against resistance
C6, C7, C8	Flexor carpi radialis	Flex wrist towards radial side
C7, C8, T1	Flexor digitorum sublimis	Resist extension at PIP joint (while you fix the proximal phalanx)
C8, T1	Flexor digitorum profundus I and II	Resist extension at the DIP joint
C8, T1	Flexor pollicis longus	Resist thumb extension at IP joint (fix proximal phalanx)
C8, T1	Abductor pollicis brevis	Abduct thumb (nail at 90 degrees to palm)
C8, T1	Opponens pollicis	Thumb touches fifth fingertip (nail parallel to palm)
C8, T1	First and second lumbricals	Extend PIP joint against resistance with MCP joint held hyperextended

Nerve Root	Muscle	Test by Asking the Patient to
Ulnar Nerve		
C7, C8	Flexor carpi ulnaris	Abducting little finger; see tendon when all fingers extended
C8, T1	Flexor digitorum profundus III and IV	Fix middle phalanx of little finger, resisting extension of distal phalanx
C8, T1	Dorsal interossei	Abduct fingers (use index finger)
C8, T1	Palmar interossei	Adduct fingers (use index finger)
C8, T1	Adductor pollicis	Adduct thumb (nail at 90 degrees to palm)
C8, T1	Abductor digiti minimi	Abduct little finger
C8, T1	Opponens digiti minimi	With fingers extended, carry little finger in front of other fingers
Nerve Root		
L4, L5, S1	Gluteus medius and minimus (superior gluteal nerve)	Internal rotation at hip, hip abduction
L5, S1, S2	Gluteus maximus (inferior gluteal nerve)	Extension at hip (lie prone)
L2, L3, L4	Adductors (obturator nerve)	Adduct leg against resistance
Femoral Nerve		
L1, L2, L3	Iliopsoas	Flex hip with knee flexed and lower leg supported (patient lies on back)
L2, L3	Sartorius	Flex knee with hip externally rotated
L2, L3, L4	Quadriceps femoris	Extend knee against resistance
Sciatic Nerve		
L4, L5, S1, S2	Hamstrings	Flex knee against resistance
L4, L5	Tibialis posterior	Invert plantarflexed foot
L4, L5	Tibialis anterior	Dorsiflex ankle
L5, S1	Extensor digitorum longus	Dorsiflex toes against resistance
L5, S1	Extensor hallucis longus	Dorsiflex hallux against resistance
L5, S1	Peroneus longus and brevis	Exert foot against resistance
S1	Extensor digitorum brevis	Dorsiflex hallux (muscle of foot)
S1, S2	Gastrocnemius	Plantarflex ankle joint
S1, S2	Flexor digitorum longus	Flex terminal joints of toes
S1, S2	Small muscles of foot	Make sole of foot into a cup

DIP, Distal interphalangeal; *IP*, interphalangeal; *MCP*, metacarpophalangeal; *PIP*, proximal interphalangeal.
From Medical Research Council. (1976). *Aids to the examination of the peripheral nervous system*. London: HMSO. Crown copyright material is reproduced with the permission of the Controller of HMSO and the Queen's Printer for Scotland.

Appendix 15

Drug Levels

Drug	Therapeutic Range
For the following drugs, blood should be taken predose:	
Carbamazepine	4–12 mg/L
Ethosuximide	40–100 mg/L
Phenobarbital	20–40 mg/L
Phenytoin	10–20 mg/L (child: 6–14 mg/L)
Primidone	As for phenobarbital
Theophylline	10–20 mg/L
For the following drugs, blood should be taken at the times indicated:	
Digoxin (8–12 hours after last dose)	0.6–2.0 µ/L; toxicity, 1.8–3.0 µg/L
Lithium (12 hours after last dose)	0.4–1.0 mmol/L
Valproate (2 hours after last dose)	50–100 mg/L

Checklist to Guide the Review of a Patient With Multiple Sclerosis

This is not a list of questions to be asked of every person with multiple sclerosis (MS) on every occasion. Rather, it is a list to remind clinicians of the wide range of potential problems that people with MS may face and which should be actively considered as appropriate. A positive answer should lead to more detailed assessment and management. Always also consider the impact that other chronic health conditions may be having on the patient and how they may interact with their MS.

Initial Question

It is best to start by asking an open-ended question such as:
'Since you were last seen or assessed, has any activity you used to undertake been limited, stopped or affected?'

Activity Domains

Then, especially if nothing has been identified, it is worth asking questions directly, choosing from the list below those appropriate to the situation based on your knowledge of the person with MS:
'Are you still able to undertake, as far as you wish, the following'?
- Vocational activities (work, education, other occupation)
- Leisure activities
- Family roles
- Shopping and other community activities
- Household and domestic activities
- Washing, dressing, and using toilet
- Getting about (either by walking or in other ways) and getting in and out of your house
- Controlling your environment (opening doors, switching things on and off, using the phone)

If restrictions are identified, then the reasons for these should be identified as far as possible considering impairments (see later) and social and physical factors (contexts).

Common Impairments

It is worth asking about specific impairments from the following list, again adapting to the situation and what you already know:
'Since you were last seen, have you developed any new problems with the following'?
- Fatigue, endurance, being overtired
- Speech and communication
- Balance and falling
- Chewing and swallowing food and drink
- Unintended change in weight
- Pain or painful abnormal sensations
- Control over your bladder or bowels
- Control over your movement
- Vision and your eyes
- Thinking or remembering
- Your mood
- Your sexual function or partnership relations
- How you get on in social situations

Final Question

Finally, it is always worth finishing with a further open-ended question:
'Are there any other new problems that you think might be due to MS that concern you'?

From: National Institute of Health and Care Excellence. (2022). *Multiple sclerosis in adults: Management. NICE guideline 220.* Available at https://www.nice.org.uk/guidance/ng220.

Appendix 17

Medical Management of Patients With Obesity

The management of patients with obesity should be approached in a holistic manner that includes advice about diet and lifestyle and taking account of the psychological factors involved in overweight and obesity.

Consideration should also be given to possible underlying medical causes of weight gain such as hypothyroidism.

Pharmacologic Management

NICE-Approved Medication	Starting Criteria	Stopping Criteria
Orlistat	BMI of: • ≥30 kg/m² or • ≥28 kg/m² with associated risk factors[a]	Continue beyond 3 months only if the person has lost 5% of their starting body weight
Liraglutide	BMI of: • ≥35 kg/m² or • ≥32.5 kg/m² in ethnic minorities known to be at higher risk from the complications of obesity and • Nondiabetic hyperglycaemia and • High risk of cardiovascular disease caused by, e.g., hypertension or dyslipidaemia and • Is prescribed in secondary care by a specialist weight loss service	—
Semaglutide	BMI of: • ≥35.0 kg/m² or • 30.0–34.9 kg/m² and meets the criteria for referral to specialist weight management services[b] • Use lower BMI thresholds (usually reduced by 2.5 kg/m²) for people from South Asian, Chinese, other Asian, Middle Eastern, Black African, or African Caribbean family backgrounds and • At least one weight-related comorbidity and • Use within a specialist weight management service	Consider stopping if <5% of the initial body weight has been lost after 6 months Use for a maximum of 2 years

[a]Associated risk factors include hypertension, cardiovascular disease, type 2 diabetes, dyslipidaemia, obstructive sleep apnoea, and nonalcoholic fatty liver disease.
[b]The criteria for referral to weight loss services include complex disease state, conventional treatment has been unsuccessful, drug treatment is being considered for someone with a body mass index (BMI) greater than 50 kg/m², or surgery is being considered.
NICE, National Institute for Health and Care Excellence.

Surgical Management

The National Institute for Health and Care Excellence advises to consider referral for bariatric surgery if:

The person has a body mass index (BMI) of 40 kg/m² or more or between 35 kg/m² and 39.9 kg/m² with a significant health condition that could be improved if they lost weight.[a]

They agree to the necessary long-term follow-up after surgery (e.g., lifelong annual reviews).

Consider referral for people of South Asian, Chinese, other Asian, Middle Eastern, Black African, or African Caribbean family background using a lower BMI threshold (reduced by 2.5 kg/m²)

Reference

National Institute of Health and Care Excellence. (2014; updated 2023), *Obesity: Identification, assessment and management. NICE clinical guideline 189*. Available at https://www.nice.org.uk/guidance/cg189.

Immunisations in Pregnancy (UK)

Immunisations Contraindicated in Pregnancy

Vaccine	Comments
Bacillus Calmette–Guérin	Live mycobacterium
Cholera (oral)	No evidence of safety; benefit unlikely to outweigh theoretical risk
Measles	Live virus; avoid pregnancy for 3 months after vaccination
Mumps	Live virus; avoid pregnancy for 3 months after vaccination
Rubella	Live virus; avoid pregnancy for 3 months after vaccination
Typhoid	Live bacterium
Ty21a	
Varicella	Live virus; consider giving varicella zoster immune globulin if exposed to chickenpox in pregnancy
Yellow fever	Live virus; give patient a written waiver if travelling to a country requiring a certificate; if risk of contracting the disease is high, the patient may choose to have the immunisation

Immunisations which may be given in pregnancy if patient and physician judge that the potential benefit outweighs the risk

That risk is theoretical. In almost all of these immunisations, there is no evidence either way. If deciding to give the immunisation, it may be thought prudent to wait until the second or third trimester in case a reaction to the vaccine were to trigger a first trimester miscarriage.

Vaccine	Comments
Diphtheria and tetanus	
Hepatitis A	The patient may choose immunoglobulin as a safer alternative
Hepatitis B COVID-19	Strongly recommended in pregnancy because of the excess risks of COVID-19 in pregnancy.
Immunoglobulin	
Influenza	The vaccine is positively indicated in pregnant females; they are more prone to pulmonary complications than nonpregnant females
Japanese encephalitis	Inactivated virus, but there is no consensus on its safety
Meningococcus	
Pneumococcus	
Pertussis	The vaccine is positively indicated in pregnancy (ideally between 16 and 32 weeks) to protect newborn babies via passive immunity
Polio (oral)	Paralysis seems more likely in pregnancy than in nonpregnant females; neonatal infection carries a high mortality rate
Rabies	
Typhoid (Vi capsular polysaccharide)	

Adapted from Centers for Disease Control and Prevention. (2008). *CDC health information for international travel*. Mosby; National Institute for Health and Care Excellence. (2008). *Antenatal care: Routine care for the healthy pregnant woman. Clinical guideline 62*. National Collaborating Centre for Women's and Children's Health. Commissioned by the National Institute for Health and Clinical Excellence. Available at https://www.nice.org.uk/guidance/ng201; and Martinez, L. (Ed.). (2002). *International travel and health*. World Health Organization.

Edinburgh Postnatal Depression Scale

Instructions for Users

1. The mother is asked to underline the response which comes closest to how she has been feeling in the previous 7 days.
2. All 10 items must be completed.
3. Care should be taken to avoid the possibility of the mother discussing her answers with others.
4. The mother should complete the scale herself unless she has limited English or has difficulty with reading.
5. The Edinburgh Postnatal Depression Scale (EPDS) may be used at 6–8 weeks to screen postnatal females. The child health clinic, postnatal check-up, or a home visit may provide suitable opportunities for its completion.

Scoring the EPDS

- Response categories are scored 0, 1, 2, and 3 according to increased severity of the symptom.
- Items marked with an asterisk are reverse scored (i.e., 3, 2, 1, and 0). The total score is calculated by adding together the scores for each of the 10 items.
- Mothers who score above a threshold 12 of 13 are likely to have a depressive illness of varying severity. Nevertheless, the EPDS score should not override clinical judgement. A careful clinical assessment should be carried out to confirm the diagnosis. The scale indicates how the mother has felt during the previous week, and in doubtful cases, it may be usefully repeated after 2 weeks. The scale does not detect mothers with anxiety neuroses, phobias, or personality disorders.

As you have recently had a baby, we would like to know how you are feeling. Please UNDERLINE the answer which comes closest to how you have felt IN THE PAST 7 DAYS, not just how you feel today. Here is an example, already completed.

I have felt happy:
Yes, all the time.
Yes, most of the time.
No, not very often.
No, not at all.

This would mean: 'I have felt happy most of the time' during the past week. Please complete the other questions in the same way.

In the past 7 days:

1. I have been able to laugh and see the funny side of things:
   As much as I always could
   Not quite so much now
   Definitely not so much now
   Not at all

2. I have looked forward with enjoyment to things:
   As much as I ever did
   Rather less than I used to
   Definitely less than I used to
   Hardly at all

3. I have blamed myself unnecessarily when things went wrong:
   Yes, most of the time
   Yes, some of the time
   Not very often
   No, never

4. I have been anxious or worried for no good reason:
   No, not at all
   Hardly ever
   Yes, sometimes
   Yes, very often

Continued

5. I have felt scared or panicky for no very good reason:
   Yes, quite a lot
   Yes, sometimes
   No, not much
   No, not at all

6. Things have been getting on top of me:
   Yes, most of the time I haven't been able to cope at all
   Yes, sometimes I haven't been coping as well as usual
   No, most of the time I have coped quite well
   No, I have been coping as well as ever

7. I have been so unhappy that I have had difficulty sleeping:
   Yes, most of the time
   Yes, sometimes
   Not very often
   No, not at all

8. I have felt sad or miserable:
   Yes, most of the time
   Yes, quite often
   Not very often
   No, not at all

9. I have been so unhappy that I have been crying:
   Yes, most of the time
   Yes, quite often
   Only occasionally
   No, never

10. The thought of harming myself has occurred to me:
    Yes, quite often
    Sometimes
    Hardly ever Never

Appendix 20

Admission Procedures for Patients With Mental Health Problems

Compulsory Admission

The team needed to complete a Section 2 or Section 3 consists of:

a. The GP or an independent Section 12 approved doctor;
b. An approved mental health professional (AMHP);
c. An approved psychiatrist (consultant or specialist registrar).

The procedure to follow for assessment of a patient who may need to be detained from home is likely to vary by local area. Some points to consider may be as follows:

- Obtain relevant information from a partner who may know the patient better.
- Review the records to assess:
  - Risk of violence;
  - Past history of outcomes of previous sections;
  - Previous responses to treatment.
- Phone the family or carer to obtain their assessment of the:
  - Current situation and urgency;
  - Need for police support;
  - Risk of violence, access to weapons.
- Contact the duty AMHP and Crisis Services:
  - Provide basic information: name, date of birth, address, past history, current problem, reason for assessment, phone number of patient, name of carer or relative at home, how to contact you in the next few hours, name of key worker, any known risk of violence or self harm.

Voluntary Admission

- If patient is known to hospital staff and a bed is available and the patient accepts admission: admission to be arranged via mental health team.
- If patient is known to hospital staff but there are no beds available: the mental health team would contact the relevant bed manager.
  - If a bed is found, arrange admission as above.
  - If a bed is not immediately available alternative arrangements to ensure the safety of the patient would be made by the mental health team, for example utilising more intensive support from Crisis services.
- If the patient not known to hospital staff: if Monday to Friday, 9 a.m. to 5 p.m. then:
  a. Check catchment area and relevant consultant or Crisis service;
  b. Contact the mental health team to request further assessment.

Early Warning Form for Use in Psychotic Illness

EARLY WARNING SIGNS

Name: ....

I am at risk of developing episodes of: ....
....

My early warning signs are (e.g., changes in sleep, eating, drinking, or mood; becoming quiet, loud, or more withdrawn):

1. ....
2. ....
3. ....

Whenever I have any of these signs, I will respond by: ....
....
....

My health worker is: ....   Phone ....

My home contact is: ....   Phone ....

My advocacy contact is: ....   Phone ....

If I have any concerns about my illness, I will contact: ....
.... immediately.

Reproduced with permission from Falloon, I. R. H., et al. (1993). *Managing stress in families: Cognitive and behavioural strategies for enhancing coping skills.* Routledge.

The Alcohol Use Disorders Identification Test

The Alcohol Use Disorders Identification Test: Interview Version

First give an explanation of the content and purpose of the questions and the need for accurate answers. Read questions as written. Record answers carefully. Begin the Alcohol Use Disorders Identification Test (AUDIT) by saying, 'Now I am going to ask you some questions about your use of alcoholic beverages during this past year'. Explain what is meant by 'alcoholic beverages' by using local examples of beer, wine, vodka, and so on. Code answers in terms of 'standard drinks'. Place the correct answer number in the box at the right.

1. How often do you have a drink containing alcohol? ☐
   (0) Never [Skip to question 9.]
   (1) Monthly or less
   (2) 2 to 4 times a month
   (3) 2 to 3 times a week
   (4) 4 or more times a week

2. How many drinks containing alcohol do you have on a typical day when you are drinking? ☐
   (0) 1 or 2
   (1) 3 or 4
   (2) 5 or 6
   (3) 7, 8, or 9
   (4) 10 or more

3. How often do you have six or more drinks on one occasion? ☐
   (0) Never
   (1) Less than monthly
   (2) Monthly
   (3) Weekly
   (4) Daily or almost daily

Skip to Question 9 if the total score for questions 2 and 3 = 0.

4. How often during the past year have you found that you were not able to stop drinking after you had started? ☐
   (0) Never
   (1) Less than monthly
   (2) Monthly
   (3) Weekly
   (4) Daily or almost daily

5. How often during the past year have you failed to do what was normally expected from you because of drinking? ☐
   (0) Never
   (1) Less than monthly
   (2) Monthly
   (3) Weekly
   (4) Daily or almost daily

Continued

6. How often during the past year have you needed a first drink in the morning to get yourself going after a heavy drinking session? ☐
   (0) Never
   (1) Less than monthly
   (2) Monthly
   (3) Weekly
   (4) Daily or almost daily

7. How often during the past year have you had a feeling of guilt or remorse after drinking? ☐
   (0) Never
   (1) Less than monthly
   (2) Monthly
   (3) Weekly
   (4) Daily or almost daily

8. How often during the past year have you been unable to remember what happened the night before because you had been drinking? ☐
   (0) Never
   (1) Less than monthly
   (2) Monthly
   (3) Weekly
   (4) Daily or almost daily

9. Have you or someone else been injured as a result of your drinking? ☐
   (0) No
   (2) Yes, but not in the last year
   (4) Yes, during the past year

10. Has a relative or friend or a doctor or another health worker been concerned about your drinking or suggested you cut down? ☐
    (0) No
    (2) Yes, but not in the past year
    (4) Yes, during the past year

Record total of specific items here: ☐

An AUDIT score in the range of 8 to 15 represents a medium level of alcohol problems in which brief interventions would be appropriate. Scores of 16 or greater represent a high level of alcohol problems with higher levels of intervention and monitoring recommended. Scores of 20 or greater suggest dependent drinking and merits further assessment.[1]

AUDIT-C uses the first three questions only. If the score is 3 or greater, then complete the full questionnaire.

---

[1] Babor, T. F., Higgins-Biddle, J. C., Saunders, J. B., et al. (2001). *Audit, the alcohol use disorders identification test: World Health Organization (WHO).* www.who.int/Alcohol_AUDIT.

The International Prostate Symptom Score

	Not at All	Less Than One Time in Five	Less Than Half the Time	About Half the Time	More Than Half the Time	Almost Always
1. Incomplete emptying Over the past month, how often have you had a sensation of not emptying your bladder completely after you have finished urinating?	0	1	2	3	4	5
2. Frequency Over the past month, how often have you had to urinate again less than 2 hours after you finished urinating?	0	1	2	3	4	5
3. Intermittency Over the past month, how often have you found you stopped and started again several times when you urinated?	0	1	2	3	4	5
4. Urgency Over the past month, how often have you found it difficult to postpone urination or felt sudden urges to urinate?	0	1	2	3	4	5
5. Weak stream Over the past month, how often have you had a weak urinary stream?	0	1	2	3	4	5
6. Straining Over the past month, how often have you had to push or strain to begin urination?	0	1	2	3	4	5

	None	Once	Twice	Three Times	Four Times	Five Times or More
7. Nocturia Over the past month, how many times did you typically get up to urinate from the time you went to bed at night to the time you got up in the morning?	0	1	2	3	4	5

(Scoring items 1–7: 0–7 = mild; 8–19 = moderate; 20–35 = severe)

Continued

Quality of Life	Delighted	Pleased	Mostly Satisfied	No Strong Feelings Either Way	Mostly Dissatisfied	Unhappy	Terrible
If you were to spend the rest of your life with urinary conditions just the way they are now, how would you feel about it?	0	1	2	3	4	5	6

Appendix 24

Body Mass Index for Adults

	Body Mass Index Range (European/ North American/White African etc) (kg/m^2)	Body Mass Index Range (Asian, Chinese, Middle Eastern, Black African, African Caribbean) (kg/m^2)
Healthy	18.5–24.9	16–22.4
Overweight	25–29.9	22.5–27.4
Obesity class 1	30–34.9	27.5–32.4
Obesity class 2	35–39.9	32.5–37.4
Obesity class 3	>40	>38.5

Central adiposity (for all ethnicities of those with a body mass index <35 kg/m^2):
- Healthy: waist-to-height ratio of 0.4 to 0.49, indicating no increased health risks
- Increased: waist-to-height ratio of 0.5 to 0.59, indicating increased health risks
- High: waist-to-height ratio of 0.6 or more, indicating further increased health risks

Appendix 25

Reference Ranges for Young Adults

Reference ranges vary according to laboratory and test method. The following are given as typical ranges, but if the laboratory performing the test gives a range that differs from these, it should be used instead. The ranges also vary according to age and gender.

Blood

Biochemistry and Immunology

Serum or Plasma

Acid phosphatase		IgG	6–13 g/L
Total	1–5 IU/L	IgM	0.5–2.0 g/L
Prostatic	0–1 IU/L	IgA	1.0–4.0 g/L
Adrenocorticotropic hormone	10–80 ng/L	Lactate dehydrogenase	70–250 IU/L
Alanine aminotransferase	5–35 IU/L	Magnesium	0.7–1.0 mmol/L
Alkaline phosphatase	30–300 IU/L	Osmolality	280–295 mOsmol/kg
Amylase	<120 IU/L	Phosphate (inorganic)	0.8–1.4 mmol/L
Asparate aminotransferase	5–35 IU/L	Potassium	3.4–5.2 mmol/L
Bicarbonate	21–26 mmol/L	Prolactin	Male: 80–400 mu/L
Bilirubin	<17 mmol/L		Females: 90–520 mu/L
Calcium	2.26–2.60 mmol/L		Postmenopausal females: 80–280 mu/L
Chloride	95–105 mmol/L	Protein	
Cholesterol	<5.5 mmol/L	Total	60–80 g/L
Complement		Albumin	35–50 g/L
C3	0.69–1.5 mg/L	PSA	0–4 ng/mL
C4	0.12–0.27 mg/L	Sodium	133–145 mmol/L
		Total thyroxine	70–140 nmol/L
Cortisol		Free thyroxine	10–26 pmol/L
9:00 a.m.	130–690 nmol/L	Free tetraiodothyronine	3–9 pmol/L
Midnight	Half the morning value	Triiodothyronine	1.2–3.0 nmol/L
Creatinine	70–130 mol/L	TSH	0.3–3.8 mu/L
Creatine kinase	<200 IU/L	Triglycerides[b]	<0.55–1.90 mmol/L
α-Fetoprotein	<10 mg/L	Urea	2.5–6.7 mmol/L

γ-Glutamyl transferase		Uric acid	
Males	11–51 IU/L	Males	0.15–0.42 mmol/L
Females	7–33 IU/L	Females	0.10–0.36 mmol/L
Glucose (fasting)	3.4–5.5 mmol/L		
Growth hormone	<5.5 mu/L	Arterial blood gases	
		pH	7.35–7.45
		PaO2	12–14 kPa
		PaCO2	4.6–6.0 kPa

aTo convert cholesterol from mmol/L into mg/dL, multiply by 39.
bTo convert triglycerides from mmol/L into mg/dL, multiply by 89.
ACTH, Adrenocorticotropic hormone; *ALT*, alanine aminotransferase; *AST*, aspartate aminotransferase; *IgA.*, immunoglobulin A, etc; *LDH*, lactate dehydrogenase; *PSA*, prostate-specific antigen; *TSH*, thyroid stimulating hormone.

Value	Reference Range
Haematology	
Haemoglobin	13.5–18.0 g/dL (males) 11.5–16.0 g/dL (females)
Mean corpuscular volume	82–98 fL
Mean corpuscular hemoglobin	26.7–33.0 pg
Mean corpuscular hemoglobin concentration	31.4–35.0 g/dL
White blood cell count	$3.2–11.0×10^9$/L
Neutrophils	$1.9–7.7×10^9$/L
Monocytes	$0.1–0.9×10^9$/L
Eosinophils	$0.0–0.4×10^9$/L
Basophils	$0.2–0.8×10^9$/L
Platelets	$120–400×10^9$/L
Reticulocytes	$25–100×10^9$/L (or <2%)
Ferritin	30–230 µg/L (males) 6–80 µg/L (females) 14–180 µg/L (postmenopausal females)

Urine	
Sodium	100–250 mmol/24 h
Potassium	14–120 mmol/24 h
Albumin – Microalbuminuria – Proteinuria	20–200 mg/L >200 mg/L
Albumin/creatinine ratio – Microalbuminuria	2.5 mg/mmol (males) or 3.5 mg/mmol (females) to 30 mg/mmol
– Proteinuria	>30 mg/mmol
Creatinine clearance	85–125 mL/min (males); 75–115 mL/min (females)
Osmolality	350–1000 mOsmol/kg

Appendix 26

Anaphylaxis

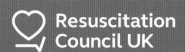 **Resuscitation Council UK**

GUIDELINES ✓ 2021

Anaphylaxis

Anaphylaxis?

A = Airway **B** = Breathing **C** = Circulation **D** = Disability **E** = Exposure

Diagnosis – look for:
- Sudden onset of Airway and/or Breathing and/or Circulation problems [1]
- And usually skin changes (e.g. itchy rash)

Call for HELP
Call resuscitation team or ambulance

- Remove trigger if possible (e.g. stop any infusion)
- Lie patient flat (with or without legs elevated)
  - A sitting position may make breathing easier
  - If pregnant, lie on left side

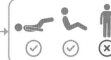

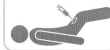

Inject at **anterolateral aspect** – middle third of the thigh

Give intramuscular (IM) adrenaline [2]

- Establish airway
- Give high flow oxygen
- Apply monitoring: pulse oximetry, ECG, blood pressure

If no response:
- Repeat IM adrenaline after 5 minutes
- IV fluid bolus [3]

If no improvement in Breathing or Circulation problems [1] despite TWO doses of IM adrenaline:
- Confirm resuscitation team or ambulance has been called
- Follow REFRACTORY ANAPHYLAXIS ALGORITHM

---

1. Life-threatening problems

Airway
Hoarse voice, stridor

Breathing
↑work of breathing, wheeze, fatigue, cyanosis, SpO_2 <94%

Circulation
Low blood pressure, signs of shock, confusion, reduced consciousness

2. Intramuscular (IM) adrenaline
Use adrenaline at 1 mg/mL (1:1000) concentration

Adult and child >12 years:	500 µg IM (0.5 mL)
Child 6–12 years:	300 µg IM (0.3 mL)
Child 6 months to 6 years:	150 µg IM (0.15 mL)
Child <6 months:	100–150 µg IM (0.1–0.15 mL)

The above doses are for IM injection **only**.
Intravenous adrenaline for anaphylaxis to be given **only by experienced specialists** in an appropriate setting.

3. IV fluid challenge
Use crystalloid

Adults: 500–1000 mL
Children: 10 mL/kg

Problems Associated With Specific Causes of Disability

Condition and Prevalence	Audiovisual	Endocrine	Psychiatric or Psychological	Central Nervous System	Cardiovascular	Musculoskeletal and Skin	Other	Inheritance
Cerebral palsy, 1:500	Visual impairment Hearing impairment		Depression Variable intellectual capacity	Epilepsy		Orthopaedic problems Neuromuscular problems	Genitourinary problems Incontinence Constipation Dental problems Recurrent aspiration Oesophagitis, gastrooesophageal reflux with or without bleeding or anaemia Swallowing or eating difficulties	
Down syndrome, 1:700	Visual impairment (multifactorial), cataracts Hearing impairment (multifactorial) Annual assessments recommended	Hypothyroidism Annual TFT recommended	Depression Alzheimer-type dementia (clinical onset uncommon before 40 years)	Epilepsy usually clonic-tonic	Congenital heart defects (present in 40%–50%)	Atlantoaxial instability Skin disorders, alopecia, eczema	Blood dyscrasias Childhood leukaemia Sleep apnoea Increased susceptibility to infections Coeliac disease	Most cases are sporadic; 4% caused by translocation involving chromosome 21 or rarely parental mosaicism
Prader–Willi syndrome, 1:10,000–25,000	Strabismus myopia	Type 2 diabetes (secondary to obesity) Hypogonadism Delayed puberty	Hyperphagia impulse control difficulties Self-injury	—	—	Scoliosis, kyphosis Hypotonia Skin picking	Infantile failure to thrive; then hyperphagia and severe obesity High tolerance to pain Decreased ability to vomit Sleep apnoea Osteoporosis Undescended testes Dental abnormalities	Atypical Most cases are sporadic

Continued

Condition and Prevalence	Audiovisual	Endocrine	Psychiatric or Psychological	Central Nervous System	Cardiovascular	Musculoskeletal and Skin	Other	Inheritance
Fragile X syndrome, 1:6000	Visual impairment (multifactorial) Hearing impairment Recurrent ear infections	—	Attention-deficit hyperactivity disorder Variable intellectual capacity Disabled in social functioning	Epilepsy Usually clonic-tonic, complex partial	Aortic dilatation, mitral valve prolapse (related to connective tissue dysplasia)	Connective tissue dysplasia Scoliosis Congenital hip dislocation	Hernias (CT (Connective Tissue) related) Abnormalities of speech and language	X-linked
Phenylketonuria, 1:10,000–20,000	—	—	Variable intellectual capacity Phobic anxiety Disabled in social functioning	Epilepsy Hyperactivity Tremor and pyramidal tract signs Extrapyramidal syndromes	—	—	Eczema	Autosomal recessive
Angelman syndrome, 1:10,000	Glaucoma	—	Easily excitable Hyperactive	Severe developmental delay Epilepsy	—	Joint contractures and scoliosis (in adults)	Speech impairment Movement and balance disorder Characteristic EEG changes	Variety of genetic mechanisms on chromosome 15
Williams syndrome, <1:20,000	Hyperacusis Strabismus	—	Variable intellectual capacity Attention-deficit problems in childhood	Perceptual and motor function reduced	Cardiac abnormalities Hypertension CVAs Chronic hemiparesis	Joint contractures Scoliosis Hypotonia	Renal abnormalities	Microdeletion on chromosome 7
Rett syndrome, 1:14,000 females	Refractory errors	—	Severe intellectual disability	Epilepsy Vasomotor instability	Prolonged QT interval	Osteopenia Fractures Scoliosis	Hyperventilation Apnoea Reflux Feeding difficulties Growth failure	Usually sporadic X-linked

Condition	Eyes/Vision	Endocrine/Hearing	Intellectual	Epilepsy/CNS	Cardiac	Skeletal	Other	Inheritance
Noonan syndrome, <1:10,000	Strabismus Refractive errors Vision or hearing impairments	—	Mild intellectual disability	Epilepsy	Pulmonary valvular stenosis ASD, VSD, PDA	Scoliosis Talipes equinovarus Pectus carinatum or excavatum	Abnormal clotting factors, platelet dysfunction Undescended tests, deficient spermatogenesis Lymphangiectasia Hepatosplenomegaly Cubitus valgus, hand abnormalities	Autosomal dominant, may be sporadic
Tuberous sclerosis, 1:6000–17,000	Retinal tumours Eye rhabdomyomatas	—	Variable intellectual capacity Behavioural difficulties Sleep problems	Cerebral astrocytomas Epilepsy	Rhabdomyomatas Hypertension	Bone Rhabdomyomata	Kidney and lung hamartomata Polycystic kidneys Liver rhabdomyomata Dental abnormalities Skin lesions	Autosomal dominant
Neurofibromatosis, 1:300	Hearing impairment (glioma affecting auditory nerve)	Various endocrine abnormalities	Variable intellectual capacity	Variable clinical phenomena depending on site of the tumours Epilepsy	—	Skeletal abnormalities, especially kyphoscoliosis	Variable clinical phenomena depending on the location of the neurofibroma Tumours are susceptible to malignant change Other varieties of tumours may be associated	Autosomal dominant

ASD, Atrial septal defect; CVA, cerebrovascular accident; EEG, electroencephalogram; PDA, patent ductus arteriosus; TFT, thyroid function test; VSD, ventricular septal defect.
Adapted from an original unpublished version by Michael Kew and Glyn Jones and reproduced with the kind permission of the University of Queensland.

Appendix 28

The Community Dependency Index[a]

Score the patient under the following nine headings. A score of less than 75 suggests moderate disability; less than 50 suggests severe disability.

Personal Toilet

5 = The client can wash hands and face, comb hair, clean teeth, and shave. Must be able to get to water and brushes without help and operate them independently.

0 = Any help or supervision needed or difficulty with personal toilet.

Feeding

10 = Independent. The client can feed themselves a meal from a tray or table when someone puts the food within reach. They must put on their own assistive device if this is needed, cut up food, spread butter, and so on. They must accomplish this in a reasonable time (that is acceptable to the client).

5 = Food must be cut for the client, or some help is necessary with the items above. Unreasonable time or effort is required if the client feeds independently.

0 = The client unable to feed themselves.

Moving From (Wheel) Chair to Bed and Return

15 = The client is independent in all phases of this activity.

Chair: The client can safely stand up from sitting in their chair (high chair allowed) without help from another person and sit down again. The client must be able to get in and out bed without help and when in bed must be able to turn and move up and down in the bed as necessary.

Or wheelchair: The client can safely approach the bed in their wheelchair, lock the brakes, lift the footrests, transfer safely to the bed, and lie down. When in bed, the client must be able to turn and move up and down the bed as necessary. The client must be able to transfer back into the wheelchair safely, including changing the position of the wheelchair for the return transfer.

10 = The client can independently sit down and stand up from chair or transfer in and out of a wheelchair but has difficulty or needs help in bed.

5 = Help or supervision is needed to ensure the client's safety in all parts of this activity, or the client performs all or parts of this activity with difficulty.

0 = The client is unable to perform this activity.

Getting On and Off the Toilet or Commode (During the Day and Night)

10 = The client is able to reach the toilet or commode area unassisted. They are able to transfer on and off the commode, fasten and unfasten clothes, prevent spoiling of clothes, and use toilet paper without help. They may use equipment or stable fittings for support if needed (e.g., rail, raised toilet seat or side of bath). If they use a commode, they must be able to position it for use, empty it, and clean it out.

5 = The client has difficulty with part of this activity, or the client needs help because of imbalance or in handling clothes, using toilet paper, or flushing the toilet.

0 = The client needs help to empty the commode or is not able to transfer.

Note: If the client can use the toilet independently during the day but has the commode at night, which someone else empties, then score 5.

Walking 50 Yards Outside the House or Using a Wheelchair

Walking

15 = The client gets in and out of the house unassisted. They can walk at least 50 yards without help or supervision outside their home. They may wear braces and prostheses and use walking aids. They must be able to reach and operate aids without help.

10 = The client has difficulty or needs minimal help or supervision in any of the above but can walk at least 50 yards.

Wheelchair

5 = The client cannot walk but can propel a wheelchair independently. They must be able to go round corners and turn around. They must be able to get in and out of the

house independently (access). They must be able to push the wheelchair at least 50 yards. If the wheelchair is used indoors, they must be able to manoeuvre to a table, bed, or toilet. Do not score for wheelchair use if the client gets a score for walking.

0 = The client is unable to walk or propel a wheelchair for 50 yards.

Dressing and Undressing

10 = The client is able to put on and remove and fasten all clothing and tie shoelaces (adaptations or aids allowed). This activity includes putting on and removing prostheses, braces, and corsets when these are prescribed. Special clothing, such as slip-on shoes or dresses that open down the front, may be used where necessary.

5 = The client has difficulty or needs help in putting on and removing or fastening any clothing. When helped, the client must do at least half the work. They must accomplish this in a reasonable time.

0 = The client needs help with all or most of dressing.

Bathing Self

5 = The client can use a bath or shower. They must be able to do all the steps involved in whichever method is used without another person helping. Verbal supervision is allowed.

0 = The client has difficulty or needs help.

Note: When the client's home does not have bathing or shower facilities, score 5 for using a bath or shower in another facility or having an all-over wash if independent. When the client has an all-over wash because they are unable to use the bath or shower, then score 0.

Ascending and Descending Stairs

10 = The client is able to get up and down stairs safely without help or supervision. They may and should use the handrails and walking aids when needed. They must be able to carry walking aids up and down the stairs if needed. If a stair lift or vertical lift is used, the client must be able to use it without help or supervision (including transfers).

5 = The client has difficulty or needs help or supervision in any one of the above items.

0 = The client unable to climb stairs.

Note: If the client does not have stairs in the house, count as 10 because they are not an obstacle to independence in the home even if they are obstacles in the community.

Continence of Bowels

10 = The client is able to control bowels and has no accidents. They can use a suppository or take an enema when necessary (e.g., spinal cord injury). They can manage external devices (e.g., colostomy).

5 = The client needs help with any of the above.

0 = The client does not have bowel control.

Continence of Bladder

10 = The client able to control their bladder day and night. Clients who wear an external device and leg bag must put them on independently, clean and empty the bag, and stay dry day and night.

5 = The client has control of their bladder but cannot get to the toilet or commode in time (e.g., because of poor mobility) or needs help with an external device.

0 = The client does not have bladder control.

ª© Professor Pamela Eakin, reproduced with permission.

Appendix 29

The Nottingham Extended Activities of Daily Living Questionnaire

Score the patient on each item on a scale of 0 to 3 in which '3' represents independent function, '2' represents alone with difficulty, '1' represents alone with help, and '0' represents unable.

Subscale	Item
Mobility	1. Do you walk around outside? 2. Do you climb stairs? 3. Do you get in and out of the car? 4. Do you walk over uneven ground? 5. Do you cross roads? 6. Do you travel on public transport?
Kitchen	7. Do you manage to feed yourself? 8. Do you manage to make yourself a hot snack? 9. Do you take hot drinks from one room to another? 10. Do you do the washing up? 11. Do you make yourself a hot drink?
Domestic	12. Do you manage your own money when you are out? 13. Do you wash small items of clothing? 14. Do you do your own housework? 15. Do you do your own shopping? 16. Do you do a full clothes wash?
Leisure	17. Do you read newspapers or books? 18. Do you use the telephone? 19. Do you write letters? 20. Do you go out socially? 21. Do you manage your own garden? 22. Do you drive a car?
	Total (0–66)

Drug Stabilities in Syringe Drivers

The following are some notes on using tables of drug mixture stabilities.
- The following tables are separated into mixtures containing two or three drugs, ordered by diamorphine first; then the other drugs in alphabetical order.
- The maximum dose for each drug in each syringe size is given. Provided the doses for every drug in the combination is less than or equal to these maximum values, then the mixture is stable for 24 hours. Above the maximum doses stated, the solution is either unstable or has not been tested, and it is not possible to say whether it is stable or not.
- All drug mixtures should be protected from light when possible.

- It is considered best practice to give dexamethasone as a bolus dose because it has a long duration of action and frequently causes compatibility problems in mixture.
- The following combinations are not stable:
  - Diamorphine, dexamethasone, and levomepromazine
  - Diamorphine, dexamethasone, and midazolam
  - Diamorphine, cyclizine, and metoclopramide
  - Octreotide and levomepromazine
  - Octreotide and cyclizine
  - Octreotide and dexamethasone
  - Diamorphine, metoclopramide, and ondansetron

Drug Combination	Maximum Dose (mg) Known to Be Stable in:							Comments
	8 mL in a 10-mL Syringe		14 mL in a 20-mL Syringe		17 mL in a 30-mL Syringe			
Two-Drug Combinations for Subcutaneous Infusion Which Are Stable for 24 Hours								
Diluent: Water for Injections BP								
Diamorphine and cyclizine	160 160[a]	If diamorphine dose >160, cyclizine dose must be no more than 80	280 280[a]	If diamorphine dose >280, cyclizine dose must be no more than 140	340 340[a]	If diamorphine dose >340, cyclizine dose must be no more than 170		If exceeding these doses, then likely to get precipitate
Diamorphine and haloperidol	800 24	400 32	—		—			If exceeding these doses, then likely to get precipitate
Diamorphine and hyoscine HBr		1200 3.2	—		—			—
Diamorphine and hyoscine butylbromide (Buscopan)		1200 160	—		—			—
Diamorphine and ketorolac		47 40	82 74		90 90			—
Diamorphine and levomepromazine (Nozinan)		400 80	700 140		850 170			Mixture can be irritant, so dilute to the largest possible volume

Continued

Drug Combination	Maximum Dose (mg) Known to Be Stable in:			Comments
	8 mL in a 10-mL Syringe	14 mL in a 20-mL Syringe	17 mL in a 30-mL Syringe	
Diamorphine and metoclopramide	1200 40	2100 70	2550 85	Mixture can be irritant, so dilute to the largest possible volume
Diamorphine and midazolam	400 16	700 28	850 34	—
Diamorphine and octreotide	200 0.9	350 1.6	425 1.9	—
Diamorphine and ondansetron	40 5	70 9	85 11	

Three-Drug Combinations for Subcutaneous Infusion Which Are Stable For 24 Hours

Diluent: Water for Injections BP

Drug Combination	8 mL in a 10-mL Syringe	14 mL in a 20-mL Syringe	17 mL in a 30-mL Syringe	Comments
Diamorphine and cyclizine and haloperidol	160 160 16	280 280 28	340 340 34	Above these doses, the mixture is likely to precipitate. Only stable if diamorphine and haloperidol are well diluted before dexamethasone is added. Use only if no other options are available
Diamorphine and haloperidol and midazolam	560 4 32	980 7 56	1190 8.5 68	—
Diamorphine and levomepromazine and metoclopramide	400 80 24	700 140 42	850 170 51	—

aMaximum recommended daily dose is 150

Reproduced with permission from Scottish Intercollegiate Guidelines Network. (2008). *Control of pain in patients with cancer. SIGN guideline 106.* Available at https://www.sign.ac.uk/our-guidelines/control-of-pain-in-adults-with-cancer/.

Suspected Cancer: Recognition and Referral[a]

Lung Cancer

OFFER URGENT CHEST RADIOGRAPHY if the patient is older than 40 years of age and has two or more of the following or ever smoked and has one or more of the following:

- Cough
- Fatigue
- Shortness of breath
- Chest pain
- Weight loss
- Appetite loss

CONSIDER URGENT CHEST RADIOGRAPHY if the patient is older than 40 years and has any of the following:

- Persistent or recurrent chest infection
- Finger clubbing
- Supraclavicular lymphadenopathy or persistent cervical lymphadenopathy
- Chest signs consistent with lung cancer
- Thrombocytosis

REFER for suspected cancer if either of the following is present:

- Chest radiography findings suggest lung cancer
- The patient is 40 years of age or older with unexplained haemoptysis

Upper Gastrointestinal Cancer

OFFER URGENT OESOPHAGOGASTRODUODE-NOSCOPY if the patient has either of the following:

- Dysphagia
- Age 55 years of age and older with weight loss and any of the following are present:
  - Upper abdominal pain
  - Reflux
  - Dyspepsia

REFER for suspected pancreatic cancer if:

- The patient is older than 40 years of age and has jaundice

CONSIDER URGENT COMPUTED TOMOGRAPHY (or ULTRASONOGRAPHY) OF THE ABDOMEN for suspected pancreatic cancer if the patient is aged older than 60 years, has weight loss, and has any of the following:

- Diarrhoea
- Back pain
- Abdominal pain
- Nausea
- Vomiting
- Constipation
- New-onset diabetes

CONSIDER URGENT REFERRAL for suspected stomach cancer if the patient has a palpable upper abdominal mass.

CONSIDER URGENT ULTRASONOGRAPHY OF THE ABDOMEN if the patient has a palpable mass consistent with an enlarged gallbladder or an enlarged liver.

Lower Gastrointestinal Cancers

REFER for suspected colorectal cancer if:

- Faecal immunochemistry test (FIT) >10 μg haemoglobin per gram of faeces.
- Offer FIT if any of the following is present:
  - Persistent change in bowel habit
  - abdominal pain and wight less and age greater than 40 etc

CONSIDER URGENT REFERRAL for suspected cancer if either of the following is present:

- Anal mass or unexplained anal ulceration
- Rectal mass

Breast Cancer

REFER for suspected cancer if either of the following is present:

- Aged 30 years and older with an unexplained breast lump with or without pain
- Aged 50 years and older with any of the following symptoms in one nipple only:
  - Discharge
  - Retraction
  - Other changes of concern

---

[a]Adapted from National Institute for Health and Care Excellence. (2015; updated 2023). *NICE guideline 12.* Available at https://www.nice.org.uk/guidance/ng12.

CONSIDER URGENT REFERRAL if either of the following is present:
- Aged 30 years and older with an unexplained lump in the axilla
- Skin changes that suggest breast cancer

Gynaecologic Cancer

REFER for suspected ovarian cancer if either of the following is present:
- Physical examination identifies ascites or a pelvic or abdominal mass (which is not obviously uterine fibroids)
- Ultrasonography suggests ovarian cancer

REFER for suspected endometrial cancer if:
- Aged 55 years and older with post-menopausal bleeding (unexplained vaginal bleeding more than 12 months after menstruation has stopped because of menopause)

CONSIDER URGENT REFERRAL for suspected endometrial cancer if age is younger than 55 years with post-menopausal bleeding.

CONSIDER URGENT REFERRAL FOR ULTRASONOGRAPHY for endometrial assessment if age 55 years and older and:
- Unexplained symptoms of vaginal discharge with any of the following:
  - Are presenting with these symptoms for the first time
  - Have thrombocytosis
  - Report haematuria
- Visible haematuria and any of the following are present:
  - Low haemoglobin levels
  - Thrombocytosis
  - High blood glucose levels

CONSIDER URGENT REFERRAL for suspected cervical cancer if the appearance of the cervix is suspicious for cancer.

CONSIDER URGENT REFERRAL for suspected cancer if any of the following are present:
- Unexplained vulval lump, ulceration, or bleeding
- Unexplained palpable vaginal mass

Urologic Cancers

REFER for suspected prostate cancer if:
- Prostate feels malignant on digital rectal examination

CONSIDER URGENT REFERRAL for suspected prostate cancer if:
- Prostate-specific antigen is raised according to age-specific thresholds

REFER for suspected bladder cancer if:
- Aged 45 years and older and have either of the following:
  - Unexplained visible haematuria without urinary tract infection (UTI)
  - Visible haematuria that persists or recurs after successful treatment of UTI
- Aged 60 years and older and have unexplained nonvisible haematuria and either dysuria or an increased white blood cell count on a blood test

REFER for suspected renal cancer if aged older than 45 years and either of the following is present:
- Unexplained visible haematuria without UTI
- Visible haematuria that persists or recurs after successful treatment of UTI

CONSIDER URGENT REFERRAL for suspected testicular cancer if there is a painless enlargement or change in shape or texture of the testis.

CONSIDER URGENT REFERRAL for suspected penile cancer if any of the following are present:
- A penile mass or ulcerated lesion when a sexually transmitted infection (STI) has been excluded as a cause
- A persistent penile lesion after treatment for a STI has been completed
- Unexplained or persistent symptoms affecting the foreskin or glans

Skin

REFER for suspected skin cancer if any of the following are present:
- A suspicious pigmented skin lesion with a weighted 7-point checklist score of 3 or more
a. Major features of the lesions (scoring 2 points each):
  - Change in size
  - Irregular shape
  - Irregular colour
b. Minor features of the lesions (scoring 1 point each):
  - Largest diameter of 7 mm or more
  - Inflammation
  - Oozing
  - Change in sensation.
- Dermoscopy suggests melanoma of the skin.

CONSIDER REFERRAL for suspected skin cancer if any of the following are present:
- A pigmented or nonpigmented skin lesion that suggests nodular melanoma
- Lesions suspicious for squamous cell carcinoma
- Lesion suspicious for basal cell carcinoma if there is particular concern that a delay may have a significant impact because of factors such as lesion site or size

Head and Neck

CONSIDER URGENT REFERRAL for suspected laryngeal cancer in people aged older than 45 years with either of the following:
- Persistent unexplained hoarseness
- An unexplained lump in the neck

CONSIDER URGENT REFERRAL for suspected oral cancer in people with any of the following:
- Unexplained ulceration in the oral cavity lasting for more than 3 weeks
- A persistent and unexplained lump in the neck
- A lump on the lip or in the oral cavity
- A red or red and white patch in the oral cavity consistent with erythroplakia or erythroleukoplakia

CONSIDER URGENT REFERRAL for suspected thyroid cancer in people with an unexplained thyroid lump.

Brain and Central Nervous System (Adults)

Urgent, direct access magnetic resonance imaging (MRI) scan of the brain (or computed tomography scan if MRI is contraindicated; to be done within 2 weeks) to assess for brain or central nervous system (CNS) cancer in adults with progressive, subacute loss of central neurologic function.

Haematologic Cancers (Adults)

REFER for suspected multiple myeloma if:
• Results of protein electrophoresis or a Bence–Jones protein urine test are suggestive of myeloma
CONSIDER URGENT REFERRAL for suspected lymphoma if:
• Unexplained lymphadenopathy or splenomegaly

Sarcoma (Adults)

CONSIDER URGENT REFERRAL if any of the following are present:
• Radiographs suggest the possibility of bone sarcoma
• Ultrasound scan findings that are suggestive of soft tissue sarcoma
• Ultrasound findings are uncertain for soft tissue sarcoma and clinical concern persists

Non–Site-Specific Symptoms (Adults)

CONSIDER URGENT REFERRAL for further investigation or assessment for anyone with unexplained:
• Weight loss
• Appetite loss
• Venous thromboembolism

Children and Young People

CONSIDER VERY URGENT REFERRAL (for an appointment within 48 hours) for suspected brain or CNS cancer in children and young people with newly abnormal cerebellar or other central neurologic function.

REFER for immediate assessment for leukaemia if there is unexplained petechiae or hepatosplenomegaly.

CONSIDER VERY URGENT REFERRAL (for an appointment within 48 hours) for specialist assessment in children and young people presenting with unexplained lymphadenopathy or splenomegaly.

CONSIDER VERY URGENT REFERRAL (for an appointment within 48 hours) for specialist assessment for sarcoma for children and young people if any of the following are present:
• Radiographs suggest the possibility of bone sarcoma
• Ultrasound scan findings are suggestive of soft tissue sarcoma
• Ultrasound findings are uncertain and clinical concern persists

CONSIDER VERY URGENT REFERRAL (for an appointment within 48 hours) for specialist assessment for neuroblastoma in children with a palpable abdominal mass or unexplained enlarged abdominal organ.

CONSIDER URGENT REFERRAL for suspected retinoblastoma for children with an absent red reflex.

CONSIDER VERY URGENT REFERRAL (for an appointment within 48 hours) for specialist assessment for Wilms tumour in children with any of the following:
• A palpable abdominal mass
• An unexplained enlarged abdominal organ
• Unexplained visible haematuria.

Non–Site-Specific Symptoms (Children)

Consider referral for children if their parent or carer has persistent concern or anxiety about the child's symptoms even if the symptoms are most likely to have a benign cause.

Appendix 32

Opioid Dose Conversion Chart

All doses are in milligrams (mg) unless otherwise stated.

Oral Opioid (24 h)		CSCI Opioid (24 h)					Subcutaneous PRN Opioid Every 4 Hours				Opioid Transdermal Patch	
Morphine	Oxycodone	Morphine	Oxycodone	Diamorphine	Alfentanil	Fentanyl	Morphine	Oxycodone	Diamorphine	Fentanyl	Fentanyl	Buprenorphine
20	10	10	5	5	500 µg	100 µg	2	1	1	12.5 µg	–	10 µg/h
30	15	15	7.5	10	1 mg	200 µg	2.5	1.5	2	25 µg	–	15 µg/h
45	20	20	10	15	1.5	300 µg	4	2	2.5	37.5 µg	12 µg/h	20 µg/h
90	45	45	20	30	3	600 µg	8	4	5	75 µg	25 µg/h	35 µg/h
140	70	70	35	45	4.5	900 µg	12	6	8	100 µg	37 µg/h	52.5 µg/h
180	90	90	45	60	6	Max. CSCI, 900 µg as limited by volume (50 µg/mL)	15	8	10	Max. PRN 100 µg as limited by volume (50 µg/mL)	50 µg/h	70 µg/h
230	115	115	60	75	7.5		20	10	12.5		62 µg/h	105 µg/h
270	135	135	70	90	9		25	12	15		75 µg/h	122.5 µg/h
360	180	180	90	120	12		30	15	20		100 µg/h	140 µg/h
450	225	225	110	150	15		35	18	25		125 µg/h	(Manufacturer's recommended maximum is 140 µg/h)
540	270	270	135	180	18		45	20	30		150 µg/h	
630	315	315	160	210	21		50	25	35		175 µg/h	
720	360	360	180	240	24		60	30	40		200 µg/h	

- The conversions stated here are only approximate and are based on manufacturers' data and other sources of data. There may be local guidelines stating different conversion ratios; these should be followed when they exist.
- When switching between opioids, it is recommended that the calculated equivalent dose of the new opioid is reduced by 25% to 50%.
- Alfentanil:fentanyl is based on 5:1. (This is the modal average taken from several different data sources; range, 3.3–6:1.)
- The fentanyl as needed (PRN) dose is calculated as 1/8 of the 24-hour dose (mean average taken from different sources; range, 1/10 to 1/6).

CSCI, Continuous subcutaneous infusion.

Index

Page numbers followed by "*f*" indicate figures, "*t*" indicate tables, and "*b*" indicate boxes.